PRINCIPLES
OF
SENSORY PHYSIOLOGY

PRINCIPLES
of
SENSORY PHYSIOLOGY

By

HENRY TAMAR

Professor of Physiology
Indiana State University
Terre Haute, Indiana

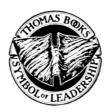

CHARLES C THOMAS · PUBLISHER
Springfield · Illinois · U.S.A.

Published and Distributed Throughout the World by
CHARLES C THOMAS • PUBLISHER
BANNERSTONE HOUSE
301-327 East Lawrence Avenue, Springfield, Illinois, U.S.A.
NATCHEZ PLANTATION HOUSE
735 North Atlantic Boulevard, Fort Lauderdale, Florida, U.S.A.

© 1972, by CHARLES C THOMAS • PUBLISHER
ISBN 0–398–02209–7
Library of Congress Catalog Card Number: 72-151879

With THOMAS BOOKS *careful attention is given to all details of*
manufacturing and design. It is the Publisher's desire to present books
that are satisfactory as to their physical qualities and artistic possibilities
and appropriate for their particular use. THOMAS BOOKS *will be true*
to those laws of quality that assure a good name and good will.

325131

Printed in the United States of America
EE-11

To The Hard-working Electrophysiologists

Preface

T he last decade has seen a burgeoning of information on the physiology of the senses. This great development of the field of sensory physiology has been accompanied by the publication of a number of excellent symposia and reviews dealing with one or two of the senses. However, sensory scientists, teachers and graduate students of sensory physiology have been keenly aware of the lack of an advanced book providing a comprehensive treatment of the breadth of their general area of interest.

Advances in sensory physiology have been so rapid, and so many specialties have developed in sensory research, that to undertake to write a work covering the entire science of sensory physiology would be far too ambitious. One can only hope to delineate the recent state of knowledge in a number of primary areas of sensory physiology and also perhaps to offer some essential background. It is to this task that the present effort is dedicated.

It is hoped that this book will serve as a nucleus for sensory physiology courses. It should give graduate and advanced undergraduate students an understanding of the nature of sensory physiology and of the important mechanisms which play a role in the operation of the senses. The reception of stimuli and the processes involved in the transmission of sensory impulses to higher centers have been emphasized over other aspects of sensory physiology, such as perception and behavioral findings.

It was felt that if the basic physiology of a number of senses was covered, it would not be too difficult for students to integrate additional material. For example, after studying the section devoted to the initial events of visual reception in Chapter V, one should be prepared to assimilate lectures on the three main types of cone receptors functional in color vision, on the action spectra of different visual pigments, and on the integration of the Young and Helmholtz theories of color vision. After reading about olfactory sensitivities (Chap. III), a lecture on the increasingly significant subject of pheromones might be in order.

Since there is still only little experimental knowledge of the initial events of olfaction, this subject has not been treated. The initial events of audition also have not been covered, because shearing forces similar to those acting on the fish lateral line seem to be involved here. The function of the lateral line is dealt with in Chapter II.

Chapter V instead consists of sections on the processes by which excitation is evoked in photoreceptors, the pacinian corpuscle, and taste cells. The initial events which take place in visual, mechanical and gustatory reception differ considerably, and their study will give one a good understanding of the various means by which excitation can be produced.

The final chapter on nervous transmission is intended to provide a review of the operation of the nervous system. Students with an inadequate background in nerve physiology may find it advisable to start their studies with this chapter.

Chapter VI also supplies information on more recently investigated aspects of nerve physiology which are pertinent to an understanding of the senses.

The references for each chapter are followed by a list of suggested reading.

This volume should prove equally useful to sensory physiologists. An attempt has been made to include in each subject section the more important recent experimental results.

Research workers could in addition benefit in terms of cross-fertilization. Processes discovered during research on one sense sometimes have their counterparts in other senses. Certain concepts may be widely applicable, and it is also well to become acquainted with other sensory receptors and organelles.

Further, this book may be of value in the applied sciences concerned with the sensory responses of man or his domestic animals, and in allied fields such as animal behavior and psychology. The mass of recent findings in sensory physiology also includes material of interest to researchers in cellular physiology, evolution and environmental physiology.

In many developing areas of sensory research, a large number of the observations cannot yet be fully integrated, and a few later ones may appear to be in conflict. It has therefore been frequently necessary to compile the findings of different investigators. Such compilation is advantageous when it permits a more complete and up-to-date presentation of a subject.

At various times during the writing the author could not avoid an arbitrary selection of subject matter or of research papers. It has also been difficult to relate some scientific information and state a number of concepts without slightly paraphrasing the words of others. Certain relationships can best be concisely and effectively expressed by the use of particular constructions or phrases, and the choice of suitable scientific terms is often very limited.

I am greatly indebted to the large number of investigators who sent me their reprints or photographs. I also wish to acknowledge the valuable contributions made by my student assistants Susan Kruzan, Linda Markee, Carol Martin and Cathy Memmer. Without their search of abstracting journals, their typing and their proofreading, the completion of this book would have been much more difficult. The Indiana State University Audio-Visual Services prepared prints for illustration, and the administration granted financial support.

Contents

PRINCIPLES
OF
SENSORY PHYSIOLOGY

Chapter I

Introduction

THE SCOPE AND NATURE OF SENSORY PHYSIOLOGY

Sensory physiology deals with the operation of the sensory systems of organisms —how the organism's receptors are stimulated by various environmental influences, how the induced excitations are transmitted to the brain or central nervous system, and how in the central portion of the nervous system the incoming sensory information is translated into perceived sensations. Sensory physiology encompasses the activities of both external receptors and purely internal receptors such as muscle spindles and crustacean myochordotonal organs. It deals both with individual receptors, such as the pressure-sensitive pacinian corpuscles and the free nerve endings which mediate pain, and with the localized masses of receptors which provide us with the special senses.

The questions the sensory physiologist may ask about any sensory system are innumerable. He may concentrate on the general or the differential sensitivities of the peripheral receptors, or any aspect of their function. He may be interested in the signal codes by which neurons transmit information about a stimulus to the brain, or he might study the spontaneous activity of sensory neurons and how it is altered by incoming signals. He may instead choose to concentrate on the electrical activity in the lower or higher relay stations of a sensory pathway, or on the signals in the final receiving centers of the brain, and attempt to elucidate the function of these levels of a sensory system. Further, he may wish to determine the nature of the perceptions elicited by certain stimuli through observation of the reactions of the whole animal.

It is clear from the above partial list of sensory problems, even before one considers the special problems posed by differences between animal groups, that there must be a multiplicity of approaches in sensory physiology. This necessary multiplicity of experimental approaches is reflected in the great variety of techniques sensory physiologists have evolved.

Thus investigation of the impulses in peripheral neurons requires methods of picking up these signals with gross electrodes or microelectrodes and amplifying, displaying and recording them. The study of brain activity may be carried out by implanting electrodes into the brain, or by recording evoked responses with electrodes located on the scalp. Peripheral nerve impulses may be correlated with brain activity, or the activity of two regions of the brain compared, by means of multichannel recording.

In the above research subjects statistical techniques often play an important role, since nervous activity may vary over a broad spectrum, and it may be necessary to establish classes of responses, find the probability distribution, and so on. Also, the averaging of responses may permit significant comparisons and thus the determination of changes produced by stimuli. In many studies involving large numbers of individual phenomena, the use of computers is vital.

The development of physical, electronic and mathematical models of biological systems has been a powerful tool in the whole area of biomedical science.

A model is a conceptual and quantitative representation of the nature and function of a real system. It is based on anatomical or experimental knowledge, requires the definition of certain components, and must have a one-to-one correspondence to the system (the principle of isomorphism). A model is valid insofar as it permits the scientist to predict or interpret the behavior of the system under various conditions. As investigation of the biological system exposes faults or inadequacies in the model, the model is modified. The structure and parameters of the model may be changed, or new conditions can be introduced. Thus a series of models may be evolved in which each later model better describes the physical principles or mathematical relationships of the system.

Many models can be modified by means of a computer.

Mathematical models, first developed by Rashevsky, are mathematical or analytical solutions for a system. Such models consist of equations which should describe the behavior of the system. Mathematical models may be topological, deterministic or probabilistic. Linear mathematical models are based on the assumption that some components of the system do not change. Nonlinear models are used to represent systems which change as they function.

Physical and mathematical models, such as those of the ear and of nerve function, have led to valuable advances. The comparison of a model with the living system can raise important questions.

The response of the whole organism to odors can be determined in simpler forms by watching their movements in the final chamber of a well-developed olfactometer, and the taste perception produced by a solution offered to birds or mammals can be studied by means of single-choice or two-choice preference tests.

However, in spite of their great variety, most of the techniques employed particularly in sensory physiology and the related areas can be categorized, according to the basic method of approach used, into electrophysiological and behavioral techniques.

Both the electrophysiological and behavioral approaches to the senses have borne fruit. Nevertheless, many areas of sensory physiology are generally marked by a relatively low ratio of developed theories and laws to the masses of specific data which have been gathered. In the fields of gustation and olfaction, repeated attempts have been made to derive general statements from the experimental data at hand, only to have additional information expose flaws in the developing concepts. Much of the experimental information obtained is highly varied, some even surprising, and it does not allow itself to be easily summarized. Neurophysiology shares these features of sensory physiology.

THE BASIC NATURE OF THE SENSORY SYSTEM

The information which must reach the brain from the receptor organs of the special senses must be highly specific, while at the same time these organs must be able to transmit types of information which vary greatly in several respects. Furthermore, the possible perceived qualities of the variety of stimuli affecting a special sense greatly exceed the number of receptor types present in the sense's organs. The brain must not only be informed of the basic type of the stimulus, but also of its peculiar quality, its average strength, the source of the stimulus within the general environment, and even of its variation with time. How is such varied information, of so many aspects, to be correctly conveyed to the brain?

Let us first deal with the identification of the basic type of stimulus by the brain.

The different receptor types in the organs of the special senses are, of course, sensitive to different stimuli. Nevertheless, the nerve impulses conveyed from them to the brain are basically alike. The chorda tympani nerve, which subserves taste in mammals, the auditory nerve, and the optic nerve, all contain some nerve fibers which transmit impulses of about the same size at approximately the same speed. Nerve fibers from these different sources may also transmit action potentials at the same frequency.

Apparently in higher organisms the brain is informed of the basic type of the received stimulus by virtue of the final destination in the cerebral cortex which a volley of nerve impulses reaches. Thus visual action potentials arrive at visual areas in the cortex, while auditory spikes reach the auditory areas of the cortex. Presumably, if we cut both the auditory and optic nerves and were able to cross them and if the fibers of the peripheral portion of the auditory nerve could "heal" with the fibers of the central portion of the optic nerve, and vice versa, it would be possible to "see" thunder and "hear" lightning.

How does the brain differentiate the several qualities of each of the various stimuli which emanate from the organs of one special sense? Such delicate identifications are made on the basis of the special "code" of impulses which originates in the receptor surface.

Gustation in higher forms is dependent upon four principal receptor types which are respectively most sensitive to sweet, salty, sour and bitter. Each receptor type can be subdivided according to which of the four basic taste qualities produces the second-largest stimulation, and so on (see Fig. 5-14). Furthermore, although in a species a majority of salt receptors, for instance, will be most sensitive to one salt, a lesser number of salt receptors will give their greatest response to another salt, and so on.

As in all the senses, for the sense of taste intensity of stimulation is denoted by the frequency of the action potentials coming from the receptors and the overall number of nerve fibers involved. The picture is further complicated by the fact that in taste, as in other senses, several receptors are innervated by branches of a single nerve fiber, and the action potentials emanating from these receptors will converge to increase the impulse frequency in the common fiber. On the other hand, the dominant receptor types are partially segregated into different regions of the tongue, this perhaps producing an approach to a spatial pattern.

It is the total "orchestra" of impulses arising from the different receptor types and their subgroups which identifies a particular taste. Thus Pfaffmann (1955) has suggested that gustatory qualities are identified by the relative quantities of nerve impulses they produce in parallel taste fibers. Erickson (1963, 1967) and Erickson, Doetsch and Marshall (1965) have tried to determine the total quantity of neural activity elicited by a taste stimulus, and have attempted to study the significant aspect of this activity, through correlation of the impulse response of many taste fibers.

In the higher ear only two basically similar receptor types are present. Here spatial patterns (the regions of the cochlea stimulated indicate pitches) and temporal patterns (characteristic changes in intensity and pitch identify certain sounds) are sufficient to fully "describe" a complex sound composed of differently varying tones.

Vision in strong light is based both upon three different kinds of cone receptors most sensitive, respectively, to blue, green, and red (color vision), and on spatial and temporal patterns. In mammals the functional organization of the visual receptors, the retinal ganglion cells and geniculate cells of the visual pathway, and cells of the visual cortex are specialized to emphasize differences in the light intensities reaching the regions of the retina. They thus produce strong spatial patterns. There are neural mechanisms in the retina for detection of movement (temporal patterns). These are especially numerous toward the periphery of the visual field.

Olfaction may be the most complex of the special senses, and is the least understood. In a macrosmatic animal large receptor sheets are available for olfaction. Several receptor types are present. The many stimuli affecting one kind of receptor may be differentiable from each other by the unique spatial pattern and temporal pattern they impose on this receptor type. A certain molecule may only reach some portions of the olfactory epithelium, and reach these areas in a particular time sequence, as indicated by experiments on the rabbit.

Thus in the most complex senses, vision and olfaction, a large number of receptors consisting of several different types may give rise to complex spatial and temporal patterns of impulses. These impulses may be considerably modified in the various relay stations of the sensory pathway leading to their final destination in the brain.

Senses Are Subjective and Differ Among Organisms

Sense perceptions are primarily the interpretations which the brain (cerebral cortex in mammals) makes of the nerve impulses which reach certain regions of it. However, the nature of a perception is also formed by processes in and by the properties of the lower levels of the sensory system. Thus the receptor itself integrates received stimuli in a series of events. These start with the development of a receptor potential in the stimulus-sensitive membrane, may involve varying states of excitability and poorly known internal potentials, and in vertebrates culminate in a generator potential which calls forth nerve impulses.

The slow accommodation of the sensory nerve fibers adjacent to certain receptors also affects the final perception. Further, receptors of the same receptor sheet may mutually inhibit one another. Receptors may also be inhibited by brain centers. Inhibitory impulses which are transmitted toward the periphery in centrifugal nerve fibers can apparently modulate afferent sensory nerve activity (see Chap. IV). Several receptors may be innervated by branches of a single afferent nerve fiber, and the action potentials called forth by their separate responses will then combine to increase the impulse frequency in the common fiber. Summation of impulses may take place at synapses in relay stations on the way to

the sites of perception, or conversely, there may be central expansion of the impulses from a restricted portion of the receptor field. In many cases significant aspects of sensory activity are emphasized at various levels of a sensory pathway by means of inhibitory influences or selectively responsive cells. Sense perceptions are therefore the subjective creations of the sensory system and brain.

Thus there can be no such thing on the part of our senses as an objective interpretation of the environment. This is also shown by the fact that groups of organisms have unique sensory environments. Separate sensory worlds exist for different animal types in respect to each of the special senses.

In regard to taste, for instance, von Frisch (1934) discovered long ago that bees respond to only nine of thirty-four substances sweet to man. Concentrations of saccharin did not affect bees, or repelled them. However, they accepted acetylsaccharose, which is bitter to man. Beidler, Fishman, and Hardiman (1955) showed that in Carnivora the ratio of the peripheral response to 0.5M potassium chloride versus that to 0.5M sodium chloride was almost the reverse of the relative responses of Rodentia to these two salts.

While the primates do not orient themselves by means of their relatively weak olfaction, macrosmatic mammals such as the bloodhound live in an environment filled with significant odors. In dogs the olfactory input takes precedence over vision in exploring the nature of the environment. Male *Bombyx mori* moths are attracted to females by the odor of a pheromone at a concentration of 0.01γ, (Karlson, 1960).

The ear of man is sensitive to sounds with frequencies between 16 cycles and 20,000 cycles per second. The range may include even 40,000 cps in childhood (von Békésy, 1957). Dogs detect frequencies of up to 50,000 cycles, and can be called with "inaudible whistles." However, some bats may hear up to 150,000 cps, and noctuid moths, which are part of their prey, can detect ultrasonic bat cries of 100,000 cps (Roeder, 1965).

Suga (1967) investigated the auditory sensitivity of three arboreal edentates of the Amazon. He discovered that the silky anteater (*Cyclopes didactylus*) hears between 600 to 62,000 cps (at 100 dB SPL), while at the same intensity the ear of sloths (*Choloepus didactylus, Bradypus tridactylus*) responds to sound between 300 to at most 30,000 cps. In these studies the threshold was defined as a microphonic with a peak-to-peak amplitude of 10μV.

Sphingid moths, unlike the *Noctuidae* and some other moth families, possess no thoracic or abdominal tympanic organs. The sphingid subfamily *Choerocampinae* instead is sensitive to acoustic stimuli by a mechanism which is localized at the labial palps. It is possible that sound-induced vibration of each labial palp excites a mechanoreceptor located close to the articulation of the palp with the cranium (Roeder, Treat and Vandeberg, 1968).

Tested choerocampinid moths showed nerve discharges after sound pulses in the range of 7 kHz to above 100 kHz. Apparently these moths are more sensitive to lower frequencies than the noctuid moths.

Suga (1968) recorded from the ventral nerve cord and the nerves serving the tympanic organ and the cercal hair sensilla of a Brazilian mole cricket (*Gryllotalpa hexadactyla*). The tympanic organ was found to respond to 100 dB sounds of less than 5,000 to 150,000 cps, while the cercal hair sensilla were sensitive to sounds between less than 100 to 1,500 cps.

In the case of vision, it is known that many insects, unlike other organisms, are responsive to ultraviolet light. A number of insect-pollinated flowers have ultraviolet-reflecting nectar guides. Also, insect ultraviolet patterns may play a role in sexual communication. The males of several neotropical butterflies of the family *Pieridae* possess wing patches which may be only poorly visible to man but which reflect ultraviolet. When viewed with the proper equipment, these male butterflies emit intense ultraviolet flickers while in flight. One species (*Eroessa chilensis*) bears orange wing markings which reflect ultraviolet only in the male (Eisner *et al.*, 1969).

In a fly, *Calliphora erythrocephala,* the spectral sensitivity curve shows maxima at 350 mμ and at 490 mμ.

The pure cone eyes of the tortoise and the snake have their sensitivity peak near 600 mμ (Granit, 1963), while the cones of other, rod-containing eyes are most sensitive to a wavelength of 560 mμ (the spectral sensitivities of the whole cone populations of rod-containing eyes are impressively uniform). The eyes of guinea pigs, bats and rats do not show the normal Purkinje shift, and if the guinea pig eye has a minimal color vision, it cannot be based on the totally absent cones.

The Danger in Relying on Our Senses

We therefore must study the senses of various animals by the eventual use of other senses, our own, which may be just as unique. This may create difficulties, as when the spectral sensitivity curve of a species is to be determined. If we attempt to equalize the intensity of stimulating lights of different wavelengths by means of a Bunsen grease spot photometer or a Lummer-Brodhun photometer, using our own eyes, we are really studying the stimulating efficacy of the different wavelengths varied in intensity according to our own spectral sensitivity curve!

We cannot use photoelectric exposure meters or the other similar photometers to achieve equal objective light intensities for the wavelengths of the spectrum, because photoelectric cells themselves show differential sensitivities. The sensitivity of photoelectric exposure meters is usually greatest in the yellow and green, and is greater to blue than to red. Their spectral sensitivity curve differs from that of the eye chiefly in that there is a much greater sensitivity to blue and violet (Dunn, 1958).

The only way to obtain objectively equal intensities of different wavelengths of light is to vary the intensities of the wavelengths until a thermopile is heated equally in unit time by all the wavelengths. Thus a pair of thermopiles could be arranged so that one receives light from a test wavelength and the other from a comparison wavelength. A monochromator could be employed to present the different test wavelengths. A variable attenuator could be used to adjust the intensity of each test wavelength until it produced the same heating of the test thermopile as is induced by the comparison wavelength on the comparison thermopile. Only equal light intensities will heat a thermopile to the same degree.

An electroretinogram (electrically recorded retinal mass effect) could then be obtained with each of the equally intense wavelengths, and a comparison of the electroretinograms would give us the spectral sensitivity curve of the organism. Alternately, in simpler species the extent of a similar response (phototaxis, etc.) by the whole organism to each of the intensity-calibrated wavelengths could be determined.

Such an equal-energy spectrum would still not suffice for an accurate comparison of the bleaching of visual purple by different wavelengths. The first step in the bleaching of visual purple is produced by the absorption of quanta of light, and wavelengths of equal intensity do not emit the same number of quanta per second. The light of a shorter wavelength contains a smaller number of quanta than the equivalent light of a longer wavelength, but each shorter-wavelength quantum has more energy. In studying the absorption spectrum of visual purple, a spectrum of equal *quantum* intensity must be used.

It is the interjection of measuring devices between the sense being studied and our own senses which marks the advance of sensory physiology. Increased quantification and better measuring devices, in fact, are the signposts of the advance of all of science.

QUANTITATIVE STIMULUS-SENSE RELATIONS

The subject of sensory physiology has its roots in an effort to quantitatively determine the smallest increase in a stimulus which can be noticed through the senses. Such measurements of stimulus intensity versus evoked response today belong in the domain of psychophysics. It was Weber who in 1846 reported that the increment by which the intensity of a stimulus had to be increased to produce a barely noticeable difference in sensation was a constant fraction of the original stimulus intensity. Thus Weber found that he could differentiate two weights placed on his hand if the ratio between them was at least 29:30. Fechner, considered the father of psychophysics, in 1860 stated Weber's finding mathematically as

$$\Delta I/I = k$$

in which ΔI, representing the stimulus increment necessary to produce a barely perceptible difference, divided by I, the intensity of the original stimulus, is equal to a constant, k.

The Weber fraction, or Weber's law, was later found to poorly fit observations at both very low and very high intensities of stimulation. Thus at higher intensities of pure tones the detectable intensity difference–original tone intensity ratios no longer provide a flat curve, which last is indicative of good agreement with Weber's law. Instead, the function for pure tones falls off rapidly, and then more slowly, with rising intensity. Weber's law therefore had to be amended.

More recently an interesting sidelight has been cast on one inadequacy of Weber's law. A number of investigators have observed that if Weber's fractions are plotted for intensity discrimination experiments with 1000 Hz pure tones for about 55 dB above the 25 dB level, an outstandingly linear function is obtained. However, while Weber's law demands that the slope of this function be unity, it actually approximates a value of 0.9. Such a deviation from the expected slope is not encountered with wideband noise or pure noise. McGill and Goldberg (1968) have offered an explanation for the deviation of the pure-tone slope in terms of mass information–flow phenomena, which entail large information losses. They suggest that in an en masse processing of the receptor response, an internal noise or information loss increases with stimulus intensity. Because the stimulus energy of pure noise has a probability distribution, its linear function has the expected slope of approximately one.

Barlow (1965) has plotted the theoretical curve relating the minimum detectable increase in quanta of light striking the human retina to the adaptation level. It is assumed that the incremental quantum to original impulse level ratio rises in direct proportion to the degree of adaptation. Barlow's curve follows the square root law at lower intensities, and Weber's law at higher intensities. Barlow suggests that neural quantization is the source of an error or noise which causes the curve to fit Weber's law at greater intensities. Thus he offers a new possible basis for experimental results which appear to follow Weber's law.

Starting from the unsatisfying Weber's law, Fechner derived the concept that sensation is proportional to the logarithm of the stimulus, or more specifically that

sensation $S = a \log_{10} I + b$

where a is a constant including the coefficient for conversion to $\log_{10}$, and b is the constant for integration. This so-called Fechner's law was based in part on the supposition that what Fechner named the *jnd*, the just noticeable difference between two stimuli, *as perceived by the subject* remains constant at all intensities of stimulation.

The discovery that sensory nerves communicate an increase in stimulus intensity to the brain by a higher frequency of nerve impulses (Adrian, 1926) was a breakthrough in sensory physiology. It opened the way for sensory physiologists to empirically prove the Fechner statement. Matthews (1931) loaded the middle toe of a frog with different weights, thus stretching a toe extensor muscle to varying degrees. This resulted in the proportionate stretching of a muscle spindle within the toe extensor. Matthews electrophysiologically recorded the frequency of the nerve impulses coming from the muscle spindle after the different loadings. He believed his results sup-

ported the Fechner statement. Other evidence that sensory response, as determined by the frequency of nerve impulses, is proportional to the logarithm of the stimulus came from research by Hartline and Graham (1932) on the eye of the horseshoe crab (*Limulus polyphemus*). They recorded the impulses in an optic nerve fiber coming from one ommatidium of the animal's eye, while stimulating the eye with light. Similar results have been obtained with single auditory nerve fibers (Galambos and Davis, 1943; Tasaki, 1954). More recently Evans and Mellon (1962) found the activity of the water receptor neuron in the chemoreceptive hair of the fly *Phormia* to be inhibited by solutions of nonelectrolytes in water according to a linear function of the logarithm of the osmotic pressure.

Over a certain range the amplitudes of the responses of monkey visual receptors are about linear with the logarithm of the stimulating light intensity (Brown and Murakami, 1967).

Indow (1966) developed a subjective scale of intensity for the four primary taste modalities, based on difference judgments. On this scale the estimated gustatory intensities are logarithmic functions of concentration, the slopes being very similar for all four basic taste qualities.

However, Fechner's "law" did not fare so well with most psychophysicists. Stevens (1936) used loudness ratios given by human subjects in developing a loudness scale in which Fechner's jnds (just noticeable subjective differences) were larger at higher than at lower sound intensities. Other investigators also negated Fechner's supposition that barely differentiable stimulus increments are perceptually always equal, and experimental data which failed to substantiate Fechner's "law" accumulated.

Stevens (1955, 1960), on the basis of studies with human subjects, using sound, light and electrical stimulation, then developed a power law to replace Fechner's "law." The power law indicates that sensation is proportional

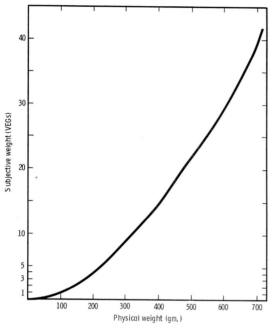

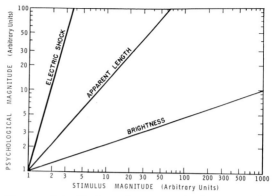

FIGURE 1-2. Estimated magnitude functions for three sensations. When plotted in log-log co-ordinates as above, Stevens' power functions produce straight lines. The slope of each line equals the value of the exponent of the function. (From Stevens, S.S.: The psychophysics of sensory function *Amer. Sci.*, *48*:226-253, 1960.)

FIGURE 1-1. Scale of subjective weight obtained by Stevens' method of magnitude estimation. Units of subjective weight (VEG's), each equal to the sensation produced by 100 grams, are plotted against actual weight. As the physical weights become greater, increasingly disproportionately large weight sensations are called forth. (From Harper, R.S., and S.S. Stevens: A psychological scale of weight and a formula for its derivation. *Amer. J. Psychol.*, *61*:343-351, 1948.)

to an exponent of the stimulus, and could be stated as

$$\text{sensation } S = a \ (I\text{-}R)^x$$

in which a is a constant with a value depending on the units used, I is the stimulus, R represents the stimulus at threshold, and x is an exponent.

The exponent x varies with the sensory system under study. It has a value of only 0.33 when light is the stimulus, is 0.6 for the odor of heptane, 1.3 for the taste of sodium chloride, and ranges up to 3.5 for electrical stimulation (Stevens, 1961).

According to Reynolds and Stevens (1960), perceived monaural loudness increases as a power function of sound pressure with an exponent of approximately 0.54, while binaural loudness rises with an exponent of about 0.6.

Using a different technique, the estimation of the linearity of loudness growth with time, Marks and Slawson (1966) also arrived at a binaural loudness exponent of 0.6. On the basis of a series of cross-modality matches between loudness and ten other types of previously studied perceptual continua, all of which produced matching functions of a power form, Stevens (1966a) suggests a value of approximately 0.64 for the exponent of the power function relating increase in perceived loudness to rise in sound pressure.

Similar cross-modality matching causes Stevens (1968) to give an exponent of approximately one for the power function for tactile vibration at 60 Hz. However, Stevens also found the exponent to vary with the frequency of stimulation. It is highest at about 30 Hz and only approximately half as large at its lowest value, near 250 Hz. Franzén (1969a) obtained a value of 0.56 for the exponent of the vibration power function during stimulation at 300 cps.

Millodot (1968) indicates a value of 1.01 for the exponent of the power function relating perceived corneal sensitivity to increasing pressure.

Stevens (1966b) determined the exponent

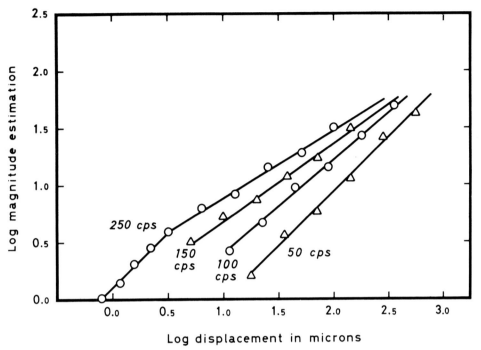

FIGURE 1-3. Estimated magnitude functions for vibratory mechanical stimuli of differing frequencies applied to the fingertip. The log-log coordinate plots show the slopes (exponents) of the power functions to vary inversely with vibration frequency. (From Franzén, O.: The dependence of vibrotactile threshold and magnitude functions on stimulation frequency and signal level. *Scand. J. Psychol., 10*:289-298, 1969.)

of the power function for perceived brightness to be lower at longer durations of the flash stimulus.

The exponent of a sensation-stimulus power function is raised over the range in which the function is being affected by a visual or auditory masking stimulus (Stevens, 1966c).

Treisman and Irwin (1967) suggest that under different conditions there may be different central measures for loudness. The loudness estimated by a more peripheral process is said to be related to the applied sound intensity according to a power function. However, the exponent of this function varies with the employed range of intensities. It has a value of about one near the absolute threshold and then falls with a rise in the general intensity.

Stevens thinks it probable that the frequently unlike ranges of exponent values obtained with the different senses reflect differences in the transducer mechanism. Thus the conversion of light energy into a generator potential would involve reduction of the steps between the widely varying levels of incoming light energies. During electrical stimulation of the fingers, the power function describing the resulting sensation is an accelerating one, with magnification of stimulus increases.

Steven's power law has stood up well in the face of empirical investigations. Rosner and Goff (1967) have replotted Matthews (1931) data in log-log coordinates, and have found it will fit a power function as well as it satisfies Fechner's logarithmic function. Other data which was used to support Fechner's statement is also amenable to reinterpretation on the basis of the power law.

Class II ganglion cells in the frog's retina are most responsive to movement, and their firing rises with increased angular velocity of the stimulus. The discharge rate of these ganglion cells has been discovered to be a power function of the angular velocity of the stimulus (Finkelstein and Grüsser, 1965).

Mountcastle and his group (1967), using monkeys, recorded the nerve impulses coming from skin receptors with slow adaptation rates upon indentation of the skin. They found that the skin indentation-discharge relation was described by a power function, and that this function matched the psychophysical (Stevens') functions obtained by similarly indenting the skin of human subjects.

Mountcastle *et al.* (1963) plotted single neuron activity in the thalamus against a stimulus of limb rotation in unanesthetized monkeys and found their values best fitted a power function. Poggio and Mountcastle (1963) obtained similar results.

Taste nerve activity too seems to be related to stimulus strength according to a power function (Sato, 1968a).

Other experiments yielded findings which fitted neither a logarithmic or a power function. Impulse frequency in some sensory nerve fibers appeared to be an S-shaped function of stimulus intensity. This was true of taste fibers (Pfaffmann, 1955) and auditory nerve fibers (Katsuki *et al.*, 1958). The potentials of certain receptors themselves, such as the pacinian corpuscle (Loewenstein, 1961) and the olfactory receptors of the frog (Mozell, 1962), also were found to be S-shaped functions of the stimulus intensity. The stimulus-receptor potential relation for the hair-plate sensilla of the honey bee (*Apis mellifica*) is described by a sigmoid curve. In *Limulus*, the eccentric cell (not the actual photoreceptor, the retinular cell) has a membrane voltage change which linearly follows the logarithm of the stimulus intensity during steady illumination (Fuortes and Poggio, 1963). This has been corroborated by Dodge, Jr., Knight and Toyoda (1968). However, at the start of responses to intermediate illumination, Fuortes and Poggio determined the voltage change to be an S-shaped function of the stimulus magnitude.

The impulse frequency in sensory axons

serving touch receptors in the skin of the toad follows stimulus intensity linearly (Lindblom, 1963).

While most recent papers suggest that S-shaped functions describe the relationship between the receptor potential and stimulus intensity, and between the sensory nerve fiber discharge and stimulus intensity, the relationship between the nerve fiber discharge and the receptor potential itself appears to be linear. Nerve impulse frequency follows the muscle spindle receptor potential linearly (Katz, 1950). Wolbarsht (1960) recorded receptor potentials from the mechanoreceptors of flies, grasshoppers, cockroaches and beetles. There was a linear relationship between the receptor potential and nerve impulse frequency until further increase in impulse frequency was prevented by the neuron's absolute refractory period. The receptor potentials also varied directly with the stimulus intensity. Morita and Yamashita (1966) found nerve impulse frequencies to be linear functions of the receptor potentials which develop in the labellar sugar receptor of the blowfly (*Phormia*). The research of Fuortes and Poggio (1963) on the eccentric cell of *Limulus* also indicates that impulse frequency follows cell membrane voltage linearly.

How are these S-shaped and linear relationships and a few unalterable logarithmic functions to be reconciled with the body of evidence supporting the Stevens power law? Earlier in this chapter mention was made of the fact that nerve impulses may be considerably modified in the various relay stations of the sensory pathway on their way to the brain. Such modifications of the trains of impulses could convert the various response-stimulus relationships to power functions by the time the nerve messages arrived at their final destination in the brain.

Rushton (1961) suggests that an exponential transformation of the impulse frequency pattern is required in the central nervous system, and that the subjective magnitude of a stimulus may be derived from an original objective entity such as repetition rate, the exponent of which has a value of 1.0. MacKay (1963) offers a matching response model to explain why sensation is a power function of the stimulus. In MacKay's model no exponential transformation would be required along the sensory pathway. The intensity of perception would instead be proportional to the level of an internal activity which would arise to balance the nerve discharge.

Melzack and Wall (1965) propose a central gate control system which would modulate afferent pain impulse activity and thus affect pain perception.

Katsuki (1961), working with cats and avoiding the use of the usual anesthetics, found that progressively higher levels of the auditory pathway showed different response-intensity functions. Until the level of the cortex, the impulse per second–decibel (intensity) relationship remained sigmoid. However, at progressively higher nervous system levels, impulse frequency rose at increasingly slower rates of differing form as the sound intensity was raised. This suggests a number of central transformations were taking place.

However, Mountcastle (1967) states that the brain is a "linear operator," and that the intensity of afferent nerve excitation is faithfully reproduced at the different relay station levels. Mountcastle can support this conclusion in part on the basis of the following procedure: curves were obtained relating the frequency of cutaneous vibration to the threshold of sensation in human subjects. Other curves were plotted relating the frequency of cutaneous vibration applied to monkeys to the beginning of a one-to-one stimulus-impulse response coming from the monkeys' vibration receptors. When the two sets of curves were compared, they fitted closely.

Talbot *et al.* (1968) report that when oscillatory stimuli of 40 or 250 cps are applied to the glabrous skin of the human hand, the subject's estimate of the magnitude of stimulation is linearly related to the amplitude of the employed sine waves. The sensation-stimulus relationships can alternatively be given in the form of power functions with exponents of about one.

The human sense of flutter vibration seems to originate in two different groups of primary afferent fibers. One of these appears to be particularly responsive to stimulus frequencies of 5 to 40 cps, seems to arise from the glabrous skin, and may be homologous to rapidly adapting afferents in the monkey. The other group of sensory fibers appears to be sensitive to a range of 60 to 300 cps, apparently originates in the deep (subcutaneous?) tissues of the hand, and may, as is probable in the monkey, innervate pacinian corpuscles.

In the monkey (*Macaca mulatta*) the first group of rapidly adapting afferents responds to near-threshold stimuli by transmitting impulse volleys at multiples of the stimulus period. As the stimulus intensity is raised, one impulse is called forth for each stimulus cycle (the authors' tuning point).

Both groups of afferent fibers continue to transmit one impulse per stimulus cycle at stimulus intensities five to ten times the intensity at the tuning point. This finding does not coincide with the near linearity of the subjective intensity estimation. Talbot *et al.* therefore hypothesize that there may be a central spatial integration of the entire input evoked by the stimulus. Vasilevskii *et al.* (1967) observed that in rabbits vibratory stimulation of an area adjacent to the original receptive field caused neurons of Area I of the somatosensory cortex to give an increased response.

Regular periodic trains of action potentials in the primary sensory fibers appear to be the basis of the perception of rhythmic oscillatory stimulation of the skin. Talbot *et al.* venture the idea that a central mechanism sensitive to the duration of the periods of the discharge trains may make the differentiation of various frequencies possible.

The analysis of single cortical neurons in the sensory receiving area of the monkey's postcentral gyrus has shown that central vibration reception is also dual. One set of neurons fires periodically in response to vibrations of up to approximately 40 cps, while another neuron population is responsive to 60 to 300 cps. The discharge of the last group of neurons does not, however, reflect the periodicity of the stimulating vibrations in the 60 to 300 cps range (Mountcastle, 1968; Hyvärinen *et al.*, 1968).

Thus the two groups of primary afferent fibers respectively transmitting impulses following flutter vibration frequencies of 5 to 40 and 60 to 300 cps seem to also be connected to two distinct populations of cortical neurons.

In the case of the neurons sensitive to vibrations of up to 40 cps, the stimulating frequency may be signaled by the temporal order of the emitted action potentials. The impulse rate of these neurons rises slowly as the stimulus intensity is increased. The cortical neurons responsive to 60 to 300 cps may reach their maximal discharge rates upon excitation with low intensity stimuli, even of human threshold intensity.

Unlike the peripheral nerve fibers, the cortical neurons exhibit no clear-cut tuning point, at which one action potential is phase-locked to one stimulus cycle, as stimulus intensity is raised (Hyvärinen *et al.*, 1968).

It is probable that a progressively greater decrease in the ratio of cortical impulses to vibrations takes place in the 60 to 300 cps range. This may well be the cause of the observed reduction in the rate of increase of perceived intensity with rising frequency of stimulation.

Further, it has been noted earlier that the Stevens' power law exponent for tactile vibration falls with increasing frequency.

An investigation of human brightness perception (Ekman and Gustafsson, 1968) has shown that at lower light intensities the estimated intensity is almost a linear function of the visual input, or the estimated intensity-input function has a slope of 0.97. However, above a transition point the slope drops to 0.58.

The impulse rate in individual sensory fibers of the dorsal nerve roots of the monkey and cat precisely mirrors the vibration frequency applied to a cutaneous tactile pad, up to and beyond a frequency of 400 cps (Lindblom and Tapper, 1967). On the other hand, the input frequency is not reproduced postsynaptically at close to 50 cps (Tapper and Mann, 1968).

Auditory nerve fiber impulses are phase-locked to (appear in synchrony with) sinusoidal stimuli at frequencies below 4,000 Hz. However, the auditory impulses do not follow the sound waves in a one-to-one relationship.

Auditory phase-locking is said to be affected by stimulus intensity, and by a second, masking stimulus (Goldberg, 1968).

In addition to transformations along the nervous pathway, other factors may contribute to the apparent conflict between peripheral observations and the validity of Stevens' power function. Thus Rosner and Goff (1967) suggest that even the use of anesthetics may play a role in producing peripheral response-intensity relations which are not power functions. The results which best confirm Stevens' power law come from the stated judgments of human subjects.

Rosner and Goff (1967) also indicate that while the receptor response may be an S-shaped function of the stimulus intensity, the nerve impulse frequency-receptor potential relationship is apparently linear.

It thus appears that much psychological data based on the use of human subjects supports the power law. Electrophysiological recordings from the brain have also furnished evidence in its favor. It is most significant that the discrepancy between these results and the variety of functions found to operate peripherally can be adequately explained.

Nevertheless, the general applicability of Stevens' power law is by no means certain.

A source of error in psychophysical loudness discrimination experiments has been brought out by Ward (1966). He reports that equal sensation levels of stimulation do not always produce equivalent loudnesses in human observers, since recruitment frequently takes place close to threshold in normal ears.

Ward urges that subjects be equated at the most comfortable sound levels.

Millodot (1969) found the sensitivity of the cornea to decrease from the center outwards to the periphery. This drop in sensitivity was greatest along the vertical meridian.

The method of magnitude estimation used in Stevens' psychophysical experiments and what is considered an improved method (Oyama-Lewis procedure) are critically examined in a paper by Oyama (1968).

Sato (1968b) views Fechner's law and Stevens' power law as special, respectively semilogarithmic and double-logarithmic expressions of a physiological activity law.

Many investigators have noted that sensory physiologists, physiological psychologists and psychophysicists attack similar problems from different directions and have much to learn from each other.

Von Békésy (1968) points out that the so-called objective observations of electrophysiologists are not necessarily more meaningful or complete than the "subjective" findings reported by psychologists. In many cases electrophysiological results are subjective in the sense that they measure only one parameter of a complex phenomenon. Furthermore, these measurements may be made with electrical apparatus that also has its limitations. Thus electrical equipment is better suited for picking up time patterns than spatial patterns.

The electrophysiologist often does not know how anesthetics affect his results, what damage has been done by operative techniques and the insertion of electrodes, what the consequences of this damage are, and so on.

On the other hand, psychophysicists may have difficulty in precisely defining the stimulus responsible for an observation. Their findings may also be influenced by integrative actions in their subjects' brains, so that extraneous stimuli may play a role. The type and degree of training of the human subjects used in psychophysical experiments presents other sources of error.

In behavioral animal experiments (physiological psychology) in which a choice of foods is offered, compensation may appear during the course of the investigation. The food selection and drinking habits of the experimental animals may undergo modification. Wild rats presented with acceptable but physiologically harmful substances have been observed to change their feeding habits (Kare, 1968).

In some behavioral animal experiments secondary stimuli considered to be of a minor nature by the investigator have been found to have a major effect. Thus chickens offered a choice of two drinking solutions have reacted to the partial opacity of one of the bottles. Experimental design also exerts an influence.

While psychophysicists do not deal with spontaneous nerve activity, electrophysiologists cannot as yet pick up the continuous response to a continuous tone.

Psychological observations not only can point the way to valuable electrophysiological investigations, but may sometimes present a fuller picture than the by necessity often more restricted electrophysiological observations. Furthermore, contradictions between psychological and electrophysiological findings may lead to new insights.

Only psychological investigations could have supplied the indications, reported by von Békésy (1967), that stimulus localization is based on the initial portion of a sensory discharge, while later impulses convey information about magnitude and stimulus quality. Electrophysiologists have not as yet developed a method for isolating a first burst of nerve impulses from later action potentials, nor are they in a position to precisely relate recorded nerve activity with different aspects of perception. The eventual perceptions evoked by peripheral sensory discharges can only be revealed by psychological methods. Such psychological studies are of the greatest importance, for it is evident that the significance of peripheral sensory discharges must usually lie in their terminal cerebral effects.

One difficulty in correlating electrophysiological results with psychological results lies in determining precisely what parameter of the neural response (perhaps an unrecorded one) gives rise to the reported sensation or, in the case of animals, to the behavioral reaction.

Frequently psychophysical and psychophysiological work can, however, complement electrophysiological research.

Borg *et al.* (1967) found a close correlation between the magnitudes of summated taste responses recorded from human chorda tympani nerves and group estimates of taste intensity when a series of concentrations of citric acid and sucrose solutions were applied to the tongue. The authors express the relationships between stimulus strength and neural or subjective cerebral response as power functions. Borg *et al.* (1967) believe that the differing exponent values of the power functions describing the taste estimates of different individuals reflect individual variations in neural response.

In a monkey's visual system the broad-band cells of the thalamus have electrophysiologically been determined to show a change in discharge only when the eye is stimulated with a sufficient intensity of any one of a group of wavelengths. These intensities correspond to the threshold intensities that have been established for these wavelengths in behavioral experiments (Werner, 1968).

Good agreement has also been obtained between psychophysical magnitude estimates and recorded evoked responses following tactile stimulation (Franzén and Offenloch, 1969).

Electrophysiology has gained much from the sister sciences of psychophysics and physiological psychology. However, it would have been a bit better for sensory physiologists, especially those recording central neuron discharges, if they had not been influenced by psychophysics until the latter's area of stimulus-response relationships could have become more mature. This is true because, during the long period of preeminence of Fechner's logarithmic formulation among psychophysicists, many sensory physiologists expected their recorded neural discharges to be loga-

rithmic functions of the stimulus intensity and in some cases interpreted their data along such lines.

It is to be hoped that the development of electrophysiology will soon be furthered by new techniques, such as the comparatively recent one of noise averaging. The Mössbauer effect, a technique of physics used in measuring minute velocities, has been successfully applied to the measurement of the very small vibrations of the ear.

For example, Gilad *et al.* (1967) have employed the Mössbauer technique to determine the relative amplitudes and examine the phases of the motions of the umbo and the end of the long process of the incus in guinea pigs. Johnstone and Boyle (1967) used the Mössbauer effect to measure the absolute amplitude of vibration of a portion of the guinea pig's basilar membrane. The maximum amplitude at 90 dB was 600 Å at 18 kHz.

The Mössbauer effect is described in an article of that name by De Benedetti (1960).

A number of articles provide a deeper insight into the subject matter discussed in this section. In the paper "To Honor Fechner and Repeal His Law," Stevens (1961) writes about Fechner's logarithmic formulation and the background and basis of his own power function. A good discussion of the techniques of magnitude estimation and cross-modality matching is given by Stevens (1967) in the paper "Intensity Functions in Sensory Systems." The aspects of psychophysical measurement and the findings of psychophysics are dealt with in "The Psychophysics of Sensory Function," by Stevens (1960). Some psychophysical results are also provided in "Transfer Functions of the Skin and Muscle Senses," by Stevens (1966d).

An excellent review of psychophysics is provided by Rosner and Goff (1967).

A discussion of the nature and goals of the sciences of psychophysics and biophysics can be found in "Biophysics and Psychophysics" by Dominguez (1965).

The interrelations between electrophysiology and psychology are ably covered in two outstanding contributions, one by von Békésy (1968) and the other by Werner (1968). The last author also extensively devotes himself to problems of measurement. Franzén (1969b), in a stimulating research report, examines some possible neurological bases for psychophysical observations.

The following pages are intended to provide a fuller picture of the structure and function of different sensory systems. The means by which suitable stimuli give rise to receptor responses are dealt with in Chapters III and V. The manner in which the afferent sensory input is modified by inhibition at the different levels of each sensory pathway is treated in Chapter IV.

REFERENCES

Adrian, E.D.: The impulses produced by sensory nerve-endings. Part I. *J. Physiol. (London)*, *61*:49-72, 1926.

Adrian, Lord E.D.: Opening Address. In Zotterman, Y. (Ed.): *Olfaction and Taste, Proceedings of the First International Symposium.* New York, Macmillan, 1963.

Barlow, H.B.: Optic nerve impulses and Weber's law. In *Sensory Receptors. Cold Spring Harbor Symposia on Quantitative Biology, 30:* 539-546, 1965.

Beidler, L.M., I.Y. Fishman, and C.W. Hardiman: Species differences in taste responses. *Amer. J. Physiol.*, *181*:235-239, 1955.

Békésy, G. von: The ear. *Sci. Amer.*, *197*:66-78, 1957.

Békésy, G. von: *Sensory Inhibition.* Princeton, Princeton U. Pr., 1967.

Békésy, G. von: Problems relating psychological and electrophysiological observations in sensory perception. *Perspect. Biol. Med.*, *11*:179-194, 1968.

Benedetti, S. de: The Mössbauer effect. *Sci. Amer.*, *202*:72-80, 1960.

Borg, G., H. Diamant, L. Ström, and Y. Zotterman: The relation between neural and perceptual intensity: a comparative study on the neural and psychophysical response to taste stimuli. *J. Physiol. (London)*, *192*:13-20, 1967.

Brown, K.T., and M. Murakami: Delayed decay of the late receptor potential of monkey cones as a function of stimulus intensity. *Vision Res.*, 7:179-189, 1967.

Burkhardt, D.: Spectral sensitivity and other response characteristics of single visual cells in the arthropod eye. *Sympos. Soc. Exp. Biol.*, *16*:86-109, 1962.

Dodge, Jr., F.A., B.W. Knight and J. Toyoda: Voltage noise in *Limulus* visual cells. *Science,* *160*:88-90, 1968.

Dominguez, J.: Biophysics and psychophysics. *Int. J. Neuropsychiat.*, *2*:78-89, 1965.

Dunn, J.F.: *Exposure Manual.* New York, John Wiley, 1958.

Eisner, T., R.E. Silberglied, D. Aneshansley, J.E. Carrel, and H.C. Howland: Ultraviolet videoviewing: The television camera as an insect eye. *Science, 166*:1172-1174, 1969.

Ekman, G., and U. Gustafsson: Threshold values and the psychophysical function in brightness vision. *Vision Res.*, 8:747-758, 1968.

Erickson, R.P.: Sensory Neural Patterns and Gustation. In Zotterman, Y. (Ed.): *Olfaction and Taste, Proceedings of the First International Symposium.* Oxford, Pergamon, 1963, pp. 205-213.

Erickson, R.P.: Neural Coding of Taste Quality. In Kare, M.R., and O. Maller (Eds.): *The Chemical Senses and Nutrition.* Baltimore, Johns Hopkins, 1967, pp. 313-327.

Erickson, R.P., G.S. Doetsch, and D.A. Marshall: The gustatory neural response function. *J. Gen. Physiol.*, *49*:247-263, 1965.

Evans, D.R., and De F. Mellon, Jr.: Electrophysiological studies of a water receptor associated with the taste sensilla of the blowfly. *J. Gen. Physiol.*, *45*:487-500, 1962.

Fechner, G.T.: *Elemente der Psychophysik.* Leipzig, Breitkopf Hartel, 1860.

Fender, D.H.: Control mechanisms of the eye. *Sci. Amer., 211*:24-33, 1964.

Finkelstein, D., and O.J. Grüsser: Frog retina: detection of movement. *Science, 150*:1050-1051, 1965.

Florey, E.: *An Introduction to General and Comparative Animal Physiology.* Philadelphia, W. B. Saunders, 1966.

Franzén, O.: The dependence of vibrotactile threshold and magnitude functions on stimulation frequency and signal level. *Quarterly Progress and Status Report*, Speech Transmission Lab., K.T.H., Stockholm, April 15, pp. 47-58, 1969a.

Franzén, O.: On spatial summation in the tactual sense. A psychophysical and neurophysiological study. *Scand. J. Psychol.,* 10:193-208, 1969b.

Franzén, O., and K. Offenloch: Evoked response correlates of psychophysical magnitude estimates for tactile stimulation in man. *Exp. Brain Res.,* 8:1-18, 1969.

Frisch, K. von: On the taste sense in bees. *Z. Vergl. Physiol.,* 21:1-156, 1934.

Fuortes, M.G., and G.F. Poggio: Transient responses to sudden illumination in cells of the eye of *Limulus. J. Gen. Physiol.,* 46:435-452, 1963.

Galambos, R., and H. Davis: The response of single auditory-nerve fibers to acoustic stimulation. *J. Neurophysiol.,* 6:39-58, 1943.

Gilad, P., S. Shtrikman, P. Hillman, M. Rubinstein, and A. Eviatar: Application of the Mössbauer Method to ear vibrations. *J. Acoust. Soc. Amer.,* 41:1232-1236, 1967.

Goldberg, J. In Wayner, M.J., and Y. Oomura: Neuronal spike trains (report on 1967 Honolulu meeting). *Science,* 160:1025-1026, 1968.

Granit, R.: *Receptors and Sensory Perception.* New Haven, Yale U. Pr., 1955.

Granit, R.: *Sensory Mechanisms of the Retina.* New York, Hafner, 1963.

Hartline, H.K., and C.H. Graham: Nerve impulses from single receptors in the eye. *J. Cell Comp. Physiol.,* 1:277-295, 1932.

Hubel, D.H.: The visual cortex of the brain. *Sci. Amer.,* 209:54-62, 1963.

Hyvärinen, J., H. Sakata, W.H. Talbot, and V.B. Mountcastle: Neuronal coding by cortical cells of the frequency of oscillating peripheral stimuli. *Science,* 162:1130-1132, 1968.

Indow, T.: A general equi-distance scale of the four qualities of taste. *Jap. Psychol. Res.,* 8: 136-150, 1966.

Johnstone, B.M., and A.J.F. Boyle: Basilar membrane vibration examined with the Mössbauer technique. *Science,* 158:389-390, 1967.

Kare, M.R.: The Functions of the Sense of Taste. Tele-lecture to I.S.U., 1968.

Karlson, P.: Pheromones. *Ergebn. Biol.,* 22:212-225, 1960.

Katsuki, Y.: Neural Mechanism of Auditory Sensation in Cats. In Rosenblith, W.A. (Ed.): *Sensory Communication.* New York, M.I.T. Pr. and John Wiley, 1961, pp. 561-583.

Katsuki, Y., T. Sumi, H. Uchiyama, and T. Watanabe: Electric responses of auditory neurons in cat to sound stimulation. *J. Neurophysiol.,* 21:569-588, 1958.

Katz, B.: Depolarization of sensory terminals and the initiation of impulses in the muscle spindle. *J. Physiol. (London),* 111:261-282, 1950.

Lindblom, U.: Phasic and static excitability of touch receptors in toad skin. *Acta Physiol. Scand.,* 59:410-423, 1963.

Lindblom, U., and D.N. Tapper: Terminal properties of a vibro-tactile sensor. *Exp. Neurol.,* 17:1-15, 1967.

Loewenstein, W.: Excitation and inactivation in a receptor membrane. *Ann. N.Y. Acad. Sci.,* 94:510-534, 1961.

MacKay, D.M.: Psychophysics of perceived intensity: a theoretical basis for Fechner's and Stevens' laws. *Science,* 139:1213-1216, 1963.

MacNichol, Jr., E.F.: Three-pigment color vision. *Sci. Amer.,* 211:48-56, 1964.

Marks, L.E., and A.W. Slawson: Direct test of the power function for loudness. *Science, 154:* 1036-1037, 1966.

Matthews, B.H.C.: The response of a single end organ. *J. Physiol. (London),* 71:64-110, 1931.

McGill, W.J., and J.P. Goldberg: A study of the near-miss involving Weber's law and pure-tone intensity discrimination. *Percept. Psychophys.,* 4:105-109, 1968.

Melzack, R., and P.D. Wall: Pain mechanisms: a new theory. *Science,* 150:971-979, 1965.

Millodot, M.: Psychophysical scaling of corneal sensitivity. *Psychon. Sci.,* 12:401-402, 1968.

Millodot, M.: Studies on the sensitivity of the cornea. *Optician,* 157:267-271, 1969.

Morita, H., and S. Yamashita: Further studies on the receptor potential of chemoreceptors of the blowfly. *Mem. Fac. Sci. Kyushu Univ. E,* 4:83-93, 1966.

Mountcastle, V.B.: Duke University Conference. In Somjen, G.G.: Sensory coding. *Science,* 158:399-405, 1967.

Mountcastle, V.B.: Neural dynamics in somethesis: peripheral encoding, central neural transformation and sensory psychophysics of flutter-vibration. Proc. Intl. Un. Physiol. Sci. Washington. *Fed. Amer. Soc. Exp. Biol.,* 6: 260-261, 1968.

Mountcastle, V.B., C.F. Poggio, and G. Werner: The relation of thalamic cell response to peripheral stimuli varied over an intensive continuum. *J. Neurophysiol.,* 26:807-834, 1963.

Mozell, M.M.: Olfactory mucosal and neural responses in the frog. *Amer. J. Physiol.,* 203: 353-358, 1962.

Oyama, T.: A behavioristic analysis of Stevens'

magnitude estimation method. *Percept. Psychophys.*, *3*:317-320, 1968.

Pfaffmann, C.: Gustatory nerve impulses in rat, cat and rabbit. *J. Neurophysiol.*, *18*:429-440, 1955.

Poggio, G.F., and V.B. Mountcastle: The functional properties of ventrobasal thalamic neurons studied in unanesthetized monkeys. *J. Neurophysiol.*, *26*:775-806, 1963.

Reynolds, G.S., and S.S. Stevens: Binaural summation of loudness. *J. Acoust. Soc. Amer.*, *32*: 1337-1344, 1960.

Roeder, K.D.: Moths and ultrasound. *Sci. Amer.*, *212*:94-102, 1965.

Roeder, K.D., A.E. Treat, and J.S. Vandeberg: Auditory sense in certain sphingid moths. *Science*, *159*:331-333, 1968.

Rosenblith, W.A. *Processing Neuroelectric Data*. Cambridge, M.I.T. Pr., 1962.

Rosner, B.S., and W.R. Goff: Electrical responses of the nervous system and subjective scales of intensity. In Neff, W.D. (Ed.): *Contributions to Sensory Physiology*. New York, Academic, 1967, vol. 2, pp. 169-221.

Rushton, W.A.H.: Peripheral Coding in the Nervous System. In Rosenblith, W.A. (Ed.): *Sensory Communication*. New York, M.I.T. Pr. and John Wiley, 1961, pp. 169-181.

Sato, M.: In Wayner, M.J., and Y. Oomura: Neuronal spike trains (report on 1967 Honolulu meeting). *Science*, *160*:1025-1026, 1968a.

Sato, M.: On some basic laws in physiological systems. *Kybernetik*, *4*:195-197, 1968b.

Stevens, S.S.: A scale for the measurement of a psychological magnitude: loudness. *Psychol. Rev.*, *43*:405-406, 1936.

Stevens, S.S.: The measurement of loudness. *J. Acoust. Soc. Amer.*, *27*:815-829, 1955.

Stevens, S.S.: The psychophysics of sensory function. *Amer. Sci.*, *48*:226-253, 1960. Also in Rosenblith, W.A. (Ed.): *Sensory Communication*. New York, M.I.T. Pr. and John Wiley, 1961, pp. 1-33.

Stevens, S.S.: To honor Fechner and repeal his law. *Science*, *133*:80-86, 1961.

Stevens, S.S.: Matching functions between loudness and ten other continua. *Percept. Psychophys.*, *1*:5-8, 1966a.

Stevens, S.S.: Duration, luminance, and the brightness exponent. *Percept. Psychophys.*, *1*:96-100, 1966b.

Stevens, S.S.: Power-group transformations under glare, masking and recruitment. *J. Acoust. Soc.*

Amer., *39*:725-735, 1966c.

Stevens, S.S.: Transfer Functions of the Skin and Muscle Senses. In DeReuck, A.V.S., and J. Knight (Eds.): *Ciba Foundation Symposium on Touch, Heat and Pain*, London, Churchill, 1966d, pp. 3-17.

Stevens, S.S.: Intensity functions in sensory systems. *Int. J. Neurol.*, *6*:202-209, 1967.

Stevens, S.S.: Tactile vibration: change of exponent with frequency. *Percept. Psychophys.*, *3*: 223-228, 1968.

Suga, N.: Hearing in some arboreal edentates in terms of cochlear microphonics and neural activity. *J. Audit. Res.*, *7*:267-270, 1967.

Suga, N.: Neural responses to sound in a Brazilian mole cricket. *J. Audit. Res.*, *8*:129-134, 1968.

Talbot, W.H., I. Darian-Smith, H.H. Kornhuber, and V.B. Mountcastle: The sense of flutter-vibration: comparison of the human capacity with response patterns of mechanoreceptive afferents from the monkey hand. *J. Neurophysiol.*, *31*:301-334, 1968.

Tapper, D.N., and M.D. Mann: Single presynaptic impulse evokes postsynaptic discharge. *Brain Res.*, *11*:688-690, 1968.

Tasaki, I.: Nerve impulses in individual auditory nerve fibers of guinea pig. *J. Neurophysiol.*, *17*:97-122, 1954.

Treisman, M., and R.J. Irwin: Auditory intensity discriminal scale. I. Evidence derived from binaural intensity summation. *J. Acoust. Soc. Amer.*, *42*:586-592, 1967.

Vasilevskii, N.N., Z.A. Aleksanyan, and S.I. Soroko: Activity evoked in cortical neurons and primary cutaneous afferent fibers by vibratory stimulation. *Fiziol. Zh. SSSR Sechenov.*, *53*:1082-1090, 1967.

Ward, W.D.: Use of sensation level in measurements of loudness and of temporary threshold shifts. *J. Acoust. Soc. Amer.*, *39*:736-740, 1966.

Weber, E.H.: Der Tastsinn und das Gemeingefühl. In Wagner, R. (Ed): *Handwörterbuch der Physiologie*. Braunschweig, Viewig, 1846, Vol. III, pp. 481-588.

Werner, G.: The Study of Sensation in Physiology: Psychophysical and Neurophysiologic Correlation. In Mountcastle, V.B. (Ed.): *Medical Physiology, 12th ed.* St. Louis, C.V. Mosby, 1968, Chapter 70.

Wolbarsht, M.L.: Electrical characteristics of insect mechanoreceptors. *J. Gen. Physiol.*, *44*: 105-122, 1960.

SUGGESTED READING

Ashby, W.R.: Mathematical models and computer analysis of the function of the central nervous system. *Ann. Rev. Physiol.*, 28:89-106, 1966.

Christensen, K.R.: Methodology in Preference Testing. In Kare, M.R., and B.P. Halpern (Eds.): *Physiological and Behavioral Aspects of Taste.* Chicago, U. of Chicago Pr., 1961, pp. 79-91.

Foerster, H. von: Computation in neural nets. *Curr. Mod. Biol.*, 1:47-93, 1967.

Granit, R.: *Receptors and Sensory Perception.* New Haven, Yale U. Pr., 1955.

Gross, C.G., and H.P. Zeigler (Eds.): *Readings in Physiological Psychology. Neurophysiology/ Sensory Processes.* New York, Harper and Row, 1969.

Hubel, D.H.: The visual cortex of the brain. *Sci. Amer.*, 209:54-62, 1963.

MacKay, D.M., *et al.*: Evoked brain potentials as indicators of sensory information processing. *Neurosciences Res. Prog. Bull.*, 7:181-276, 1969.

Ogawa, H., M. Sato, and S. Yamashita: Multiple sensitivity of chorda tympani fibres of the rat and hamster to gustatory and thermal stimuli. *J. Physiol. (London)*, 199:223-240, 1968.

Perkel, D.H., and T.H. Bullock: Neural coding. *Neurosci. Res. Prog. Bull.*, 6:221-348, 1968.

Roeder, K.D.: Moths and ultrasound. *Sci. Amer.*, 212:94-102, 1965.

Rosner, B.S., and W.R. Goff: Electrical Responses of the Nervous System and Subjective Scales of Intensity. In Neff, W.D. (Ed.): *Contributions to Sensory Physiology.* New York, Academic, 1967, vol. 2, pp. 169-221.

Stevens, S.S.: The psychophysics of sensory function. *Amer. Sci.*, 48:226-253, 1960. Also in Rosenblith, W.A. (Ed.): *Sensory Communication.* New York, M.I.T. Pr. and John Wiley, 1961, pp. 1-33.

Stevens, S.S.: To honor Fechner and repeal his law. *Science*, 133:80-86, 1961.

Stevens, S.S.: Intensity functions in sensory systems. *Int. J. Neurol.*, 6:202-209, 1967.

Werner, G.: The Study of Sensation in Physiology: Psychophysical and Neurophysiologic Correlation. In Mountcastle, V.B. (Ed.): *Medical Physiology, 12th ed.* St. Louis, C.V. Mosby, 1968, Chapter 70.

Whitfield, I.C.: Coding in the auditory nervous system. *Nature*, 213:756-760, 1967.

A Survey of the Receptors

Receptors are end organs which are specialized to inform the brain of external or internal changes. These sensory end organs vary greatly in their degree of structural complexity and in the level of sophistication of their adaptation to their function. Also, the immense variation in the specific external and internal stimuli to be monitored has resulted in the development of a multitude of differing types of receptors.

The division of such a spectrum of structures along arbitrary lines is usually unsatisfactory; therefore, sensory receptors do not readily lend themselves to practical classification. The receptors covered in this chapter under Types and Locations are treated according to a scheme which represents a compromise. In the first portion of Types and Locations, the important receptor types are arranged according to their basic structure, but this is followed by a division of receptors along the lines of location into exteroceptors and interoceptors.

The last method of classification is most suitable for the examination of certain specialized receptor types. Among these are included insect visceral stretch receptors, thermal and chemoreceptors of the brain, the chemoreceptors of the carotid body, and the pressure receptors of the aorta.

The muscle spindle, the crustacean stretch receptor and the labyrinth of the vertebrate ear have been subjected to an unusually large amount of research. Findings resulting from some of this research have elucidated aspects of receptor function in general. A separate section of this chapter is therefore devoted to each of these three sensory structures.

A discussion of the nervous innervation of some receptors follows types and locations.

TYPES AND LOCATIONS

Free Nerve Endings

A sensory end organ may be only a free afferent nerve ending, such as a nociceptor which mediates pain or a trigeminal ending for common chemical sense.

Such free nerve endings are the most numerous receptors in man, and at the body surface are found both in the epithelium and the dermis of the skin. In monkeys, pigs, cats and rats, free terminals are not too frequent in the epidermis of hairy skin, but are encountered in high numbers in the epidermis of the glabrous, thickened skin of the nose, as well as in the epithelium of the nasal and oral cavities.

Sea robins (*Prionotus carolinus*) also possess free nerve endings. These teleost fish have separated anterior fin rays carrying knoblike evaginations that act as mechanoreceptors (Bardach and Case, 1965). The knob epidermis is innervated by nerve fibers which bear free terminal swellings and pass around the outermost epidermal cells (Scharrer, 1963).

The free nerve endings of man's skin are primarily sensitive to pain and temperature change, show great differences in axoplasmic content and cholinesterases, and may be the terminations of any type of axon (Cauna, 1966). However, these endings usually arise from medium or small myelinated axons. Nociceptors are widely branched and their receptive fields overlap.

In the corium of the domestic cat's foot pad are found both simple free endings and arborized endings (Malinovský, 1966a). Such endings also exist in mammalian and avian joint capsules. The dentine canals of permanent mammalian teeth contain single tapered nociceptor terminals, the endings of branches from a pulp sensory axon, which are responsive to heat, touch and chemicals (Frank, 1966) and have a steady normal impulse rate of 10/sec (Scott, Jr., 1968). The free branched endings of thin myelinated (see Chap. VI) nerve fibers function as cold receptors in the tongue of the cat (Zotterman, 1959). Numerous subdivided free nerve endings, each expanded subdivision giving rise to many delicate branching processes, are the warmth receptors in the facial pits of pit vipers (Bullock, 1959).

The facial pits of some pythons and boas also detect changes in environmental radiant heat. The Australian python's (*Morelia spilotes*) facial pits are innervated by free axons of the trigeminal nerve. In some cases these axons, like their counterparts in pit vipers, have palmate endings. In others subterminal axonal swellings give rise to filaments which in the skin surface again enlarge into conical forms. The last in turn give rise to delicate, short filaments (Warren and Proske, 1968). The axons in question show a spontaneous discharge which rises in frequency if a warm object approaches and falls in frequency in proximity to a cold object.

Ice brought to within 30 cm of Crotalidae pits immediately and completely suppresses the spontaneous discharge (Goris and Nomoto, 1967).

Goris and Nomoto (1967), recording electrophysiologically from the pit membrane supramaxillary nerves of oriental Crotalidae, observed that the response to infrared changed from the continuous tonic to phasic when the level of stimulation exceeded the normal, "bearable" limits. The phasic response consisted of an "on" burst of spikes followed by cessation of the response during the remainder of a maintained stimulus, and an "off" burst after the end of stimulation. The latent period preceding the "off" burst was proportional to the duration of the stimulus.

The pit membrane lacked any unusual absorptive capacities for infrared, and seems only to provide mechanical support for the sensitive nerve endings.

Bullock and Barrett (1968) examined five families of snakes, and found that of these only the Boidae, the boas and pythons, and the Crotalidae, the pit vipers, are sensitive to radiant heat. All investigated species of the last two families have such sensitivity, even if they do not possess facial or labial pits. Electrophysiological records were obtained from branches of the trigeminal nerve. The Boidae, in which warmth receptors evolved separately, appear to have somewhat lower sensitivity and to possess receptive areas which are less suited for the discrimination of direction. The threshold sensitivity of two boas in terms of caloric flux is 1.3×10^{-3} calories CM^2SEC^{-1}, that known for pit vipers 3.15×10^{-4} calories $CM^2 SEC^{-1}$. The responses may show depression and a subsequent rise and fall.

Encapsulated Nerve Endings

More complex receptors consist of nerve endings surrounded by other tissue. Shantha, Golarz and Bourne (1968) state that the capsules of pacinian and Herbst corpuscles, muscle spindles, end bulbs of Krause, and Meissner's corpuscles are continuations of the perineural epithelium surrounding the nerve fibers innervating these receptors.

Enveloped end organs in the skin, because of their relatively greater depth, are not as subject to pain and temperature stimulation as are the free nerve endings. However, mechanical deformation of the overlying tissues is easily transmitted to them.

The pacinian corpuscle is found, among other locations, subcutaneously and in the deepest layers of the dermis, at a greater depth than the other cutaneous sense organs. It may be sensitive to higher frequency vibration (or at least pressure changes) or may monitor changes in local blood supply (Sinclair, 1967). The pacinian corpuscle is an unusually large receptor and is 0.5 to 0.7 mm across and about 1 mm in length. It consists of an afferent nerve ending with terminal branches bearing end bulbs, surrounded by thirty odd interconnected lamellae of squamous epithelial cells which are less than 1μ thick. The outer layers of these cells are continuous with the perineural epithelium investing the innervating nerve fiber (Shantha veerappa and Bourne, 1963). The endoneurium and myelin sheath of the nerve fiber both enter the corpuscle, but then terminate together so that the distal portion of the nerve fiber is left bare. A node of Ranvier is found along the curved portion of the axon within the proximal part of the corpuscle. Immediately outside of the corpuscle another node of Ranvier constricts the axon's myelin sheath, and such nodes are spaced close to 0.25 mm apart along the course of the nerve fiber.

Cherepnov (1968a, b) observed the inner core of the cat's pacinian corpuscle to be composed of the processes of lamellar cells. The somas of these cells are located in the part of the corpuscle where the nerve fiber's myelin sheath ends. The inner core cell processes contain a large number of vacuoles having a diameter of 250 to 600 Å. In the functional corpuscle all these vacuoles, which are evenly distributed throughout the inner core, release their contents into the capsular fluid.

The inner core of the corpuscle is divided into two symmetrical portions by a thin space (Cherepnov, 1968a), which is occupied by the elliptical nerve ending (Pease and Quilliam, 1957).

The sensory nerve ending has the shape of an elliptical cylinder within the inner core. Beyond the last the nerve fiber is round, and has a diameter of 4μ to 11μ (Il'Inskii, Volkova and Cherepnov, 1968).

The nerve ending in the pacinian corpuscle contains many mitochondria and also small, spherical structures the significance of which is not yet understood (Loewenstein, 1960a).

Cherepnov (1968a) noted round, vesicle-containing structures in the inner core of the cat's pacinian corpuscle.

Sensory corpuscles resembling pacinian corpuscles have been described from the skin of the nasal-mouth zone of cattle by Hebel and Schweiger (1967). Using electron microscopy, they identified collagenous fibrils between the lamellae of the corpuscles and characterized the lamellae as composed of connective tissue. The distal portion of the sensory nerve ending of this corpuscle sends out fingerlike projections, and at the bases of the last mitochondria, vesicles, granules and fibrils are massed.

Hebel and Schweiger thus do not corroborate the observations of Shantha, Golarz and Bourne (1968) that the outer lamellae of such types of corpuscles are continuations of the perineural epithelium.

Merkel's disks and the lancetlike endings and lamellated corpuscles of vibrissae have also been found to have fingerlike sensory projections (Andres, 1966b), and it appears possible that the last will be observed in additional sense receptors.

Pacinian-type corpuscles show a differential distribution in the skin of the domestic cat (*Felix domestica*). They are most numerous in the area of the sulcus labii maxillaris, less so in the nasal and upper lip regions, and least frequent in the foot pad (Malinovský, 1966c).

Encapsulated corpuscles with split axons are described from the foot pad of the cat by Malinovský (1966a). Such types of corpuscles with branched axons are most common in the foot pad, and much less frequent in the cat's facial regions (Malinovský, 1966c). They may contribute to the more delicate mechanoreception required to distinguish the variety of mechanical stimuli acting on the foot pad (Malinovský, 1966b).

Merkel's disks are touch receptors in the hairy skin of man (and lower animals) and in such skin are found at the tip of deep epidermal processes. In Merkel's disk a specialized epidermal cell surrounded by a basement membrane is contacted by a large, flat nerve ending (Cauna, 1966).

Meissner's corpuscles respond to touch in the papillary ridges of the hairless glabrous skin of man's feet and hands. They are also present in the hairless skin, such as that of the lips, of a large number of animals. These receptor organs are composed of flat laminar cells formed into a column which is innervated by nerve endings (Cauna, 1966). The whole corpuscle is surrounded by a highly developed basement membrane and an elastic capsule.

The existence and anatomy of Ruffini's organ, believed to be a heat receptor, is in doubt. Ruffini's organ has been considered an "expanded tip," rather than an encapsulated organ.

Krause's end bulbs are generally credited with sensitivity to cold, and are located in the dermis of mucosa-cutaneous border zones. According to Winkelmann (1960), they are composed in man of a loose ball of myelinated and unmyelinated fibers, and the concentrated tissue which surrounds these nerve elements is not clearly formed into a capsule. However, in lower mammals Winkelmann (1960) observed a cellular capsule, and in these organisms it enclosed a central nerve.

Kellner (1966) instead reports Krause's end bulbs in man to be surrounded by a capsule composed of several delicate connective tissue lamellae. He found these receptors to further contain a well-developed capillary network within their connective tissue envelope.

Transitional receptors between Meissner's corpuscles and Krause's end bulbs have been found in the human skin (Kellner, 1966), and simpler corpuscular end organs exist in the tongue and the hairless regions of the genitalia. There seems to be an entire spectrum of cutaneous end organs.

Malinovský (1966a) found many gradations and similarities among the split and indented sensory corpuscles of the foot pad of the domestic cat (Fig. 2-1). He tends to agree with the view that there is a spectrum of developmental levels leading in a continuous line from the most primitive free endings to the pacinian corpuscle.

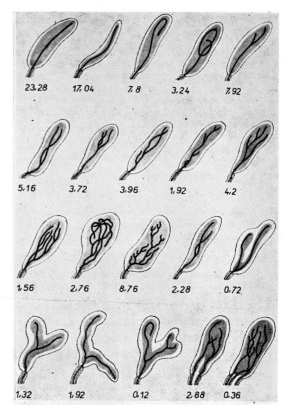

FIGURE 2-1. Structural variability among the corpuscles of the cat's foot pad. The percentage of occurrence is given beneath each type. (From Malinovský, L.: Variability of sensory nerve endings in foot pads of a domestic cat [*Felis ocreata* L., *F. domestica*]. *Acta Anat.*, 64:82-106, 1966 [Karger, Basel/New York 1966].)

Siminoff and Kruger (1968) have identified two types of myelinated afferent fibers in the hind limb of the alligator. These innervate receptors that appear to resemble the mechanoreceptors of mammalian glabrous skin. One category of fibers gives only "on" and "off" discharges on displacement of the scales or claws and thus seems to serve phasic receptors. This group of fibers has the lower thresholds. The second type of afferent fibers adapts slowly and indicates the magnitude of applied force or cutaneous movement.

On the snout of the mole (*Talpa*) sense organs known as Eimer's organs produce very small elevations. In each Eimer's organ there are many geometrically arranged unmyelinated nerve endings. Deeper in the organ lies a group of Merkel's disks, and in the dermis below the Eimer's organ, a lamellated end organ.

The dermis of the mole's snout generally contains pacinian-type corpuscles and large myelinated nerve plexuses, and seems to have

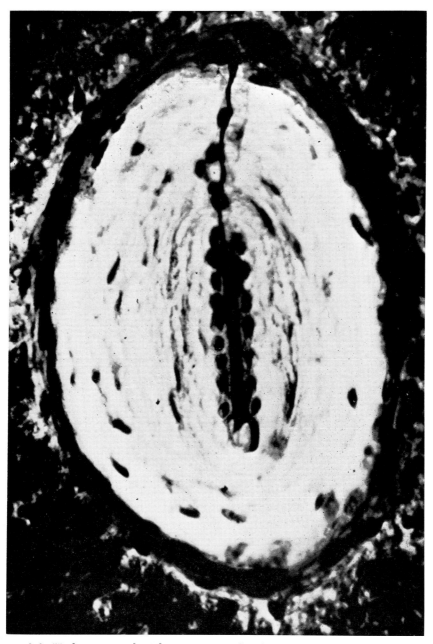

FIGURE 2-2. Herbst corpuscle. The outer capsule, the middle core composed of longitudinal lamellae and the inner core can be differentiated. In the inner core a row of nuclei can be seen on each side of the internal nerve ending. The last terminates in a vesicle of approximately 10μ diameter. (From Quilliam, T.A., P. Graziadei, and J. Armstrong: Recettori cutanei. *Rassegna medica e culturale*, 41:31-41, 1964. Courtesy G. Gondoni, Editor.)

important sensory functions (Quilliam, Graziadei and Armstrong, 1964).

Pinkus plates are especially common in the abdominal skin of the mole. These highly vascularized skin elevations, also observed in the hairy skin of man and the cat, contain receptors of the type of Merkel's disks (Quilliam, 1966). The disk receptors are typically associated with a single large myelinated fiber (Mann and Straile, 1965). Every Pinkus plate seen by Mann and Straile was associated with either a sensory hair follicle or a vibrissa follicle.

Ducks possess lamellated corpuscles known as Herbst corpuscles, which are presumably sensitive to vibration, immediately under the surface of their bills, in the connective tissue of their skin and mucosa, and in their joint capsules. In the duck (*Anas*) there is located on each side of the internal nerve ending a row of six to ten nuclei, and these rows join distally around the axon ending, which is enlarged there (Fig. 2-2). A more elongated form of Herbst corpuscle found in other birds may contain rows of up to thirty nuclei each. A third and less common type of Herbst corpuscle not found in ducks but present in chickens (*Gallus*) has a low number of nuclei, which are not ordered into rows. The capsule of this type is formed by a low number of lamellae (Malinovský, 1967).

Polacek *et al.* (1966) examined thousands of encapsulated bird corpuscles, and observed that these formed a continuous series of transitions from very simple corpuscles of a paciniform type to the composite Herbst corpuscles. The simplest forms included various elongated, thin and bent corpuscles. A few split corpuscles and some arranged like beads on a single axon were seen. Axons also showed peculiarities within some corpuscles, such as a wavy course, doubling back, or several bifurcations.

Encapsulated corpuscles are much more numerous in the joint capsules of birds than in those of mammals. Among bird joints the highest concentration of corpuscles is met in the wing joints. The joint corpuscles are mostly aligned parallel to the joint capsule surface.

A corpuscle of the pacinian type, but with transversely oriented lamellae in the intermediate core, has been reported from a woodpecker's beak (*Dendrocopus*) (Quilliam, Graziadei and Armstrong, 1964).

Just below the duck's bill surface lie Grandry corpuscles, of still undetermined function. Grandry corpuscles consist of a nerve disk bordered on each side by a satellite cell. All three structures are encompassed by a thin capsule. On entering the corpuscle, the nerve fiber loses its myelin sheath.

Generally lamellated corpuscles are found in lower layers of connective tissue than Grandry's corpuscles. Spraylike nerve endings that lie among auxiliary cells have been described from the joint capsules of mammals and birds.

Specialized Sensory Neurons

On the other hand, a receptor may be a specialized nerve cell, such as the sensory neurons subserving specific taste modalities in insects.

Also in insects the dendrite of a sensory neuron may curl around the base of a chitinous hair to form a simple touch receptor. Similar arrangements are present in still lower animal phyla. An insect dendrite may be attached internally to a softer section of cuticle subject to torsion, to form a scolopidium.

Pabst and Kennedy (1967) have described a new type of crustacean mechanoreceptor neuron from the crayfish (*Procambarus*). This receptor initiates reflex suppression of the tonic efferent discharge to the abdominal flexor muscles and the swimmerets. The mentioned mechanoreceptor neurons are unusual in that their cell bodies lie along the proximal portions of the segmental nerves. The bipolar, or less commonly tripolar, bodies of the neurons are located along the first and second nerve roots of the abdominal ganglia and within several millimeters of each ganglion. The neuron cell bodies, which normally form groups, each give rise to highly branched dendrites which innervate widely separated areas of the inner surface of the abdominal ventral cuticle. Innervation of cuticular hypodermis at the sites of superficial flexor muscle insertion and in the bases of appendages is particularly frequent. A single receptor's sensory field may extend over the ventral surface of two adjoining abdominal segments. Impulses are transmitted at an average speed of 0.6-0.8 meters/sec in dendrites, and an action potential originating in any dendritic branch spreads to the others by axon reflex. The dendrites commonly terminate in end bulbs having a distal "peg." The receptors are most sensitive to weak pressure on the cuticle.

It is estimated that fifty to one hundred such mechanoreceptors may be present in the abdomen of a crayfish.

Sensory Hairs

Mammalian tactile hairs function by means of large areas of contact between nerve branches and the epithelial cells of the hair root sheath (Cauna, 1966).

The vibrissae of mammals such as the rat, cat, rabbit and mole (*Talpa*) may be more specialized. These vibrissae are thought capable of transmitting pressure waves produced by their owner's approach to objects. In this way cats and moles may become aware of objects and prey in total darkness (Quilliam, Graziadei and Armstrong, 1964).

Vibrissae have been reported to possess directional sensitivity (Fitzgerald, 1940), perhaps by virtue of the differential excitation of some of their straight lancet sensory endings (Andres, 1966b). Less than 5 per cent of a cat's vibrissae have a spontaneous discharge, and their adaptation is slow.

Andres (1966a, 1966b), using optical and electron microscopes, has made a thorough investigation of the structure of rat, cat and rabbit vibrissae.

The vibrissa hair root is surrounded by blood sinuses, a proximal spongy sinus and a distal ring sinus (Fig. 2-3). These sinuses have developed from the capillary network of ordinary hair follicles.

In the outermost layer of the root sheath's distal thickening are located Merkel's disks. These sensory cells give rise to fingerlike processes, 0.3μ thick and 2μ to 3μ long, which contain predominantly axially oriented, delicate filaments. The basal cells surrounding the Merkel's disks have vesiculated membranes, this vesiculation being heaviest on the sides adjacent to the sense cells and their associated platelike nerve endings.

In the inner hair follicle myelinated nerve fibers terminate in sensory endings shaped like thick lancets. The flat sides of these lancetlike endings are covered by Schwann cells with heavily vesiculated plasma membranes (the vesiculation is greatest adjacent to the endings). However, the free edges of each ending and the midline of its tip give rise to fingerlike processes which are 0.5μ to 3.5μ long (Fig. 2-4). These processes, which appear to attach the sensory endings to the connective tissue, may be the site of origin of the receptor potential. Bending of the hair should lead to movement of the connective tissue and result in stretching of the receptor membrane.

In the lancet endings, as in the Merkel's disks, are found an axial bundle of neurofilaments and microtubules as well as mitochondria. In the outer layer of an ending are located vesicular bodies (also in the Merkel's disks) and delicate filaments. The last also run axially through the fingerlike processes (Fig. 2-4).

The endings can be subdivided into straight lancet terminals, branched lancet terminals and circular lancet terminals. The straight terminals are located at the level of the distal thickening of the root sheath, branched terminals are found external to the root sheath's proximal thickening, and circular terminals have only been observed in the sinus hairs of the rat (Fig. 2-3).

In the inner hair follicle, at the level of the proximal thickening of the root sheath, there are encapsulated corpuscles (Fig. 2-3). These contain a lancetlike sensory ending jutting out between, and surrounded by, cellular lamellae. Andres (1966b) suggests that the corpuscles, through stretching of the fingerlike processes on their sensory endings, may be responsive to blood pressure changes in the spongy sinus.

In the rat's sinus hairs the endings of unmyelinated fibers are also present.

Nilsson and Skoglund (1965) have investi-

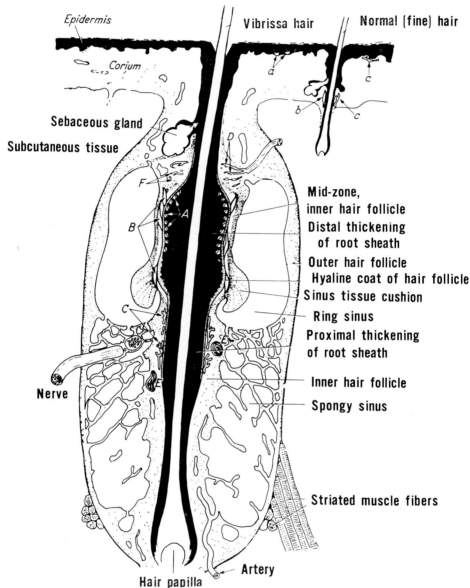

FIGURE 2-3. Diagrammatic longitudinal section of a vibrissa hair from the upper lip of the rat. The hair root and follicle have been considerably shortened in the lower portion of the drawing. The receptor structures are represented in their proper locations by enlarged symbols. (A) Merkel's disks, (B) straight lancet-shaped terminals, (C) branched lancet-shaped terminals, (D) circular lancet-shaped terminals, (E) encapsulated corpuscles. The respective receptors at the normal lip hair (upper right) have been labeled with the equivalent lower case letters. (Adapted from Andres, K.H.: Über die Feinstruktur der Rezeptoren an Sinushaaren. Z. *Zellforsch.*, 75:339-365, 1966 [Berlin-Heidelberg-New York, Springer].)

gated tactile hairs located at the wrist of the cat's foreleg, hairs which resemble the vibris- sae surrounding the mouth. As in vibrissae, a sizeable blood sinus is found in the follicles

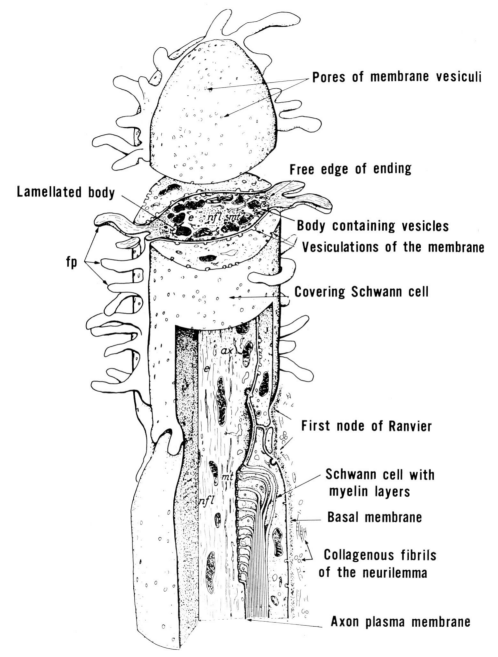

FIGURE 2-4. In depth representation of a straight lancet-shaped terminal in a vibrissa. The terminal's main portion (*e*) has been shortened. The axoplasm (*ax*) is shown to contain neurofilaments (*nfl*), microtubules (*mt*), a reticulum and mitochondria. At its free edges the ending bears fingerlike processes (*fp*). (Adapted from Andres, K.H.: Über die Feinstruktur der Rezeptoren an Sinushaaren. Z. *Zellforsch.,* 75:339-365, 1966 [Berlin-Heidelberg-New York, Springer].)

of these tactile hairs. Around each follicle there are five to thirteen pacinian corpuscles.

The nerve endings of the majority of wrist tactile hairs produce a spontaneous discharge. Bending a hair may result in a frequency of as many as 250 impulses/sec, but this early response discharge quickly falls to an impulse rate of 20-40/sec, which is maintained for a few minutes. The tactile hairs, like vibrissae, adapt much more slowly than the pacinian corpuscles. No clear-cut directional sensitivity was noted.

Nilsson and Skoglund review previous hypotheses that the blood sinus enclosing the hair root may increase the hair's sensitivity to vibration, or may permit control of sensitivity. They then suggest that the nearby pacinian corpuscles may monitor pulsations or other parameters of the blood sinus.

The trichobothria, delicate hairs on the cuticle of some arthropod groups, seem to be air current receptors. In the spider *Tegenaria* the hair ends proximally, below the body surface, in a bilobed (tarsus) or trilobed (tibia) helmet-shaped structure which encompasses two or three neurons (Görner, 1965). Each neuron is activated only by hair displacement in one direction. The excitation of a neuron seems to result from deformation due to its being inclined over the edge of the helmet structure. The impulse frequency is determined both by the direction and by the angular velocity of displacement.

The sensilla (hairs) of the cervical hair plates of insects act as position receptors in joints. In the honeybee (*Apis mellifica*) these sensilla and also campaniform sensilla were stimulated if a cap at the base of the hair was compressed. This cap, probably composed of the protein resilin, encloses a special outer segment of a dendrite (part of a bipolar neuron). Thus compression of the terminal portion of the nerve fiber's outer segment can be assumed to be the specific stimulatory action (Thurm, 1964).

Desert locusts possess wind-receptor hairs on their head. A single neuron's dendrite is eccentrically connected to each hair, and the hairs point forward at some angle of curvature. The response obtained is greatest if the wind comes from the direction into which the hair is pointed (Camhi, 1967). Accommodation is slow.

Vibration Receptors

Sensory neurons may further act as vibration receptors.

This is exemplified by the subgenual organs, found in the tibia of some insect groups, and composed of neurons spanning the space between tracheae and the exoskeleton. These neurons are stimulated by vibrations of 100 to 10,000 cps (Autrum and Schneider, 1948).

The lyriform organ of the vibration receptors of spiders is located proximally to the tarsal-metatarsal joints of the legs. It consists of a series of parallel surface chambers which give the appearance of slits and are each connected by a small opening to an internal vessel. In the case of every surface chamber a terminal nerve filament, essentially lacking in internal structure, runs from the end bulb of a bipolar sense cell through the small inner opening of the chamber unto a chamber wall (Salpeter and Walcott, 1960). These vibration receptors are sensitive to frequencies of 20 to over 45,000 cps and respond to a threshold displacement of the spider leg tip of 25 Å. The spider's vibration organs are stimulated by prey movements in the web, but the separate tuning of individual chambers to specific frequencies does not hold true for vibrations transmitted through the strands of the web (Walcott and Salpeter, 1966). The spider's courtship is also dependent on the vibration receptors.

An arachnid sense organ, consisting of a single chamber opening on the tarsus, has been shown electrophysiologically to be sound sensitive. In this one-slit sense organ a nerve terminal is found at the outer membrane rather than on the chamber wall as in the lyriform organ (Levi and Dondale, 1968).

Arachnid slit sense organs are all considered to be mechanoreceptors (Barth, in Levi and Dondale, 1968).

Sensory Epithelial Cells

The olfactory cells and retinal rods and cones of vertebrates represent highly evolved and specialized primary sense cells (sensory neurons) and possess long central processes. New visual cells cannot develop to replace lost ones.

However, a receptor may also be a spe-cialized sensory epithelial cell (a secondary sense cell) which is in intimate contact with one or more afferent nerve fibers, as in the case of taste receptors. Secondary sense cells may be defined as modified epithelial cells.

In fish the secondary sense cells for taste have been described as being as sensitive as the primary sense cells for olfaction (Glaser,

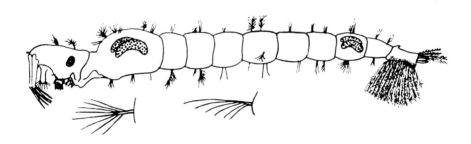

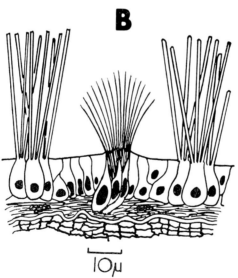

FIGURE 2-5. Vibration receptors in aquatic invertebrates. A. The *Chaoborus* mosquito larva. Shown in detail below are the branched bristles which are presumed to respond to water vibration. B. A group of cilia (center), each of which apparently originates in a separate sensory neuron, and two bunches of setae that are believed to be touch receptors, from the chaetognath *Spadella*. The cilia are thought to be vibration receptors and alternate with groups of setae around the periphery. Both the *Chaoborus* larva and *Spadella* show directional sensitivity to vibration. (From Horridge, G.A.: Some Recently Discovered Underwater Vibration Receptors in Invertebrates. In Barnes, H. [Ed.]: *Some Contemporary Studies in Marine Science.* London, George Allen and Unwin, and New York, Hafner, 1966, pp. 395-405.)

1966). However, in most vertebrates olfaction (by primary sense cells) is far keener than gustation (by secondary sense cells). Man may detect some substances by smell when their concentration is only 1/3,000 of that needed for tasting them.

Let us examine the distribution of secondary sense cells in the animal kingdom and learn something of the types of receptor organs in which they may play a role.

Hair Cells

Hair cells present in statocysts may in different phyla be secondary sense cells or primary sense cells. Hair cells are found in the statocysts of most phyla possessing these mechanoreceptor organs of equilibration, and statocysts already appear in the Coelenterata. In arthropods, however, the statocysts contain chitinous hairs innervated by sensory neurons (Cohen, 1960).

The hair cells of statocysts are stimulated by a shearing force produced by a change in position of the statolith, a mass with a greater specific gravity than the statocyst fluid. Such stimulation takes place when the organism ceases to move in a horizontal plane.

Maturana and Sperling (1963) recorded nerve impulses from the statocyst of *Octopus vulgaris*. They obtained no spontaneous discharge but got a unidirectional response to angular acceleration (counterclockwise). The octopus statocyst, significant in posture and equilibrium, also responds to low-frequency vibration which is not airborne.

Receptors sensitive to currents of water (rheoreceptors) are found throughout the animal kingdom, but they are primary sense cells in invertebrates (Hoar, 1966), while the lateral line receptors of vertebrates are secondary sense cells.

In ctenophores, chaetognaths, and on the claws and carapace of the lobster there are sensory neurons ending in nonmotile cilia or bristles which act as vibration receptors. This is probably also true of some coelenterates. The *Chaoborus* mosquito larva bears several types of branched bristles (Fig. 2-5A) which appear to be vibration receptors (Horridge, 1966). Some of these receptors, probably by virtue of their being organized into groups or their having a fan of bristles, provide directional sensitivity.

The whirligig water beetle (*Gyrinus substriatus*) has directional sensitivity to surface waves and other vibrations. Surface waves with an amplitude of a few micrometers call

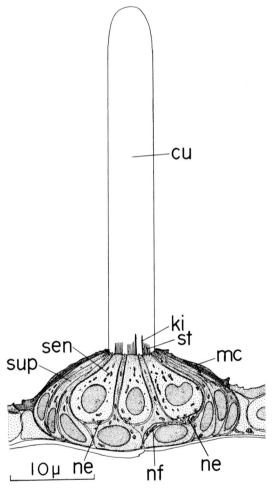

Figure 2-6. Diagrammatic section of a free neuromast in a teleost larva. Cupula (*cu*), kinocilium (*ki*), stereocilium (*st*), sense cell (*sen*), supporting cell (*sup*), mantle cell (*mc*), nerve ending (*ne*), nerve fiber (*nf*). (From Iwai, T.: Structure and Development of Lateral Line Cupulae in Teleost Larvae. In Cahn, P. [Ed.]: *Lateral Line Detectors.* Bloomington, Indiana U. Pr., 1967, pp. 27-44.)

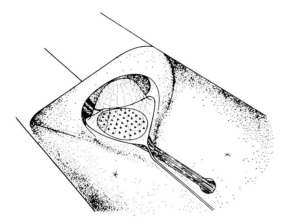

FIGURE 2-7. A canal neuromast. This organ, consisting of an oval sensory area covered by a domelike cupula, lies on the floor of the lateral line canal. The cupula also covers a zone of mantle cells which encompasses the sensory area. (From Flock, Å.: Transducing Mechanisms in the Lateral Line Canal Organ Receptors. In *Sensory Receptors. Cold Spring Harbor Symposia on Quantitative Biology,* 30:133-145, 1965.)

forth a response, and the last increases with frequency. Stimulus reception is based on the vibration produced between the flagellum, which extends outwards above the water, and the pedicellus on each antenna (Rudolph, 1967).

Even a protozoan, *Halteria bifurcata,* has been reported to be sensitive to water movement or vibration, possibly through its bifurcated bristles (Tamar, 1968).

The vibration receptors described above variously initiate feeding or escape responses.

Aquatic vertebrates possess secondary sense cells in their neuromasts (sensory hillocks). The last may be free neuromasts (Fig. 2-6), found on the body surface of aquatic amphibia and fish, or canal neuromasts (Fig. 2-7), located within the lateral line system present in most fish. The secondary sense cells or hair cells generally each bear a bundle of sensory hairs composed of one kinocilium and thirty to forty stereocilia. However, the hair cells of the salamander *Necturus maculosus* carry only a kinocilium. Aronova (1967) describes the pike kinocilium as mobile and its stereocilia as not so. The cilia extend from the

surface of the hair cells into a cupula of gelatinous, mucoid material which overlies the sensory area of each neuromast. While the cupulae of free neuromasts, such as those of the clawed frog *Xenopus laevis,* are often elongated and project out into the water environment (Fig. 2-6), the cupulae of canal neuromasts, which last may have oval, disk-shaped sensory areas as in the burbot (*Lota vulgaris*), are frequently dome shaped (Fig. 2-7). The mucoid cupulae contain a network of microfibrils and are attached by these microfibrils to the hair cell cilia (Flock, 1967).

Tester and Kendall (1968) report that in sharks there is a continuous replenishment of the mucoid material composing the mound-shaped cupulae over the canal neuromasts. The supporting cells of the neuromast epithelium, which constantly produce the mucoid matter, are themselves also continually replaced. Aronova (1967) noticed a concentration of mitochondria and a considerable number of secretory granules in the apical portions of pike supporting cells.

The neuromast hair cells most frequently appear to be mechanoreceptors sensitive to water currents (Dijkgraaf, 1963). The hair cells have been variously described as sensitive to pressure fluctuations, pressure changes (Kuiper, 1967) and displacement. Flock (1966) states that these secondary sense cells are primarily displacement detectors and are responsive to movements of the order of Angstrom units. Harris and van Bergeijk (1962) found the hair cells to react to displacement by nearby sources of vibration instead of to pressure.

The origin of the hair cell response is the shearing force produced by movement of the base of the cupula, where the cilia are located. The microfibrils attached to the cilia may transmit the extent of displacement to these sensory structures. A consequent suitable motion of the cilia then probably gives rise to a hair cell graded potential.

In the hair cells of the lateral line of *Necturus* the receptor potential has been observed to not exceed a peak-to-peak amplitude of

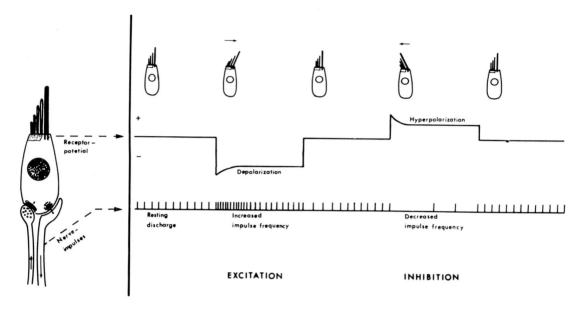

FIGURE 2-8. Hypothesized effect of direction of stimulation on the response of hair cells. Movement of the cilia toward the position of the kinocilium is considered to result in a negative potential and an increased impulse discharge. If the cilia are displaced in a direction away from the position of the kinocilium, it is thought that a positive potential appears and the impulse rate falls. Flock believes that the asymmetric location of the kinocilium may be related to this directional sensitivity. (From Flock, Å.: Ultrastructure and Function in the Lateral Line Organs. In Cahn, P. [Ed.]: *Lateral Line Detectors.* Bloomington, Indiana U. Pr., 1967, pp. 163-197.)

$800\mu V$ (Harris, Frishkopf and Flock, 1970).

The hair cells also display directional sensitivity. This may be related to the off-center position of the kinocilium among the stereocilia (Fig. 2-13) and even to the asymmetric structure of the kinocilium itself. If the cilia are moved from the direction of the stereocilia toward the kinocilium, the result is excitation (Fig. 2-8). A movement in the reverse direction has an inhibitory effect (Flock, 1967).

Deep-sea fish and cave fish are provided with a highly developed cephalic lateral line system, and cave fish also have an unusually large number of free neuromasts.

The mudminnow (*Umbra limi*) responds to a small water current directed at a portion of its lateral line system at a rate of 1.6 mm/sec (Schwartz and Hasler, 1966). The considerably larger end organs of the lateral line of the clawed frog (*Xenopus laevis*) have been

shown electrophysiologically to individually react to a threshold water current of 0.2 mm/sec (Görner, 1963).

Fish have been found to respond to both water pressure and velocity. Pressure is more significant at higher noise levels, such as 400 dB, and velocity at lower levels of stimulation (Cahn, Wodinsky and Siler, 1967).

Lorenzinian Ampullae

In a number of fish the cells of the lateral line system are situated at the bottom of Lorenzinian ampullae, which are tubes filled with a jellylike material. Here the sense cells possess only a single cilium.

Loewenstein (1960b) has found the Lorenzinian ampullae of elasmobranchs to be sensitive to hydrodynamic pressure, but their function is nevertheless not certain. Murray

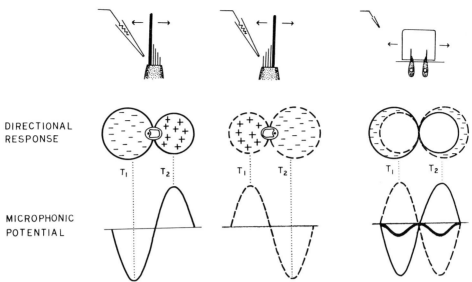

FIGURE 2-9. Hypothesized origin of the double frequency of canal neuromast microphonics (alternating potentials). Flock has suggested that the direction in which a hair cell's cilia are displaced by a stimulus determines whether depolarization or hyperpolarization will result. Since neighboring hair cells have their kinocilia located at opposite (rostral or caudal) ends of the cell, a vibratory stimulus first displacing the cupula in a certain direction will evoke depolarization in some cells and hyperpolarization in others (T_1, lower left and lower middle). During the ensuing rebound of the cupula the reverse effect will be called forth in each cell (T_2, lower left and lower middle). The microphonic produced by the interaction of many hair cells is equivalent to the sum of the opposed potentials. This makes it a distortion product with double the stimulus frequency (lower right). (From Flock, Å.: Ultrastructure and Function in the Lateral Line Organs. In Cahn, P. [Ed.]: *Lateral Line Detectors.* Bloomington, Indiana U. Pr., 1967, pp. 163-197.)

(1965) discusses the high sensitivity of these organs to mechanical and electric stimuli as well as to changes in salinity.

Murray (1967) stresses that the short nerve pathways in the ampullae are of equal length. This could be of significance in determining the time relations of mechanical stimuli. The fact that the ampulla tubes point in different directions could make it possible for elasmobranchs to detect voltage gradients in the water. In this connection Murray states that the ampullae appear suited for the detection of small external stimuli and that imposing a potential difference of $1\mu V$ across their sensory epithelium produces a response.

Dijkgraaf (1967) reports elasmobranchs to have a minimum threshold to electrical gradients of $0.01\mu V/cm$. Furthermore, he offers evidence for involvement of the ampullae of Lorenzini. Thus a threshold of $3\mu V/cm$ for electric stimulation between the spiracle and the first gill slit was raised tenfold by cutting the nerves from this region's ampullae. Even higher thresholds were obtained by eliminating impulses from all the ampullae of Lorenzini.

Murray (1967), although he allows for differentiation between ampullae in certain species, leans toward an electroreceptive function. Dijkgraaf (1967) is even more positive in this regard.

Various natural phenomena could lead to stimulating electric fluxes. The combined muscle action potentials of prey organisms have been shown to provide an adequate electrical stimulus by Dijkgraaf, and salinity changes could also give rise to electrical stimuli.

Pierau and Meissner (1966) stress the possibility of different functions by localized ampullae and report temperature reception akin to that of homoiotherms by the ampullae of two dogfish shark (*Scyliorhinus canicula*). However, Loewenstein (1961) reports that if the pressure of the ampulla is lowered below the level required for excitation, no temperature can elicit a response. Warm temperatures only enhance the responses to pressure.

Electroreceptors

Of unusual interest are the lateral line receptors of mormyrid and gymnotid fish, which act as electroreceptors. Lissmann (1963) has studied the function of such receptors, found in capsules in the skin tubes of the head and sides of *Gymnarchus niloticus*. In nature the observed cells apparently respond to changes in the amplitude of a continuous stream of 300 electric pulses per second emanating from the electric organ in the tail of the fish. Objects in the water affect the amplitude of the pulses, and a single sensory pore's nerve discharge should be able to indicate a 3×10^{-15} ampere current change.

Hagiwara *et al.* (1962) found the lateral line nerve fibers of three species of gymnotids to have a nerve impulse train threshold of 5-30 mV/cm. An added nerve impulse in each train was elicited by a 1 to 10 per cent (50μV-$1,000\mu$V/cm) rise in the voltage of the applied pulses. Increasing the length of the applied pulses to beyond 3 to 4 msec did not call forth additional impulses per train. Apparently the receptors' integration time constant is lower than 3 to 4 msec.

Gymnotid and mormyrid fish have been shown to possess two principal kinds of electroreceptors: tonic and phasic (Bennett, 1967; Suga, 1967). Bennett describes the ampullary receptors as tonic and those which are tuberous and whose cavities are apparently closed as phasic. Both receptors contain receptor cells; the cells of the ampullary receptor are seated in the sides of the ampulla, while the tuberous receptor's cells protrude into this re-

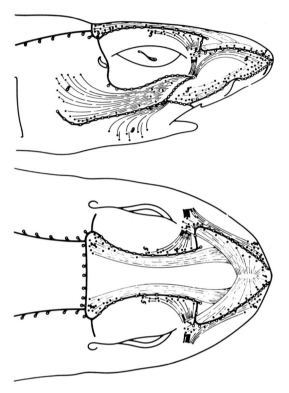

FIGURE 2-10. The location of some sensory structures on the head of a dogfish (*Scyliorhinus canicula*). The black dots represent ampullae of Lorenzini, the thick black lines, lateral line canals, and the empty circles symbolize external openings of the canals. Lateral view (top) and dorsal view (bottom). (From Dijkgraaf, S.: Biological Significance of the Lateral Line Organs. In Cahn, P. [Ed.]: *Lateral Line Detectors*. Bloomington, Indiana U. Pr., 1967, pp. 83-95 [Courtesy of S. Dijkgraaf].)

ceptor's internal cavity.

The tonic, ampullary receptors are sensitive to low-frequency electric stimuli, while the tuberous receptors are only reactive to higher frequencies. Suga indicates that the tonic receptors report the continued existence of a stimulus, while the phasic receptors respond to a stimulus change. The phasic, tuberous fibers (receptors) are reactive to the electric pulses produced by the fish, and are sensitive to objects which modify the fish's self-created electric field (Fig. 2-12A).

Different tuberous nerve fibers seem not to

be responsive at any one time to the same aspect of the phasic receptor response to the fish's electrical discharge.

The tonic, ampullary fibers (receptors) do not require the production of electric pulses by the fish to respond with a new rate of spontaneous discharge to a silver plate (Fig. 2-12C). However, the tuberous fibers (receptors) are dependent on the fish's discharge for such responses. Suga suggests that the ampullary receptors are not as significant as the tuberous receptors in reporting changes produced by the fish's pulses in the electric field.

Bennett (1967) also discusses a third type of receptor organ, of tuberous nature, in mormyrids. It contains two kinds of receptor cells, which seem to give rise to two types of phasic responses.

The three receptor organ types of *Gnathonemus petersii*, a mormyrid fish with relatively low electric emission, cover the head of the fish. They are also distributed along its dorsal and ventral surfaces up to the tail region (Bennett, 1965).

Minkoff, Clark and Sachs (1967) found *G. petersii* to generate biphasic electric pulses at four speeds with intervals such as 200 and 300 msec. The pulses showed a cyclical pattern, and their rate rose with increasing water speed.

Harder, Schief and Uhlemann (1967) found *G. petersii* to react to electric stimulation with an increased pulse frequency (as from 15 Hz to 30-40 Hz). Sometimes this increase in frequency was preceded by a pause in the fish's electric pulse emission. The most sensitive specimens responded to a threshold field intensity of approximately 0.7 mV/cm, applied to a restricted body region. The area between the eye and the gill slit had the greatest sensitivity.

If the entire body of *G. petersii* was in a homogeneous field, the threshold intensity was 0.2-0.5 mV/cm. *Gymnarchus niloticus* was first stimulated at an a.c. frequency of 800 Hz if its whole body lay in a field of 20 mV/cm.

G. petersii showed equal sensitivity both to changes in its own electric field and to externally imposed fields.

If external electric pulses of a frequency close to the electric discharge frequency of *Eigenmannia* are applied to this gymnotid fish, it shifts its frequency upwards or downwards (Watanabe and Takeda, 1963). This has been interpreted as an attempt on the part of the fish to avoid interference with its own discharge-receptor system.

Granath *et al.* (1967) investigated the frequency and electric field sensitivities of *Stenarchus albifrons*, a weakly electric gymnotid

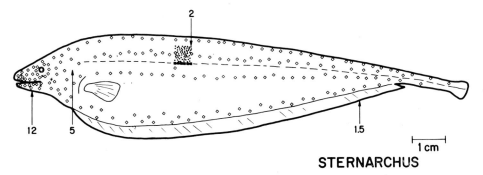

STERNARCHUS

FIGURE 2-11. Lateral line sense organs in *Sternarchus albifrons*, a gymnotid fish. The dashed lines and black squares represent canal neuromasts and the diamonds ampullae. Dots are used to indicate the density of tuberous electroreceptors in an area of 5 mm². The number of tuberous electroreceptors per millimeter squared is given at four locations. In any area the tuberous electroreceptors are much more numerous than the other lateral line organs. In gymnotid fish tuberous electroreceptors are found on all body regions. (From Szabo, T.: Sense organs of the lateral line system in some electric fish of the Gymnotidae, Mormyridae and Gymnarchidae. *J. Morphol., 117*:229-250, 1965.)

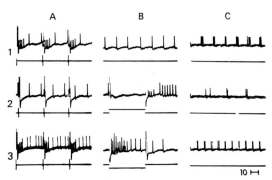

FIGURE 2-12. Tuberous and ampullary fiber responses (*Gymnotus carapo*). The larger spikes in *A1-3,* and the impulses in *B1* and *C1-3* are ampullary, while the smaller spikes in *A1* (4 per electric discharge) and *A3* (3 per electric discharge) are tuberous responses. The fish's electric discharge is recorded in the lower traces of *A1-3.* The placement of a plastic plate into the fish's vicinity affected the tuberous discharge but not the ampullary discharge (*A1-3*). The tuberous impulse rate, latency and spike interval varied (there is no tuberous response in *A2*). An artificial, head-positive electric pulse suppressed the ampullary response, but the last increased afterwards, and there was a tuberous fiber phasic "off" response (*B2*). A head-negative pulse had the opposite effects (*B3*). A silver plate could cause the spontaneous discharge of the ampullary fiber (*C1*) to either fall (*C2*) or rise (*C3*). Electric organ discharges temporarily ceased before *B* and *C*. (From Suga, N.: Electrosensitivity of Specialized and Ordinary Lateral Line Organs of the Electric Fish, *Gymnotus carapo.* In Cahn, P. [Ed.]: *Lateral Line Detectors.* Bloomington, Indiana U. Pr., 1967, pp. 395-409.)

having a discharge frequency of 600 to 1,000 Hz at 23°C. They used a.c. fields as stimuli and food as a reward to condition the fish, and found it was most sensitive to frequencies near its own discharge rate at 23°C. There was a secondary sensitivity peak around the frequencies of the second harmonic of the discharge. Responses are obtained with this species to a total range of 30 to 3,000 Hz (Howe, Jr. *et al.,* 1966). The fish were also most sensitive to approximately 0.2µV/cm (at 700 Hz), and should be able to detect each other at the distance of three meters (Howe, Jr. *et al.,* 1966).

Clark and Granath (1967) report *Gymnotus carapo* to emit a signal of 10 mV/cm and 2 msec duration, at a natural rate of 40 Hz. The response threshold was 0.04µV/cm (2 specimens). A lamp decreased the sensitivity of the fish to stimulating pulses by a factor of 10, and the addition of substances to the water could cause a loss of sensitivity. *Gymnotus carapo* ceased to emit its own signals on the initiation of stimulating pulses, until it became "used" to the latter.

The gymnotid fish *Sternopygus sp.* has been observed to continuously discharge electrical signals at an unvarying rate, ranging from 85 to 140 per second in different specimens (Bullock and Chichibu, 1965). One of three types of lateral line sensory fibers changed its phase in relation to other fibers and the electric organ, and in a permanent relationship to the position changes of an object. Thus a movement of 1 cm resulted in a 2 msec phase shift, and the position of an object was therefore "coded" in phase.

Perhaps in mormyrid and gymnotid fish electric scanning of the environment plays a role in navigation, feeding and even communication.

Work on the lateral line system is reviewed in the book *Lateral Line Detectors,* edited by P. H. Cahn (1967).

Beyond the structures mentioned above, fish seem only to have free nerve endings in their skin.

Auditory Receptors

Auditory receptors cannot clearly be categorized as secondary sense cells. The inner and outer hair cells of the organ of Corti are separated from their afferent nerve fibers by a small synapse, and some workers view these cells as specialized neurons. The receptors of the ear are covered in Chapter IV.

Ciliated Receptors—General

Photoreceptors have long been considered ciliated receptors. The disks in the outer segments of vertebrate rods and cones have been observed to develop by invaginations of the ciliary membrane (Eakin, 1965). The hair cells of the vertebrate organ of Corti are also known to be ciliated receptors, and have both stiff stereocilia and a motile kinocilium (Vinnikov, 1965). Insect auditory cells too bear a flagellum. Furthermore, the distal ends of vertebrate and insect olfactory cells possess one or more flagella, and the taste cells of invertebrates show a kinocilium. The kinocilium of vertebrate taste cells has instead evolved into a shaft structure (Vinnikov, 1965). Similar structures of ciliary or flagellar origin can be demonstrated in the receptors of the special senses of many other animal groups.

It is therefore also correct to consider gustatory, olfactory, auditory and visual receptors as ciliated receptors.

Crustacean stretch receptors too are said to contain cilia (Salpeter and Walcott, 1960).

Exteroceptors and Interoceptors

Receptors may also be classified according to location as exteroceptors and interoceptors.

The exteroceptors include the distance receptors, those for olfaction, audition and vision, and also taste. Another group of exteroceptors is found in the undulations of the mammalian dermis. These include the touch receptors: tactile hairs, Merkel's disks and Meissner's corpuscles. Also in the dermis are Ruffini's organs(?) and Krause's end bulbs.

Pacinian corpuscles are found not only in and under the skin, but also signal pressure in joints to indicate closure, and are found in the mesenteries of some species, such as the house cat, where they may respond to the dilations of blood vessels. Loewenstein (1960a) took advantage of this last location to study the function of the pacinian corpuscle.

Pacinian corpuscles are also located in the pleura, the pancreas, lymph nodes, muscles, tendons and periosteum, and along nerve trunks and blood vessels. Shantha veerappa and Bourne (1966) have reported a pacinian corpuscle from the inferior surface of the olfactory bulb of the squirrel monkey (*Saimiri sciurea*). The corpuscle was situated between the leptomeninges covering and the nerve fiber layer.

Free nerve endings for pain also are found not only just beneath the skin but in the viscera as well. Paravascular sensory nerves, which accompany blood vessels everywhere, end in free-branching, pain-sensitive terminals close to capillaries and venules (Lim, 1967). Lim reports such endings to actually be chemoreceptors for pain substances.

The interoceptors may be subdivided into proprioceptors, the semicircular canals, and visceral receptors.

The proprioceptors are represented by the Golgi tendon organs, located primarily at tendomuscular junctions, and the muscle spindles. The lyriform organs of scorpions respond to cuticular tensions (Pringle, 1955) and thus are proprioceptors, and the same may be true of the tibial slits of spiders.

Visceral receptors, in addition to free nerve endings and pacinian corpuscles, include encapsulated, branched nerve endings in or under mucous membranes which respond to distension of these membranes.

In the blowfly (*Phormia regina*) two visceral stretch receptors have been located, which respond to stretching (in life by peristalsis) of the foregut. These two receptors, which help to regulate feeding, are typical insect bipolar neurons (Gelperin, 1967). Stretch receptors in the body wall are even more significant in the control of feeding (Dethier and Gelperin, 1967).

Further visceral receptors are the hypothalamic osmoreceptors, mammalian and possible reptilian brain thermoreceptors (Cabanac, Hammel and Hardy, 1967), receptors in the hypothalamus and the midbrain which are sensitive to changes in indole compound concentrations (Fraschini *et al.*, 1968), and the chemoreceptors and pressoreceptors of the aortic arch and carotid bodies of vertebrates.

Evidence of the existence of brain chemoreceptors was found by Tanaka and Yamasaki (1965a, b), who obtained central excitation upon introducing morphine, tubocurarine and other chemical agents into the cerebrospinal fluid of rabbits. Previous intraventricular or intracisternal injection of anesthetics pre-

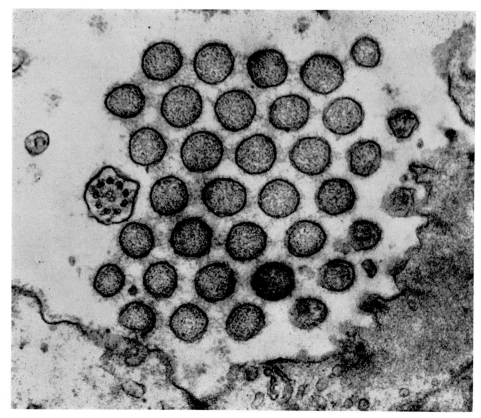

FIGURE 2-13. Cross-section through the cilia of a lateral line hair cell. The kinocilium (internal 9 + 2 fiber pattern) lies on the left periphery, and the other round sections are stereocilia. The last show a stepwise reduction in length with increasing distance from the kinocilium. There is a fibrillar network between the mucoid cupula and the cilia (*Lota vulgaris,* ×53,000). (From Flock, Å.: Transducing mechanisms in the lateral line canal organ receptors. In *Sensory Receptors. Cold Spring Harbor Symposia on Quantitatve Biology, 30:*133-145, 1965.)

vented this excitation. It appears possible that the drugs produced a release of histamine, which then stimulated the receptors.

Tanaka, Kimishima and Yamasaki (1965) review the histological literature which indicates the presence of cerebrospinal fluid receptors within the brain. Bipolar neurons of an apparently sensory nature, with bodies or processes which extend either to the ependymal layer of the third ventricle or to the cavity of the third ventricle itself, have been reported by several sources from frogs, reptiles and mammals (Fig. 2-14). Sensory nerve endings at the lumen of the cerebral aqueduct, or at its ependymal layer, have also been described by a number of investigators from reptiles and mammals. Further sensory terminals have been seen in the pia mater.

Cozine and Ngai (1967) used unanesthetized midcollicular decerebrate cats to show that chemosensitive receptors are located on the ventrolateral surface of the medulla oblongata. Application of procaine to these receptors was followed by reduced ventilation and a decrease in CO_2 sensitivity. However, the partial maintenance of ventilation and CO_2 sensitivity points to the existence of other such central chemoreceptors, perhaps lying deeper in the brain.

There have been a number of anatomical

and physiological studies on the carotid chemoreceptors.

DeKock and Dunn (1966) report that the carotid body of the cat contains sinusoids and two types of receptor cells and nerve innervations. It appears likely that the two nerve fiber types of these authors are afferent and efferent fibers. The nerve fibers show considerable spiraling, the type I cells possess long processes, and the type II cells have highly folded cell membranes.

Ishii and Oosaki (1966) performed an electron microscopic study of the carotid body of the toad. They observed the oval, abundant chemoreceptor cells, which appear to be equivalent to mammalian type I cells, to contain cytoplasmic vesicles of 600 to 1,400 Å. Highly osmiophilic granules, which were considered to resemble catechol, were present in the vesicles (Fig. 2-15). Duncan and Yates (1967), using cats, found that the appearance of the granules in the vesicles of type I carotid body cells varied with the fixative employed. Although Duncan and Yates still believed the granules to be composed of catecholamines (norepinephrine?), they noted that the administration of reserpine did not cause the disappearance of these granules in carotid bodies fixed with glutaraldehyde. This last observation caused Duncan and Yates to suggest that in the vesicles of type I cells catecholamines might be bound differently than they are in the vesicles of sympathetic nerve endings and the adrenal medulla.

Eyzaguirre and Zapata (1968a, b) provide abundant physiological evidence that the carotid chemoreceptor transmitter substance is acetylcholine. They used the Loewi effect, showing that stimulation of an "upstream donor" cat carotid body enhances the sensory discharge from a "downstream detector" cat carotid body (1968b). The Loewi effect was magnified by eserine, reduced by hexamethonium, and prevented by mecamylamine or acetylcholinesterase. Eyzaguirre and Zapata (1968a) performed further tests with such sub-

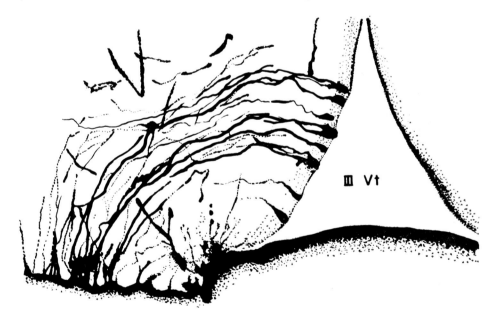

FIGURE 2-14. Possible periventricular brain receptors. Mannen observed these bipolar neurons in the rabbit's brain. The cell somas lie in the ependymal layer and adjacent to the cavity of the third ventricle. Long fibers run from the somas into deeper regions of the brain. (From Tanaka, K., K. Kimishima, and T. Yamasaki: Studies on the intraventricular chemoreceptors. 3. Anatomical considerations. *Yonago Acta Med.,* 9:186-189, 1965.)

stances as choline, hemicholinium-3, morphine sulphate, atropine and acetylcholine. Eyzaguirre, Koyano and Taylor (1965) report the cat carotid body to contain 20µg to 30µg of acetylcholine per gram of tissue.

Ishii and Oosaki (1966) found the chemoreceptor cells to be served by two types of nerve ending. One kind of nerve terminal was devoid of vesicles and was presumably afferent (Fig. 2-16). The other type contained numerous transparent, small vesicles, of an average diameter of 400 Å, and many mitochondria (Fig. 2-17). This nerve ending therefore appeared to be presynaptic, or the termination of efferent axons.

Mammalian carotid bodies, and also the carotid body of the toad, respond to a lack of oxygen. Biscoe, Sampson and Purves (1967) dissected single chemoreceptive afferent fibers from the sinus nerve of the cat to establish that the discharge-oxygen tension curve for each fiber has the form of a rectangular hyperbola. When the partial pressure of oxygen was reduced from 150-250 mm Hg to 25-50 mm Hg, the impulse rate of single fibers rose from 0.5-5/sec to 20-25/sec. There was no threshold oxygen tension, the fibers firing even at an oxygen partial pressure of 650 mm Hg. The discharge of single fibers rose with greater partial pressures of carbon dioxide and with a fall in pH (within the 6.9-7.6 range).

Eyzaguirre and Zapata (1968a) believe that low pH's act by increasing the release or by decreasing the breakdown of the transmitter substance produced by the chemoreceptor cells, or both. An increased external hydrogen ion concentration may act by causing greater retention of intracellular hydrogen ions, and these could further the release of acetylcholine or inactivate intracellular cholinesterase.

Duncan and Yates (1967) think it likely that the type I cells are the receptors for partial pressures of gases and for hydrogen ion concentration.

The aortic baroreceptors of rats have also been the subject of physiological studies. In normal rats these baroreceptors cease to fire

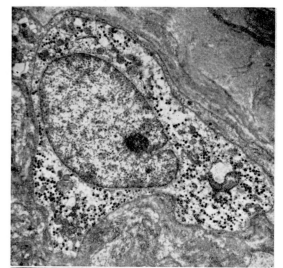
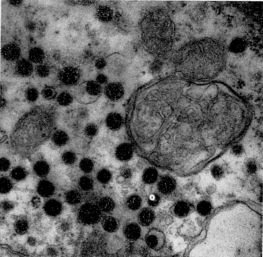

FIGURE 2-15. Chemoreceptor cell in the carotid body of the toad (*Bufo vulgaris*). The cell (top) has numerous granule-containing vesicles in its cytoplasm (approximately ×5,600). In an enlarged portion of the cytoplasm (bottom), it can be seen that a clear zone usually remains beyond the periphery of the intensely osmiophilic granules but beneath the vesicular membrane (approximately ×25,000). (From Ishii, K., and T. Oosaki: Electron microscopy of the chemoreceptor cells of the carotid labyrinth of the toad. *Nature*, *212*:1499-1500, 1966.)

when the blood pressure is sufficiently lowered, and they give a steady discharge when it is adequately raised. In chronically hypertensive rats the aortic baroreceptors continue to in-

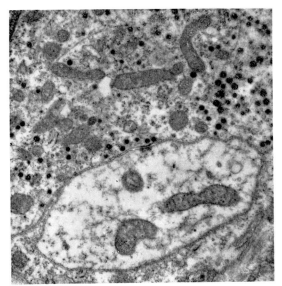 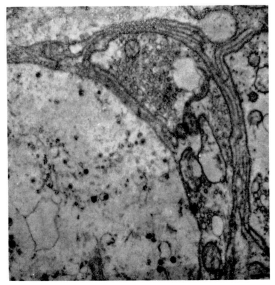

FIGURE 2-16. Apparently afferent nerve ending serving a carotid chemoreceptor cell. Above the ending, which lacks vesicles, lies a portion of the receptor cell. Granule-containing vesicles are concentrated in the receptor cytoplasm near the nerve terminal, in which three mitochondria are seen (approximately ×17,500). (From Ishii, K., and T. Oosaki: *Nature*, *212*:1499-1500, 1966.)

FIGURE 2-17. Suspected efferent nerve ending innervating a carotid chemoreceptor cell. The nerve ending exhibits a concentration of synaptic vesicles near its zone of contact with the receptor cell, which lies below and to the left (approximately ×20,000). (From Ishii, K., and T. Oosaki: *Nature*, *212*:1499-1500, 1966.)

hibit the vasomotor centers, but undergo an upwards shift of the range at which they discharge (Krieger and Marseillan, 1966).

Pressure receptors may also be present in the pulmonary artery, heart, and in the vessels of the kidney and adrenal gland (Niijima and Winter, 1968).

In the dog, osmoreceptors have been indicated in body interstitial spaces near capillaries.

NERVE INNERVATIONS

Some receptor types may have distinct kinds of nervous innervation. Thus it has been reported that touch (Meissner's corpuscles, Merkel's disks) is subserved by large myelinated (see Chap. VI) nerve fibers. The nerve fibers transmitting pain have been described as either small myelinated fibers conducting at 15-20 meters/sec, or small unmyelinated fibers conducting impulses at 2 meters/sec or less (Gasser, 1943).

Collins, Nulsen and Shealy (1966), by antidromic (see Chap. VI) electrophysiological recording from cooperative human subjects, were able to correlate sensation with sural nerve fiber size. They identified the small delta and C fibers as pain transmitters. Peripheral unmyelinated fibers carried poorly localized, strong pain, while myelinated fibers mediated well-localized pain (and touch). The larger beta and gamma fibers subserved only touch.

Three groups of myelinated afferents appear to be sensitive to skin vibration (Mountcastle *et al.*, 1967). One group, which fires when tiny puffs of air are blown at the skin, is thought to serve the pacinian corpuscles. A second group of fibers, which ends in the dermal ridges, transmits a high-frequency discharge upon stepwise depression of the skin. This discharge drops to a lower but steady rate in 100 to 200 msec. A third set of myelinated afferents, also terminating in the dermal ridges, follows changes in weak stimulation only irregularly or in submultiples, in terms of impulse frequency. It may subserve human sensitivity to oscillations between 2 to 40 cps.

Burgess and Perl (1967) studied the responses mediated by afferent fibers from the skin of the cat's hind limb. Fibers with an impulse velocity of 6-37 meters/sec reacted only to injurious mechanical skin stimulation, especially to pinching with serrated forceps and to cutting. Injurious heat or cold and acid had no effect on these nociceptors. These fibers normally had receptive fields of 2-5 cm $\times$ 1-2.5 cm, with separated responsive spots of less than 1 mm diameter. The slowest fibers tended to have the highest threshold of stimulation.

Perl *et al.* (1967) are quoted as getting results such as the above from apparently small myelinated fibers of carnivores and primates. These were "fast" pain fibers of the skin.

Fibers of a similar or somewhat larger size, with a similar receptive field, had greater sensitivity and fired on moderate pressure. They accommodated more slowly than the nociceptors. The conduction velocities of these fibers ranged from those of the above nociceptors upwards to 51 meters/sec. The fibers with the highest conduction velocities also had the lowest thresholds (Burgess and Perl, 1967).

Afferent fibers with the previously described type of receptive field generally had a higher threshold for stimulation than the other skin mechanoreceptors.

Most of the very small myelinated axons innervated hair receptors and primarily had conduction speeds of 14-22 meters/sec.

Findings indicating that the smallest nerve fibers are nonspecific in the sensations they convey have also been made. Thus Lele and Weddell (1956) showed that the very small fibers serving the cornea transmit touch and temperature sense as well as pain. Douglas and Ritchie (1957) found the C fibers to respond to touch. Iggo (1959, 1960a, b) reported C fiber discharges after temperature and touch stimulation, and Casby *et al.* (1963) described all fibers of a peripheral nerve as giving discharges after a full range of stimuli.

However, it appears possible to conclude that pain is mediated only by the smaller nerve fibers.

It has also been stated that impulses signaling a drop in temperature travel in bigger myelinated fibers and small unmyelinated fibers, whereas only small, unmyelinated fibers transmit the impulses indicating increased warmth. In dogs, cats and rats cold responses from the hairy facial region are transmitted by myelinated A_p fibers and the unmyelinated C fibers. Some additional C fibers fire only on a rise in temperature. In primates all skin regions are served by both A_p "cold" fibers and C "cold" fibers, as well as by C "warm" fibers (Iggo, 1963).

Kenshalo and Gallegos (1967) recorded impulses from single fibers of the radial and saphenous nerves of monkeys. They found some discharged if any of from two to eight 1 mm points distributed over up to 1.7 cm^2 of skin surface was cooled.

It seems there is at least some differential cutaneous nerve fiber innervation for the different types of sensation.

THE MUSCLE SPINDLE—AN EXAMINATION

The muscle spindle is a proprioceptor which monitors the degree of relaxation or stretching of the surrounding muscle fibers. It determines the nature of the slower and more delicate muscle movements, and it is the afferent terminal of the myotatic reflex. Its importance is shown by the fact that in numerous cat muscles the total afferent and efferent spindle innervations exceed the number of normal motor nerve fibers. The muscle spindle has a complex structure, and its function is not yet fully understood.

Muscle spindles have a length of several millimeters.

The Structure of the Amphibian Muscle Spindle

The frog muscle spindle is composed of

parallel bundles of intrafusal muscle fibers which lie in a fluid-filled space incompletely encompassed by a connective tissue envelope, the inner capsule. Beyond the inner capsule lies a second space which is in turn surrounded by a few layers of connective tissue lamellae, the outer capsule. The last may enter between and partially separate the intrafusal fiber bundles in their central portions (Karlsson *et al.*, 1966). This separate encapsulation of every intrafusal fiber bundle in and near its central sensory (reticular) portion (Fig. 2-18) may have a functional significance. The capsules may also play a role in stabilizing the composition of the spindle's internal fluid.

Each intrafusal muscle fiber consists of polar motor regions at either end and a central sensory region. Karlsson *et al.* (1966) have divided the central sensory region into a middle sensory reticular region and two peripheral sensory compact regions (Fig. 2-18).

Sensory Innervation

The intrafusal fibers are innervated by both sensory nerves and two types of motor nerves. The sensory fibers are biphasically distributed in the central sensory region, with the highest concentrations between each sensory compact region and the medial sensory reticular region (Katz, 1961; Karlsson *et al.*, 1966). The high number of fibers in these two zones may be the result of third-order or fourth-order nerve branching. After losing their myelin sheaths, the sensory nerves terminate in nerve bulbs (up to 2μ-3μ) which are joined by thinner links (Fig. 2-18). Katz (1961) hypothesized that the bulbs are the site of transduction of the mechanical energy of intrafusal fiber contraction to the electrical energy of the nerve impulse. The sensory nerve fibers appear to be of only one type.

The sensory reticular region of an intrafusal fiber is considered to be noncontractile, and it and its nerve endings should be stretched when the polar motor regions and sensory compact regions contract. A dynamic portion of the frog spindle response is thought to emanate from the nerve endings on the reticu-

lar region (Katz, 1961). Those sensory nerve endings near the junctions between the compact regions and the reticular region which overlie more numerous myofibrils and are not subject to so much stretch would provide a static part of the response. Similarly, the few intrafusal fibers lacking a reticular region would only add to the magnitude of the static response.

Motor Innervation

The polar motor regions of an intrafusal fiber are innervated by efferent fiber branches. Karlsson *et al.* (1966) observed intracapsular motor nerve endings (Fig. 2-18), and noticed that motor innervations extended into the sensory compact regions.

The two kinds of efferent (fusimotor) fibers are branches of large and small efferent fibers supplying the surrounding normal muscle fibers. They have terminals on the intrafusal fibers which are similar to the skeletomotor endings of their mother fibers. The large (over 5μ) efferent fibers innervate rapidly-contracting (twitch) extrafusal muscle fibers, while the small (2μ-5μ) efferent fibers end on slow (tonic) extrafusal muscle fibers which contract upon nonpropagated depolarizations. The stimulation, at a sufficient frequency, of a large efferent fiber caused a spindle sensory fiber to show an immediate rise in impulse rate. The cessation of efferent fiber stimulation resulted in a drop of the spindle afferent fiber's discharge to beneath the starting frequency. Similar stimulation of a small efferent fiber produced a gradual rise and slow poststimulatory fall in the spindle afferent fiber's discharge, and the last did not drop below the original level. There may be two different types of intrafusal fibers (Matthews, 1964). It also appears that a single intrafusal muscle fiber can be served by two or more efferent fibers.

Satellite Cells

Up to 50μ-long fusiform satellite cells were seen by Karlsson *et al.* (1966) immediately adjacent to the intrafusal fibers, especially along their sensory zones (Fig. 2-18). Ten to fifteen such cells were located around some

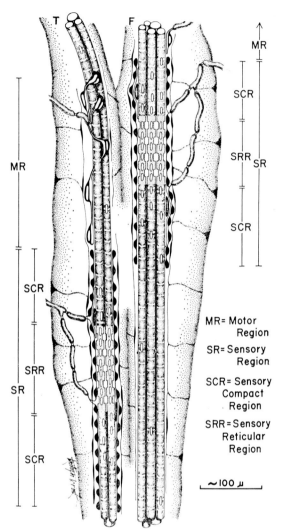

FIGURE 2-18. The structure of the frog muscle spindle. Two intrafusal muscle fibers, consisting respectively of three fibers (*T*) and five fibers (*F*), have been drawn. In their sensory reticular regions (*SRR*) the fibers have the largest number of nuclei, which are arranged there in central rows, and a complex, regular folding of the plasma membranes. In the sensory regions (*SR*) the linked sensory nerve bulbs are indicated as lines of linked black beads. The motor regions (*MR*) possess motor nerve endings, which are symbolized by larger blank beads. In the sensory compact regions (*SCR*) fusiform satellite cells are shown in close contact with the intrafusal fibers. Each intrafusal muscle fiber bundle lies within an inner capsule in its sensory region (*SR*). However, the inner capsule may end be-

yond the sensory region. The outer capsule (stippled) may enter between fiber bundles in the sensory reticular region. (From Karlsson, U., E. Andersson-Cedergren, and D. Ottoson: Cellular organization of the frog muscle spindle as revealed by serial sections for electron microscopy. *J. Ultrastruct. Res.*, 14:1-35, 1966 [Academic Press].)

intrafusal fibers. Satellite cells were also in close contact with sensory nerve endings. These satellite cells may fulfill a function similar to that of glia cells.

The long axis of muscle spindles is parallel with that of the surrounding muscle fibers.

The Structure of the Mammalian Muscle Spindle

The mammalian muscle spindle shows considerably more complexity than the amphibian spindle.

Within the connective tissue sheath of the typical mammalian spindle lie two kinds of intrafusal muscle fibers, the nuclear-bag fibers and the nuclear-chain fibers. The first show a concentration of nuclei in their central region, where the fiber widens. In the nuclear-chain fibers the nuclei instead form only a single line (Fig. 2-19). The nuclear-chain fibers are usually thinner and shorter than the nuclear-bag fibers and often outnumber them. At their ends the nuclear-chain fibers are joined to the nuclear-bag fibers (Boyd, 1962).

The two intrafusal muscle fiber types differ in contractility. While nuclear-chain fibers behave like rapidly contracting (twitch) extrafusal fibers, the nuclear-bag fibers more closely resemble slow (tonic) extrafusal fibers (Boyd, 1966; Smith, 1966). Nuclear-bag fibers respond with but a small contraction (Bessou, Laporte and Pagès, 1968), and shorten maximally only after repeated excitation.

A number of investigators have reported the presence in mammalian spindles of a third, intermediate kind of fiber (Matthews, 1964).

Rabbit spindles only possess nuclear-bag fibers, but intrafusal fiber dimorphism already exists in primitive insectivores.

Sensory Innervation

The mammalian spindle is clearly served by sensory fibers of two different kinds. In each spindle a single large afferent fiber (12μ-20μ) gives rise to a primary ending composed of spirals which, at least usually, wind around the central regions of the nuclear-bag and nuclear-chain fibers. Another, smaller afferent fiber (4μ-12μ) ends in spirals and sprays on the nuclear-chain fibers and often has a few sprays on the nuclear-bag fibers (Fig. 2-19). This secondary ending, however, never touches the central widenings, the nuclear bags, of the nuclear-bag fibers, nor does it send spirals around these fibers. In a typical cat spindle the secondary afferent ending is approximately 400μ long, and its parts are adjacent and distal to those of the primary afferent ending.

The mammalian spindle apparently differs from the amphibian spindle in being innervated by two types of sensory nerves.

Motor Innervation

The motor fibers are thin and myelinated, and enter the spindle together with the afferent fibers.

Some investigators have reported the existence of two motor nerve systems in the mammalian spindle. Boyd (1962) states that the small γ_1 efferent (fusimotor) fibers innervate only the nuclear-bag intrafusal fibers. These nerve fibers are said to give rise to end plates on both polar portions of the nuclear-bag fibers. Boyd describes even more minute γ_2 fusimotor fibers as having diffuse endings located only on nuclear-chain intrafusals (Fig. 2-19). The diffuse γ_2 endings are spread over those portions of the central halves of the nuclear-chain fibers which are not covered by sensory terminations. However, Barker (Barker and Cope, 1962) is of the opinion that both types of intrafusal fibers are served by the branches of individual γ_1 and γ_2 axons.

Barker (1967) differentiates between two kinds of spindle motor end plates. One type, the p 1 plate, is similar to the extrafusal end plates and degenerates more quickly when its nerve fiber is cut. The other, p 2 plate is big-

ger, has no nucleated sole plate, and is composed of knobs and rings. In cats p 2 plates and diffuse endings are found at both spindle poles.

Barker (1967) states that no motor ending is found on only one kind of intrafusal muscle fiber. Also, no motor ending is exclusively innervated by the axons of one group.

Other research workers have corroborated the existence of motor end plates and motor diffuse endings and have also shown that both the end plates and the diffuse endings are found on both kinds of intrafusal fibers. The diffuse endings lie nearer to the central portions of the fibers than the end plates (Lennerstrand, 1968).

In his later work Boyd (Boyd and Davey, 1966) primarily distinguishes between thick and thin γ fusimotor fibers. Since transmission speed varies directly with nerve fiber size, it is also interesting to note that Matthews and Westbury (1965) and Bessou, Emonet-Dénand and Laporte (1965) deal with fast and slow fusimotor fibers in, respectively, the frog spindle and the cat spindle. Granit (Barker and Boyd, 1966) no longer considers the division of the spindle motor nerves into γ_1 and γ_2 groups as useful.

An important division of the γ fusimotor fibers into static and dynamic groups has also been made. It has been suggested that the dynamic fibers correspond to Boyd's γ_1 fibers, and the static fibers to Boyd's γ_2 fibers. However, the dynamic and static fusimotor fibers have been reported to have similar conduction velocities, and should hence also have about the same fiber diameters (Brown, Crowe and Matthews, 1965).

A portion of those γ fusimotor fibers of the cat spindle which terminate in end plates are branches of motor fibers also serving normal, extrafusal muscle fibers. The mentioned fusimotor fibers have the "dynamic" action to be described later (Bessou, Emonet-Dénand and Laporte, 1965).

A number of studies indicate that larger motor nerve fibers, of the small α type, also innervate mammalian spindles. Such α fusi-

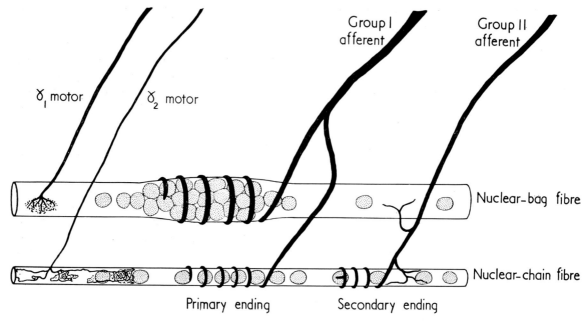

FIGURE 2-19. Structural diagram of the central portion of the mammalian muscle spindle. The concentration of nuclei in the central widening of one of the nuclear-bag fibers, the centrally located spirals of the primary afferent ending, and the secondary afferent ending's innervation of mainly the nuclear-chain fibers are illustrated. The γ_1 motor fibers terminate with end-plates on the polar portions at each end of the nuclear-bag fibers. Each γ_2 motor fiber gives rise to several diffuse trail endings on the central halves of the nuclear-chain fibers. (From Matthews, P.B.C.: Muscle spindles and their motor control. *Physiol. Rev., 44:*219-288, 1964.)

motor fibers have been found in flexor muscles, (Green and Kellerth, 1966; Haase, Meuser and U Tan, 1966) and transmit impulses at higher speeds than the γ fibers.

The Physiology of the Muscle Spindle

The chief function of the muscle spindle lies in its control of muscle tension and contraction through spinal reflex arcs. There is also a strong nervous connection between spindles and the cerebellum, the portion of the brain concerned with refined muscle movements, coordination and equilibrium.

Excitation of the primary afferent endings of spindles is conveyed through the Ia sensory fibers leading from these endings to the α motor neurons serving the spindle-containing muscle and its synergists. This pathway, which includes only the single synapse between the Ia sensory axons and the α motor neurons, composes the afferent half of a simple reflex arc. Impulses from the primary afferent endings also inhibit the motor neurons of antagonistic muscles.

The full effects of the impulses called forth in the secondary afferent endings may not yet be known. However, it has been determined that the impulses transmitted from these endings through group II sensory fibers excite motor neurons serving flexor muscles, even if the secondary endings themselves lie in spindles located in an extensor muscle. The actions of secondary endings include autogenetic inhibition.

Impulses generated in either primary or secondary afferent endings may also exert an inhibitory action on the central axon endings of certain other first-order afferent neurons (presynaptic inhibition).

The spindle primary afferent endings can

discharge in synchrony with quite high rates of vibration, particularly when excited by fusimotor discharges. This is not true of the secondary endings.

The monosynaptic reflex arc connecting the primary afferent ending of a spindle with the extrafusal fibers of the same muscle makes possible the postural or myotatic reflex.

The myotatic reflex is elicited by the stretching of a muscle due to gravity or the contraction of the antagonistic muscle. The lengthening of the muscle is apparently accompanied by a lengthening of the intrafusal spindle fibers, and the extent and rate of stretching of the central regions of these fibers determines the level of stimulation of the overlying primary afferent ending. The frequency of the impulse discharge reaching the α motor neurons through their sensory synapses produces a proportionate efferent discharge, which is transmitted to the extrafusal muscle fibers. The whole muscle responds to the magnitude of this efferent discharge with an appropriate degree of contraction, which in turn results in a drop to normal levels of the impulse discharge emanating from the primary ending. The degree of muscle contraction thus is determined by the extent of previous stretching. Contraction is not reduced by the action of antagonistic muscles because of the concomitant inhibition of the motor neurons of these muscles.

Contraction of the extrafusal muscle fibers to a length shorter than that of the intrafusal fibers results in a pause in the muscle spindle's discharge. This discharge pause may in turn lead to a cessation of α motor neuron activity. The spindle is said to be unloaded when its discharge is interrupted.

When a continuous stretch is exerted upon a muscle, as is true in a standing man of the postural quadriceps femoris group which extends the lower leg, the described reflex circuit produces a constant series of contractions by different scattered extrafusal fibers. This results in muscle tonus.

Muscle spindles exert control over at least all but the faster, stronger muscle contractions and also control steady states.

The reflex arc from the primary ending to the extrafusal muscle fibers is sufficiently long to involve a significant time delay. Also, there is an interval between muscle fiber stimulation and contraction. The total time delay could be sufficient to cause the response to be out of step with a changing stimulus, which can result in oscillations. Such a lack of sufficient stimulus-response correlation and consequent oscillations can be prevented by sensitivity to the rate of change of a stimulus, so that the system can correct for a projected magnitude of stimulation. The primary ending has such sensitivity, for it responds not only to muscle stretch but also to the velocity at which the muscle lengthens (Matthews, 1964). Perhaps the primary ending compensates for the time delay of the spindle reflex arc and thus enhances the functional accuracy of movements.

Static γ fusimotor activity may be maintained for one second or longer after it is elicited. Such lasting activity may contribute to the smoothness of muscle movements.

How does the muscle spindle operate when a new degree of maintained muscle tonus is called for, as on a standing man shifting his weight to one leg, or when a delicate voluntary contraction is required?

The achievement of such adjustments appears to be the function of the γ fusimotor nerve fibers innervating the spindle's intrafusal muscle fibers. According to one view, for the initiation of a small voluntary contraction, impulses from higher nervous centers pass down the γ fusimotor axons. These γ impulses reach and produce the shortening of the two contractile polar portions of each intrafusal fiber. The central section of each intrafusal fiber, which is noncontractile and is innervated by the spindle's single primary afferent ending, is stretched because of the contractions on both its sides. This causes an increased impulse discharge to be transmitted from the primary ending to the α motor neurons, just as if all of each intrafusal fiber had been stretched during muscle lengthening, and results in muscle contraction. The contraction of the surrounding extrafusal fibers is accompanied by shortening of the spindle, and the proper degree of shortening of a whole intrafusal fiber can compensate for the extent of stretching being undergone by its central portion due to contraction of its sides. In this manner a certain amount of γ fusimotor activity can bring about that degree of muscle contraction which will cause the discharge of the primary afferent ending of each spindle to once again drop to the normal level. It must be remembered that many spindles act to determine a muscle's state of contraction.

Conversely, if the mentioned muscle is now to be relaxed and allowed to lengthen, a reduction in γ fusimotor input will lead to a relaxation of the polar portions of the involved intrafusal fibers. Consequently the primary ending output will fall. A subnormal level of spindle afferent activity will result in a proportionately reduced α motor neuron discharge; therefore, the muscle will lengthen until spindle activity once more rises to normal levels.

It has been further suggested that γ fusimotor fiber impulses bring about changes in comparative structural viscosities and elasticities between the central and polar portions of intrafusal fibers (Matthews, 1964; Toyama, 1966).

Many investigators have observed the γ fusimotor neurons to discharge spontaneously. This spontaneous discharge should affect the sensitivity and activity level of the afferent endings, or is equivalent to a "γ bias."

Considerable evidence has accumulated for the existence of an alpha-gamma linkage. By this is meant the excitation, from higher centers, of γ fusimotor neurons along with the α skeletomotor neurons during muscle action, and conversely, the inhibition of both sets of neurons at about the same time by brain centers (Granit, 1968). Muscle contraction would be initiated directly by the brain, rather than being brought about by way of the gamma loop, as indicated in the previously given explanation.

Such an alpha-gamma linkage would mean

that during muscle contraction, when impulses pass down the α motor axons to the extrafusal muscle fibers, there is also increased fusimotor excitation of the intrafusal spindle fibers. That this is really the case was indicated by Critchlow and Euler (1963). They reported that in respiration the spindles in the external intercostal muscles gave off a discharge during the contraction of these muscles when it might have been expected that the spindles' impulse rate would fall. This spindle discharge could be abolished by paralyzing the γ fusimotor fibers with cocaine. It has been suggested that the external intercostal spindles cease their discharge and inspiration ends when the intrafusal muscle fibers undergo a degree of relaxation equivalent to that of the extrafusal fibers.

Kukkonen (1968) also found the spindles of the external intercostal muscles to show increased activity during inspiration. However, this greater activity was noted in denervated muscles, whose γ motor innervation had been severed. The inspiratory spindle discharge could therefore not be due to γ fusimotor impulses. Kukkonen instead ascribed the increased spindle discharge to stimulation by the passive stretching of the external intercostals during expansion of the chest.

Filaretov (1968) investigated an increase in the stretch receptor discharge from the abdominal muscles during expiration. He observed this rise in discharge to be facilitated by the γ motor system. Other abdominal muscle stretch receptors fired primarily at inspiration, possibly because of passive stretching of the muscles.

Many of the fusimotor impulses which do travel to the external intercostal muscles are initiated by the respiratory center.

Corda *et al.* (1966) found an external intercostal γ fusimotor discharge which was tonic and not synchronized with the respiratory cycle. This discharge originated from the cerebellum and was linked with myotatic chest α reflexes.

The alpha and gamma discharges to the external intercostals are believed to be linked by interneurons in the spinal cord.

According to Granit (1968), the alpha-gamma linkage is automatic, or higher centers cannot initiate a γ fusimotor discharge alone. However, the γ fibers have lower thresholds than the α fibers, and gamma loop activity may be sufficiently early to allow spindle afferent impulses to appear ahead of the γ-linked α motor activity.

During contraction of the external intercostal muscles, their spindles are highly sensitive to increases in muscle load (Corda *et al.*, 1965). Granit (1968), through the concept of automatic load compensation, reduces the gap between the explanation of fusimotor function given earlier in this section and the large body of evidence for an alpha-gamma linkage. Granit believes that γ fusimotor impulses, or at least the static γ fibers contributing to a length servomechanism, automatically modify the α-output to produce the best load compensation. Thus the earlier discussion of fusimotor function could be essentially integrated with the facts of alpha-gamma linkage by allowing for an activation of the α motor neurons about the same time that the fusimotor discharge is started. Now, instead of initiating contraction, the fusimotor discharge, together with the effect of muscle load and thus extrafusal contraction on the spindle, determines the impulse activity in the spindle afferents. This afferent discharge will then act correctively on the α motor neurons to determine the extent of contraction.

The γ fusimotor discharge, by way of primary afferent ending excitation, is easily capable of producing a discharge of the α skeletomotor neurons. Fusimotor activity can call forth motor neuron impulses despite concomitant contraction by the extrafusal muscle fibers, autogenetic inhibition by the secondary afferent endings and inhibitory action on the part of Golgi tendon organs (Granit, Kellerth and Szumski, 1966). Intrafusal contraction presumably exceeds extrafusal contraction, or there would be a pause in the spindle discharge.

In the face of the two inhibitory actions listed above, which hyperpolarize the α motor neuron membrane, γ fusimotor excitation elicited a motor neuron discharge of approximately 25 impulses/sec at threshold. Gamma loop excitation of the primary afferent endings of the spindles produces a proportionate discharge, over a wide range, of the α motor neurons. The maximal α motor response is obtained at four times the threshold for its excitation by the gamma loop. A maximum γ fusimotor discharge may call forth a spindle impulse rate of 300-400/sec (Crowe and Matthews, 1964a).

The activity of α motor neurons over a considerable range directly reflects the sum of all the discharges reaching these neurons. Thus stretching a muscle to a certain extent always increases the α motor neuron discharge by a certain number of impulses.

According to some authorities, a change in muscle tonus may be initiated primarily by the appropriate excitation of γ fusimotor neurons, whereas the higher centers probably activate both γ fusimotor neurons and α motor neurons to produce the slower, weaker striated muscle contractions. The same workers believe that a sudden, strong conscious contraction may be carried out chiefly through the agency of α motor neurons. However, Granit (1968) thinks it likely that the neural organization for rapid movement involves a linkage between α fibers and the dynamic type of γ fusimotor fibers.

Another view of the γ fusimotor innervation sees in these fibers a means of restoring the impulse activity of the spindle to normal levels during a prolonged contraction or after a new tonus level has become established. In this way the spindle could maintain its sensitivity and continue its function. However, the concept that the γ fusimotor fibers provide a method of initiating muscle movement, which is the basis of the explanations of γ fusimotor fiber function given earlier, seems to be generally favored.

The transmitter released at the γ fusimotor axon terminals is apparently acetylcholine.

Mavrinskaya (1967) has found high nonspecific esterase activity in the motor endings of developing human muscle spindles.

The mechanism of the spindle is complicated by the fact that γ fusimotor activity may result in an increase of the secondary afferent ending discharge which is as great as that produced in the primary ending discharge. Also, it has been observed that the γ fusimotor fiber discharge can increase the frequency of the impulses emanating from the primary ending in response to greater muscle length. Thus the fusimotor discharge may influence the level at which the spindle reflex arc operates and change the gain of the stretch reflex loop (Matthews, 1964). By affecting the dynamic (velocity) response of the primary ending, the γ fusimotor fibers may affect the degree of compensation for the spindle reflex arc's time delay. Precisely how fusimotor activity raises spindle sensitivity is still undetermined.

Matthews (1967) does not believe there is sufficient evidence that the gain of the stretch reflex loop is large enough to permit it to, by itself, maintain a proper muscle length through the servomechanism.

The reason for the innervation of the intrafusal fibers by two kinds of γ fusimotor fibers has been an important question of spindle physiology.

It was found that γ fusimotor fibers can be divided into two functional types, the dynamic fibers and the static fibers. Any fusimotor fiber, whether dynamic or static, has the same action on all spindles which it innervates. Dynamic fiber activity greatly increases a spindle's response to the rate of muscle stretching without producing nearly as much of an increase in the afferent discharge at an unchanging muscle length. On the other hand, static fiber activity significantly increases the afferent impulse rate at a constant muscle length but has no effect on or elicits a reduction in the response to velocity of stretch (Crowe and Matthews, 1964a, b). Schäfer and Henatsch (1968) obtained similar results and emphasize a considerable increase in the spontaneous discharge

during static fiber stimulation. On subtracting the spontaneous discharge, static fiber activity can only be said to lower the sensitivity to rate of stretch, while dynamic fiber activity raises it. Static fiber activity dominated the response of primary endings to muscle contraction (Lennerstrand, 1968).

The discharges of some primary endings have been observed to be more regular when they are affected by dynamic rather than by static fusimotor impulses (Jansen and Rudjord, 1965).

While dynamic γ fusimotor activity essentially affects only the primary afferent ending discharge, static fiber activity modifies both the primary ending and the secondary ending discharge (Brown, Engberg and Matthews, 1967). In agreement with this last finding, Lennerstrand (1968) considers static γ fusimotor activity to act chiefly through the nuclear-chain fibers, and believes the dynamic γ fusimotor axons to preponderantly innervate the nuclear-bag fibers (Fig. 2-20). Secondary afferent endings have a lower sensitivity to rate of stretch.

The observations of Bessou, Laporte and Pagès (1968) indicate that apparently static γ fusimotor axons produce very rapid contractions and dynamic γ fusimotor axons slower contractions. However, these authors are not prepared to join Smith (1966) in suggesting that nuclear-chain intrafusal fibers give rise to the static effects and nuclear-bag fibers to the dynamic effects. This hesitancy is based on as yet unexplained variations in the responses to γ axons and on the belief that only direct optical observations can determine which intrafusals are excited by which fusimotor fibers.

Appelberg, Bessou and Laporte (1966) corroborate the results of the above investigations by reporting that cat static fusimotor fibers but not dynamic fibers stimulate the secondary afferent endings. After reviewing the already stated view (Crowe and Matthews, 1964b) that dynamic γ fibers end on nuclear-bag intrafusal fibers and static γ fibers on nuclear-chain intrafusals, Appelberg, Bessou and Laporte offer the following interpretation of their observations: dynamic fusimotor fibers, perhaps acting through the diffuse equatorial trail endings, call forth weak and localized intrafusal contractions. These contractions are just able to raise the discharge rate of the primary afferent endings at an unchanging muscle length. The secondary endings are not excited, since the contractions can only produce stretches which are subthreshold for them.

The static fusimotor fibers, perhaps by way of the plate endings, produce strong twitch contractions. These more powerful contractions, acting through nuclear-chain fibers or through nuclear-bag fibers linked to nuclear-chain fibers, stimulate the secondary endings.

A number of previous papers are cited in support of this last explanation of fusimotor function.

Lennerstrand (1968) hypothesizes that it could be the chief function of the dynamic γ fibers to provide γ fiber bias for the primary afferent ending (bring the sensitivity and discharge rate to the proper level). In the frog muscle spindle additional afferent responses to near-subthreshold stretches have been observed to be brought about by spontaneous intrafusal contractions (Jahn, 1968a).

The static γ fibers would provide the input leading to a suitable degree of muscle contraction or supply the guiding input for the spindle reflex arc servomechanism. When a muscle is stretched, stimulation of the static γ fibers raises the afferent spindle discharge, and it then remains at this higher level (Crowe and Matthews, 1964a).

However, there is also another school of thought on the nature of the two kinds of γ fusimotor nerve fibers. Schäfer and Henatsch (1968) do not view the two γ fusimotor fiber types as separately controlling the dynamic and the static sensitivity of the spindle. Instead, the dynamic γ fibers are seen as improving the spindle's differential sensitivities, while the static γ fibers are thought to turn the spindle into a less sensitive trigger organ for α motor neuron activity (Henatsch and Schäfer, 1967).

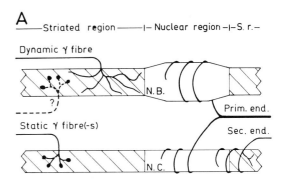

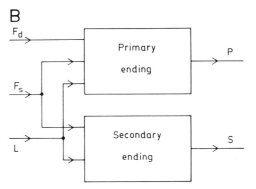

Figure 2-20. A. Functional diagram of mammalian muscle spindle innervation. It is indicated that the dynamic γ fusimotor fibers act on the nuclear-bag fibers and that there is an extensive innervation of the nuclear-chain fibers by static γ fusimotor fibers. A static γ fusimotor fiber innervation of nuclear-bag fibers is hypothesized. Dynamic γ fibers are shown to have trail endings, and static γ fibers plate endings. The diagram basically incorporates the views of Crowe and Matthews (1964a) and Boyd (1962) rather than those of Schäfer and Henatsch (1968), based on Barker (1967). B. Scheme of mammalian spindle operation. The static fusimotor discharge (F_s) and the muscle length (L) determine the output (S) from the secondary afferent ending and, in conjunction with dynamic fusimotor impulses (F_d), the output (P) from the primary afferent ending. (From Lennerstrand, G.: Dynamic Analysis of Muscle Spindles in the Cat. Stockholm, Nobel Institute for Neurophysiology, Karolinska Institutet, 1968.)

Schäfer and Henatsch (1968) call the dynamic fibers γ-trail fibers and the static fibers γ-plate fibers, according to their supposed terminations. Plate endings and the more diffuse trail endings seem to be found on both nuclear-bag and nuclear-chain intrafusal fibers. Schäfer and Henatsch allow only for quantitative differences in the activity mediated through one versus the other of the two intrafusal fiber types by the agency of each kind of γ fusimotor neuron.

In contradiction to Schäfer and Henatsch (1968), Barker (1967) considered his p 1 motor end plate to be dynamic.

A number of investigators have found that brain centers act differently on the two types of γ fusimotor fibers. Such differential action also occurs during certain reflexes.

The α fusimotor fibers innervating flexor muscles are dynamic in nature.

There is also some evidence that skeletomotor α fibers may act on spindles by electrical cross-excitation (the ephaptic effect).

Jahn (1968b) studied both the spontaneous afferent discharge of the frog muscle spindle and spontaneous contractions of its intrafusal muscle fibers.

Jahn (1968c) also worked on the features of muscle spindle stretch which play a role in evoking responses. Jahn (1968d) further investigated the excitability of frog muscle spindles by varied stretches at different time intervals after conditioning. A comparison was made of the effects of conditioning by spontaneous afferent action potentials and by afferent action potentials evoked with imposed stretches.

The effect of cerebellar influences on spindle reactivity was examined by Gilman and McDonald (1967a, b). They observed that cerebellectomy, and to a lesser degree section of the superior cerebellar peduncles, produced a rise in the threshold for a maintained discharge in response to stretch. Also, there was a lowering of the impulse frequency after

progressive static muscle stretch. After the operative procedures, spindle primary endings whose afferent fibers had high conduction speeds were less responsive to static stretch than endings with low-velocity fibers. Maximum response levels to external stimuli were not affected. The authors suggest two reflex mechanisms, one enhancing the response to continuous stretch, and the other making for fast changes in spindle responses in the absence of further muscle stretch.

Gilman (1968) obtained evidence for contralateral cerebellar influences on spindle facilitation. Both sides of the cerebellum appear to send facilitatory effects to some spindle endings.

McDonald and Gilman (1968) deal with the consequences of demyelination to spindle function.

It has been shown that the development of the muscle spindle and also its maintenance are dependent on the presence of the sensory nerves, and to a lesser extent of the motor nerves, which innervate it. This requirement is similar to the dependence exhibited by taste buds on their sensory innervation. The taste buds of the rat deteriorate when their nerve supply is cut.

As is true of taste cells, the terminals of the fusimotor fibers undergo periodic breakdown and are continuously replaced. At any one time as many as 20 to 40 per cent of the spindle's motor terminals may be deteriorating. New terminals sprout from the fusimotor axons (Barker, 1967).

The review article "Central Nervous System: Motor Mechanisms," by Eldred and Buchwald (1967), contains a valuable section on spindle physiology. Granit (1968) lucidly expresses his views on some aspects of spindle function in a review of spindle physiology.

THE CRUSTACEAN STRETCH RECEPTOR—AN EXAMINATION

The Alexandrowicz stretch receptor or crustacean stretch receptor was first described from the lobsters *Homarus* and *Palinurus* by

Alexandrowicz in 1951. This phasic-tonic receptor is found in two pairs in each abdominal segment of lobsters and crayfish and monitors the stretch of the dorsal abdominal extensor muscles which results from abdominal flexion. The crustacean stretch receptor thus fulfills a role analogous to that of the muscle spindle in vertebrates. Like the muscle spindle, the crustacean stretch receptor has been the subject of numerous physiological studies.

The Structure of the Crustacean Stretch Receptor

Florey and Florey (1955) performed an anatomical examination of the abdominal stretch receptors of the crayfish *Astacus fluviatilis*. They found these stretch receptors to differ significantly in several respects from those of *Homarus* and *Palinurus*, including efferent innervation.

In the crayfish each receptor organ includes two receptor muscles which in their zone of sensory innervation are enclosed in a common connective tissue capsule. The two receptor muscle bundles are composed of striated muscle fibers that are much thinner than the fibers of the superficial muscles. The medial muscle bundle has finer striations, and its myofibrils are thinner and more closely grouped than those of the lateral muscle bundle. In the zone of sensory innervation the fibers of each bundle spread apart, noticeably increasing the diameter of the bundle (Fig. 2-21). The sensory innervations themselves contribute to this enlargement.

Sensory Innervation

Each muscle bundle, the lateral as well as the medial, has its own sensory neuron innervation. The two neuron cell bodies are very near to the muscle bundles (Fig. 2-21). The cell bodies elongate and gradually constrict proximally to form the sensory axons, and these axons therefore have an unusually large diameter. Distally each sensory neuron cell body gives rise to dendrites whose terminations lie on the muscle fibers. The form, direction and branching of the dendrites is highly constant among specimens.

The dendrites of the sensory neuron serving the lateral muscle bundle fall into three systems, which together may overlie more than 500µ of the lateral muscle bundle's length. Upon reaching the innervated muscle fiber, a dendrite divides, and the resulting branches go off in opposite directions with the long axis of the fiber at right angles to the mother dendrite. This arrangement has the form of a T. In a preparation the terminal branches appear as wavy lines, but they may be drawn straight when their muscle fiber stretches.

The three or four dendrites of the sensory neuron serving the medial muscle bundle go off from the cell body in more or less the same general direction. The branching distal portions of these dendrites are collected in one area. In this area a mass of short nerve endings travel in all directions with no relation to the directions of the muscle fibers.

The difference in the manner in which the terminal dendritic branches of the two sensory neurons innervate the fibers of their muscle bundles may be correlated with a difference in response of these two neurons. Since the end branches of the lateral muscle neuron run parallel with their muscle fibers, any stretch of the muscle fibers will effect a stretch of the nerve branches. On the other hand, since the medial neuron endings run in various directions, an initial period of muscle fiber stretching is required to bring these endings into a plane with the muscle fibers and make them subject to stimulation by further stretching. The lateral neuron discharges at a constant frequency during constant stretch, even if the latter is weak. The medial neuron responds only after the extent of muscle stretch crosses a relatively high threshold, provided that the velocity of stretch is sufficient.

The midportions of the muscle bundles, where they are heavily innervated by sensory dendrites, are stiffer and more elastic than the bundle's polar regions (Wendler, 1963).

Motor Innervation

Florey and Florey (1955) found one large (7µ-10µ) motor fiber to innervate the medial muscle bundle. This fiber bifurcates near the medial muscle sensory neuron, the two branches passing in opposite directions along

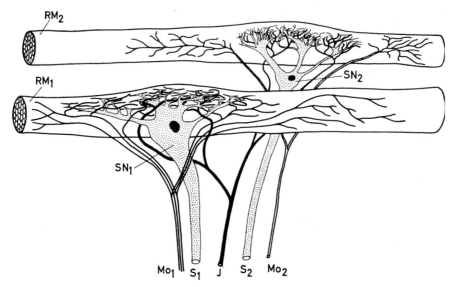

FIGURE 2-21. Diagram of the abdominal stretch receptor organ of the crayfish *Astacus fluviatilis*. (RM_1) lateral muscle bundle, (RM_2) medial muscle bundle, (SN_1) and (SN_2), sensory neurons respectively serving the lateral and medial muscle bundles, (MO_1) thin fibers, probably the motor innervation of the lateral muscle bundle, (MO_2) motor fiber innervating the medial muscle bundle, (*J*) inhibitory fiber sending two branches to each sensory neuron. (From Autrum, H.: Nonphotic Receptors in Lower Forms. In Field, J. (Ed.): *Handbook Of Physiology*, Washington, American Physiological Society, 1959, vol. 1, section 1, pp. 369-385; and Burkhardt, D.: Die Sinnesorgane des Skeletmuskels und die nervöse Steuerung der Muskeltätigkeit. *Ergebn. Biol.*, *20*:27-66, 1958 [Berlin-Göttingen-Heidelberg, Springer].)

the medial muscle bundle. Each of the two main branches then divides further to serve the individual muscle fibers. No comparable fiber innervates the lateral muscle bundle in the crayfish.

However, in the lobster *Homarus* there are two large motor fibers, each serving one muscle bundle.

In the crayfish another large (5μ-10μ) nerve fiber bifurcates twice to innervate each of the two sensory neurons with two branches (Fig. 2-21). Its terminal branchings spiral around the dendrites of the sensory neurons and end among the sensory neuron terminations. It has been proven to inhibit the sensory neurons (Kuffler and Eyzaguirre, 1955).

There are also a few thin fibers which innervate the lateral muscle bundle. These fibers branch repeatedly, bundles of their branches

also running to the superficial muscles. Final subdivisions, which have diameters of 1μ to 3μ close to the lateral muscle bundle, pass on to innervate the entire surface of this muscle bundle. The thin fibers probably represent the motor innervation of the lateral muscle bundle. Since in one preparation a thin fiber serving the lateral muscle bundle in addition supplied the lateral sensory neuron, these fibers may also bring about neural excitation.

In the case of the lateral muscle bundle, the motor innervation is thus probably spread over the entire surface of the bundle, whereas the medial muscle bundle has no motor endings in its sensory zone. Therefore, motor discharges cause the lateral muscle bundle's sensory zone to contract like the remainder of the bundle. However, the sensory zone of the medial muscle bundle is stretched during a motor discharge because only the regions on both sides of the sensory zone contract.

Kuffler (1954) observed that efferent activity did not result in cessation of the stretch receptor's afferent discharge. Instead, efferent impulses always promoted an increase in the frequency of the sensory discharge.

The Physiology of the Crustacean Stretch Receptor

Eyzaguirre and Kuffler (1955) observed that stretching the dendrites of the crayfish stretch receptor's lateral sensory neuron gives rise to a generator potential in the dendrites. Stretch produces a sustained dendritic depolarization of great magnitude which extends into the cell body and axon but decreases in size with distance. The mentioned depolarization apparently develops in the distal arborizations of the dendrites, and the bigger dendritic branches are not affected by the stretching of their muscle bundle. The distal terminations of the dendrites thus are the site of transduction of the mechanical energy of stretch into electrical energy.

Eyzaguirre and Kuffler (1955), as well as Florey (1955), reported that the nerve impulses of the lateral muscle bundle's sensory neuron are initiated in its dendrites or cell body. Edwards and Ottoson (1958), who used the lobster, suggest that the nerve impulses of the lateral sensory neuron originate in its axon. The last researchers admit that their electrodes may have produced a pressure block which could have prevented impulse initiation in the cell body. However, they tend to discount this possibility.

The disagreement between Edwards and Ottoson (1958) and the earlier investigators in regard to the site of origin of the nerve impulse brings to mind a similar difference in findings concerning the action potential of the pacinian corpuscle (see Reception by the Pacinian Corpuscle, Chap. V).

Rusinov and Ezrokhi (1967) observed that the number of somatic spikes may be larger or smaller than the number of axonal impulses. Nakajima and Onodera (1969a) showed that the portion of the axon with a greater diameter, at some distance from the cell soma (at a minimum of 0.4-1.0 mm from the nucleus), cannot produce maintained discharges (Fig. 2-22). These workers indicate that the condition of the soma at least influences the frequency of discharge.

It has been determined that while the lateral muscle bundle's sensory neuron adapts slowly to stimulation, the medial neuron adapts rapidly. Thus, when Nakajima (1964) applied constant moderate currents to "slow" and "fast" neurons, the former continued to fire impulses for longer than the observation period of 3 minutes, while the "fast" neurons ceased to fire within 30 seconds (Fig. 2-23). The rapidly adapting, medial neuron also has a higher threshold for nerve impulses, and produces only high-frequency discharges. The action potentials of the slowly adapting, lateral neuron are usually of a greater amplitude than those of the medial neuron, but in this respect one encounters an overlap between the two neuron groups (Nakajima and Onodera, 1969a).

Eyzaguirre and Kuffler (1955) attributed the different adaptation rates of the two sensory neurons to different rates of decrease on the part of their generator potentials. They in turn correlated these different decay rates of the potentials with the unlike attachment of the neurons' dendrites to their respective muscle bundles. However, Krnjević and van Gelder (1961) discounted the effects of such mechanical factors as the mode of dendrite attachment. Their results instead drew attention to differences in the electrical membrane properties of the two neurons as the proper explanation for the unlike adaptation rates. Nakajima (1964) showed that the rates of decline of the generator potentials of the two receptor neurons were essentially the same. The generator potentials of both "slow" and "fast" neurons dropped similarly quickly from their initial peaks, and then decayed equally slowly during continued stretch (Fig. 2-24). Nakajima (1964) stated that the difference in the neurons' adaptation rates is probably due to differences in the properties of their

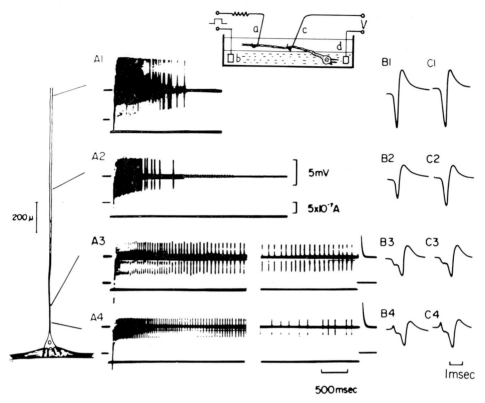

FIGURE 2-22. Action potentials elicited by stimulating the axon of a slowly adapting neuron at various distances from the cell soma. In the experimental preparation illustrated at the top, the stimulating currents flow from the extracellular electrode *a* to *b*. The resulting action potentials are recorded by electrodes *c* and *d*. In each A record the action potentials are shown in the upper trace, and the flow of current by the downward deflection below. *A1* — stimulation at 1.6 mm from the neuron nucleus; *A2*, 1.1 mm; *A3*, 0.23 mm; and *A4*, 0.14 mm. Maintained discharges were called forth only at *A3* and *A4* (the gaps equal about 110 sec). B records — action potential obtained by constant current stimulation on a faster time base. C records — action potential produced by stretching the muscle bundle. Records from the same location are identically numbered. (From Nakajima, S., and K. Onodera: *J. Physiol. [London]*, *200*:161-185, 1969a.)

electrically excitable membrane components.

Nakajima and Onodera (1969a) could not explain the difference in adaptation rate on the basis of a single attribute of the electric properties of the membrane. Also, no adequate differences in the passive properties of the membranes were found.

Nakajima and Onodera (1969a) suggest that changes in the membrane's sodium or potassium permeability could be responsible for adaptation. The electrogenic sodium pump

(see The Resting Potential in Nervous Transmission, Chap. VI) of the neuron membrane might also play a role in adaptation. The electrogenic sodium pump produces the posttetanic hyperpolarization of the slowly adapting neuron (Nakajima and Takahashi, 1966). In the last the electrogenic sodium pump has an action similar to that of a constant hyperpolarizing current passing through the cell membrane.

How ionic permeabilities and movements

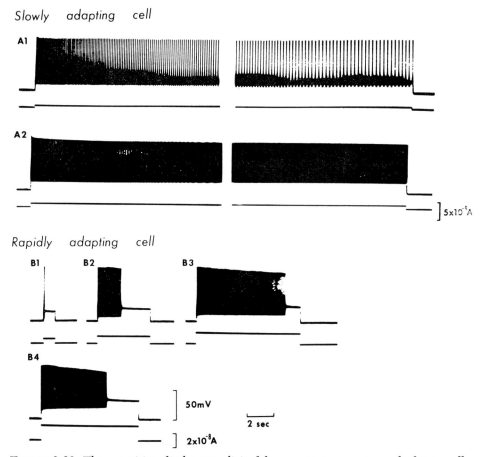

FIGURE 2-23. The repetitive discharges elicited by constant currents applied intracellularly. The slowly adapting neuron responded with a maintained discharge for the duration of the current (The gaps in *A1* and *A2* represent about 40 sec). The rapidly adapting neuron reacted with only short-term discharges to various current intensities. (Adapted from Nakajima, S., and K. Onodera: *J. Physiol. [London], 200*:161-185, 1969a.)

may be involved in the difference in adaptation rate of the two neurons cannot yet be determined. Perhaps several factors play a role. These may not be identical for adaptation after both high-frequency and lower frequency discharges.

Both receptor neurons showed a similar current-voltage relationship.

The total adaptation rate of each neuron is determined by two components, the rate of decline of the generator potential (generator adaptation) and the rate of adaptation of the impulse-generating membrane mechanisms (spike adaptation). In the slowly adapting neuron it is generator adaptation which appears to form the more significant segment of total adaptation, while spike adaptation seems more important in the "fast" neuron (Nakajima and Onodera, 1969b).

The above investigators (1969b) further reported that the size of the generator potential elicited by a unit stress or strain of the innervated muscle bundle was approximately the same for both receptor neurons. Also, the tension changes in the medial and lateral muscle bundles after stretch took a similar time course.

About 70 per cent of the decline of the

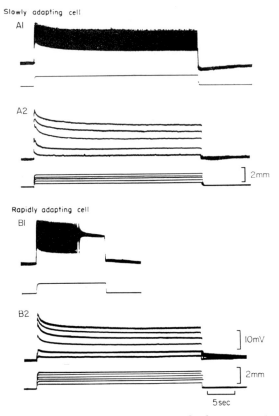

Slowly adapting cell

A1

A2

] 2mm

Rapidly adapting cell

B1

B2

] 10mV

] 2mm

5 sec

FIGURE 2-24. Receptor neuron discharges and generator potentials elicited by constant muscle stretches. *A1* and *B1*, evoked discharges in normal saline (only a lower portion of the action potentials is shown in *A1*); *A2* and *B2*, the generator potentials, upon application of tetrodotoxin, called forth by the muscle bundle elongations indicated in the lowest traces. In A the muscle bundle's resting length was 3.8 mm, in B, 5.5 mm. The generator potentials of both neuron types have a similar time course. (From Nakajima, S., and K. Onodera: *J. Physiol. [London],* 200:187-204, 1969b.)

generator potential (generator adaptation) in the slowly adapting neuron is a consequence of the viscoelastic nature of the lateral muscle bundle.

Dissimilarities between the two muscle bundles may partially underlie the different levels of stimulation at which their sensory neurons respond. The lateral muscle bundle normally has a taut appearance, while the "fast" neuron's medial muscle bundle, when

not contracted, is coiled and slack. Perhaps partly for this reason stronger stretches are needed to activate the "fast" neuron (Eyzaguirre and Kuffler, 1955). Krnjević and van Gelder (1961) suggest that the unusually low coefficient of elasticity and the noticeably lesser resistance to stretch of the medial muscle bundle may be factors. Furthermore, the medial bundle is approximately 20 per cent longer than the lateral bundle. This last feature alone would make a greater extension of the medial bundle necessary in order to achieve an equivalent tension change per unit area. The slowly adapting neuron is twice as sensitive as the "fast" neuron to the same muscle elongation (Nakajima and Onodera, 1969b).

The listed attributes of the muscle bundles, as well as the differing arrangement of their innervating sensory dendrites, may be responsible for the higher threshold of the medial "fast" neuron.

Efferent impulses to the stretch receptor initiate contraction of the innervated muscle bundle(s), and this contraction in turn leads to an afferent discharge. A motor discharge is effective in provoking sensory impulses only if the receptor is subjected to a certain degree of stretch. Greater initial stretch increases the number of sensory impulses elicited by a given motor discharge. If motor stimuli follow each other at sufficiently short intervals, they summate to produce increased afferent discharges (Kuffler, 1954).

In the lobster impulse activity in the motor fiber to the medial muscle bundle elicits rapid, twitchlike contractions in that bundle. These contractions result in single or grouped afferent impulses. Motor activation of the lateral muscle bundle causes it to undergo a slow, tonic contraction. Such a slow contraction can be graded by altering the frequency of motor stimulation, and this effect is visible under the microscope. The sensory discharge of the "slow" neuron rises comparatively smoothly. Maximum motor stimulation of the lateral bundle appears to produce a maintained, nonfluctuating degree of tension and discharge (Kuffler, 1954).

While the medial bundle develops a contraction fusion frequency of close to 50/sec during motor fiber excitation, the lateral bundle has a fusion frequency of only 5/sec.

In the medial muscle bundle a contraction, even if restricted, is associated with propagated spikes. This is not true of the lateral bundle. The last instead shows multiple, localized graded contractions, preceded only by end-plate potentials, all along the fiber.

The stretch receptor can be excited both by stretch and by motor activity acting through muscle bundle contraction. In general, changes in the frequency and/or duration of motor stimulation can, over a considerable range, compensate for variations in stretch to keep the sensory discharge at a certain level (Kuffler, 1954). The motor fibers of the crustacean stretch receptor can thus maintain its discharge and sensitivity in a manner somewhat similar to the "γ bias" and load compensation actions proposed for the γ fusimotor fibers of the muscle spindle. When the abdomen is extended, motor fiber activity produces sufficient contraction of the receptor muscle bundles to keep them at the proper tension.

The crustacean stretch receptor normally fires impulses at a low rate, being spontaneously active.

Kuffler (1954) believed the lobster's "slow" neuron discharge to contribute to the maintenance of tail positions, since this discharge remains proportional to the degree of abdominal stretch or flexion for long periods. On the other hand, the lobster's medial (fast) receptor appears to be more sensitive to rapid abdominal movements.

Borsellino, Poppele and Terzuolo (1965) found that the lobster stretch receptor's output is proportional in amplitude to the input and that this receptor also exhibits the other characteristics of linear behavior. The transfer function of the stretch receptor's "slow" neuron could be fully described within the context of linear behavior. The stretch receptor's transducer function could be interpreted in terms of a resonating second-order system.

Brown and Stein (1966) studied the impulse discharge from the crayfish (*Astacus*) stretch receptor following stepwise increases in the length of the slowly responding lateral muscle bundle. They reported the impulse discharge to be a linear function of both length and tension. Evidence was obtained that the discharge was called forth by tension, corroborating a similar finding by Wendler (1963). After a step stretch, impulse frequency fell with time according to a power function. This form of response decay following a stimulus is shown by a variety of mechanoreceptors. The discharge also increased as a power function of the velocity of stretch when the muscle was pulled to a constant length. The stretch receptor can thus provide information about both velocity of muscle stretch and muscle length (or more specifically tension). Upon rapid stretching there is a burst of impulses, which decays to a lower but maintained frequency-signalling muscle length.

In the midportion of the lateral bundle, the zone of heavy sensory innervation, length and tension fall after stretches like the discharge does, and to a maintained level (Wendler, 1963).

Mellon, Jr. (1968), reports that the stretch receptor discharge follows muscle length linearly, but tension logarithmically. However, Krnjević and van Gelder (1961) emphasize that the tension-discharge relationship is linear. Wendler (1963) also found the discharge to be a linear function of tension.

Kuffler and Eyzaguirre (1955) studied the inhibitory action of the large nerve fiber innervating the dendrites of the two sensory neurons. By stimulating this fiber close to the "fast" neuron, it was possible to investigate its inhibitory effect on the dendrites of the lateral "slow" neuron. This technique involved the antidromic passage of impulses to the point of first bifurcation of the fiber. While thus stimulating inhibitory impulses, the membrane potential of the affected dendrites could be lowered or raised by using stretch and impressed currents. Kuffler and Eyzaguirre

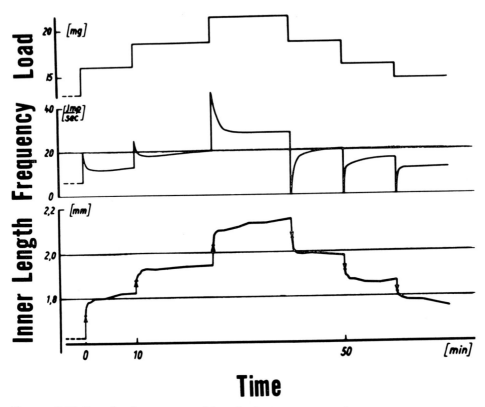

FIGURE 2-25. Impulse frequency and length during a series of tension increases. Top, mechanical tension in milligrams; middle, discharge frequency in impulses per second; bottom, length in millimeters of the portion of the lateral muscle bundle innervated by the sensory neuron. The time is given in minutes after the start of the experiment. Stepwise changes were made in muscle tension, and there was no interference with length adjustments by the muscle. The arrows in the bottom graph indicate the beginnings of the length adjustments which occurred subsequent to tension changes and continued for some time. It can be seen that impulse frequency rises to a peak (falls to a minimum) during a tension step, but then undergoes a sizeable decrement (increase). The last, and the time required for this decrease (increase), vary directly with the level of muscle tension. These results resemble those obtained with stepwise stretching, but the present changes in impulse rate are less marked and their time constant greater. Wendler (1963) considers adaptive processes acting on the generator potential of the sensory neuron to be responsible for the decrease in impulse rate. A postdecrement rise in impulse frequency may be due to the late stretching of the muscle. (Adapted from Wendler, L.: Über die Wirkungskette zwischen Reiz und Erregung. Z. *Vergl. Physiol.*, 47:279-315, 1963 [Berlin-Göttingen-Heidelberg, Springer].)

(1955) showed that the inhibitory potentials act only on the dendrites and oppose the development of the generator potentials called forth in the dendrites by stretch. The inhibitory potentials prevent dendritic depolarization from exceeding a certain limit and thus make it impossible for the generator potential

to reach the threshold for the initiation of nerve impulses.

It was found that the inhibitory fiber acts to bring the sensory neuron's membrane potential to an equilibrium value. This equilibrium value is not far from the resting membrane potential of the neuron; therefore, if a large

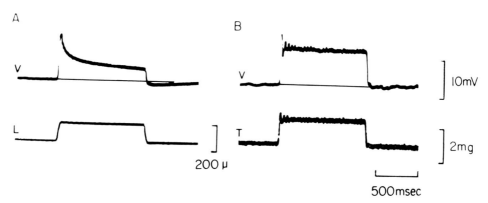

FIGURE 2-26. "Slow" (lateral) neuron generator potentials under length and tension clamping. A(V), generator potential during the length clamp shown in A(L); B(V), generator potential during the tension clamp illustrated in B(T). Resting muscle length 1.6 mm, A(L) baseline at a stretch of 0.4 mm, B(T) baseline at a tension of 0.4 mg; tetrodotoxin. The generator potential declines noticeably during length clamping but shows little decline during a tension clamp. Thus the neuron is shown to respond to muscle tension. (From Nakajima, S., and K. Onodera: *J. Physiol. [London]*, *200*:187-204, 1969b.)

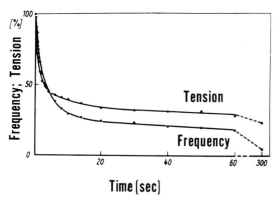

FIGURE 2-27. Values for impulse frequency and muscle tension after a step increase in muscle stretch. Frequency and tension are given in percentages, and the differences between the original frequency and tension and their respective peak levels were assigned values of 100 per cent. Time is measured in seconds after the applied stretch. The frequency and tension curves are largely parallel. However, the tension curve flattens out before the frequency curve does, pointing to the action of adaptive processes on the generator potential. (Adapted from Wendler, L.: Über die Wirkungskette zwischen Reiz und Erregung. Z. Vergl. Physiol., 47:279-315, 1963 [Berlin-Göttingen-Heidelberg, Springer].)

change has been effected in the membrane potential, inhibitory potentials appear to restore the resting potential.

The inhibitory potentials' equilibrium value, at which they reversed their action on the membrane potential, differed among neurons. Most commonly the inhibitory equilibrium value was about 5 mV lower than the resting potential (Fig. 2-28).

Inhibition could thus depolarize the neuron or have a polarizing effect, according to the direction in which the membrane potential had been shifted previously. The farther the neuron's membrane potential is shifted in either direction from the inhibitory potentials' equilibrium value, the greater will be a subsequent inhibitory potential.

Inhibitory action is not affected by the value of the equilibrium point, provided this value is sufficiently far from the level of depolarization which is the threshold for impulse initiation. Every inhibitory fiber potential acts to temporarily "fix" the dendrite membrane potential at a certain value, and a continuous inhibitory discharge can thus maintain a particular membrane potential.

Inhibitory fiber activity may block all afferent stretch receptor impulses or only lower the stretch receptor's discharge rate. The inhibitory potentials have a comparatively strong effect and can within milliseconds block the activity engendered by excitatory stimuli of large magnitude.

Kuffler and Eyzaguirre, on the basis of some of their results, suggest that the inhibitory potentials act on the dendrite membrane by increasing its electrical conductance. They speculate that increased membrane permeability to potassium and chloride ions, and perhaps even reduced permeability to sodium ions, could be brought about by an inhibitory transmitter substance. Increased dendritic conductance produced by inhibitory potentials may also prevent the spread of current from the dendrites to the neuron's cell body and thus block nerve impulses.

The inhibitory neurons of the crayfish are stimulated to fire when this organism swims backward by strongly flexing and extending its abdomen. This prevents the stretch receptors from discharging during the stretching of the extensor muscles and thus reducing the extent of the swimming movements.

The inhibitory nerve fiber transmits its impulses comparatively slowly. The inhibitory potentials produced in the dendritic membrane reach their maximum amplitude in approximately 2 msec and drop exponentially to the original membrane potential in around 30 msec. Following repetitive inhibitory activity, there often occurs a delayed secondary polarization phase. It may represent a mechanism for extending the period of the inhibitory effect.

Gamma-aminobutyric acid (GABA) has been obtained from crustacean inhibitory nerve fibers. Since this compound has the effect produced by stimulating the inhibitory fibers, it could be the transmitter substance released by the inhibitory axon terminals.

The crustacean stretch receptor's motor fiber(s) resemble the γ fusimotor innervation of the mammalian spindle. In addition, there is parallelism between the actions of the slow lateral and fast medial muscle bundles present

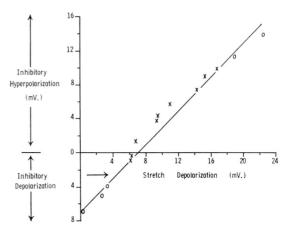

FIGURE 2-28. Size of the inhibitory potential at various membrane potential amplitudes in the "fast" (medial) sensory neuron. Abscissa: Degrees of membrane depolarization elicited by stretch. Zero represents the resting membrane potential. Ordinate: Inhibitory potential values. The line denoting the relation between the two potentials has a slope of 45 degrees and crosses the abscissa at close to 6.4 mV. This crossing point represents the inhibitory potential's equilibrium value. The inhibitory potential counteracts any membrane potential shifts from this equilibrium level, exerting a depolarizing effect if membrane depolarization drops below 6.4 mV. (Adapted from Kuffler, S.W., and C. Eyzaguirre: Synaptic inhibition in an isolated nerve cell. *J. Gen. Physiol.*, 39:155-184, 1955.)

in the crustacean receptor and the functions of the two kinds of intrafusal muscle fibers found in the mammalian spindle. It can be said that in general structure and function the crustacean stretch receptor is similar to the mammalian muscle spindle.

The crustacean stretch receptor is also innervated by the described inhibitory fiber. This inhibitory innervation should provide a means for peripheral modulation of the stretch receptor discharge. The muscle spindle has no analogous inhibitory input. Although the effect of inhibitory discharges on the crustacean receptor's "slow" neuron has been investigated, the functional significance of the crustacean stretch receptor's inhibitory input has not yet been clarified.

Giacobini and Jongkind (1968) determined that glycogen breakdown is required to maintain the impulse activity of the "slow" neuron of the crayfish stretch receptor. The pentose shunt is also involved.

The crustacean stretch receptor represents a useful physiological system for further experimentation. Its constituent parts are accessible, can be isolated, and their structure can be examined microscopically. The parts of the stretch receptor are subject to direct observation while they are active. The sensory neurons can be brought to a desired degree of depolarization by means of an easily controllable mechanism, the application of the proper amount of muscle bundle stretch. The sensory impulse discharge increases linearly with stretch. Also, the receptor sensory neurons are large enough to permit the insertion of electrodes into various regions of these cells. Such intracellular recording makes it possible to determine potential changes in different parts of the neuron.

It is usually preferable to record intracellularly from the lateral, "slow" neuron, because it responds to weaker stretches. Thus mechanical stresses which might damage the preparation can be avoided.

An additional advantage for studies of nerve physiology is conferred by the inhibitory input, which represents another mechanism for modification of the neurons' membrane potential.

Furthermore, the crustacean stretch receptor, since it contains a slowly adapting neuron next to a rapidly adapting neuron, offers an opportunity to compare the effects of the various factors involved in adaptation (generator adaptation vs. spike adaptation, etc.).

Extracellular recording from an isolated stretch receptor can be continued for many hours with little variation in response.

THE VERTEBRATE LABYRINTH, EXCLUDING THE COCHLEA—AN EXAMINATION

The membranous labyrinth (internal ear) developed from an anterior part of the lateral line canal system. Like the remainder of the lateral line system found in fish and amphibia, it contains groupings of hair sense cells whose cilia project into an overlying matrix. Much as the hair cells of the lateral line, labyrinthine hair cells are stimulated by the shearing forces resulting from the weight or movement of the overlying matrix (see hair cell response, p. 33, Types and Locations).

The membranous labyrinth is so constructed that responses are produced in its three different portions by respectively three distinct forces. These are gravitational pull, rotational and linear movements, and—in the case of the cochlea—airborne vibration. The labyrinth is therefore involved in postural reflexes and in rotation and angular and linear acceleration of the head.

The Structure of the Labyrinth

The vertebrate labyrinth is composed of epithelial spaces and tubes. It includes two larger sacs, a dorsal utriculus and a ventral sacculus.

In man the utriculus is an ovoid, somewhat flattened sac which is held in place by connective tissue and the innervating nerve. The sacculus (2.2 mm wide and 2.6 mm long) is also ovoid and is similarly attached, but is smaller than the utriculus (Anson, Harper and Winch, 1967).

The sacculus gives rise to another chamber, the lagena. The lagena becomes the cochlea in mammals. Reptiles and birds possess both a lagena and a cochlea.

There are also three semicircular ducts, in man the upper, vertical superior duct, the middle, horizontal lateral duct, and the inferior, vertical posterior duct. Each of these semicircular ducts is at right angles to all the others, and they connect to an enlarged part of the utriculus known as the vestibule. There is a swelling, the ampulla, at one end of every semicircular duct. The semicircular ducts run within bony semicircular canals of the same names. In man the ducts are only one-third the diameter of the containing canals.

Inside each ampulla there is a shelflike structure or crest, the crista, on which there are grouped sensory hair cells and supporting cells. The crista is homologous to the neuromast of the lateral line. The cilia of the crista's hair cells project into a gelatinous matrix, the cupula. The last does not touch against the sensory epithelium; there exists instead a subcupular space filled with a clear, viscous substance produced by the supporting cells (Lowenstein, 1967). The cupula is long enough to reach to the opposite side of the ampulla. The cupula is moved by the internal fluid of the labyrinth, the endolymph, whenever this fluid is thrown by inertia toward one or the other end of the canal. Cupular movement then exposes the cilia of the hair cells to shearing forces and initiates a response.

In the utriculus, sacculus and lagena, the masses of hair sense cells and supporting cells form oval, thickened areas called maculae. These maculae have a curved surface. In man the macula of the utriculus measures 2.3 x 2.1 mm, and the macula of the sacculus 2.2 x 1.2 mm (Anson, Harper and Winch, 1967). The cilia of the hair cells of a macula project into a gelatinous material in which lie embedded crystals, granules or an organized structure of aragonite or calcite. Both of these last substances are crystalline forms of calcium carbonate. A mineral concretion of such composition surrounded by a gelatinous matrix is known as an otolith. The weight and movements of an otolith produce shearing forces which act on the cilia of the underlying hair cells to bring about a response.

In the human utriculus and sacculus there are a number of otoliths of different sizes.

The otoliths of some fish are described in a paper by Morris and Kittleman (1967). The otolith of the fish *Micromesistius poutassou* grows in an organized, rhythmic fashion and in proportion to the growth of the fish's head (Bas and Morales, 1966). Some elasmobranchs are unusual in using sand grains obtained from the external environment as otoliths.

Thus in fish and mammals the labyrinth contains six separate groupings of sense cells —one each in the utriculus, sacculus and lagena, and three more in the ampullae of the semicircular ducts. Reptiles and birds have an additional, seventh mass of sense cells, since they possess both a lagena and a cochlea.

In fish and amphibia the labyrinth contains only one type of hair sense cell, the type II cell, which is cylindrical in form. Birds and mammals also have another kind of labyrinthine hair cell, the flask-shaped type I cell (Wersäll, Flock and Lundquist, 1965).

The mature hair cells of the labyrinth, with the exception of those of the cochlea, are, like the hair cells of the lateral line, endowed with stereocilia and a kinocilium (Fig. 2-30).

Each hair cell has a denser cuticular plate beneath the plasma membrane facing the lumen of the labyrinth. On one side of the cuticular plate, where it is incomplete, a centriole gives rise to the kinocilium. The kinocilium has the typical ciliary organization of two central fibers and nine peripheral fibrils.

The stereocilia instead each contain only a single, fibrillar axial core. This axial core below the cuticular plate gives rise to a line of microtubules, which runs toward the nucleus, where it bifurcates (Fig. 2-30). In the ammocoete larva one of the resulting two rows of microtubules continues down to the synaptic region in the base of the cell (Lowenstein and Osborne, 1964). The rods of the rat retina contain a similar, presumably microtubular, organelle (Mountford, 1964), as do frog tadpole lateral line receptors (Jande, 1966). It appears likely that the bifurcated line of microtubules plays a role in transduction (Jande, 1966; Wersäll, Gleisner and Lundquist, 1967).

Olney (1968) describes a structure which seems to be identical with the microtubular organelle, the synaptic spindle, from the photoreceptor terminals of the mouse retina. This organelle has been seen in guinea pig visual receptors, but Olney did not find it in the rabbit retina. Heist, Mulvaney and Landis (1967) and Okano, Weber and Frommes (1967) found rootlets similar in appearance to the microtubular organelle to extend from the basal

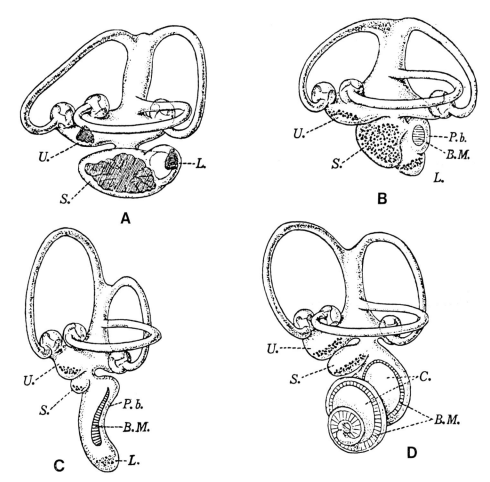

FIGURE 2-29. The labyrinth of several vertebrates: A, The typical fish; B, the turtle; C, the bird; D, the mammal. The utriculus (U), sacculus (S), lagena (L), papilla basilaris ($P.b.$), basilar membrane ($B.M.$), cochlea (C), semicircular ducts and ampullae can be identified. (From Frisch, K. von: Über den Gehörsinn der Fische. *Biol. Rev.*, *11*:210-246, 1936.)

bodies of dog olfactory receptor cells. However, the first group of investigators did not see such rootlets in the olfactory cells of rabbits, cats and frogs.

Lowenstein (1967) has failed to observe the mentioned microtubular organelle in the hair cells of the ray (*Raja clavata*).

The stereocilia adjacent to the kinocilium are longest, and the length of the stereocilia gradually decreases with distance from the kinocilium.

The hair cells of the ampulla of the horizontal semicircular canal generally each have their kinocilium on the side nearest to the utriculus. The hair cells of the ampullae of the two vertical semicircular canals normally each have their kinocilium on the side closest to the canal (Fig. 2-31). As a consequence of these orientations, the kinocilium is usually on that side of the hair cell which faces the direction in which the cupula is displaced during its first excitatory movement.

In the maculae of the utriculus and sacculus, sensory cell groups differ in orientation. In the utriculus the hair cells along the edge of the macula show a reversed orientation. These hair cells at the macular periphery therefore have the opposite orientation from the other

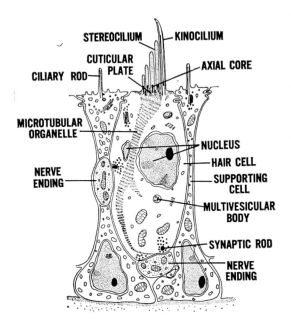

FIGURE 2-30. Diagrammatic representation of a hair cell from a crista of the ammocoete labyrinth. The microtubular organelle can be seen to extend from the cuticular plate to the synaptic region at the base of the cell. Its microtubules have an average periodicity of 130μm, and it bifurcates near the nucleus. (Adapted from Lowenstein, O., and M.P. Osborne: Ultrastructure of the sensory hair-cells in the labyrinth of the ammocoete larva of the lamprey, *Lampetra fluviatilis. Nature, 204:* 197-198, 1964.)

hair cells, which are oriented outwards in the form of a fan. In the saccule the hair cells face in opposite directions on either side of a line running near the middle of the macula's long axis (Fig. 2-31).

The structural orientation of the hair cells of the ampullae, utriculus and sacculus can be correlated with the directional functional properties of these cells. The dislocation of a hair cell's stereocilia toward its kinocilium results in depolarization, while movement away from the kinocilium produces hyperpolarization.

The lumen of the membranous labyrinth contains a fluid, endolymph. The membranous labyrinth itself lies in a space filled with perilymph and bounded by connective tissue or bone. Thus, the space between the endo-lymph-containing semicircular ducts and their considerably larger bony canals is filled with perilymph.

The perilymph has a much greater volume than the endolymph. While mammalian peri-lymph contains large amounts of sodium and chloride ions, and less potassium ions, mam-malian endolymph has more potassium ions than sodium ions (Fernández, 1967).

Since the endolymph is found beyond the surface of the hair cells, its composition may affect the development of depolarization in the hair cells. A similar problem exists in the case of taste receptor cells, since their apices are exposed to the fluid which happens to fill the oral cavity at the time. Perhaps in both cases depolarization of the receptor cell does not involve the cell apex but rather lower cell regions which are effectively sealed off from the ions beyond the apical cell surface.

Mucopolysaccharides beyond the hair cells have been mentioned as possibly being in-volved in the depolarization mechanism.

In higher vertebrates the bony shell border-ing the perilymph-filled cavities in which the membranous labyrinth lies is known as the bony labyrinth. Along the cavities the surface layer of bone, which is harder than the re-maining bone tissue, is lined with periosteum and an external delicate epithelioid layer.

In addition to being applied to an enlarged portion of the utriculus, the term *vestibule* has also been used to designate the older sacs and canals of the labyrinth. The expression vestibule can thus mean all parts of the laby-rinth exclusive of the auditory apparatus.

Sensory Innervation

The labyrinthine hair cells are secondary sense cells. The dendrites of myelinated, bi-polar neurons form synapses with the hair cells. The dendritic terminations on the type II cells, the only kind of hair cells present in fish and amphibia, take the form of numerous small, club-shaped endings at the cell's base. In the case of the type I cells, present in birds and mammals, a dendritic fiber forms a cup or chalice around most of the cell to synapse

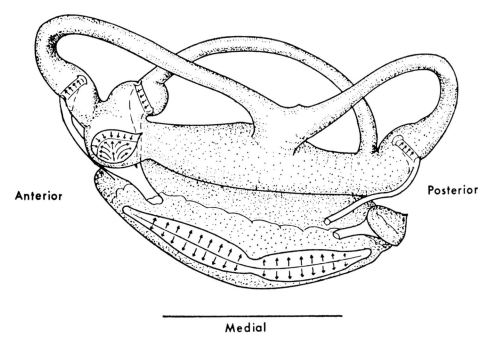

Medial

FIGURE 2-31. Diagram of a typical fish labyrinth to indicate the orientation of the hair cells. The arrows point in the direction of the asymmetric location of the kinocilium on the hair cell's surface. The horizontal semicircular canal and its ampulla lie behind the vertical semicircular canals. On the anterior side (left) the utriculus is seen below two ampullae. The sacculus is medial (bottom). (From Wersäll, J., L. Gleisner, and P.-G. Lundquist: Ultrastructure of the Vestibular End Organs. In De Reuck, A.V.S., and J. Knight [Eds.]: *Myotatic, Kinesthetic and Vestibular Mechanisms.* London, Churchill, 1967, pp. 105-120.)

with it. Occasionally two or three type I cells will be partially enveloped by such a dendritic chalice.

The type II cells show a great deal of afferent convergence, including more extensively branched dendritic systems. In the lamprey "candelabra" fibers may innervate many labyrinthine sense cells (Wersäll, Gleisner and Lundquist, 1967, Discussion).

The hair cells contain synaptic vesicles, indicating that transmission across the afferent synapse is chemical. There is a good possibility that the transmitter substance is cholinergic. In the cytoplasm near the afferent synapse, the hair cells also have synaptic bodies. However, it has been suggested that transmission from the type I cells may also be electrotonic.

The dendritic fibers of the bipolar, afferent neurons which innervate the ampullae, utriculus and sacculus form the vestibular division of the vestibulocochlear nerve. The cell bodies of these afferent neurons are located in the vestibular ganglion (Scarpa's ganglion), which lies at the bottom of the internal acoustic meatus.

Motor Innervation

There is also an efferent innervation of the labyrinthine hair cells. The efferent nerves terminate differently on various kinds of hair cells (branched endings, terminal boutons), but the efferent endings always have numerous synaptic vesicles. Acetylcholine may be the transmitter stored in these vesicles. Across the synapse from the efferent ending, the hair cell cytoplasm, next to the plasma membrane, usually contains a flat sac (synaptic sac).

There may also be efferent synapses with

the afferent dendrites.

The efferent nerve fibers mostly originate from cells in the lateral vestibular nucleus and from a group of cells located in the vicinity of this nucleus. Some efferent fibers also arise from the reticular substance.

The Physiology of the Labyrinth

The different portions of the labyrinth are specialized in their function.

The cupula in the ampulla of each semicircular duct is displaced when the endolymph moves in relation to the duct. This occurs only when a rotation of the head and duct, in the plane of the duct, is accelerated or slowed. During steady motion the endolymph moves together with the duct and does not change its location within it.

However, when rotation in the plane of a duct is initiated or when such rotation is accelerated, inertia causes the endolymph to move relative to the duct structures. This relative endolymphatic movement is in the direction opposite to the one in which the head is being turned. Therefore, the cupula is also displaced in a direction opposite to that of the turning, and the discharge from the underlying hair cells is affected accordingly.

The displacement of the cupula ends when head rotation reaches a steady rate. The effects of the earlier inertia quickly dissipate because the cupula-endolymph system acts like an excessively damped, spring-loaded torsion pendulum (Lowenstein, 1967). Therefore, the fluid and the cupula regain their original position as soon as a change in rate of movement is terminated.

When head rotation is slowed or stopped, inertia once more comes into play. Now the endolymph continues in the direction of the turning relative to the duct, and the cupula is displaced in the direction of the previous head rotation. This also brings about a change in the discharge of the hair cells.

Thus it is apparent that the discharge of the hair cells in the ampulla of a semicircular duct is affected only by a change in the rate of movement of the duct. Also, during an ac-

celerating or decelerating rotation the endolymph and cupula are displaced exclusively by the vector which is exerted in the plane of the duct.

The cupula of a semicircular duct may be considered to be relatively rigidly coupled with the endolymph.

The afferent nerves innervating the cristae of the semicircular duct ampullae typically transmit an impulse discharge when the hair cells are not being stimulated. This resting discharge apparently originates in the hair cells and exhibits a very high degree of regularity.

The spontaneous discharge doubles the opportunities for response available to the hair cells. They may not only give off an increased discharge but may also respond with varying decreases in their resting discharge. The spontaneous discharge perhaps also gives rise to a suitable level of vestibular tonus (Lowenstein, 1967).

When the cupula over a crista is displaced, the resulting effect depends on whether the produced shearing force dislocates the stereocilia of each hair cell toward the kinocilium or in the opposite direction. Movement toward the kinocilium, since it results in depolarization, leads to a greater discharge. Movement away from the kinocilium produces hyperpolarization and a fall in the sensory discharge. Therefore, the orientation of the hair cells in any semicircular duct determines whether a certain rate change in a head rotation will increase or decrease the discharge from the said hair cells. Displacement of the horizontal duct cupula toward the utriculus is followed by an increased discharge, as is displacement of the vertical duct cupulae away from the utriculus. On the other hand, movement of the horizontal duct cupula away from the utriculus results in a drop of the horizontal duct's hair cell discharge to below the resting level.

Over a sizeable range a rise in an ampullar hair cell discharge, if called forth by an acceleration, is a linear function of that acceleration.

The majority of vestibular neurons (which are connected to hair cells) each show a rise in activity if there has been angular acceleration in one direction and, conversely, a drop in their discharge if angular acceleration has taken place in the opposite direction. However, a type of vestibular neuron, type III, has been found which gives off a greater discharge after angular acceleration in both one and the opposite direction. The type III neurons are stimulated by activity from ampullar hair cells.

Groen, Lowenstein and Vendrik (1952) describe differences in spontaneous discharge and responses between sensory units in the horizontal duct ampulla of the ray (*Raja clavata*).

It is the function of the highly specialized semicircular ducts to provide information about changes in the rate of head rotation, or about angular acceleration and deceleration, in the three planes of space.

Manni and Desole (1966) warmed and cooled the semicircular canals of guinea pigs while electrophysiologically recording from the oculomotor nuclei. They obtained a lasting increase in the discharge rate or rhythmic responses. Warm stimulation of the lateral duct's ampulla evoked a different response from that produced by warming the superior ampulla.

In decerebrate cats, with only the ipsilateral labyrinth functional, the gamma lumbar motor neurons show a maximum phasic response 0.5 seconds after head rotation. The intensity of this response is determined entirely by the angular velocity of head rotation. This indicates that this phasic motor neuron response is called forth by afferent discharges from the semicircular duct ampullae (Poppele, 1967).

In contrast to the semicircular ducts, the otolith organs (the maculae of the utriculus, sacculus and lagena) most likely are reactive to both static and dynamic stimuli. These organs are believed to be chiefly responsive to linear acceleration of the head. Such acceleration can be interpreted as the acceleration of gravity. Recordings from primary afferent neurons show that the hair cells of the otolith organs really possess the specific directional sensitivity indicated by their structural orientation.

It appears that the directionally sensitive otolith organ cells in a general manner exhibit simple trigonometric resolution of experimental linear acceleration. However, the shape of the waveform of the response of these hair cells and also the observed direction of sensitivity seem to be dependent on the nature of the dynamic stimulus. The form of the dynamic stimulus can thus modify the basic response (Milsum and Jones, 1967).

Reflex electromyograms, electrophysiological recording from the utricular nerve, and studies of the positioning of the utricular and saccular maculae in space have shown that the utriculus and sacculus, acting together, are responsive to linear acceleration in any direction. The utricular macula, as well as the saccular macula, is most sensitive to linear acceleration in a direction vertical to itself. A linear acceleration of about 9 cm/sec^2 is reported to be the threshold for response by the otolith organs (Sasaki, 1967).

Pressure appears to be the best stimulus for the utriculus, but traction is also effective.

The maculae of the utriculus and sacculus seem to closely duplicate each other's function. This presumably makes the organism's sensitivity to linear acceleration in any direction possible (Sasaki, 1967).

Ikoma *et al.* (1967), by electrically stimulating the utricular macula and recording from the reticular formation of the brain stem, obtained evidence that otolith responses are transmitted through the reticular formation. The spontaneous discharge of the reticular formation could rise or fall after stimulation of the utricular macula.

Azzena, Giretti and Deriu (1967), upon stimulating the labyrinth thermically, observed activity in the oculomotor nuclei, reticular formation, red nuclei and the gray substance below the aqueduct.

In decerebrate cats, with the contralateral labyrinth destroyed, alpha and gamma lumbar motor neurons show tonic responses to head rotation. The amplitude of these tonic responses is dependent on the degree of angular head movement. This indicates that the tonic responses are a consequence of otolith organ discharges (Poppele, 1967).

Normal gravitational pull also acts on the hair cells of the utricular macula by way of the shearing forces resulting from the weight distributions of the utricular otolith(s). In vertebrates the utriculus therefore plays an important role in orientation in space and in the initiation of postural reflexes.

Fish orient themselves according to both light and gravity. If their only exposure to light is from a source at their side, they will lean in the direction of this light source. The pull of gravity on the otolith of each utriculus of such a fish, when that fish is swimming at an angle toward a light, can be resolved into two vectors. A shearing vector acts sideways, parallel with the surface of the otolith. A second vector, pressure, acts directly vertically. The shearing vector V is related to gravity G and to the angle from the vertical f of the fish according to the equation $V = G \sin f$.

An experimental fish can be placed in a centrifuge in which it is exposed to side light entering at an unchanging angle, while the gravitational forces acting on it may be varied. If the fish is subjected to greater gravitational pull or if G is increased the fish accordingly changes its angle from the vertical (f) so that the value of the shearing force V, the product of G and sine f, remains unchanged. On the other hand, the pressure vector is allowed to vary (Schöne, 1967). This represents further evidence that the macular hair cells of the utriculus are stimulated by the shearing force exerted by the otolith.

In a fish under the above stimuli the shearing force remained near 0.76 g.

Werner and Whitsel (1968) recorded electrophysiologically from squirrel monkeys to show that primary afferent vestibular nerve fibers, during steady head positions, exhibit noticeably regular discharge intervals. These fibers, which innervate the utricular and sac-cular maculae, seem to be "stato-receptor" elements which report unchanging head positions. Various head positions provoke different discharge rates. By combining a proper roll (coronal plane) and pitch (sagittal plane) a zone of maximum discharge and a zone of almost no impulse discharge can be demonstrated for every afferent fiber. In intermediate positions the impulse rate is a monotonic function of the angular head position (and thus the position of a macula).

The variation in fiber discharge rate with head position should be correlated with variations in the shearing force acting on the utricular or saccular macula. Werner and Whitsel suggest that in the case of the saccular macula only the vector of the shearing force directed toward the base of the skull is effective. In the utricular macula a shearing force acting in a medial direction is believed to be stimulating.

Werner and Whitsel (1968) also recorded from a good number of afferent fibers which were responsive to steady motion. They compare these fibers with the "out-of-position" labyrinthine receptors of the thornback ray (Lowenstein and Roberts, 1949).

The function of the sacculus in higher vertebrates has been less fully studied than that of the utriculus. The sacculus and lagena are organs of hearing in lower vertebrates. The lagena gave rise to the cochlea of higher forms, and, as mentioned previously, is absent in mammals.

The labyrinthine hair cells are characterized by a wide dynamic range of response. They also show slow adaptation.

Lowenstein (1967) indicates that much is not yet known about the transduction of mechanical to electrical energy which takes place in hair cells. It has also not yet been possible to get intracellular electrophysiological recordings from hair cells.

Discharges from the labyrinth may be correlated with nystagmus, a reflex flicking of the eyes. Nystagmus occurs both during acceleration and deceleration of rotation, but its direction in each of the two processes is the opposite. In nystagmus, during acceleration, the eyes move ahead and then remain on a visible object or point until, due to the rotation of the head, it leaves the field of view. The eyes then once more jump ahead and fix on a new locus. Nystagmus thus consists of a fast (phasic) jumping-ahead phase and a slow (tonic) return phase.

During rotation in light, the slow return movement of the eyes has more or less the speed of the rotation. This is true because the eyes are fixed on a visible object. However, in darkness the slow phase is entirely dependent on the labyrinthine discharge. It will then have a velocity only proportional to the magnitude of the stimulus. The labyrinth alone cannot cause the slow phase to equal the speed of the rotation; it only stimulates a slow-phase velocity of 30 to 80 per cent of the rotational velocity.

The speed of the slow phase is the aspect of nystagmus which is most closely related to labyrinthine activity, whether the last occurs in response to rotation or to caloric stimuli. In fact, the velocity of the slow phase is used clinically to gauge the condition of the nonauditory labyrinth. Some investigators think of the phasic portion of nystagmus as primarily a central correction.

The directional and temporal aspects of nystagmus can be related to complex discharges of the labyrinth. These labyrinthine responses stem from both the semicircular ducts and the otolith organs (Eviatar and Goodhill, 1968). In addition, central factors and inhibitory effects are involved in nystagmus. Eviatar and Goodhill (1968) describe nystagmus as a multifaceted kinetic complex and as a rotatory oscillatory complex.

Eviatar and Goodhill used multiple channel electronystagmography. They observed that the otolith organs gave rise to the nystagmus components in the vertical and diagonal channels. Nystagmic responses appeared in the horizontal channel upon stimulation of the anterior vertical semicircular duct.

Nystagmus persists after deceleration ends because of the effects of inertia.

In normal subjects, with the eyes fixating a light, the threshold for nystagmus is a constant angular (rotational) acceleration of the order of $1°-2°/sec^2$. Fixation of a visible point inhibits vestibular nystagmus. In total darkness the normal thresholds vary from $0.1°-0.2°/sec^2$ (Henriksson, Johansson and Östlund, 1967, Discussion).

If nystagmus is to be observed visually, rather than by electronystagmography, some inhibition must be allowed for. However, inhibition can be reduced to a minimum by use of Frenzel's spectacles. These powerful lenses make it impossible for a subject to see his environment and fixate on a point. At the same time the magnifying action of Frenzel's spectacles facilitates the study of nystagmus.

Nystagmic responses are greatly altered by the weightlessness of space flight. The absence of a gravity effect on the otolith organs may modify the response to the input from the semicircular ducts.

In addition to angular acceleration and deceleration, caloric stimulation, or the production of a temperature change, may be used to initiate nystagmus. Since the horizontal semicircular duct is close to the ear drum and within a bony canal, its temperature will be changed by cooling or heating the external auditory meatus. Maximum responses are obtained by filling the outer ear with water at $30°C$ (for cooling) or at $44°C$ (for heating). Cold water causes the tonic phase of nystagmus to travel toward the contralateral side, while hot water causes the tonic phase to be directed toward the ipsilateral side (Jongkees, 1967).

The discharge of the vestibular neurons is highly irregular in unanesthetized monkeys. The fluctuations in the discharge rate of these neurons has been related to the frequency of concomitant nystagmus (Werner and Whitsel, 1968).

Papers dealing with nystagmus include a report by Nagle (1967) that brief caloric stimulation may elicit nystagmic responses in one eye which differ from those in the other.

Yamanaka and Bach-Y-Rita (1968) correlate fast and slow fiber activity in the abducens nerve with the phases of nystagmus. Miller II and Graybiel (1964) presented material on otolith function and nystagmus at the International Vestibular Symposium held at the graduate school of medicine, University of Pennsylvania.

REFERENCES

Andres, K.H.: Die Feinstruktur der sensiblen Endapparate gerader, zirkulärer und verzweigter Terminalfasern am Sinushaar. *Naturwissenschaften,* 8:204, 1966a.

Andres, K.H.: Über die Feinstruktur der Rezeptoren an Sinushaaren. *Z. Zellforsch.,* 75:339-365, 1966b.

Anson, B.J., D.G. Harper, and T.R. Winch: The vestibular system. *Arch. Otolaryng.,* 85:497-514, 1967.

Appelberg, B., P. Bessou, and Y. Laporte: Action of static and dynamic fusimotor fibres on secondary endings of cat's spindles. *J. Physiol. (London),* 185:160-171, 1966.

Aronova, M.Z.: Electron microscopic study of lateral line organs in pike. *Arkh. Anat.,* 52:30-40, 1967.

Autrum, H., and W. Schneider: Vergleichende Untersuchungen über den Erschütterungssinn der Insekten. *Z. Vergl. Physiol.,* 31:77-88, 1948.

Azzena, G.B., M.L. Giretti, and P.L. Deriu: Convergence of labyrinthine and cerebral nystagmogenic impulses on brain-stem units. *Exp. Neurol.,* 19:401-411, 1967.

Bardach, J.E., and J. Case: Sensory capabilities of the modified fins of squirrel hake (*Urophycis chuss*) and searobins (*Prionotus carolinus* and *P. evolans*). *Copeia,* 2:194-206, 1965.

Barker, D.: The Innervation of Mammalian Skeletal Muscle. In de Reuck, A.V.S., and J. Knight (Eds.): *Myotatic, Kinesthetic and Vestibular Mechanisms.* Ciba Foundation Symposium. London, Churchill, 1967, pp. 3-15.

Barker, D., and I.A. Boyd: Signed Contributions to the Discussion on Muscle Spindles. In Granit, R. (Ed.): *Muscular Afferents and Motor Control.* Nobel Symposium I. Stockholm, Almquist and Wiksell, 1966, pp. 115-119.

Barker, D., and M. Cope: The Innervation of Individual Intrafusal Muscle Fibres. In Barker, D. (Ed.): *Symposium on Muscle Receptors.* Hong Kong, Hong Kong U. Pr., 1962, pp. 263-269.

Bas, C., and E. Morales: Crecimiento y desarrollo en *Micromesistius (Gadus, Merlangus) poutassou.* I. Desarrollo del otolito. *Inv. Pesq.,* 30:179-195, 1966.

Bennett, M.V.L.: Electroreceptors in mormyrids. In *Sensory Receptors. Cold Spring Harbor Symposia On Quantitative Biology,* 30:245-262, 1965.

Bennett, M.V.L.: Mechanisms of Electroreception. In Cahn, P.H. (Ed): *Lateral Line Detectors.* Bloomington, Indiana U. Pr., 1967, pp. 313-393.

Bessou, P., F. Emonet-Dénand, and Y. Laporte: Motor fibres innervating extrafusal and intrafusal muscle fibres in the cat. *J. Physiol. (London),* 180:649-672, 1965.

Bessou, P., Y. Laporte, and B. Pagés: Frequency-grams of spindle primary endings elicited by stimulation of static and dynamic fusimotor fibres. *J. Physiol. (London),* 196:47-63, 1968.

Biscoe, T.J., S.R. Sampson, and M.J. Purves: Stimulus response curves of single carotid body chemoreceptor afferent fibres. *Nature,* 215:654-655, 1967.

Borsellino, A., R.E. Poppele, and C.A. Terzuolo: Transfer functions of the slowly adapting stretch receptor organ of Crustacea. In *Sensory Receptors. Cold Spring Harbor Symposia on Quantitative Biology,* 30:581-586, 1965.

Boyd, I.A.: The structure and innervation of the nuclear bag muscle fibre system and the nuclear chain muscle fibre system in mammalian muscle spindles. *Phil. Trans. Roy. Soc. London, Ser. B,* 245:81-136, 1962.

Boyd, I.A.: The behaviour of isolated mammalian muscle spindles with intact innervation. *J. Physiol. (London),* 186:109-110P, 1966.

Boyd, I.A., and M.R. Davey: The Distribution of Two Types of Small Motor Nerve Fibre to Different Muscles in the Hind Limb of the Cat. In Granit, R. (Ed.): *Muscular Afferents and Motor Control.* Nobel Symposium I. Stockholm, Almquist and Wiksell, 1966, pp. 59-68.

Brown, M.C., A. Crowe, and P.B.C. Matthews: Observations on the fusimotor fibres of the tibialis posterior muscle of the cat. *J. Physiol. (London)*, 177:140-159, 1965.

Brown, M.C., I. Engberg, and P.B.C. Matthews: Fusimotor stimulation and the dynamic sensitivity of the secondary ending of the muscle spindle. *J. Physiol. (London)*, 189:545-550, 1967.

Brown, M.C., and R.B. Stein: Quantitative studies on the slowly adapting stretch receptor of the crayfish. *Kybernetik*, 3:175-185, 1966.

Bullock, T.H.: Initiation of Nerve Impulses in Receptor and Central Neurons. In Oncley, J.L. (Ed.): *Biophysical Science—A Study Program*. New York, John Wiley, 1959, pp. 504-514.

Bullock, T.H., and R. Barrett: Radiant heat reception in snakes. *Communic. Behav. Biol., A, 1*:19-29, 1968.

Bullock, T.H., and S. Chichibu: Further analysis of sensory coding in electroreceptors of electric fish. *Science, 148*:664-665, 1965.

Burgess, P.R., and E.R. Perl: Myelinated afferent fibres responding specifically to noxious stimulation of the skin. *J. Physiol. (London), 190*: 541-562, 1967.

Cabanac, M., T. Hammel, and J.D. Hardy: Tiliqua scincoides: temperature-sensitive units in lizard brain. *Science, 158*:1050-1051, 1967.

Cahn, P.H. (Ed.): *Lateral Line Detectors*. Proceedings Of A Conference Held At Yeshiva University, New York, April 16-18, 1966. Bloomington, Indiana U. Pr., 1967.

Cahn, P.H., J. Wodinsky, and W. Siler: A Signal Detection Study on the Acoustico-lateralis System of Fishes. Paper presented at A.A.A.S. meeting, New York, Dec. 30, 1967.

Camhi, J.M.: Locust Aerodynamic Setae: Sensory and Interneuron Responses. Paper presented at A.A.A.S. meeting, New York, Dec. 30, 1967.

Casby, J.U., R. Siminoff, and T.R. Houseknecht: An analogue cross-correlator to study naturally induced activity in intact nerve trunks. *J. Neurophysiol., 26*:432-448, 1963.

Cauna, N.: Fine Structure of the Receptor Organs and Its Probable Functional Significance. In de Reuck, A.V.S., and J. Knight (Eds.): *Ciba Foundation Symposium on Touch, Heat and Pain*. London, Churchill, 1966.

Cherepnov, V.L.: Ultrastructure of the inner core of the Pacinian corpuscles (cat). *Zh. Evol. Biokhim. Fiziol., 4*:91-96, 1968a.

Cherepnov, V.L.: Effect of mechanical stimulation on ultrastructure of the internal bulb of Pacinian bodies. *Dokl. Acad. Nauk SSSR, 178*:947-948, 1968b.

Clark, W.L., and L.P. Granath: A Measure of the Threshold Sensitivity of *Gymnotus carapo* to Electric Fields. Paper presented at A.A.A.S. meeting, New York, Dec. 30, 1967.

Cohen, M.J.: The response patterns of single receptors in the crustacean statocyst. *Proc. Roy. Soc. [Biol.], 152*:30-49, 1960.

Collins, W.F., F.E. Nulsen, and C.N. Shealy: Electrophysiological Studies of Peripheral and Central Pathways Conducting Pain. In Knighton, R.S., and P.R. Dumke (Eds.): *Pain*. Boston, Little, Brown, 1966.

Corda, M., G. Eklund, and C. von Euler: External intercostal and phrenic motor responses to changes in respiratory load. *Acta Physiol. Scand., 63*:391-400, 1965.

Corda, M., C. von Euler, and G. Lennerstrand: Reflex and cerebellar influences on α and on "rhythmic" and "tonic" gamma activity in the intercostal muscle. *J. Physiol. (London), 184*: 898-923, 1966.

Cozine, R.A., and S.H. Ngai: Medullary surface chemoreceptors and regulation of respiration in the cat. *J. Appl. Physiol., 22*:117-121, 1967.

Critchlow, V., and C. von Euler: Intercostal muscle spindle activity and its γ motor control. *J. Physiol. (London), 168*:820-847, 1963.

Crowe, A., and P.B.C. Matthews: The effects of stimulation of static and dynamic fusimotor fibres on the response to stretching of the primary endings of muscle spindles. *J. Physiol. (London), 174*:109-131, 1964a.

Crowe, A., and P.B.C. Matthews: Further studies of static and dynamic fusimotor fibres. *J. Physiol. (London), 174*:132-151, 1964b.

DeKock, L.L., and A.E.G. Dunn: An electron microscope study of the carotid body. *Acta Anat. (Basel), 64*:163-178, 1966.

Dethier, V.G., and A. Gelperin: Hyperphagia in the blowfly. *J. Exp. Biol., 47*:191-200, 1967.

Dijkgraaf, S.: The functioning and significance of the lateral-line organs. *Biol. Rev., 38*:51-105, 1963.

Dijkgraaf, S.: Biological Significance of the Lateral Line Organs. In Cahn, P.H. (Ed.): *Lateral Line Detectors*. Bloomington, Indiana U. Pr., 1967, pp. 83-95.

Douglas, W.W., and J.M. Ritchie: Non-medullated fibers in the saphenous nerve which signal touch. *J. Physiol. (London), 139*:385-399, 1957.

Duncan, D., and R. Yates: Ultrastructure of the carotid body of the cat as revealed by various fixatives and the use of reserpine. *Anat. Rec.,* 157:667-682, 1967.

Eakin, R.M.: Evolution of photoreceptors. In *Sensory Receptors. Cold Spring Harbor Symposia on Quantitative Biology,* 30:363-370, 1965.

Edwards, C., and D. Ottoson: The site of impulse initiation in a nerve cell of a crustacean stretch receptor. *J. Physiol. (London),* 143:138-148, 1958.

Eldred, E., and J. Buchwald: Central nervous system: motor mechanisms. *Ann. Rev. Physiol.,* 29:573-606, 1967.

Eviatar, A., and V. Goodhill: Vector electronystagmography: a method of localizing nystagmic impulses within the vestibular system. *Ann. Otol.,* 77:264-274, 1968.

Eyzaguirre, C., H. Koyano, and J.R. Taylor: Presence of acetylcholine and transmitter release from carotid body chemoreceptors. *J. Physiol. (London),* 178:463-476, 1965.

Eyzaguirre, C., and S.W. Kuffler: Processes of excitation in the dendrites and in the soma of single isolated sensory nerve cells of the lobster and crayfish. *J. Gen. Physiol.,* 39:87-119, 1955.

Eyzaguirre, C., and P. Zapata: Pharmacology of pH effects on carotid body chemoreceptors *in vitro. J. Physiol. (London),* 195:557-588, 1968a.

Eyzaguirre, C., and P. Zapata: The release of acetylcholine from carotid body tissues. Further study on the effects of acetylcholine and cholinergic blocking agents on the chemosensory discharge. *J. Physiol. (London),* 195: 589-607, 1968b.

Fernández, C.: Biochemistry of labyrinthine fluids. *Arch. Otolaryng.,* 86:222-233, 1967.

Filaretov, A.A.: Proprioception of abdominal muscles during respiration. *Fiziol. Zh. SSSR Sechenov.,* 54:39-46, 1968.

Fitzgerald, O.: Discharges from the sensory organs of the cat's vibrissae and the modification in their activity by ions. *J. Physiol. (London),* 98:163-178, 1940.

Flock, Å.: Ultrastructure and Function in the Lateral Line Organs. In Cahn, P.H. (Ed.): *Lateral Line Detectors.* Bloomington, Indiana U. Pr., 1967, pp. 163-197.

Florey, E.: Untersuchungen über die Impuls-Entstehung in den Streckrezeptoren des Flus-

skrebses. *Z. Naturforsch. [B],* 106:591-597, 1955.

Florey, E., and E. Florey: Microanatomy of the abdominal stretch receptors of the crayfish (*Astacus fluviatilis* L.). *J. Gen. Physiol.,* 39: 69-85, 1955.

Frank, R.M.: Ultrastructure of Human Dentine. In *Calcified Tissues.* Proc. Europe Symp., 3. New York, Springer-Verlag, 1966, pp. 259-272.

Fraschini, F., B. Mess, F. Piva, and L. Martini: Brain receptors sensitive to indole compounds: Function in control of luteinizing hormone secretion. *Science,* 159:1104-1105, 1968.

Gasser, H.S.: Pain-producing impulses in peripheral nerves. *Res. Publ. Ass. Res. Nerv. Ment. Dis.,* 23:44-62, 1943.

Gelperin, A.: Stretch receptors in the foregut of the blowfly. *Science,* 157:208-210, 1967.

Giacobini, E., and J.F. Jongkind: Pentose shunt enzymes in the crustacean stretch receptor neuron after impulse activity. *Acta Physiol. Scand.,* 73:255-256, 1968.

Gilman, S.: A crossed cerebellar influence on muscle spindle primaries. *Brain Res.,* 8:216-219, 1968.

Gilman, S., and W.I. McDonald: Cerebellar facilitation of muscle spindle activity. *J. Neurophysiol.,* 30:1494-1512, 1967a.

Gilman, S., and W.I. McDonald: Relation of afferent fiber conduction velocity to reactivity of muscle spindle receptors after cerebellectomy. *J. Neurophysiol.,* 30:1513-1522, 1967b.

Glaser, D.: Untersuchungen über die absoluten Geschmacksschwellen von Fischen. *Z. Vergl. Physiol.,* 52:1-25, 1966.

Goris, R.C., and M. Nomoto: Infrared reception in oriental crotaline snakes. *Comp. Biochem. Physiol.,* 23:879-892, 1967.

Görner, P.: Untersuchungen zur Morphologie und Elektrophysiologie des Seitenorgans vom Krallenfrosch (Xenopus laevis). *Z. Vergl. Physiol.,* 47:361-388, 1963.

Görner, P.: A proposed transducing mechanism for a multiply-innervated mechanoreceptor (trichobothrium) in spiders. In *Sensory Receptors. Cold Spring Harbor Symposia on Quantitative Biology,* 30:69-73, 1965.

Granath, L.P., H.G. Sachs, and F.T. Erskine III: Electrical sensitivity of a weakly electric fish. *Life Sci.,* 6:2373-2377, 1967.

Granit, R.: The functional role of the muscle

spindle's primary end organs. *Roy. Soc. Med. Proc., 61*:69-78, 1968.

Granit, R., J.O. Kellerth, and A.J. Szumski: Intracellular recording from extensor motoneurons activated across the gamma loop. *J. Neurophysiol., 29*:530-544, 1966.

Green, D.G., and J.O. Kellerth: Postsynaptic versus presynaptic inhibition in antagonistic stretch reflexes. *Science, 152*:1097-1099, 1966.

Groen, J.J., O. Lowenstein, and A.J.H. Vendrik: The mechanical analysis of the responses from the end-organs of the horizontal semicircular canal in the isolated elasmobranch labyrinth. *J. Physiol. (London), 117*:329-346, 1952.

Haase, J., P. Meuser, and U Tan: The convergence of fusimotor alpha-impulses on de-efferentiating flexor spindles in the cat. *Pflügers Arch. Ges. Physiol., 289*:50-58, 1966.

Hagiwara, S., K. Kusano, and K. Negishi: Physiological properties of electroreceptors of some gymnotids. *G. Neurophys., 25*:430-449, 1962.

Harder, W., A. Schief, and H. Uhlemann: Zur Empfindlichkeit des schwachelektrischen Fishes *Gnathonemus petersii* (Gthr. 1862) (Mormyriformes, Teleostei) gegenüber elektrischen Feldern. *Z. Vergl. Physiol., 54*:89-108, 1967.

Harris, G. G., and W.A. van Bergeijk: Evidence that the lateral-line organ responds to the near field displacements of sound sources in water. *J. Acoust. Soc. Amer., 34*:1831-1841, 1962.

Harris, G.G., L.S. Frishkopf, and Å. Flock: Receptor potentials from hair cells of the lateral line. *Science, 167*:76-79, 1970.

Hebel, R., and A. Schweiger: Zur Feinstruktur und Funktion sensibler Rezeptoren. *Zbl. Veterinaermed. [A], 14*:15-25, 1967.

Heist, H.E., B.D. Mulvaney, and D.J. Landis: Odor Sensing Cell Ultrastructure by Electron Microscopy. Final report to Air Force Office of Scientific Research, Contract No. AF49 (638)-1618. Presented by Honeywell, Inc., Corporate Research Center, Hopkins, Minn., 1967.

Henatsch, H.D., and S.S. Schäfer: Fusimotor-sensor and fusimotor-trigger functions: A reinterpretation of the dual control of mammalian muscle spindles. *Brain Res., 6*:385-387, 1967.

Henriksson, N.G., G. Johansson, and H. Östlund: New Techniques of Otoneurological Diagnosis. II. Vestibulo-spinal and Postural Patterns. In de Reuck, A.V.S., and J. Knight (Eds.):

Ciba Foundation Symposium On Myotatic, Kinesthetic And Vestibular Mechanisms. London, Churchill, 1967, pp. 231-237.

Hoar, W.S.: *General and Comparative Physiology.* Englewood Cliffs, Prentice-Hall, 1966.

Horridge, G.A.: Some Recently Discovered Underwater Vibration Receptors in Invertebrates. In Barnes, H. (Ed.): *Some Contemporary Studies In Marine Science.* London, George Allen and Unwin, 1966, pp. 395-405.

Howe Jr., D.W., F.T. Erskine, and L.P. Granath: Threshold sensitivity of *Sternarchus albifrons* to electric fields. *Amer. Zool., 6 (Abst. 80),* 1966.

Iggo, A.: Cutaneous heat and cold receptors with slowly conducting (C) afferent fibres. *Quart. J. Exp. Physiol., 44*:362-370, 1959.

Iggo, A.: A Single Unit Analysis of Cutaneous Receptors With C Afferent Fibers. In Wolstenholme, G.E.W., and O'Connor, M. (Eds.): *Pain and Itch: Nervous Mechanisms. Ciba Foundation Study Group No. 1, March 1959.* Boston, Little, Brown, 1960a.

Iggo, A.: Cutaneous mechanoreceptors with afferent C fibres. *J. Physiol. (London), 152*:337-353, 1960b.

Iggo, A.: An electrophysiological analysis of afferent fibers in primate skin. *Acta Neuroveg. (Vienna), 24*:225-240, 1963.

Ikoma, H., H. Makino, M. Yamada, and H. Sasaki: Changes in the activity of the brain stem reticular formation in the cat, following electrical stimulation of the utricle. *Yonago Acta Med., 11*:150-158, 1967.

Il' Inskii, O.B., N.K. Volkova, and V.L. Cherepnov: Structure and function of Pacini's corpuscles (cat). *Fiziol. Zh. SSSR Sechenov., 54*: 295-302, 1968.

Ishii, K., and T. Oosaki: Electron microscopy of the chemoreceptor cells of the carotid labyrinth of the toad. *Nature, 212*:1499-1500, 1966.

Jahn, S.A.A.: The excitability of frog's isolated muscle spindles during repetitive stretches. *Acta Physiol. Scand., 73*:418-426, 1968a.

Jahn, S.A.A.: Spontaneous afferent discharges and spontaneous intrafusal contractions in isolated muscle spindles of the frog. *Acta Physiol. Scand., 72*:350-365, 1968b.

Jahn, S.A.A.: Response of isolated muscle spindles to single transient stretches. *Acta Physiol. Scand., 72*:441-455, 1968c.

Jahn, S.A.A.: Excitability of the frog's muscle spindle to transient stretches following spontaneous and evoked afferent action potentials. *Acta Physiol. Scand., 73*:176-185, 1968d.

Jande, S.S.: Fine structure of lateral-line organs of frog tadpoles. *J. Ultrastruct. Res., 15*:496-509, 1966.

Jansen, J.K.S., and T. Rudjord: Fusimotor activity in a flexor muscle of the decerebrate cat. *Acta Physiol. Scand., 63*:236-246, 1965.

Jongkees, L.B.W.: The Examination of the Vestibular Organ. In Zotterman, Y. (Ed.): *Progress in Brain Research. Sensory Mechanisms.* Amsterdam, Elsevier, 1967, vol. 23, pp. 155-168.

Karlsson, U., E. Andersson-Cedergren, and D. Ottoson: Cellular organization of the frog muscle spindle as revealed by serial sections for electron microscopy. *J. Ultrastruct. Res., 14*:1-35, 1966.

Katz, B.: The termination of the afferent nerve fibre in the muscle spindle of the frog. *Phil. Trans. Roy. Soc. London, Ser. B, 243*:221-240, 1961.

Kellner, G.: Über ein vaskularisiertes Nervenendkörperchen vom Typ der Krauseschen Endorgane. *Z. Mikr. Anat. Forsch., 75*:130-144, 1966.

Kenshalo, D.R., and E.S. Gallegos: Multiple temperature-sensitive spots innervated by single nerve fibers. *Science, 158*:1064-1065, 1967.

Krieger, E.M., and R.F. Marseillan: Neural control in experimental renal hypertension. The role of baroreceptor and splanchnic fibers. *Acta Physiol. Lat. Amer., 16*:343-352, 1966.

Krnjević, K., and M. van Gelder: Tension changes in crayfish stretch receptors. *J. Physiol. (London), 159*:310-325, 1961.

Kuffler, S.W.: Mechanisms of activation and motor control of stretch receptors in lobster and crayfish. *J. Neurophysiol., 17*:558-574, 1954.

Kuffler, S.W., and C. Eyzaguirre: Synaptic inhibition in an isolated nerve cell. *J. Gen. Physiol., 39*:155-184, 1955.

Kuiper, J.W.: Frequency Characteristics and Functional Significance of the Lateral Line Organ. In Cahn, P.H. (Ed.): *Lateral Line Detectors.* Bloomington, Indiana U. Pr., 1967, pp. 105-121.

Kukkonen, M.I.: Role of chest-wall receptors in regulation of respiration. *Fiziol. Zh. SSSR Sechenov., 54*:213-219, 1968.

Lele, P.P., and G. Weddell: The relationship between neurohistology and corneal sensibility. *Brain, 79*:119-154, 1956.

Lennerstrand, G.: *Dynamic Analysis of Muscle Spindles in the Cat.* A publication of the Nobel Institute for Neurophysiology, Karolinska Institutet, Stockholm, Brogenhardt Tryckeri AB, 1968.

Levi, H.W., and C.D. Dondale: Arachnology meeting. *Science, 161*:1033, 1968.

Lim, R.K.S.: Pain mechanisms. *Anesthesiology, 28*:106-110, 1967.

Lissmann, H.W.: Electric location by fishes. *Sci. Amer., 208*:3, 50-59, 1963.

Loewenstein, W.R.: Biological transducers. *Sci. Amer., 203*:98-108, 1960a.

Loewenstein, W.R.: Mechanisms of nerve impulse initiation in a pressure receptor (Lorenzinian Ampulla). *Nature, 188*:1034-1035, 1960b.

Loewenstein, W.R.: On the specificity of a sensory receptor. *J. Neurophysiol., 24*:150-158, 1961.

Lowenstein, O.: Functional Aspects of Vestibular Structure. In de Reuck, A.V.S. and J. Knight (Eds.): *Ciba Foundation Symposium on Myotatic, Kinesthetic and Vestibular Mechanisms.* London, Churchill, 1967, pp. 121-128.

Lowenstein, O., and M.P. Osborne: Ultrastructure of the sensory hair-cells in the labyrinth of the ammocoete larva of the lamprey, *Lampetra fluviatilis. Nature, 204*:197-198, 1964.

Lowenstein, O., and T.D.M. Roberts: The equilibrium function of the otolith organs of the thornback ray (*Raja clavata.*) *J. Physiol. (London), 110*:392-415, 1949.

Malinovský, L.: Variability of sensory nerve endings in foot pads of a domestic cat (*Felis ocreata L., F. domestica*). *Acta Anat., 64*: 82-106, 1966a.

Malinovský, L.: The variability of encapsulated corpuscles in the upper lip and tongue of the domestic cat (*Felis ocreata L., F. domestica*). *Folia Morph. (Prague), 14*:175-191, 1966b.

Malinovský, L.: Variability of sensory corpuscles in the skin of the nose and in the area of sulcus labii maxillaris of the domestic cat. *Folia Morph. (Prague), 14*:417-429, 1966c.

Malinovský, L.: Die Nervenendkörperchen in der Haut von Vögeln und ihre Variabilität. *Z. Mikr. Anat. Forsch., 77*:279-303, 1967.

Mann, S.J., and W.E. Straile: Tylotrich (hair) follicle: Association with a slowly adapting tactile receptor in the cat. *Science, 147*:1043-1045, 1965.

Manni, E., and C. Desole: Responses of oculomotor units to stimulation of single semicircular canals. *Exp. Neurol., 15*:206-219, 1966.

Matthews, P.B.C.: Muscle spindles and their motor control. *Physiol. Rev., 44*:219-288, 1964.

Matthews, P.B.C.: Vibration and the Stretch Reflex. In de Reuck, A.V.S., and J. Knight (Eds.): *Ciba Foundation Symposium on Myotatic, Kinesthetic and Vestibular Mechanisms*. London, Churchill, 1967, pp. 40-50.

Matthews, P.B.C., and D.R. Westbury: Some effects of fast and slow motor fibres on muscle spindles of the frog. *J. Physiol. (London), 178*: 178-192, 1965.

Maturana, H.R., and S. Sperling: Unidirectional response to angular acceleration recorded from the middle cristal nerve in the statocyst of *Octopus vulgaris. Nature, 197*:815-816, 1963.

Mavrinskaya, L.F.: Development of muscle spindles in man. *Arkh. Anat., 53*:42-49, 1967.

McDonald, W.I., and S. Gilman: Demyelination and muscle spindle function. *Arch. Neurol., 18*:508-519, 1968.

Mellon, Jr., D.: *The Physiology Of Sense Organs*. San Francisco, W. H. Freeman, 1968.

Miller, II, E.F., and A. Graybiel: Otolith function as measured by ocular counterrolling. *Trans. Int. Vestib. Symp., Grad. Sch. Med.*, U. Penn. NAVSCOLAVNMED 6000/1(REV. 6-64).

Milsum, J.H., and G.M. Jones: Trigonometric resolution of neural response from the vestibular otolith organ. *Digest 7th Int. Con. Med. Biol. Engineering*, Stockholm, sess. 12-8, 1967.

Minkoff, L.A., W.L. Clark, and H.G. Sachs: Interspike Interval Analysis of the Discharge of a Weakly Electric Mormyrid Fish. Paper presented at A.A.A.S. meeting, Dec. 30, New York City, 1967.

Morris, R.W., and L.R. Kittleman: Piezoelectric property of otoliths. *Science, 158*:368-370, 1967.

Mountcastle, V.B., W.H. Talbot, I. Darian-Smith, and H.H. Kornhuber: Neural basis of the sense of flutter-vibration. *Science, 155*:597-600, 1967.

Mountford, S.: Filamentous organelles in receptor-bipolar synapses of the retina. *J. Ultrastruct. Res., 10*:207-216, 1964.

Murray, R.W.: Receptor mechanisms in the ampullae of Lorenzini of elasmobranch fishes. In *Sensory Receptors. Cold Spring Harbor Symposia on Quantitative Biology, 30*:233-243, 1965.

Murray, R.W.: The Function of the Ampullae of Lorenzini of Elasmobranchs. In Cahn, P.H. (Ed.): *Lateral Line Detectors*. Bloomington, Indiana U. Pr., 1967, pp. 277-293.

Nagle, D.W.: An unusual vestibular nystagmus elicited from normal subjects. *Ann. Otol., 76*: 447-454, 1967.

Nakajima, S.: Adaptation in stretch receptor neurons of crayfish. *Science, 146*:1168-1170, 1964.

Nakajima, S., and K. Onodera: Membrane properties of the stretch receptor neurones of crayfish with particular reference to mechanisms of sensory adaptation. *J. Physiol. (London), 200*: 161-185, 1969a.

Nakajima, S., and K. Onodera: Adaptation of the generator potential in the crayfish stretch receptors under constant length and constant tension. *J. Physiol. (London), 200*:187-204, 1969b.

Nakajima, S., and K. Takahashi: Post-tetanic hyperpolarization and electrogenic Na pump in stretch receptor neurone of crayfish. *J. Physiol. (London), 187*:105-127, 1966.

Niijima, A., and D.L. Winter: Baroreceptors in the adrenal gland. *Science, 159*:434-435, 1968.

Nilsson, B.Y., and C.R. Skoglund: The tactile hairs on the cat's foreleg. *Acta Physiol. Scand., 65*: 364-369, 1965.

Okano, M., A.F. Weber, and S.P. Frommes: Electron microscopic studies of the distal border of the canine olfactory epithelium. *J. Ultrastruct. Res., 17*:487-502, 1967.

Olney, J.W.: An electron microscopic study of synapse formation, receptor outer segment development, and other aspects of developing mouse retina. *Invest. Ophthal., 7*:250-268, 1968.

Pabst, H., and D. Kennedy: Cutaneous mechanoreceptors influencing motor output in the crayfish abdomen. *Z. Vergl. Physiol., 57*:190-208, 1967.

Pease, D.C., and T.A. Quilliam: Electron microscopy of the Pacinian corpuscle. *J. Biophys. Biochem. Cytol., 3*:331-347, 1957.

Perl, E.R., *et al.*: In G.G. Somjen: Sensory coding. *Science, 158*:399-405, 1967.

Pierau, F.K., and H.D. Meissner: Die Temperaturempfindlichkeit isolierter Lorenzinischer

Ampullen. *Helgoländer Wiss. Meeresunters.,* 14:381-391, 1966.

Polacek, P., A. Sklenska, and L. Malinovský: Contribution to the problem of joint receptors in birds. *Folia Morphol.,* 14:33-42, 1966.

Poppele, R.E.: Response of gamma and alpha motor systems to phasic and tonic vestibular inputs. *Brain Res.,* 6:535-547, 1967.

Pringle, J.W.S.: The functions of the lyriform organs of arachnids. *J. Exp. Biol.,* 32:270-278, 1955.

Quilliam, T.A.: The mole's sensory apparatus. *J. Zool., (London),* 149:76-88, 1966.

Quilliam, T.A., P. Graziadei, and J. Armstrong: Skin receptors. *Rass. Med. E. Cult.,* 41:31-41, 1964.

Rudolph, P.: Zum Ortungsverfahren von *Gyrinus substriatus* Steph. *Z. Vergl. Physiol.,* 56:341-375, 1967.

Rusinov, V.S., and V.D. Ezrokhi: Local and propagating excitation in different parts of stretch receptor neurons in crustaceans. *Fiziol. Zh. SSSR Sechenov.,* 53:777-783, 1967.

Salpeter, M.M., and C. Walcott: An electron microscopical study of a vibration receptor in the spider. *Exp. Neurol.,* 2:232-250, 1960.

Sasaki, H.: The function of the otolith organs. *Yonago Acta Med.,* 11:133-140, 1967.

Schäfer, S.S., and H.D. Henatsch: Dehnungsantworten der primären Muskelspindel-Afferenz bei elektrischer Reizung und natürlicher Innervation der beiden fusimotorischen Fasertypen. *Exp. Brain Res.,* 4:275-291, 1968.

Scharrer, E.: Intraepithelial nerve terminals in the free finrays of the searobin, *Prionotus carolinus* L. *Anat. Rec.,* 145:367-368, 1963.

Schöne, H.: Gravity Orientation Under Water. In Burkhardt, D., W. Schleidt, and H. Altner (Eds.): *Signals in the Animal World.* Transl. by K. Morgan, New York, McGraw-Hill, 1967.

Schwartz, E., and A.D. Hasler: Superficial lateral line sense organs of the mudminnow (*Umbra limi*). *Z. Vergl. Physiol.,* 53:317-327, 1966.

Scott, Jr., D.: Aspirin: action on receptor in the tooth. *Science,* 161:180-181, 1968.

Shantha, T.R., and G.H. Bourne: New observations on the structure of the Pacinian corpuscle and its relation to the perineural epithelium of peripheral nerves. *Amer. J. Anat.,* 112:97-109, 1963.

Shantha, T.R., and G.H. Bourne: Pacinian cor-

puscle on the olfactory bulb of the squirrel monkey. *Nature,* 209:1260, 1966.

Shantha, T.R., M.N. Golarz, and G.H. Bourne: Histological and histochemical observations on the capsule of the muscle spindle in normal and denervated muscle. *Acta Anat.,* 69:632-646, 1968.

Siminoff, R., and L. Kruger: Properties of reptilian cutaneous mechanoreceptors. *Exp. Neurol.,* 20:403-414, 1968.

Sinclair, D.: *Cutaneous Sensation.* London, Oxford U. Pr., 1967.

Smith, R.S.: Properties of Intrafusal Muscle Fibres. In Granit, R. (Ed.): *Muscular Afferents and Motor Control.* Nobel Symposium I. Stockholm, Almquist and Wiksell, 1966, pp. 69-80.

Suga, N.: Electrosensitivity of Specialized and Ordinary Lateral Line Organs of the Electric Fish, *Gymnotus carapo.* In Cahn, P.H. (Ed.): *Lateral Line Detectors.* Bloomington, Indiana U. Pr., 1967, pp. 395-409.

Tamar, H.: Observations on *Halteria bifurcata* sp. n. and *Halteria grandinella. Acta Protozool.,* VI:175-184, 1968.

Tanaka, K., K. Kimishima, and T. Yamasaki: Studies on the intraventricular chemoreceptors. III. Anatomical considerations. *Yonago Acta Med.,* 9:186-189, 1965.

Tanaka, K., and T. Yamasaki: Studies on the intraventricular chemoreceptors. I. Vasopressor effect of morphine introduced into the cerebrospinal fluid. *Yonago Acta Med.,* 9:178-180, 1965a.

Tanaka, K., and T. Yamasaki: Studies on the intraventricular chemoreceptors. II. Central excitatory effects of tubocurarine and other substances introduced into the cerebrospinal fluid. *Yonago Acta Med.,* 9:181-185, 1965b.

Tester, A.L., and J.I. Kendall: Cupulae in shark neuromasts: composition, origin, generation. *Science,* 160:772-774, 1968.

Thurm, U.: Mechanoreceptors in the cuticle of the honey bee: fine structure and stimulus mechanism. *Science,* 145:1063-1065, 1964.

Toyama, K.: An analysis of impulse discharges from the spindle receptor. *Jap. J. Physiol.,* 16:113-125, 1966.

Vinnikov, J.A.: Fine structure of the taste bud. *J. Ultrastruct. Res.,* 12:328-350, 1965.

Walcott, C., and M.M. Salpeter: The effect of molting upon the vibration receptor of the spider (Achaearanea tepidariorum). *J. Morph.*, *119*:383-392, 1966.

Warren, J.W., and U. Proske: Infrared receptors in the facial pits of the Australian python *Morelia spilotes. Science, 159*:439-441, 1968.

Watanabe, A., and K. Takeda: The change of discharge frequency by a-c stimulus in a weak electric fish. *J. Exp. Biol., 40*:57-66, 1963.

Wendler, L.: Über die Wirkungskette zwischen Reiz und Erregung (Versuche an den abdominalen Streckreceptoren des Flusskrebses). *Z. Vergl. Physiol., 47*:279-315, 1963.

Werner, G., and B.L. Whitsel: The activity of afferent nerve fibers from the vestibular organ and of neurons in the vestibular nuclei of unanesthetized primates. Arlington, Va., AF-AFOSR-66-1005 B, Air Force Office of Scientific Research, 1968.

Wersäll, J., Å. Flock, and P.-G. Lundquist: Structural basis for directional sensitivity in cochlear and vestibular sensory receptors. 115-132. In *Sensory Receptors. Cold Spring Harbor Symposia on Quantitative Biology, 30*:115-132, 1965.

Wersäll, J., L. Gleisner, and P.-G. Lundquist: Ultrastructure of the Vestibular End Organs. In de Reuck, A.V.S., and J. Knight (Eds.): *Ciba Foundation Symposium On Myotatic, Kinesthetic And Vestibular Mechanisms.* London, Churchill, 1967, pp. 105-116.

Winkelmann, R.K.: *Nerve Endings in Normal and Pathologic Skin.* Springfield, Charles C Thomas, 1960, p. 195.

Yamanaka, Y., and P. Bach-Y-Rita: Conduction velocities in the abducens nerve correlated with vestibular nystagmus in cats. *Exp. Neurol., 20*:143-155, 1968.

Zotterman, Y.: Thermal sensations. In Field, J. (Ed.): *Handbook of Physiology.* Washington, American Physiological Society, 1959, Vol. I, sect. 1, pp. 431-458.

SUGGESTED READING

Burkhardt, D., W. Schleidt, and H. Altner: *Signals in the Animal World.* Transl. by K. Morgan. New York, McGraw-Hill, 1967.

Cahn, P.H., (Ed.): *Lateral Line Detectors. Proceedings Of A Conference Held At Yeshiva University, New York, April 16-18, 1966.* Bloomington, Indiana U. Pr., 1967.

Carthy, J.D., and G.E. Newell (Eds.): *Invertebrate Receptors, Symposia of the Zoological Society of London, 23.* London and New York, Academic, 1968.

Case, J.: *Sensory Mechanisms.* New York, Macmillan, 1966.

De Reuck, A.V.S., and J. Knight (Eds.): *Myotatic, Kinesthetic and Vestibular Mechanisms, Ciba Foundation Symposium.* London, Churchill, 1967.

Eldred, E., and J. Buchwald: Central nervous system: motor mechanisms. *Ann. Rev. Physiol., 29*:573-606, 1967.

Florey, E.: *An Introduction to General and Comparative Animal Physiology.* Philadelphia, W. B. Saunders, 1966.

Granit, R.: The functional role of the muscle spindle's primary end organs. *Roy. Soc. Med. Proc., 61*:69-78, 1968.

Hoar, W.S.: *General and Comparative Physiology.* Englewood Cliffs, Prentice-Hall, 1966.

Kenshalo, D.R. (Ed.): *The Skin Senses, Proceedings of the First International Symposium.* Springfield, Charles C Thomas, 1968.

Sensory Receptors. *Cold Spring Harbor Symposia On Quantitative Biology,* Vol. 30, 1965.

Sinclair, D.: *Cutaneous Sensation.* London, Oxford U. Pr., 1967.

Chapter III

The Function of Receptors

THE GENERAL MECHANISM OF THE RECEPTOR RESPONSE

The response of a receptor can probably best be divided into three stages. The first of these might broadly be said to consist of initial events—how the stimulus first affects the receptor, and how this effect results in a depolarization of the receptor membrane and the development of what some investigators have differentiated as the receptor potential. The development of this potential change as a consequence of stimulus action also forms the subject matter of receptor transduction—how receptors convert various types of stimulus energy into electrical energy.

Abrahamson and Ostroy (1967) deal with the molecular change, the cis-trans isomerization of retinal, which is the immediate effect produced by a light stimulus in visual receptors. They then speculate that in other classes of receptors the first action of the proper stimulus may be to bring about a major molecular reconfiguration. Thus a taste-stimulating molecule may complex with a protein molecule in the surface membrane of a gustatory receptor to produce an important configurational change. Perhaps similar molecular amplifications are the first results of stimulation in mechano-, presso-, and thermo-receptors.

However, in mechanoreceptors the stretching of the cell membrane alone appears to satisfy the requirements for an effective initial stimulus action.

The second stage of the receptor response might be described as made up of the formation of generator currents from the receptor potential and the development, as a result of the conduction of these generator currents to the central and proximal portions of the receptor, of the generator potential. The generator current precedes and gives rise to the generator potential. The generator potential may be said to be located at or extend over the site of nerve impulse formation.

The differentiation of the receptor potential from the generator potential, however, is valid only on the basis of a type of receptor structure. Thus in rat taste cells the true receptor membrane is thinner than the rest of the cell plasma membrane—it measures only 90 Å as compared to 120 to 130 Å for the rest of the plasma membrane—and is localized at the distal end of the elongated taste cell (Farbman, 1965). In this cell the electrical change (generator currents) emanating from the receptor potential in the distal receptor membrane must travel over much of the length of the taste receptor to reach the receptor's proximal portion where "mesaxons" surround nerve fibers. Only the (generator) potential developing proximally can produce nerve impulses.

The differentiation of the two potentials loses its meaning when the functional receptor is structurally homogeneous and receives stimuli around its entire periphery, as is true of the 600μ-800μ-long unmyelinated nerve ending in the pacinian corpuscle. Therefore Loewenstein (1960, 1961a, b) speaks only of the generator current or the generator potential in the pacinian corpuscle.

Insect mechano- and chemo-reception, which take place through bipolar neurons, may be simpler than other receptor activity in that here the receptor potential and the generator potential may be identical (Dethier, 1962). This was indicated by the work of Wolbarsht (1958), who studied a receptor potential in insect mechanoreceptors which Dethier considers as either also being the generator potential or being associated with the generator potential. Morita (1959), using insect chemoreceptors, found a slow potential that he concluded was a generator potential. He did not differentiate between the receptor potential and the generator potential, and they appear to be identical in this chemoreceptor.

Wolbarsht (1965) differentiates only between a receptor potential and an impulse potential (nerve impulse) in the insect chemosensory neuron. He defines the receptor potential as the nonpropagated change in the potential across the sensory membrane of the dendrite tip which is produced by a stimulus.

Hodgson (1967) judges that if several insect chemosensory neurons contribute to a general, maintained initial potential, or if inhibition is involved, such a potential should be described as a receptor potential. However, Hodgson agrees that under some circumstances such slow insect potentials show the closest resemblance to normal generator potentials.

The generator potentials recorded from insect chemosensory hairs are slow, negative potentials. They may be stimulated by substances such as sodium chloride and sucrose, and increase in magnitude with the stimulus concentration.

The generator potential which can be evoked by a certain stimulus is a linear function, over a wide range, of the resting potential of the stimulated membrane.

The third and final stage of the receptor response then could encompass the generation of nerve impulses by the generator potential.

Nerve impulses are first produced by a generator potential when its amplitude reaches a threshold. The frequency of the nerve impulses is dependent on the rate of increase and on the amplitude of the generator current within the limits imposed by the durations of the absolute and relative refractory periods of the nerve fiber. With increasing amplitude of the generator potential, the nerve impulses appear earlier in the nerve's relative refractory period until the absolute refractory period sets a final limit on impulse frequency. Until the interval between nerve impulses becomes equivalent to the absolute refractory period, impulse rate varies directly with the size of the generator potential. Under normal stimu-

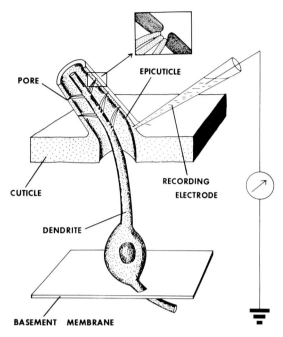

FIGURE 3-1. Structure of an insect olfactory hair and method of recording from its sensory neuron. Branches of the bipolar neuron's dendrite contact the air at pores. The axon joins the antennal nerve and runs to the deutocerebrum. The recording microelectrode is usually forced through the epicuticle, while the reference electrode's tip is placed into the hemolymph space. (Adapted from Boeckh, J., K.E. Kaissling, and D. Schneider: Insect olfactory receptors. In *Sensory Receptors. Cold Spring Harbor Symposia on Quantitative Biology*, 30:263-280, 1965.)

lation the rate of increase of the generator current remains within limits.

If the receptor cell is not a neuron, but a specialized cell which is intimately related to a neuron through a synapse, the receptor's generator potential may cause the release of a substance which will lower the membrane resistance of the neuron. Such lowered resistance is linked to an increase in membrane permeability and will result in the development of an action potential or impulse in the neuron. A probably similar process involving the release of a chemical agent occurs at synapses between neurons.

Fuortes (1959) observed a resistance drop in the membrane of the eccentric cell (nerve cell) of the *Xiphosuran (Limulus)* ommatidium when light reached the nonnervous, photoreceptor retinular cells. Such a resistance drop is not produced by an electric current. Adolph (1964) noticed small, random, continuous fluctuations in potential of probably the dendrite membrane of the *Xiphosuran* eccentric cell. He hypothesized that these fluctuations, which can be recorded from dark-adapted cells, result from the continuous release of small quantities of a transmitter by the retinular cells. A continuous release of transmitter substance packets has been observed at nerve cell synapses (Katz, 1961). Adolph further suggested that light stimulation of the retinular cells acts to raise the quantity of released transmitter to a level sufficient to initiate nerve impulses. This is also analogous to the process at nerve synapses.

Fuortes and Yeandle (1964) found miniature conductance in the membranes of *Xiphosuran* retinular cells to occur at random under steady illumination. Random miniature conductance "bumps," most likely elicited by single quanta of light, have also been recorded from the retinula cells of the locust (Scholes, 1964). These "bumps" reached amplitudes of as much as 1 mV, and differed from nerve impulses by their great duration. The small visual cell conductance increases had latent periods of between 100 to 150 msec.

Dodge, Jr., Knight and Toyoda (1968), by recording from *Limulus polyphemus*, observed that the eccentric cell generator potentials develop by the summation of numerous separate brief increases in the membrane conductance of the visual (retinular) cells. These conductance fluctuations are apparently each engendered by the absorption of one photon, have a considerable duration in relation to the membrane time constant, and vary noticeably in average size during normal activity.

Greater light intensity increases the rate of the receptor conductance fluctuations or "bumps," reduces their duration and lowers their amplitude. The last falls more or less according to the inverse square root of the light intensity. This reduction in amplitude in response to increased light intensity appears to be the chief basis of light adaptation.

The rate of the "bumps" does not remain entirely proportional to light intensity as the latter is raised, suggesting a drop in quantum efficiency.

Fuortes and Hodgkin (1964) and Pinter (1966) stimulated individual *Xiphosuran* ommatidia with light flashes while recording the generator potentials of their eccentric cells. They found that a model assuming the operation of a linear filter with close to ten successive steps of exponential decay was in substantial agreement with their experimental results. Marimont (1965) advanced a model divided into many compartments as better suiting the results of Fuortes and Hodgkin.

Some of the results obtained on the "bumps" of the *Xiphosuran* (*Limulus*) ommatidium are summarized in a review by Wolbarsht and Yeandle (1967).

If the frog's tongue is covered with acetylcholine or cholinesterase, the glossopharyngeal nerve's taste responses are changed. Inhibitors of acetylcholine or cholinesterase have a similar effect. These findings have been used as evidence that acetylcholine plays a role in initiating taste nerve impulses (Landgren *et al.*, 1954; Rapuzzi and Pedrini, 1963; Sakai, 1964). However, Duncan's observations (1964) on frogs' tongues perfused with the specific cholinesterase inhibitor 62C47 and the specific pseudocholinesterase inhibitor iso-OMPA, as well as his results with low concentrations of the general cholinesterase inhibitors physostigmine and neostigmine, indicate instead that acetylcholine does not cross the gap between the secondary taste cells of vertebrates and the subjacent nerve fibers. Duncan suggests that another chemical transmitter may be released by vertebrate taste cells or that transmission may be electrical.

If acetylcholine is injected intravenously, it enhances gustatory excitation but does not affect spontaneous activity. Acetylcholine supplied intravenously is believed to exert its action by way of the central nervous system and the sympathetic nerves (notes in Halpern, 1967).

Evidence that nonnervous receptor cells release a chemical transmitter which affects the innervating neurons is seen in the high concentration of vesicles in the synaptic region of the outer hair cell of the cochlea (Spoendlin, 1966). In the hair cells of lateral line organs, there is a grouping of vesicles around a dense synaptic body in the zone of synaptic contact with an afferent nerve ending (Flock, 1967). Vesicles are also numerous in the bases of visual rods (Sjöstrand, 1958). The chemoreceptor cells of the carotid body contain a large number of vesicles (Ishii and Oosaki, 1966). Such clear-cut evidence of a transmitter is not found in taste cells, although flattened membranous sacs observed in other locations also often lie in the region of the taste receptor adjacent to nerve processes (Farbman, 1965).

Gray and Watkins (1965) could not find aggregations of vesicles on the inside of either the presynaptic membrane of rat taste cells or the postsynaptic afferent axon membrane. However, a scattering of vesicles, including larger forms, was seen in both the taste cell and the afferent axon. Gray and Watkins suggest that in the absence of synaptic vesicle aggregations, transmission, even if not quantal, may still be chemical. They noted dense projections in the presynaptic taste cell membrane. These projections may help a transmitter to bridge the synapse.

Several investigators have become convinced that the taste cell's membrane and its afferent nerve fiber are always separated by a synaptic space. This last observation makes the presence of a chemical transmitter quite likely.

In Merkel's disks, cytoplasmic granules (800-1400 Å) surrounded by membranes are concentrated at the portion of the plasma membrane adjacent to the synapse. However, vesicles as such have not been demonstrated. The granules appear to dissolve at the synapse (Andres, 1966a).

Between Merkel's disks and the adjacent flattened afferent nerve endings, there are synaptic membrane contacts measuring 250 to 300 mμ (Andres, 1966a).

In gymnotid and mormyrid electric fish the transmission of excitation from the electroreceptors to their afferent nerve fibers also appears generally to be chemically mediated. However, there are indications that the large phasic electroreceptors of mormyrids are electrotonically coupled to their afferent nerve endings (see Chap. VI) or that in this case there exists a junction with electric transmission (Bennett, 1967).

Observations on nerve endings show that depolarization, even if due to localized external electric pulses, causes an unusually high number of vesicles to release their contents to the outside of the cell plasma membrane within a short period of time. It is very likely that in most nonnervous receptor cells generator potentials are responsible for a similar sizeable release of a chemical transmitter into the synapse with an adjoining afferent nerve fiber.

Lowenstein (1967) suggests that, since the spontaneous discharge recorded from afferent vestibular fibers is surprisingly regular and protracted, the unstimulated hair sense cells may release a neurotransmitter at a significant and reasonably constant rate. This may make it possible for mechanical stimulation to cause a rise or a fall in the quantity of released transmitter substance. Thus a normal, spontaneous liberation of a transmitter may provide the choice of directionality of response available to hair cells and could therefore have an important functional role.

In the chemoreceptive neurons of the blowfly (*Phormia regina*), the initiated nerve impulses pass antidromically over the area of receptor potential generation in the dendrite. A similar process occurs in the pacinian corpuscle, where the nerve impulse develops immediately proximally to the site of origin of the receptor potential and passes back over the receptor membrane of the nerve ending.

Wolbarsht and Hanson (1965) studied the cause of the diphasic impulses recorded from the labellar chemoreceptor of the blowfly. This chemoreceptor consists of a hollow hair which extends from a sac that contains three to five sensory neurons. The dendrites of the chemosensory neurons (one neuron is a mechanoreceptor) run toward the hair, enter it through a constriction at its base, and then pass up the lumen of the hair to the opening at its tip, where the dendrites can be acted upon by chemical stimuli.

In the described chemoreceptor neurons the impulse develops proximally to the level of the chemosensory hair's lumen, either in the cell body or perhaps in the proximal portion of the dendrite. The impulse then not only travels toward and down the axon, but is also propagated distally (antidromically) up the dendrite and over the site of generation of the receptor potential, near the tip of the dendrite. The impulse is recorded as positive at first, while traveling only through the dendritic membrane, but after moving more distally and passing the constriction at the base of the chemosensory hair, it escapes into the lumen of the hair and gives rise to a negative phase. Therefore the recorded impulse is diphasic.

On the other hand, in the mechanoreceptor hairs of a group of insects, elicited impulses do not pass back over the area of development of the receptor potential, and only a positive impulse is recorded (Wolbarsht, 1960).

It is well known that cells which actively propagate excitation, such as the neuron and the striated muscle fiber, must release energy in connection with this activity. This energy is mostly used in restoring and maintaining the resting potential of the cell membrane. It follows that receptors, particularly because they conduct generator currents and give rise to the generator potential, must also release considerable internal energy as a consequence of their function.

That this is true was shown some time ago by von Békésy (1960) when he moved tiny steel balls placed on the basilar membrane of the cochlea of the inner ear by means of a magnet. The resulting deformations of the basilar membrane produced potentials the electrical energy of which greatly exceeded the mechanical energy supplied by the moving steel balls.

That receptors release considerable energy is also evidenced by the concentrations of mitochondria found in many receptors. Thus visual receptors have concentrations of mitochondria in those portions of their inner segments closest to their outer segments (Dowling, 1967b). Vertebrate olfactory receptors, which are neurons, contain numerous mitochondria in their distal, sensory dendrites (Heist, Mulvaney and Landis, 1967; Bannister, 1965). Large numbers of mitochondria are located in the synaptic regions of the cochlea's outer hair cells, indicating that in these auditory structures the mitochondria play a role in transmitter production (Spoendlin, 1966). Carotid chemoreceptor cells also have abundant mitochondria (Ishii and Oosaki, 1966). Taste cells do not possess many mitochondria (Farbman, 1965).

Yur'Eva (1967) disconnected the process of phosphorylation from respiration in frog taste cells by means of 2, 4-dinitrophenol or thyroxin. This eliminated taste responses and produced a decrease in spontaneous activity. Subsequent administration of a combination of ATP (adenosinetriphosphate) and EDTA (ethelenediaminetetra-acetic acid) restored taste responses.

The administration of small quantities of ATP to normal taste receptors produced a slight increase in their responses. However, if larger doses of ATP were supplied, the taste responses were reduced.

It therefore appears that the normal function of taste cells requires an expenditure of energy and that this energy is supplied by ATP.

In view of the above findings a study of the receptor response could include the energy cycles of the receptor.

Metabolic energy has been directly implicated in the development of the receptor potential in the photoreceptors of *Limulus polyphemus*. There is evidence that this visual receptor potential is not produced by an increase in cell membrane permeability. Instead, the receptor potential seems to result from the change produced by light in a current generator located in the membrane (Smith, Stell and Brown, 1968). This current generator in turn appears to be an electrogenic sodium pump which participates in the formation of the resting membrane potential and which is affected by some consequence of light stimulation (Smith, Stell, Brown, Freeman and Murray, 1968).

The action of electrogenic sodium pumps has previously been reported to be responsible for hyperpolarization of the membranes of nerve cells and nerve fibers. Electrogenic sodium pumps have also been found to be operative in muscle fibers, and such a pump even contributes to the membrane potential of *Neurospora*. The authors named above are the first to provide evidence that an electrogenic sodium pump is the basis for the receptor potential in a nonnervous receptor. However, it is quite likely that electrogenic sodium pumps are involved in the formation of other receptor potentials.

Fuller discussions of the role and operation of electrogenic sodium pumps will be found in the visual reception section of the chapter on initial events and in the chapter on nervous transmission.

Receptors can be grouped according to whether their generator potentials and the consequent impulse frequencies quickly reach a high peak and show an equally rapid decline, or whether they have a slowly rising but also long-drawn-out response to stimuli. Receptors of the first type are termed *phasic*, whereas those of the second type are known as *tonic*. Phasic-tonic receptors show an initial peak of response, which quickly declines (perhaps in some 10 to a few hundred milliseconds) to a lower but long-lasting level of response.

The antennal receptor specific for the sexual attractant in the moth *Antheraea* is phasic, its response being high but short lived, while the muscle spindle is an example of a tonic receptor. Mechanoreceptors on the claspers of male blowflies and on the anal plates of female blowflies are slowly adapting tonic receptors, as are Pinkus plates and vibrissae. The hake (*Urophycis chuss*) has both tonic proprioceptors and phasic proprioceptors on its pelvic fins (Bardach and Case, 1965).

The extremely specific carbon dioxide receptor of the honeybee is phasic-tonic. On stimulation it jumps to a high peak of response which may produce up to 700 impulses/sec, but then quickly declines to a low response level which, however, may last as long as one hour (Boeckh, Kaissling and Schneider, 1965). Evans and Mellon (1962a, b) found labellar water and salt receptors of the blowfly to be phasic-tonic.

Vertebrate olfactory receptors also appear to be phasic-tonic (Shibuya and Shibuya, 1963).

Wolbarsht (1960) differentiates two types of insect mechanoreceptors: those which respond only to a varying stimulus (phasic), and those which also continue to produce impulses during constant stimulation, sometimes for as much as twenty minutes, and are thus tonic. Wolbarsht names the first type velocity-sensitive, and the second kind pressure-sensitive. A reduction of the stimulus causes a drop in the receptor potential of a pressure-sensitive receptor, but produces a new receptor potential in a velocity-sensitive receptor. The velocity-sensitive receptors on the wing of flies may fire as many as 600 impulses/sec. Phasic receptors which respond both to the application and the reduction of a stimulus have also been found in the skin of toads and cats. These "on-off" receptors include the pacinian corpuscle.

Single-cell olfactory discharges in the toad *Bufo vulgaris Jap.* may be of an "on," "on-off," or "off" character (Takagi and Omura, 1963).

The latent periods of insect olfactory receptors, on sufficiently high stimulation, extend from 5 to 10 msec, and in a few cases to as much as 30 to 80 msec. Pacinian corpuscles show latencies of 0.5 to 3.0 msec.

The first stage of the receptor response will be dealt with in greater detail, in terms of those receptors which have yielded the most information, in the fifth chapter.

ADAPTATION

After receptors reach their maximum level of response to a stimulus, their response begins to decrease in magnitude. This reduction in discharge, known as adaptation, may continue to the level preceding the response.

There is no generally accepted, more specific definition of adaptation, and the term is often used interchangeably with accommodation, sensory fatigue and habituation. Hahn (1968a) employs a more restricted definition, using adaptation to mean changes in the characteristics of a sense system resulting from an altered stimulus. He excludes the rapid decrement of the pacinian corpuscle's generator potential, because this is due to the unchanged viscoelastic properties of the capsule of the corpuscle.

When the speed with which an object sinks into the skin falls below the threshold for stimulation, the termination of excitation cannot be ascribed to adaptation. Rather, excitation ceases because the stimulus has become inadequate. This illustrates a benefit of Hahn's definition.

Receptors differ in their rate of adaptation to a stimulus, or, as the term is defined here, in the rate of their approach to the resting condition. This partially forms the basis of their division into tonic and phasic types.

The observed adaptation of secondary-cell receptors to stimuli has two aspects. One arises from the nonnervous structure and physiology of the receptor and from the nature of surrounding elements, while the other is based on the electrochemical properties and structure of the nerve endings innervating the receptor.

The Role of Nonnervous Structures and the Environment

The adaptation of all nonneuronal receptors is to a greater or lesser extent determined by the nature of the receptor itself, irrespective of its innervation. Often the relations of the receptor to its environment also play a significant role.

Mechanoreceptors

Among mechanoreceptors the function of the pacinian corpuscle has been studied most thoroughly. In the pacinian corpuscle a nonmyelinated nerve ending is surrounded by a capsule consisting of lamellae, their connections and an interlamellar fluid. This combination of elastic elements (the lamellae and connections) and a viscous element (the interlamellar fluid) only poorly transmits low stimulus frequencies and the elastic forces arising from steady pressure. The capsule thus acts as a filter for the static features of a mechanical stimulus; only a large proportion of the viscous force produced during dynamic compression reaches the central nerve ending, and pressure there is highly dependent on the velocity of compression (Loewenstein and Skalak, 1966).

The relatively rapid adaptation of the pacinian corpuscle, or its phasic response, are therefore partially attributable to the capsule (see Reception by the Pacinian Corpuscle, Chap. V). When the corpuscle is mechanically stimulated, the capsule causes the generator potential to be short, as has been shown by stripping the lamellated capsule from the inner nerve ending (Loewenstein and Mendelson, 1965). The generator potential of a complete pacinian corpuscle falls to zero in approximately 6 msec, while the generator potential of an exposed nerve ending may persist for 70 msec after the initiation of a continued stimulus.

The time course of adaptation in the mammalian muscle spindle is also largely determined by the mechanical properties of the receptor (Lippold *et al.*, 1960). A viscoelastic theory of mechanoreceptor adaptation has been tested with models and experiments on rat and frog cutaneous receptors (Catton and Petoe, 1966).

Wendler (1963) sees a parallel between the adaptation processes of the phasic pacinian corpuscle and those of the tonic crustacean stretch receptor. Thus, while the pacinian corpuscle has an elastic filter in the lamellae and interconnections of its capsule, in the crustacean stretch receptor a similar role is played by the elastic, reversible stretch components of the muscle. Wendler considers a primary difference between the two adaptation processes to be one of time span; what occurs in only a few milliseconds in the pacinian corpuscle requires several minutes in the crustacean stretch receptor.

In the case of cutaneous tactile receptors, the application to the skin of vibrotactile stimuli appears to mitigate the adapting effect of the intervening tissues which is so marked when static pressure is employed. Research by Hahn (1968b) on the adaptation of pacinian corpuscles and other cutaneous mechanoreceptors suggests that the mechanical properties of the skin tissues overlying the receptors have little role in the adaptation to sinusoidal, vibrotactile stimuli.

A good discussion of mechanoreceptor adaptation can be found in *The Physiology Of Sense Organs*, by Mellon, Jr. (1968).

Gustatory Receptors

Taste receptors may show a high degree of adaptation. Borg *et al.* (1967), by electrophysiologically recording from the chorda tympani nerve, determined that in man the adaptation to 0.2M sodium chloride is complete; the impulse discharge in the chorda tympani falls to zero.

This is not true of the rat, in which the low concentration of sodium chloride present in the saliva continuously elicits impulse activity. This discharge can be eliminated by rinsing the rat's tongue with distilled water.

Previous to the operative procedure and recording, Borg *et al.* performed psychophysical tests on their patients. They obtained periods of 79, 90 and 122 seconds for complete subjective adaptation to 0.2M sodium chloride. Two human subjects have also reported complete adaptation to 0.15M sodium chloride in 50 and 54 seconds (Bujas, 1953).

Borg *et al.* (1967) consider their neural adaptation times to agree reasonably well with the psychophysical results. They conclude that the complete adaptations reported by human subjects may reflect the decrease to zero of taste nerve activity.

Hahn (1949) found taste adaptation to be a linear function of the stimulus concentration. Adaptation, as observed in the form of a rise in taste threshold, also varies almost linearly with the period of stimulation. The taste threshold increases continuously with the period of stimulus application even at threshold levels (von Békésy, 1965).

In a study of taste adaptation, Yur'eva (1968) recorded from the glossolingual nerve of the frog while applying taste solutions to its tongue. Stimulation was terminated by washing the tongue with Ringer's solution, to which the frog's taste receptors are nonreactive.

The frog's peripheral response to taste stimuli was found to last as long as 10 to 20 minutes. Thus, when 3 per cent sodium chloride was dripped onto the tongue, the nerve discharge fell from an initial 100 impulses/sec to 60 impulses/sec after 3 minutes. Impulse activity reached the normal, spontaneous level only after 12 minutes.

If the interval between successive taste stimulations is 3 to 5 minutes, there is a consecutive reduction in the magnitude of the initial discharge, and in the length of the response, as a series of stimulations are carried out. Even with intervals of 10 to 15 minutes the duration of the response steadily decreases —when 3 per cent sodium chloride was employed, it fell from an initial 14 minutes to 4 minutes upon the fourth stimulation.

Cutting off the blood supply to the tongue results both in a precipitous drop in the initial magnitude of the response and in a large reduction of its duration. On clamping of the tongue arteries the time span of the response to 5 per cent sodium chloride fell to about a quarter of the normal.

Perfusion of the tongue with Ringer's solution not only resulted in the maintenance of a high initial response after repeated stimulations but also, in a remarkably uniform manner, even doubled or tripled the duration of the response. There was then only a quite slow decrease in impulse frequency. Conversely, the termination of perfusion produced rapid and complete adaptation.

The results of the blood supply and perfusion experiments suggest to Yur'eva that during a taste response metabolites accumulate in the synaptic gap between a gustatory receptor and the innervating sensory nerve ending, this interfering with the transmission of excitation across the synapse.

One candidate for such a metabolite is ATP, which is essential for the gustatory receptor response. When the taste receptor cells are stimulated for a prolonged period, the energy-releasing ATP should be used in larger quantities, and it (or its breakdown products) could gather in the synapse. Yur'eva (1968) observed that perfusion of the frog's tongue with an ATP solution (1×10^{-6} to 1×10^{-4} gm/1), instead of Ringer's solution, shortens the duration of the taste response to 5 per cent sodium chloride.

Yur'eva points out that ATP or a similar substance interferes with the action of the transmitter acetylcholine in the frog heart and the edentate heart, probably by competing for receptor sites.

Numerous observations prove that taste solutions having concentrations below the threshold level can produce adaptation. This is evidence that gustatory adaptation is at least in part the result of changes in the taste receptor cells, exclusive of their nervous innervation. Since subliminal stimuli do not bring about an increase in the frequency of taste nerve fiber impulses, the nervous system cannot be involved in subthreshold adaptation.

McBurney and Pfaffmann (1963) reported that adaptation of the human tongue to a subthreshold solution of 0.000069M sodium chloride raised the taste threshold for sodium chloride above its lowest, water-adapted level (0.00014M sodium chloride). Hahn (1949) used adaptation to a solution of 0.9 threshold concentration to elevate the threshold for this kind of solution. Von Békésy (1965) deter-

mined that if the human tongue is exposed to a barely subthreshold concentration of an acid solution for two minutes, the threshold is elevated.

An important influence in the immediate environment to which the gustatory receptors of higher vertebrates are continuously adapted is the saliva (Pfaffmann, 1965a). Thus taste thresholds are determined by the composition of the saliva, and the magnitude of taste responses are affected by it. When a continuous rinse of water is run over the tongue, the sodium chloride threshold drops to less than 1/100 of its saliva-adapted value. The sodium chloride dissolved in the saliva appears to adapt the gustatory receptors much in the same way as an applied solution (McBurney and Pfaffmann, 1963).

McBurney and Pfaffmann (1963) found the threshold for sodium chloride to be a function of adapting sodium chloride over a large range of adapting concentrations.

After the tongue has been adapted to a sufficient concentration of sodium chloride or acid, the application of a subadapting concentration of the same substance, or of water, evokes an antitaste. Thus a concentration of sodium chloride below the adapting concentration produces a sensation of sour, bitter, or a combination of both in different human subjects. A sweet taste has been attributed to water after adaptation to acid has taken place.

The strength of anti-tastes increases as the adapting concentration is made greater. Since human saliva has a sodium chloride concentration close to the lower limit of the adapting concentrations which may be used to later call forth antitastes, water typically seems flat or almost tasteless (Bartoshuk, McBurney and Pfaffmann, 1964). The other substances in the saliva as well may produce adaptations which contribute to the failure of water to evoke a clear taste in man.

The magnitude of antitastes also rises with dilution below the adapting concentration, so that after the application of a sufficiently concentrated solution water provokes the strongest antitaste (Bartoshuk, McBurney and Pfaffmann, 1964). Antitastes may become so intense that they equal or exceed the normal sensation called forth by the same stimulus following a water rinse (Bartoshuk, McBurney and Pfaffmann, 1964; Pfaffmann, 1965b).

Electrophysiological recordings from the cat have produced similar results (Pfaffmann, 1965b). In rats stimulated with sodium chloride, the subsequent application of a subadapting concentration evokes a sizeable transient drop in taste impulse frequency, after which there is a rise to a new steady level. This last maintained impulse rate is lower than that called forth by the original, adapting stimulus.

According to Bartoshuk, McBurney and Pfaffmann (1964), and Pfaffmann (1965b), the contrasting antitastes provoked by more dilute concentrations following adaptation may be analogous to the negative consecutive images met in vision. Research is needed on the manner in which adaptation is responsible for the appearance of antitastes.

Neurophysiological studies on the rat (Beidler, 1961) indicate that there is no peripheral cross-adaptation to monovalent salts.

Electrophysiological recordings have shown that in a single organism the course of adaptation to different taste substances varies. Oakley and Benjamin (1966) state that even the adaptations to unlike chemicals recorded from a single taste fiber may take dissimilar forms. They suggest that such differential adaptation in one taste unit may develop from initial receptor events rather than from later processes common to all the evoked taste responses. Thus taste adaptation may have to be considered in the formulation of taste theories.

Von Békésy (1965) reports that in man there are also large individual differences in taste thresholds. He further considers it likely that differences in adaptation rates may be revealed to an even greater extent in taste judgments.

In the blowfly (*Phormia regina*) the labellar taste hairs adapt within 5 to 20 seconds, but rarely stop firing. When the taste receptors of the oral papillae are adapted, they continue to discharge impulses at a steady rate for a number of minutes (Dethier and Hanson, 1965).

The tarsal taste receptors usually adapt more quickly than the labellar receptors and normally finally cease firing. However, certain tarsal receptors have been known to maintain a low rate of discharge for up to 15 minutes (Dethier and Gelperin, 1967).

Auditory Receptors

The inner and outer hair cells of the organ of Corti, the auditory receptors, are not unequivocally secondary sense cells. They are regarded as specialized neurons by a number of investigators.

The adaptation observed in audition may involve adaptation of the hair cells themselves to stimulation by shearing forces acting on their stereocilia. Auditory adaptation may also arise from processes occurring at the synapses between the hair cells and the innervating nerve fibers.

A very low degree of adaptation is met in audition. Thus when the ear is stimulated with a 200 cps tone at threshold intensities for 15 minutes, no change in the threshold is observed (von Békésy, 1947). Adaptation appears only at higher sound pressure levels, perhaps 100 to 10,000 times the threshold intensity.

Tsuiki (1965) and Wittich (1966), in psychophysical experiments involving the simultaneous loudness-balance method, found that the degree of loudness adaptation varies with sound intensity. According to Tsuiki, who exposed one ear to an intermittent tone and the other to a continuous tone, the increase in loudness adaptation with rising sound intensity is described by a negatively accelerated curve which approaches an asymptote at an intensity of 60 dB.

Hood (1950) suggests that the increase in loudness adaptation with intensity is due to the rise in the number of hair cells which are involved.

Kiang (1965) electrophysiologically recorded from fibers of cat auditory nerves while stimulating with tone bursts having a duration of 50 msec and a frequency of 10/sec. He observed that at moderate stimulus levels (50-70 dB) impulse activity reached a plateau 30 msec after the start of stimulation.

If the stimulus instead consisted of single, long tone bursts, the impulse frequency sometimes even changed many minutes after stimulus initiation. In the two units tested with extremely long tone bursts of their own characteristic frequency and of, respectively, 50 and 70 dB intensity, the response reached a steady rate after 13 minutes. This final, maintained discharge frequency of, respectively, about 70-100 impulses/sec and 80-120 impulses/sec still markedly exceeded the frequency of spontaneous activity.

Kiang (1965) did not observe any responses to fall to or below the rates of spontaneous activity as a result of adaptation.

Psychophysical experiments indicate that during a maintained, unvarying tone the response ceases to decline after a few minutes, when it seems to reach an asymptote (Tsuiki, 1965; Egan, 1955). Hood (1950) found loudness adaptation to all his tested intensities to be essentially complete after 3.5 minutes.

Adaptation produces the most extensive reduction in loudness shortly after the initiation of stimulation (Tsuiki, 1965; Wittich, 1966). According to Egan (1955), the perceived loudness of a constant noise of 90 dB, of any frequency between 100 to 5,000 cps, drops markedly during the first minute. However, adaptation was seen to continue during the remaining test period of six minutes.

The time course of intensity adaptation determined by psychophysical experiments is not basically at variance with the development of adaptation as observed by electrophysiological means in single units.

Matsnev and Yakovleva (1967), using 132 human subjects, found the increase in auditory threshold produced by adaptation to vary between 5 and 10 dB.

Olfactory and Visual Receptors

Since olfactory and visual receptors are primary sense cells, or essentially highly evolved sensory neurons, they are covered in a final section.

The Role of the Nerve Endings

Many nerve endings associated with receptors accommodate only very slowly to the receptor response (generator potential), as compared to the accommodation of nerve fibers to direct stimulation. This suggests specialization of these sensory nerve endings, which are of the typical, branching type.

The mammalian muscle spindle has been known to fire 300 action potentials per second for extended periods.

Granit (1955) has offered three possible explanations as to how sensory nerve endings may be capable of long-continued discharges. One is that sensory nerves may normally be on the point of firing and have autorhythmicity, a tendency to resonance. Another suggestion is based on the fine, unmyelinated terminal arborizations of the concerned sensory fibers, which appear to be present in most sense organs. Even if some of the end branches have adapted to the generator potential, others could give rise to, perhaps, only local potentials, which, on meeting at the point of union of the branches, would sum to produce a propagated impulse in the undivided nerve fiber. Katz (1950a, b) has provided evidence for this concept. He found spontaneous local potentials in terminal sensory nerve branchings which summed to produce a nerve impulse. Thirdly, Granit writes of the possible spreading of the generator potential to neutralize accommodation.

Some sensory nerve endings have been discovered to be capable of rapid adaptation.

Mechanoreceptors

Wendler (1963) has found evidence for an adaptation process or for a dynamic reduction in excitation in the generator potential of the sensory neurons in the crustacean stretch receptor. This generator potential decrements even when an unchanging tension is maintained in the stretch receptor by continuously increasing its length. When the length and tension of the receptor are allowed to fall, the generator potential rises again.

Florey (1957a, b) observed similar adaptation of the generator potential when he stimulated the crustacean stretch receptor with acetylcholine or an inhibitory agent (factor I). The generator potential was directly evoked by these chemical substances. This precluded a contribution to the observed decrease of the generator potential by changes in the receptor muscle.

Thus in the crustacean stretch receptor the transduction of mechanical into electrical energy appears to involve processes which decrement with time. These processes presumably take place in the dendrites (Wendler, 1963).

On the basis of their work on pacinian corpuscles, Nishi and Sato (1968) have suggested that one process contributing to the decline of receptor potentials is a delayed rise in the permeability of the sensory neuron membrane to potassium ion. In one of their experiments these investigators noted that during a maintained stimulus a decrease in the receptor potential was followed by hyperpolarization.

Loewenstein and Mendelson (1965) and Ozeki and Sato (1965) have noted that the nerve ending in the pacinian corpuscle fires only a few impulses at most, even when it develops a lasting generator (receptor) potential. The characteristics of the nerve ending could thus prevent a tonic response by the pacinian corpuscle, even if the capsule did not suffice to restrict the duration of the generator potential to about 6 msec. A generator potential of such short duration normally gives rise to just one nerve impulse.

Krnjević and van Gelder (1961) indicate that the unlike adaptation rates of the two sensory neurons in the crustacean stretch receptor are chiefly due to different electrical membrane properties (see Crustacean Stretch Receptor, Chap. II).

Adaptation in Primary Sense Cells

Olfactory Receptors

The olfactory receptors of vertebrates, like those of insects, are specialized sensory neurons. Therefore, adaptation can only have a nervous aspect in these receptors.

There have been some investigations of adaptation in olfactory receptors.

Boeckh, Kaissling and Schneider (1965) stimulated the specific sexual attractant receptor of the honeybee (*Apis mellifica*) with the sexual attractant, 9-keto-2-decenoic acid. They observed that directly following a 100μg stimulus, a 1μg stimulus evokes no response, indicating adaptation. Recovery takes a few seconds, as shown by receptor responses at that time.

Similar adaptation was observed when the less effective caproic acid was the stimulus.

Stimulation with the sexual attractant followed by use of caproic acid, or vice versa, again produced normal adaptation. However, such an absence of selective adaptation may reflect the accommodation occurring somewhere along the sensory neurons (the dendrites or the area of impulse generation), rather than provide information about the receptor molecules.

In man certain odorants, such as camphor and cloves, produce cross-adaptation. Presumably these odorants excite the same sensory neurons.

When olfactory receptors are subjected to prolonged excitation, the response consists of an initial peak which drops to a plateau phase. The decline of the receptor potential from its original peak to the plateau level represents the degree of adaptation undergone by the receptor cells. When the applied stimulus is of low intensity, the plateau phase may have only 50 per cent of the amplitude of the initial peak.

The plateau phase of the receptor potential may virtually remain at a constant level throughout a prolonged period of moderate stimulation (Ottoson and Shepherd, 1967).

The olfactory system has been described as slowly adapting.

Visual Receptors

Visual systems can operate and adapt over a very extensive range of light intensities. At all these intensity levels the primary process of light adaptation occurs quite rapidly; it does not require more time than impulse transmission across a synapse. Most of the process takes place within 0.1 second.

Vertebrate light adaptation, or the increase in threshold or loss of sensitivity, as a whole has little relationship to the amount of visual pigment bleached. Instead, it is almost completely dependent on the intensity of the stimulating light. There is no significant bleaching of visual pigment until the intensity of the light stimulus is 5 or 6 log units above the threshold for the appearance of the electroretinogram. Furthermore, at a normal light intensity the bleaching of half of the pigment produces a rise in threshold of only 0.3 log units, compared to the total 4 to 5 log unit elevation of adaptation.

In vertebrate dark adaptation, or the recovery of sensitivity, both a slow and a rapid process may be observed. The slow process reflects the regeneration of bleached visual pigment, and predominates when most of the pigment has been bleached. It has been named photochemical adaptation. The rapid process, which is the only one to be observed after sufficiently low light intensities, is largely over in several seconds. The rapid process is known as neural adaptation, and is apparently the reverse of the process of light adaptation.

Bleached visual pigment provokes impulse activity, and this activity has been equated with the existence of an afterimage. Barlow and Sparrock (1964) have shown that the increase in sensitivity during photochemical dark adaptation is paralleled by the fading of the afterimage.

In the photochemical process the log threshold recovers, together with rhodopsin, with an exponential time constant of 6 minutes.

During photochemical dark adaptation of the rods of the frog retina, the threshold of the ERG falls with the decrease in the amount of metarhodopsin (Donner and Reuter, 1967). This pigment drops gradually after bleaching.

Dowling (1967a), in an extensive and excellent discussion of vertebrate visual adaptation, presents experimental evidence from several investigators that light adaptation is not cen-tered in the visual receptors. Also, the drop in sensitivity upon light stimulation does not involve the retinal ganglion cells or centrifugal fibers from higher levels of the visual pathway (see Vertebrate Retina, Chap. IV).

Barlow and Andrews (1967) provide experimental evidence which leads them to believe as well that visual adaptation precedes summation, which first occurs in the retinal ganglion cells.

The b-wave of the vertebrate electroretinogram is the first visual phenomenon to undergo clear-cut adaptation. A rise in background light intensity is followed by an increase in the log threshold of the b-wave. The increase in this log threshold is a linear function of the rise in light intensity, and the function approaches a slope of 1.

Since the b-wave is thought to develop in the bipolar cell layer of the retina, Dowling (1967a) believes that adaptation primarily takes place at the level of the bipolar cells. These cells have reciprocal synapses with amacrine cells, and Dowling suggests that an inhibitory feedback to the bipolar cells could produce adaptation.

Dowling (1967a) even ventures the view that inhibitory feedback mechanisms may be responsible for adaptation in other sensory systems. He points to the presence of reciprocal synaptic connections in the arthropod eye and the olfactory bulb.

Not all retinal ganglion cells show similar light adaptation. At stronger light intensities the majority of "on" center ganglion cells undergo complete adaptation, while "off" center cells usually are even depressed, and often stop firing. The great reduction in the activity of "off" center ganglion cells on maintained light stimulation may be chiefly responsible for the reduced optic nerve discharge during illumination (Arduini and Pinneo, 1962).

It has been found in the goldfish retina that a ganglion cell's response threshold to illumination of a portion of its receptive field can be elevated by throwing light on another section of the receptive field (Easter, 1968). A like observation has been made on the cat retina

(Sakmann, Creutzfeldt and Scheich, 1969). By means of a psychophysical experiment Westheimer (1967) has shown that the level of adaptation of a group of human visual receptors is affected by the illumination of other areas of the retina. The above findings indicate that an adaptation pool, as described by Rushton (1965), determines the sensitivity of portions of a receptive field.

Easter (1968) also learned, through recording from goldfish retinal ganglion cells, that, by extending a concentric area of adapting illumination considerably beyond a test spot, the threshold of the last could be raised further. The sizeable area (hundreds of microns across) of the receptive field which could contribute to the adaptation of a small spot within this area suggests that horizontal or amacrine cells may play a role in such adaptation. The involved adaptation pool is not as extensive as the receptive field of a ganglion cell.

Brown and Watanabe (1965) reported that the type of interaction between light-adapted visual receptors differs from that which occurs between dark-adapted receptors.

There have also been many investigations of arthropod visual receptor adaptation.

In invertebrates visual adaptation bestows the benefit of enabling the photoreceptors to respond to additional, intense light stimuli superimposed on a maintained illumination. Adaptation, by reducing the membrane potential to a lower level, increases the dynamic range of a receptor and does not allow it to become saturated.

Naka and Kishida (1966) suggest that the reduced sensitivity produced in the eye of the honeybee (*Apis mellifica*) drone by a maintained light stimulus arises from the characteristics of the retinula (visual receptor) cell membrane. The sensitivity of the drone photoreceptor returns to the preadaptation level or frequently even exceeds it several seconds after the end of an intense adapting light stimulus. This observation is in accord with the concept that adaptation develops in the receptor's cell membrane rather than through the visual pigments.

Naka and Kishida (1966), like Dowling (1967a), consider visual adaptation to result from some sort of feedback acting on the receptor cell membrane. Fuortes and Hodgkin (1964) have hypothesized that a feedback mechanism produces adaptation in *Limulus* and have developed a model for this feedback, which is analyzed by Marimont (1965). Fuortes and Hodgkin (1964) postulate that their feedback mechanism increases time resolution and lowers gain when light stimuli depolarize the cell.

A sensory feedback could explain the adaptation which follows each input increment in the eyes of *Limulus* and the wolf spider, even after a period of light adaptation (Pinter, 1966). Also, when stimuli of great intensity and duration are applied to originally dark-adapted *Limulus* eyes, the receptor potentials initially overshoot. This overshoot is attributed by Marimont (1965) to an excessive delay in the lowering of the gain (sensitivity) by the operation of a feedback mechanism.

A fleeting decrease in the extent of the response of the drone photoreceptor, which immediately follows the cessation of a light stimulus, could be due to a delayed feedback effect.

However, De Voe (1966) reports that the Fuortes-Hodgkin feedback model does not account for the phase leads of responses over stimuli (sinusoidal modulations of the adapting light) which are met at low frequencies in the wolf spider eye. Pinter (1966) had difficulty in applying the feedback model to the potentials evoked in both the light- and dark-adapted states of a *Limulus* ommatidium.

Extracellular recordings from the eyes of locusts (*Locusta*) jibe with those obtained from single retinula cells of other insects in showing insect light adaptation, like olfactory adaptation, to consist of an original large on-transient potential change which gradually falls to a plateau. As the intensity of the light stimulus is elevated, the plateau phase ceases to rise beyond a certain (saturation) level (Burtt, Catton and Cosens, 1966).

Ruck (1964) has suggested that the plateau

portion of the light response represents the generator potential of the retinula (arthropod visual receptor) cells. The slow part of the light response has been found to be far more resistant than the transient to anoxia, an indication that it is not of nervous but of receptor cell origin. Also, unlike the transient, the slow component survives destruction of the optic lobe.

Light stimulation of the locust eye also results in an original rapid rise in threshold, with a subsequent fast but not complete recovery. The last leads to a plateau, which is the level of the light-adapted threshold. On return to darkness the threshold falls rapidly at first, and then more gradually, to sink to the dark-adapted level (Fig. 3-2).

The potential changes of dark adaptation differ from the synchronous threshold changes in that the potential overshoots the normal level of dark adaptation and then drops back to this level (Fig. 3-2).

An equation describing dark adaptation in *Limulus* was developed by Hartline (1929). Variations of this equation have been found applicable to changes in the electroretinogram, the neural discharge and the ommatidial potential of the horseshoe crab eye. Hartline's equation can be stated as

$$R = m \left[\log S - F(t) \right]$$

in which R is the amplitude of response, S represents the intensity of a stimulus of unvarying duration, F(t) is a function of time which decreases monotonically with time and reaches a value of zero on total dark adaptation, and m denotes a function which increases monotonically with [log S − F(t)].

The curve describing the light adaptation of the ommatidial potential is determined, over a considerable range, by the product of the adapting light intensity and the light duration. This is also true of the curve for adaptation based on the nerve impulses emanating from the ommatidia.

Light adaptation may produce linear incremental responses in the wolf spider eye.

De Voe (1966) has developed a mathematical model for the nonlinear responses of the

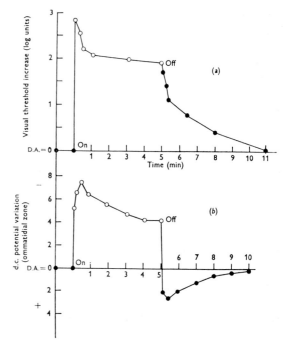

FIGURE 3-2. Effect of light adaptation (empty circles) and subsequent dark adaptation (filled circles) on (a) visual threshold and (b) ommatidial potential in the locust eye. (From Burtt, E.T., W.T. Catton, and D.J. Cosens: Electrical Potential Field in Eye and Optic Lobe of Locust: Potential Variations and Changes in Visual Threshold During Light- and Dark-adaptation. In Bernhard, C.G. [Ed.]: *The Functional Organization of the Compound Eye*. Long Island City, Pergamon, 1966, pp. 219-230.)

light-adapted wolf spider eye.

Since the process by which the bleaching of visual pigments leads to depolarization of the visual receptor membrane is not yet fully known, visual adaptation at the receptor level also cannot yet be completely understood.

The development of a curve for dark adaptation in the retinular (visual receptor) cells of *Limulus* is made more difficult by small, nonpropagated potentials. These are seen after an interval following the eye's exposure to a strong adapting light. Also, subsequent to intense light adaptation of the arthropod eye, a marked, lasting hyperpolarization takes place.

Wolbarsht and Yeandle (1967) devote a

section of their review paper to visual adaptation in the horseshoe crab, while Creutzfeldt and Sakmann (1969) in a review discuss vertebrate visual adaptation. Granit (1963) deals with light adaptation and dark adaptation in a chapter of his book *Sensory Mechanisms of the Retina.*

Central Adaptation

It should be remembered that adaptation also occurs at the various relay stations of a sensory pathway. The adapting processes at the synapses of a sensory system, which may collectively be designated as central adaptation, cause perceptual adaptation to have a substantially longer time course than receptor adaptation.

Thus the cortical potentials evoked by auditory and tactile stimuli undergo slow declines long after the frequency of the impulses in the auditory and somatosensory nerves has reached a steady state. A similar phenomenon can be observed in respect to temperature perception. The thresholds for taste perception are largely determined centrally; they have been found to fall when the stimulated area of the tongue is increased. The long-maintained plateau level of the olfactory receptor potential also points to an important role for central adaptation in olfaction.

It has been possible to study the adaptation of individual neurons in the thalamus during electrical stimulation of afferent tactile nerve fibers in the skin (Rose and Mountcastle, 1959). While at the periphery of the gustatory system there is no cross-adaptation between sodium chloride and other monovalent salts (Beidler, 1961), such cross-adaptation does take place in the nucleus fasciculus solitarius of the medulla oblongata, at a higher level of the gustatory pathway (Halpern, 1967).

Discussion

It should be clear from the preceding material that adaptation may take different forms and may occur at several levels of each sensory pathway. The accommodation which takes place in nerve fibers is part of the subject matter of Chapter VI.

While in some sensory systems peripheral adaptation is of outstanding significance and largely determines the central sensory input, in other systems central adaptation may have an equally important role.

It appears evident that many peripheral receptor structures and sensory nerve endings have evolved to produce such adaptation as will result in activity that is appropriate to the needs and well-being of the organism.

Burkhardt (1960, 1961), in two general papers dealing with the properties, physiology and functional groupings of receptors and sense organs, treats the various processes which contribute to the limitation or decrement of afferent sensory activity. According to Burkhardt's general scheme, stimuli, which may be modified by specialized external organs, are first subjected to attenuation in the transforming elements of the receptor. This attenuation may be produced by two different processes—a dynamic stimulus reduction and a lowering of receptor sensitivity. Centrifugal activity from peripheral neurons or higher levels of the sensory pathway may contribute to the effects which modify the stimulus in the external structures of the receptor.

Excitation is aroused in the sensory nerve endings of the receptor, or in afferent fiber endings, by the effective stimulus that reaches these nervous structures. The sensory nervous terminations may be subject to adapting influences which are similar to those acting on outer receptor tissues.

Finally, sensory impulses, after being transmitted from the peripheral nervous terminations to the various centers of each sensory system, are affected by central adaptation.

The role of efferent influences will be examined in Chapter IV.

STRUCTURES OF UNDETERMINED FUNCTION

It is recognized that many aspects of receptor function, including the various mechanisms whereby the energy of the stimulus is transduced to electrical energy, are not adequately understood. This lack of knowledge is evidenced by the existence of structures of unknown function which are largely peculiar to sense cells. Among these are microtubular organelles (see The Structure of the Labyrinth, Chap. II), lamellated bodies, and synaptic rods. The last two will be treated at length below.

Lamellated Bodies

Auditory Hair Cells

The outer hair cells of the organ of Corti each possess a system of rounded lamellar bodies, also known as Hensen bodies (Fig. 3-4A). These lamellar bodies are located in, or less commonly below, the infracuticular zone of the outer hair cells (Engström, 1967a). They are usually found in the central cytoplasm of their cell zone (Fig. 3-3).

The lamellar bodies, which Engström (1967b) believes to originate from the Golgi body, envelop a central core of slightly granular cytoplasm and sometimes include several thin membranes which border lamellae.

The shape and size of the lamellar bodies differ in various species. While they form relatively flat groupings of disconnected membranes in the squirrel monkey, they are frequently rounded in the guinea pig. The system of lamellar bodies is most pronounced in the guinea pig. In the cat and the rat the membranes are less noticeable and lack the concentric arrangement. The system of lamellar bodies is concentric in man (Kimura *et al.*, 1964).

An apparently premature attempt has been made to assign to the system of lamellar bodies a role in the formation of cochlear microphonics. It was suggested that mechanical distortion of the lamellae might lead to cellular potentials (Spoendlin, 1959).

Disconnected membrane lamellae are also located beyond the inner surface of the cell plasma membrane of each outer hair cell (Fig. 3-3). They vary considerably among individual cells. There are few, or only a single layer of these lamellae in the human,

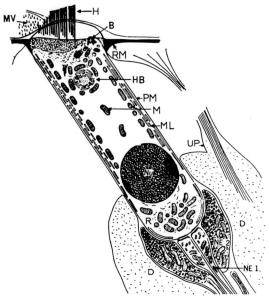

FIGURE 3-3. Diagram of an outer hair cell of the cochlea. (*H*) Stereocilia, (*B*) basal body or kinocilium, (*HB*) lamellar body, (*PM*) cell plasma membrane, (*ML*) disconnected submembrane lamellae, (*M*) mitochondrium, (*Nu*) nucleus, (*R*) body of Retzius, containing numerous mitochondria, (*NE1*) afferent nerve ending, (*NE2*) efferent nerve ending, (*D*) Deiters' cell, from which a phalangeal process (*UP*) extends to the surface of the organ of Corti. There this process bears microvilli (*MV*), (*RM*) reticular membrane. (From Engström, H.: The morphology of the normal sensory cells. Collegium O. R. L. A. S. Lyon [Table Ronde], *Acta Otolaryng.*, 63, Suppl. 5-19, 1967.)

squirrel monkey, cat and rat, but the submembrane lamellae are generally highly developed (exposing a large surface area) in the guinea pig. In either case, the layer adjoining the inner surface of the plasma membrane lines the last along the entire periphery of the cell, except for the portion beyond the afferent synapse (Engström, 1967b).

In the guinea pig the submembrane lamellae reach their highest number of layers (6-7) only some distance above the nucleus. The submembrane lamellae may have considerable functional importance (Engström, 1967a). Perhaps they act in the maintenance of a potential gradient or as insulators (Spoendlin, 1966).

Sometimes the rounded lamellar bodies of a cell are in close contact with the submembrane lamellae.

Mitochondria are closely associated with both the cell's system of rounded lamellar bodies and the submembrane lamellae (Fig. 3-3, Fig. 3-4A). This indicates that energy-consuming processes occur at these lamellae.

There are no lamellar bodies and only poorly developed submembrane lamellae in the inner hair cells.

Koitchev (1969) subjected guinea pigs and rats to sound stimulation (95 dB, 2,000 Hz for guinea pigs, 5,000 Hz for rats) for 30 minutes. He reports this causes the Hensen bodies in the hair cells of the lower spirals of the cochlea to change in appearance. There are also changes in the orientation and appearance of the membranes of the endoplasmic reticulum, and the mitochondria are redistributed.

Sinus Hairs (Vibrissae)

In the root sheaths of mammalian sinus hairs there are a good number of Merkel's discs. The last are served by afferent nerve fibers which contain, immediately beneath the constriction of the first node of Ranvier, a structure reminiscent of concentric lamellar bodies (Andres, 1966a).

Visual Receptors

Matsusaka (1967) has published a paper dealing with the lamellated bodies in the basal portion of the accessory cone of the chicken. These spherical lamellated bodies, located at the synapse, are about 0.7μ across. Their internal structure may consist of concentrically arranged paired membranes, although it varies and sometimes packed masses of paired membranes are seen. Dense materials and vesicles are found between loosely arranged lamellae, and in some cases a group of vesicles is only surrounded by a few concentric membranes.

At times two connected lamellar bodies are met (Fig. 3-4C).

The lamellated bodies are often observed to be in contact with a tubular network and with the endoplasmic reticulum.

Incubation of the lamellated bodies with saliva results in the loss of their internal structure. This indicates that the lamellated bodies contain carbohydrate, and they probably also include much lipid.

Rounded lamellated bodies have been reported from the presynaptic cytoplasm of rabbit visual receptors (Grignolo *et al.*, 1966). A circular membrane structure has also been seen in the visual cells of the gray squirrel.

Rabbit retinal pigment epithelium cells, which had undergone degeneration upon exposure to sodium iodate, have been found to contain concentric membrane layers having the appearance of lamellated bodies (Grignolo *et al.*, 1966). Perhaps these concentric layers were formed by the repeated rolling of the cell membrane. Degenerated pigment epithelium cells also exhibited large round membrane-bounded bodies containing a granular cytoplasm.

Brammer and White (1969) reared mosquitoes (*Aedes aegypti*) in the absence of vitamin A and B-carotene. The photoreceptor cells of these specimens did not contain the multivesicular bodies typical of arthropod visual cells. The formation of these multivesicular bodies is related to the specialized activity of arthropod photoreceptors, and reflects the state of visual cell function. Normally the multivesicular bodies may remove products or wastes of visual activity.

The affected photoreceptors also differed from their healthy counterparts in containing massed endomembranes at their proximal ends. Continuous illumination produced a more profuse development of these endomembranes. The membranes, which were composed of closed cisternae, seemed at first to have an association with the nucleus.

The rhabdomeres (pigment organelles) of the abnormal photoreceptors did not exhibit any effect, except that some had a smaller size.

Taste Receptors

Lamellated, electron-dense bodies were seen in the presumed taste cells of the rat's fungi-

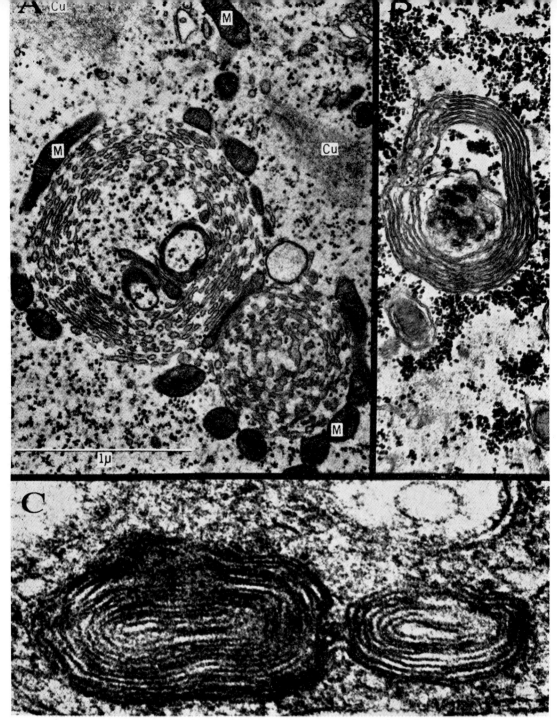

FIGURE 3-4. Lamellated bodies in different sense organs. A. In the infracuticular region of an outer hair cell of the cochlea. (*M*) Mitochondria, (*Cu*) extensions of the cuticle. B. In a supporting cell of mouse (*Mus*) olfactory mucosa. This lamellated body, in the cytoplasm below the nucleus, consists of smooth-surfaced membranes. Numerous glycogen granules lie in the vicinity. C. In the presynaptic cytoplasm of an accessory cone of the chick (*Gallus*) retina. These two lamellated bodies were joined together. (A. From Engström, H.: The ultrastructure of the sensory cells of the cochlea. *J. Laryng., 81*:687-715, 1967. B. From Fig. 12, Frisch, D.: Ultrastructure of mouse olfactory mucosa. *Amer. J. Anat., 121*:87-120, 1967. C. From Matsusaka, T.: Lamellar bodies in the synaptic cytoplasm of the accessory cone from the chick retina as revealed by electron microscopy. *J. Ultrastruct. Res., 18*:55-70, 1967 [Academic Press].)

form papillae by Farbman (1965). They were approximately 0.8µ-1.0µ in diameter and irregular in shape. The contained lamellae formed randomly arranged parallel bundles, and showed cross-striations with a period of 35 to 40 Å. Such lamellated bodies had not been previously reported from taste cells.

Other investigators have described similar entities as lysosomes.

A second kind of cell identified by Farbman (1965) in the taste buds may be of a supporting type. Farbman considered it likely that this cell functions in the development and maintenance of the taste pore.

The above cell sometimes contained membrane-surrounded groups of vesicles. There were also thick, double membranes which each enclosed a translucent area. Within the double membranes vesicles and moderately dense material were present.

Nemetschek-Gansler and Ferner (1964) demonstrated that in the rabbit Farbman's "taste pore" cells hold small, crowded vacuoles, each of which has an inclusion. The last is frequently composed of concentric layers.

Like the taste cells, the "taste pore" cells occasionally exhibited a flattened, membrane-bordered sac near the synapse with a nerve process (Farbman, 1965). In taste cells such sacs are not always restricted to the synaptic region. The sacs are also present in cochlear hair cells.

Dense bodies were in addition seen in a nerve process serving a "taste pore" cell by Farbman, and were also reported from axons under rabbit taste buds by Murray and Murray (1967).

Murray and Murray (1967) examined taste buds in the foliate papillae of rabbits. They consider the equivalent of Farbman's (1965) rat taste cells to be supporting cells and the cells most like Farbman's "taste pore" cells to be the true taste cells. Although Murray and Murray observed some larger droplets, which they thought might be lysosomes, in both kinds of cells, they failed to find lamellated bodies in the rabbit.

Olfactory Receptors

In the olfactory cells of the mouse one to several electron-dense lamellated bodies are located in the perikaryon (cell body) near the Golgi apparatus. Each lamellated body is surrounded by a trilaminar membrane, and its internal lamellae are cross-striated with a period of about 30 Å (Frisch, 1967).

Heist, Mulvaney and Landis (1967) performed an electron microscopic study of rabbit olfactory epithelium. They observed the bipolar olfactory receptor cell to contain multivesicular bodies in its distal portion, but below the dendrite.

The frequent presence of concentric lamellar structures was demonstrated. In some cases groups of rings lay within a single body. Two connected ring structures within a single membrane-bounded entity were also observed. In addition, bodies containing parallel, straight lamellae or lamellae having both straight and curved sections were seen.

The mentioned lamellae-containing units were positioned either close to the nuclear and plasma membranes or next to the endoplasmic reticulum and the Golgi complex.

Heist, Mulvaney and Landis suggest that the observed, variously shaped lamellae may be the cristae of mitochondria. They point out that concentric cristae formations resembling some of their lamellae have been reported from a number of animal and plant sources.

Large numbers of mitochondria are concentrated in the olfactory cell's dendrite, below its terminal swelling, as is the case in the dog (Okano, Weber and Frommes, 1967). These mitochondria also possess a relatively high number of cristae. The possibility is raised that the olfactory cell mitochondria play a role in transduction. They may also contribute to electric potential changes through enzymatic activity and their function in ion transport.

In the midportion of the olfactory cells of dogs, cats and rats large, high-contrast lysosomes were met by Andres (1966b). In adult animals these lysosomes contained lamellar membrane layers that apparently included lipid constituents. Multivesicular bodies were located near the Golgi apparatus and in the olfactory dendrite. Okano, Weber and Frommes (1967) also found multivesicular bodies in the dog's olfactory dendrite, below the terminal vesicle. The oval multivesicular bodies, about 0.6μ x 1.2μ, held 40 to 130 small vesicles.

Bronshtein and Ivanov (1965) found the olfactory receptors of the lamprey to possess, in their perikaryons, large spherical bodies containing fibrillar masses.

The supporting cells of the mouse olfactory epithelium show some resemblance to its receptor cells in possessing microvilli and branching processes. The olfactory supporting cells of other animals are also equipped with microvilli.

Masses of lamellae and loose whorls of lamellae were demonstrated by Frisch in respectively the apical and basal portions of the supporting cells (Fig. 3-4B). However, these lamellae consist of smooth-surfaced membranes and appear to be derived from the agranular endoplasmic reticulum. There are also dense bodies in the basal parts of the supporting cells.

Andres (1966b) describes the supporting cells of the olfactory epithelia of dogs, cats, and rats as containing a multiple-layered, lamellar, agranular endoplasmic reticulum in their distal halves. He also found ergoplasmatic layers close to the nucleus.

Multivesicular bodies of a smaller size (0.2μ x 0.5μ) than those in the olfactory receptor dendrites were seen in the supporting cells of the dog by Okano, Weber and Frommes (1967). Smooth- and rough-surfaced reticular membranes were also present.

The supporting cells of the lamprey's olfactory mucosa exhibit a concentric endoplasmic reticulum (Bronshtein and Ivanov, 1965).

Heist, Mulvaney and Landis (1967) report multivesicular bodies from the supporting cells of the rabbit olfactory epithelium.

An electron microscopic study by Graziadei

(1966) did not reveal lamellated structures in the olfactory receptors or supporting cells of the mole (*Talpa*).

The Bowman's glands of the mouse olfactory mucosa are composed in part of electron-dense dark cells. The electron-density of these cells results from a very high content of osmiophilic smooth-surfaced membranes. The smooth-surfaced membranes, which form the agranular endoplasmic reticulum, often appear as concentrated whorls around mitochondria (Frisch, 1967). Thus the dark cells of Bowman's glands also contain entities which bear a superficial resemblance to lamellated bodies.

The smooth-surfaced endoplasmic reticulum seems to be involved in the formation of lipid substances and in carbohydrate metabolism.

Neurons

Certain neurons too have been described as containing a lamellar type of structure. Among these findings are the reports of lamellated bodies in the proximal and distal endings of transsected axons and in the regenerating end bulbs of axons by Blumcke and Niedorf (1965) and Blumcke, Niedorf and Rode (1966). These lamellated bodies are chiefly disc shaped, have regular, compacted layers, and are composed of lamellae 40 to 45 Å in diameter. They are often found in the company of multivesicular bodies which the authors consider thin-walled, cytoplasm-enclosing lamellated bodies in cross-section.

The lamellated bodies appear before the mitochondria and the endoplasmic reticulum in the vicinity undergo degeneration. The mentioned investigators therefore do not consider it likely that the lamellated bodies originate from the membranes of either mitochondria or the endoplasmic reticulum. Instead, they suggest that the axonal lamellated bodies may develop from lipid aggregations which form as a consequence of metabolic changes. The lamellated bodies are particularly numerous at nodes of Ranvier.

The lamellated bodies behind the growing end bulbs of regenerating axons dissolve as the axoplasm differentiates.

Discussion

The related observations on lamellated bodies in receptor cells show that much still remains to be learned of the ultrastructure of receptor cells.

Lamellated bodies are present in secondary sense cells as well as in bipolar neurons such as the olfactory receptors.

It is significant that in the case of the olfactory and gustatory systems lamellated bodies, as well as other organelles, are found both in the sense cells and their supporting cells. This most likely is indicative of common cell origins. However, Murray and Murray (1967) have gone so far as to suggest that the supporting cells of the olfactory and gustatory systems are in reality additional types of sense cells. Just as there are rods and cones in the retina, and outer and inner hair cells in the cochlea, there may be two kinds of olfactory receptors and two types of taste cells.

The reported findings on lamellated bodies indicate that species differences exist in respect to these organelles.

Glycogen granules are frequently met in the cytoplasm of sense cells and supporting cells, often also in the proximity of the lamellated membrane bodies.

Synaptic Rods

Synaptic rods are found in different sense cells and are primarily present in such cells.

Synaptic rods (bars) are surrounded by synaptic vesicles. Also, in labyrinthine hair cells and certain mechanoreceptors there seem to be structural connections between the responsive surface of the cell and the synaptic rod located near the synapse with the afferent nerve fiber. Thus in the labyrinthine hair cells of the ammocoete larva, a line of microtubules runs from the apical hairs to the synaptic region at the base of the cell (see Fig. 2-30).

These relationships suggest that the rods play some role in the formation, storage, or release of the chemical transmitter substance. A function in the conversion of electrical into chemical energy is possible.

In hair cells the synaptic rod is believed to mark the active site of the afferent synapse.

Labyrinthine Hair Cells

Synaptic rods or bodies surrounded by synaptic vesicles are normally found in the bases of vestibular hair cells, close to the synapse. In fish and amphibians these synaptic bodies are globular or ovoid (Fig. 3-5). In mammals a bar (cross-section) or small plate is present (Fig. 3-5), and it rests against the synaptic membrane (Wersäll, Flock and Lundquist, 1965). The synaptic rods of mammalian labyrinthine and auditory hair cells have also been described as small round masses, rings (probably the microscopic appearance of hollow spheres), and large laminas, in all cases bordered by a single layer of synaptic vesicles.

In addition, in fish and amphibians a line of dark globules or thickenings is located at portions of the hair cell's synaptic membrane.

Synaptic rods are also found in the bases of lateral line hair cells, and in the sense cells of fish electroreceptors (Lissmann, 1963). These last cells too are a part of the acousticolateral system.

Auditory Hair Cells

Like the labyrinthine hair cells, the inner and outer hair cells of the organ of Corti have, at their synaptic membranes, synaptic rods fringed by vesicles. In mammals the rods contact the synaptic membrane at one end, as is true in mammalian vestibular hair cells (Wersäll, Flock and Lundquist, 1965).

Echandia (1967) observed only focal thickenings of the cytoplasm at the afferent synapses of cat outer hair cells. He could not discern the synaptic rods described from the guinea pig and squirrel monkey. Echandia's work corroborates Spoendlin (1966), who found neither synaptic vesicles or rods in the cat's outer hair cells.

Engström (1967a) reports that sometimes supporting cells in the organ of Corti contain bodies resembling synaptic rods.

Visual Receptors

The basal portions of vertebrate retinal

cones may contain several synaptic rods. This is the case in the cones of the ground squirrel *Citellus* (Hollenberg and Bernstein, 1966).

On the other hand, vertebrate visual rods typically have only a single synaptic rod in their basal processes. Several synaptic rods were observed in some human retinal rods by Missotten (1960).

Matsusaka (1967) studied the synaptic rod of the accessory cone of the chicken retina by means of electron microscopy. He found the synaptic rod to have at the membrane a base (the arciform density) shaped like a three-pronged fork. Deeper in the cell each of three layers of the rod was 70 Å wide and consisted of a light space bordered on each side by a darker layer. The three layers were separated by less dense spaces, also 70 Å wide. The total width of this synaptic rod was 350 Å (Fig. 3-5).

Dowling and Boycott (1965) reported the bipolar cell axons in the inner plexiform layer of the retina to possess synaptic rods. Such bipolar cell synaptic rods typically point in between two postsynaptic processes with which the cell is making contact.

Olney (1968a) traces the development of synaptic rods and other synaptic structures in the neonatal mouse retina. The synaptic rods of the bipolar cell axons penetrating the inner plexiform layer at first have an ovoid shape but then elongate to the adult form.

In the mouse retina some photoreceptor terminals (the beta type) have between five and ten synaptic rods. During their formation the synaptic rods of photoreceptors are first seen not far from the cell nucleus as small, amorphous densities. Even at this stage they are already surrounded by synaptic vesicles. The synaptic rods later seem to move as a cluster down the axonal portion of the receptor toward the synapse. Rods which had reached the synapse were noticeably larger than those seen at earlier stages (Olney, 1968b).

Olney (1968b) found no indications in bipolar cells of a formation of synaptic rods in the central portion of the cell, or of any mi-

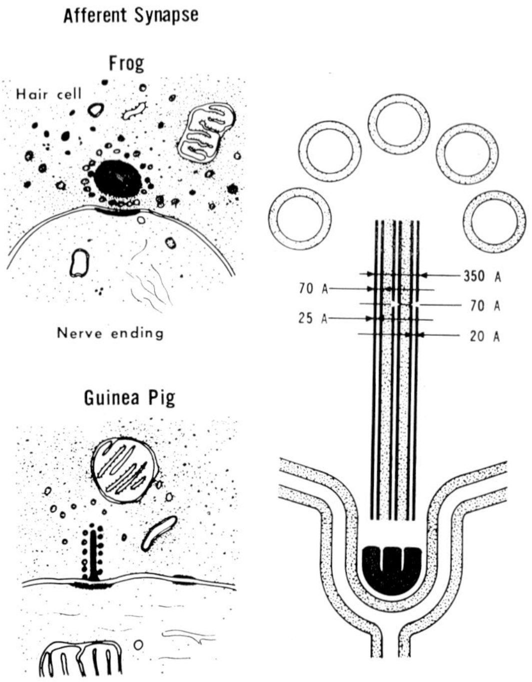

FIGURE 3-5. Diagrammatic representations of synaptic rods. Upper left, ovoid synaptic body at the afferent synapse of a hair cell in the labyrinth of the frog. Bottom left, synaptic bar at the afferent synapse of a hair cell in the labyrinth of the guinea pig. In both drawings the thickening of the afferent nerve ending's plasma membrane in the zone of contact is shown. (From Wersäll, Flock, and Lundquist: Structural basis for directional sensitivity in cochlear and vestibular sensory receptors. In *Sensory Receptors. Cold Spring Harbor Symposia on Quantitative Biology, 30*: 115-132, 1965.) Right, cross-section of the synaptic rod in the presynaptic cytoplasm of the accessory cone of the chick (*Gallus*) retina. The rod consists of three dense layers and two intervening spaces. The arciform density (black) forms the rod's base. Circles at the diagram's top represent synaptic vesicles. (From Matsusaka, T.: Lamellar bodies in the synaptic cytoplasm of the accessory cone from the chick retina as revealed by electron microscopy. *J. Ultrastruct. Res., 18*: 55-70, 1967 [Academic Press].)

gration of the rods to their final locations at synaptic sites. The fully developed synaptic rods of bipolar cells were sometimes observed to have an arciform density.

Taste Receptors

Farbman (1965) does not mention the synaptic rod in his paper on the electron microscopy of the rat taste bud. Murray and Murray (1967) noted only isolated and indefinite indications of synaptic rods during their examinations of rabbit taste buds by electron microscopy. However, Murray and Murray did not employ specialized techniques for the demonstration of synaptic structures.

Gray and Watkins (1965), in an electron microscope study of rat taste buds, observed only dense projections internal to the synaptic membranes of taste cells. These projections appear to be coiled or curled filaments, and may be associated with the movement of a transmitter substance into the synaptic cleft. The dense projections have not been related to synaptic rods and are not surrounded by massed vesicles. They resemble similar structures at synapses in the vertebrate central nervous system and thickenings at parts of the synaptic membrane of fish and amphibian lateral line receptors.

Olfactory Receptors

Vertebrate olfactory receptor cells are really bipolar neurons whose long, thin axons only synapse with secondary neurons, the mitral cells, in the glomeruli of the olfactory bulbs.

Therefore, any olfactory receptor synaptic rods must be sought in the olfactory bulb glomeruli. Here the olfactory cell axons form synapses exclusively with the dendrites of the secondary neurons (axo-dendritic synapses).

De Lorenzo (1963) observed synaptic vesicles near the terminals of olfactory axons. There were also synaptic membrane thickenings. However, no reports were obtained of the presence of a synaptic rod in any part of the olfactory receptor cell.

Discussion

Synaptic rods have been found to have unlike predominant forms in some different classes of vertebrates. It also appears that there are species differences in respect to these structures. The application of electron microscopy to the study of synaptic rods should clarify the significance of such differences. It may also provide information leading to the determination of rod function.

The observation of structures resembling synaptic rods in supporting cells within the organ of Corti (Engström, 1967a) need not cast doubt on the function of the rods. Supporting cells share a number of distinctive organelles with the respective receptor cells, possibly because of a common origin.

SENSITIVITIES

It is generally assumed that the first sensory system to appear in the animal kingdom was the common chemical sense, which is sensitive to a large variety of noxious agents.

In higher animals the common chemical sense is dependent on the free endings of the trigeminal nerves.

From the common chemical sense there may have developed general receptors, with a broad range of sensitivities, and these in turn may have given rise to more specialized, specific receptors.

Chemical receptors are present in primitive animal groups, such as jellyfish (*Scyphozoa*). These coelenterates possess elongated sensory neurons, named palpocils, which have special-

ized tips. In *Hydra* the palpocils have been observed to bear a unique cilium at their tip, presaging the ciliary structures possessed by the later gustatory, olfactory, auditory and visual receptors.

The receptors of some senses have evolved to become extremely sensitive to their type of stimulus. Man perceives a flash of light when but 5 quanta of light are absorbed by the same number of dark-adapted visual rods in his eye. Hecht accordingly deduced that 1 quantum of light will cause a dark-adapted retinal rod to initiate nerve impulses. Similarly, man can respond to ⅓ trillionth of an ounce of mercaptan mixed with a normal nasal inspiration of air, although this quantity of mercaptan cannot be detected in the chemistry laboratory. According to the calculations of DeVries and Stuiver (1961), eight or fewer molecules of a mercaptan will produce threshold excitation in a human olfactory cell. A bitter taste can be clearly discerned if 10^{15} molecules of strychnine are applied to the tongue, and the human palate has an even greater sensitivity to the bitter modality. Auditory sensations can result from vibrations with subatomic amplitudes. The human ear and the subgenual organs of insects are responsive to vibrations of 4×10^{-10} cm (Autrum, 1959).

Generally receptors are structured to be highly sensitive to only one main type of stimulus. Thus in the chemoreceptive hairs of the blowfly (*Phormia regina*), one sensory neuron is sensitive to sugars and a few additional carbohydrates, another primarily to monovalent salts, a third only to water, and a fourth to mechanical stimuli. A fifth sensory neuron, which is not found in all labellar chemoreceptive hairs, responds to anions (Steinhardt, 1966).

The blowfly's sugar-sensitive neuron is highly responsive to d-fructose, d-glucose, d- and l-arabinose, sucrose, l-sorbose and inositol. The last is the only polyhydric alcohol with a ring structure, as is found in the more stimulating sugars. Other polyhydric alcohols do not produce responses. The sugars d-mannose and d- and l-xylose evoke little response, and lactose and cellobiose, none. The sugar neuron has a small action potential, and in the sheep blowfly (*Lucinia cuprina*) shows a minimum latent period of 5 msec (Hodgson, 1957, 1961, 1965).

The neuron responsive to salts has a less specific reactivity, produces larger impulses, and in the sheep blowfly may show a latent period of less than 1 msec. While the salt neuron is reactive to monovalent salts, it is not sensitive to the divalent calcium chloride. Acids and alcohols also stimulate the salt neuron, but only at supraphysiological concentrations that may have an irreversible action (Hodgson and Roeder, 1956; Hodgson, 1961).

The anion-sensitive neuron carries impulses of considerably lesser amplitude, but somewhat greater duration, than those picked up from the salt neuron.

Whereas the impulse activity of the sugar-sensitive neuron produces positive responses, that of the salt-sensitive neuron usually causes avoidance behavior. The anion-sensitive neuron appears to always initiate avoidance behavior (Steinhardt, 1966).

The sugar-sensitive neuron of the tarsal chemoreceptive hair of the butterfly *Vanessa indica* responds only to sucrose, d-glucose, and d-fructose from among a large number of sugars (Takeda, 1961).

Receptors of extreme specificity, which respond to primarily one stimulating substance, are found in the male common silk moth, *Bombyx mori*. Its antennal receptors react "all or none" to bombykol, a complex alcohol which is the sexual attractant of the species (Dethier, 1967a). It appears the moth's nervous system may come close to detecting the adsorption of a single bombykol molecule on an olfactory receptor cell. The male moth's responses to bombykol isomers are noticeably lower, and related compounds such as cycloheptanon and terpineol elicit only weak responses. It is interesting that the female moth shows not only weak or rare responses to bombykol, but even gives a relatively stronger response to terpineol and linalool (Boeckh, Kaissling, and Schneider, 1965).

In the larva of *Bombyx mori* one receptor tested with carbohydrates and inositol was reactive only to the latter (Ishikawa, 1963). Inositol is found in the leaves eaten by this larva.

Highly specific receptors have also been discovered in a different caterpillar. They respond only to glucosides found in the food plants (*Cruciferae*).

A receptor in the Colorado potato beetle (*Leptinotarsa decemlineata*) is highly excited by two alkaloid glycosides, tomatin and solanin, which are found in leaves usable by the beetle (Stürckow, 1959).

The males of many species of euglossine bees have been reported to be attracted to particular orchid species primarily by pure compounds present in the fragrance of these orchids (Dodson *et al.*, 1969).

Honeybee (*Apis mellifica*) drones respond best to the sexual attractant of the queen bee, 9-keto-2-decenoic acid, which has the formula

$$CH_3 - \underset{\underset{O}{\|}}{C} - (CH_2)_5 - CH = CH - COOH$$

This substance further prevents workers from raising new queens and stimulates cluster formation during swarming. The bee sexual attractant excites the olfactory receptors of drones, workers and queens.

Perhaps the most specific receptor known is the carbon dioxide receptor of the antennae of the honeybee (*Apis mellifica*). Only carbon dioxide stimulates this receptor at reasonable concentrations (Lacher, 1964). Electrophysiological recordings show the bee's carbon dioxide receptor to have the extremely high threshold of 10^{15} molecules/cc of air.

The stimulation of specific receptors results in highly stereotyped behavior on the part of the organism.

In the case of specific receptors certain stimulating molecules may be more effective than others. Thus the honeybee's receptor for 9-keto-2-decenoic acid has been found electrophysiologically to give a threshold response when this compound reaches a concentration of 10^8 molecules/cc of air, while 10^{12} molecules/cc of caproic acid call forth an equivalent response (Boeckh, Kaissling and Schneider, 1965). Amoore *et al.* (1969) have correlated the effectiveness of a series of ketones and nonketones on a specific receptor of an ant with the molecular shapes of these substances. However, it is still not understood how, in so many cases, a less suitable molecule, when it is present in greater concentration, can elicit a degree of excitation equivalent to that provoked by the most effective compound.

Primitive, although highly specific receptors for food substances, which do not function in concert with the normal filtering and neural coding mechanisms, are found in coelenterates.

In *Hydra littoralis* external receptors specific for reduced glutathione, a tripeptide, are probably numerous on the tentacles. These receptors interact only with molecules possessing the main tripeptide chain of glutathione. They are not excited by asparthione, which differs from glutathione only in the absence of one methylene group. The thiol group is not required for linkage with the receptor, but the α-amino portion of the glutamyl structure of glutathione seems to be necessary (Lenhoff, 1968).

The marked affinity of the described receptor for glutathione is shown by the low value, 10^{-6}M, of the dissociation constant.

Chemical groups suspected of participating in the glutathione-receptor interaction of *H. littoralis* are examined in Gustatory Reception, Chapter V.

The gastrozooids of the Portuguese man-of-war (*Physalia physalis*) also show an extremely strong reaction to glutathione.

Hydra also possesses tyrosine-specific receptors in its digestive cavity. These enteroceptors do not respond to other natural amino acids, and the hydroxyl, α-amino and α-carboxyl groups of tyrosine are required for excitation (Lenhoff, 1968).

The colonial hydroid *Cordylophora lacustris* responds to the amino acid proline and almost as well to azetidine-2-carboxylic acid, a ring composed of four chemical groups. The receptors in question seem to be specifically reactive to the imino portion of heterocyclic α-imino acids which have not been altered, by substitution or unsaturation, in a manner affecting the imino acid group.

An actinian coelenterate, *Boloceroides sp.*, appears to have receptors that respond only to n-α-amino butyric acids which branch at the β-carbon. This organism is reactive to the amino acid valine.

A sea anemone has been noted to respond to glutamine but not to glutathione, glutamic acid or asparagine (Lenhoff, 1968).

Evidence for specific chemosensitive "receptor" sites has been obtained at a still lower level of evolution. Studies on the bacterium *Escherichia coli* indicate that this organism has a minimum of five distinct types of chemo-receptive sites for organic molecules. These "receptor" sites respond respectively to galactose, glucose, ribose, aspartate and serine. The galactose "receptor" sites apparently also interact with the galactose analog D-fucose, and the glucose-sensitive structures with the glucose analogs 2-deoxyglucose, α-methyl glucoside and L-sorbose. The "receptor" sites for the amino acid aspartate are also reactive to glutamate (Adler, 1969).

Further investigations suggest that there are also specific receptive structures for fructose, as well as for maltose and for trehalose.

Full competitive inhibition has been observed between galactose and D-fucose, and between the amino acids aspartate and glutamate (Adler, 1969).

The specific sensitivities of normal receptors are only partially determined by the nature of the receptor or the sensitive nerve ending itself.

First, surrounding structures may act as filters to enhance the specificity of the receptor. Thus the cornea, aqueous humor, lens and vitreous humor of the eye give the wavelengths of visible light easy passage but protect the visual receptors, the rods and cones, from chemical and normal mechanical stimuli. The sensory nerve ending of the pacinian corpuscle is not stimulated by the constant, unvarying components of a mechanical stimulus by virtue of the filtering effect of the laminar capsule (Mendelson and Loewenstein, 1964).

There may also be present sense organ structures which channel a greater quantity of the stimulus to the receptors. The peculiar structures of the pinna of the ears of some bats are a case in point. The nature of the tympanic membrane, auditory ossicles, and so on, of the ear also affects the sensitivities shown by the auditory receptors, the hair cells of the organ of Corti.

There is in addition a filtering effect produced by the bat pinna structures in that they permit determination of the direction from which a sound originates (Schwartzkopff, 1966).

Norberg (1968) studied the functional significance of a marked vertical asymmetry of the external auditory meatuses of an owl (*Aegolius funereus* Linné, Strigiformes). For this purpose time and intensity measurements were made of the auditory differences produced between the two ears of an artificial owl head by direction and frequency (2,500-16,000 cps) of sound.

Norberg found that in order to determine the direction of origin of a normal sound in the horizontal and vertical planes, an owl having symmetrical ear apertures would have to make two separate judgments at different positions of the head along a right-left line. The vertical asymmetry of the owl's external ears (Fig. 3-6) theoretically obviates the necessity of turning the head around its longitudinal axis.

The distance between the owl's ears is sufficient for interaural time differences to contribute to directional hearing. A sound will produce no interaural time differences only when it comes from certain clearly defined directions which are perpendicular to the axis between the centers of the two ear apertures.

The sensitivities of a sensory system may be heightened by an increase in the number of receptor cells. Thus certain male moths (*Saturniidae*, etc.) which locate the females of their species by following a sexually attractive odor have much more extensively branched antennae than their female counterparts. These highly branched antennae may bear as many as 250,000 olfactory sensilla, each containing several receptor cells. Of the more than 150,000 sensory neurons in the subdivided portion of each antenna of the male polyphemus moth (*Telea polyphemus*), about 60 to 70 per cent are specifically sensitive to the sex attractant emitted by the female, close to 20 per cent are excited by other odorous substances, and the remainder react to different sensory stimuli (Schneider, Lacher and Kaissling, 1964). The resultant high number of sex-attractant receptors increases the likelihood of a molecule of the sexual attractant making contact with a sensitive receptor's sur-

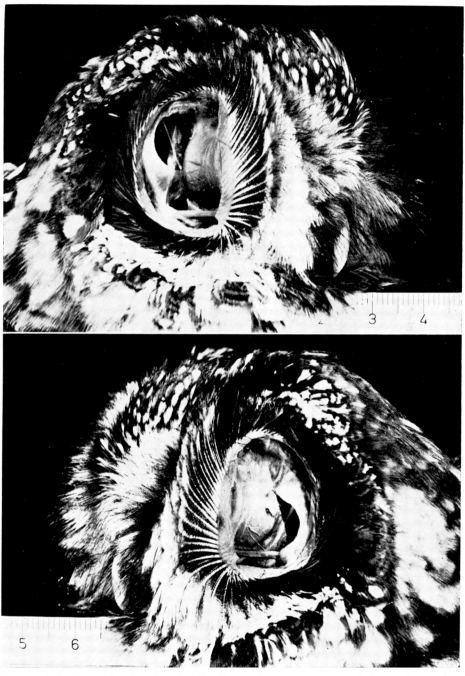

FIGURE 3-6. The right (top) and left (bottom) ear apertures of the owl *Aegolius funereus* (Linné). The bilaterally asymmetrical position of the exposed ear apertures of the skull can be noted in reference to the bilaterally symmetrical jugal bars and scleral rings. A centimeter scale is provided. On the average the left ear aperture is 6.3 mm lower than the right. (Courtesy of Dr. Åke Norberg, University of Gothenburg, Sweden.)

face during a limited period (Schwartzkopff, 1966).

The males of *Bombyx mori* are attracted by bombykol at a concentration of only 0.01 γ. Schneider, Kasang and Kaissling (1968) indicate that these male moths may have a behavioral response threshold to bombykol of 1.4×10^4 molecules/cc^3, at an air current velocity of 57 cm/sec and a stimulus duration of 2 seconds. At threshold each sensitive receptor hair should not adsorb an average of more than one molecule. This does not mean, however, that a single bombykol molecule can call forth a receptor response.

The apparent sensitivities and responses of a receptor further depend on the nervous elements within or behind it.

In the pacinian corpuscle the number of repetitive impulses, and thus the duration of the response, is partly controlled by the electrochemical makeup of the internal nerve ending (Mendelson and Loewenstein, 1964).

It is not yet known how much specificity is bestowed on receptor systems by the central nervous system. The central nervous system may also act as a filtering agent, and eliminate divergent responses produced by stimuli related to the one proper for the receptor.

Therefore, on several bases a receptor is usually much more sensitive to its proper stimulus than to other environmental factors. The eye, for instance, has a much lower threshold for stimulation by light than it does for stimulation by electricity or mechanical pressure. Furthermore, as indicated by the law of specific nerve energies (Mueller's law), the last two named types of stimulation will still produce a perception of light (as would be expected from the termination of the visual pathway in the visual areas of the cortex). The perception of a strong circle of light, called a phosphene, can be produced in total darkness by turning the eye medially and pressing with a finger on the eyeball.

If the chemosensory hair of a blowfly (*Phormia regina*) is subjected to a sufficient degree of mechanical stimulation, the normal behavioral taste response, extension of the proboscis, will follow (Hodgson and Roeder, 1956).

However, in the last few decades the total application of Mueller's law, with its implication of high receptor sensitivity to only one type of stimulus, has been opened to question.

Hensel and Zotterman (1951) found afferent nerve fibers (8μ-10μ in diameter) in the house cat's tongue which carried impulses not only after a low level of stimulation of the tongue by pressure, but also after low stimulation by cooling.

Sato (1963) recorded from single nerve fibers of the cat's chorda tympani nerve, which mediates taste from the anterior portion of the tongue. He found that 50 per cent of the fibers carried responses to warming, cooling and also to several types of taste stimuli, and that another 30 per cent transmitted impulses on both cooling and different taste stimuli. These results indicate that taste receptor cells may also be sensitive to temperature, since taste fibers only innervate taste-type receptors in taste buds.

Nagaki *et al.* (1964) also report the majority of the cat's chorda tympani fibers to respond to both gustatory and thermal stimuli, and similar results have been obtained with the rat and hamster (Ogawa, Sato and Yamashita, 1968).

In the hamster the majority of single chorda tympani fibers have been observed to respond to more than one taste quality and also to cooling or warming. One type of fiber responded to sucrose and warming, while another kind was highly reactive to sour (HCl), bitter (quinine) and cooling, and in some cases also gave good responses to the salty quality (NaCl) (Yamashita *et al.*, 1967b).

In the rat also many single chorda tympani fibers were seen to respond strongly to HCl, quinine and cooling (Yamashita *et al.*, 1967a).

A good number of the rat's chorda tympani fibers were observed to have a spontaneous impulse rate of under 2/sec, and spontaneous activity was especially marked in cold-sensitive fibers. The correlation between the magnitude of cold responses and the rate of spontaneous activity was highly significant, indicating that the observed spontaneous activity might even be a continuous response to the ambient temperature.

Spontaneous activity was also noted in the warm-sensitive fibers of the hamster and was positively correlated with the possession of a broad spectrum of gustatory sensitivities by a taste unit.

The spontaneous activity of the rat's salt fibers can be reduced by rinsing water over its tongue (Pfaffmann, 1965a).

Yamashita *et al.* (1967a) found a rat chorda tympani unit in which cooling enhanced the response to 0.1M sodium chloride solution but had no effect alone. This indicates that in this case the stimulating effects of low temperature and salt summed, suggesting the possibility of both temperature and salt sensitivity on the part of a single receptor cell.

In the frog glossopharyngeal nerve fibers respond to both taste solutions and warmth.

Emmers (1966) recorded responses from single thalamic neurons of the cat to both taste and cold stimuli applied to the tongue. Responses to intermittent cooling were continuous, but cold prevented taste responses. However, in this case interaction at various nervous system levels, including between "thermal" and "gustatory" thalamic neurons, was quite possible.

On the other hand, few of the squirrel monkey's (*Saimiri sciureus*) thalamic neurons respond to both gustatory stimulation and cooling, and no thalamic response to warming has been noted (Benjamin, 1963).

Bullock and Faulstick (1953) recorded from afferent fibers serving the rattlesnake's facial pit and found they discharged after both touch and heat stimulation of the pit. Bullock and Diecke (1956) obtained similar results.

Great caution must be exercised in attributing sensitivity to basically diverse types of stimuli to a receptor.

In the pacinian corpuscle, which is specific for mechanical stimuli, the rate of rise and the amplitude of the generator potential elicited by mechanical stimulation, and therefore often also the frequency of the emitted nerve impulses, vary directly with temperature. Apparently in the pacinian corpuscle increased ion conductance by the receptor membrane, which leads to the development of a generator potential, is limited by an energy barrier. Membrane conductance is therefore greatly enhanced by a rise in temperature. However, high temperatures cannot themselves initiate a reduction in the electrical resistance of the membrane and an increase in membrane conductance, and thus stimulate the pacinian corpuscle (Ishiko and Loewenstein, 1961).

One must therefore distinguish between an effective stimulus and a factor which can enhance or reduce the response to such a stimulus. A method of making such a distinction consists of lowering the suspected effective stimulus to subphysiological levels while one attempts to stimulate the receptor with the other, apparently stimulating, agent (Loewenstein, 1961a).

It should be kept in mind that the branches of a single nerve axon may innervate several different receptors. Therefore, the fact that nerve impulses can be recorded from a single axon on the application of different types of stimuli to the region innervated by the axon need not mean that individual receptors have multiple sensitivities.

The extent of the specificity of a receptor should also be evaluated in terms of the threshold intensities of the different apparent stimuli required for excitation. Further, it may be possible to differentiate between apparent stimuli on the basis of the spatial summation needed to call forth a response (Loewenstein, 1961a).

The sensitivity of receptors to more than one fundamental type of stimulus would entail the necessity of a mechanism somewhere along the sensory pathway by which the different impulse codes produced in response to different stimulus types could be carried to different parts of the brain.

A practical addition to the subject of receptor specificity consists of the question of the specificity of the function of the receptor in nature. It may not normally be exposed to more than one type of stimulus.

It is also interesting to examine receptors which react to stimuli of only one basic type but show a broad range of sensitivities within that limit. Mechanisms exist in such receptors which enable the organism to differentiate between qualitatively unlike stimuli.

Receptors showing responses to a broad range of stimuli belonging to one main type have been named generalists, to differentiate them from the previously treated specific receptors called specialists (Boeckh, Kaissling and Schneider, 1965). At least many of these generalists show spontaneous activity, and each receptor cell has a stable and individual response spectrum which overlaps that of other receptors. Such receptor cells may also differ in overall sensitivity as well as in specific threshold levels. Many generalists respond to a large number of substances. Apparently in a generalist cell a number of different receptor molecule types are distributed on the surface membrane, and individual receptors may carry different types and proportions of receptor sites.

It is sometimes possible to group generalists into types according to the stimuli which elicit the strongest responses, but it may not be certain that the unique responses of the cells have been discovered. The multitude of gradations in weaker responses which characterizes the peculiar response spectrum of each cell defies the further classification of many generalist types.

Findings of the above nature have been obtained with the olfactory receptors of the frog *Rana pipiens* (Gesteland *et al.*, 1963) and with insect olfactory receptors (Lacher, 1964; Schneider, Lacher and Kaissling, 1964; Boeckh, Kaissling and Schneider, 1965; Schoonhoven and Dethier, 1966). Similar response spectra have been recorded from mammalian taste fibers (Erickson, 1963).

In the blowfly (*Phormia regina*) there are different sweet receptor sites, probably on the same sensory neuron, which interact with unlike molecular configurations (Evans, 1963). Thus fructose and mannose act on one receptor site, and glucose on another.

In the hamster each taste cell is responsive to substances representing three or all four of the basic taste modalities (Kimura and Beidler, 1961). In the cat only four out of twenty-six investigated single chorda tympani taste fibers fired after just one stimulus, while in the frog over 90 per cent of the taste fibers were reactive to two or more of nine applied chemicals. Three frog fibers were responsive only to water. Out of 114 single taste fibers tested in the carp (*Cyprinus carpio*) 14 reacted only to sodium chloride and 3 only to acetic acid.

Ogawa, Sato and Yamashita (1968) have found evidence in rats and hamsters that taste fibers which seem to be specific for one or a special group of substances at low test concentrations may show more general sensitivities at higher stimulus concentrations. Thus a sucrose-sensitive taste fiber was hardly reactive to 0.1M sodium chloride but responded well to 0.5 and 1M sodium chloride. It appears quite possible that at different levels of stimulus concentration the ratios between the responses to certain compounds could be markedly different, especially if these substances act on unlike receptor sites.

Some generalists may discriminate between qualitatively different effective stimuli by responding with the normal increase in impulse frequency to some but reacting with a drop in impulse rate of spontaneous origin to others. The latter response is known as inhibition, whereas the well-known former response is called excitation.

Investigations on insect olfactory receptors have shown that while an increase in impulse frequency, excitation, is accompanied by depolarization, inhibition involves hyperpolarization of the receptor membrane. The excitatory potential quickly reaches a peak and recovers rapidly, but it takes the inhibitory potential ten times as long to fully develop. The inhibitory hyperpolarization shows no clear peak and has a slower recovery. The inhibitory responses also have a considerably higher threshold than the excitatory responses.

Some substances have been shown to excite certain insect receptors and inhibit others in the same specimen.

Inhibition was demonstrated in the mechanoreceptors of the cercal hairs of the cockroach (*Periplaneta americana*) by Nicklaus (1965). Bending the hairs in one direction resulted in excitation, while bending in the opposed direction reduced the impulse frequency.

Also in the case of the hair cells of lateral line organ neuromasts, the direction in which the cilia are bent determines whether excitation or inhibition takes place. When the stereocilia are bent toward the kinocilium, a negative potential develops in the hair cell and gives rise to nerve impulses. Displacement in the opposite direction produces a positive cell potential (hyperpolarization) accompanied by a drop in the resting discharge (Flock, 1967).

Boeckh (1962, 1967) studied inhibition in the olfactory receptors of carrion beetles. In *Necrophorus* mercaptan, homologous fatty acids with a 6 to 10 atom carbon chain and amines elicited an increased impulse frequency, while impulses were inhibited by 3 or 4 carbon fatty acids and cycloheptanone. The receptors of *Thanatophilus* gave a positive response to carrion, 4 to 7 carbon aldehydes, hexenol, mercaptan and amylacetate and were inhibited by cycloheptanone.

Dicarboxylic amino acids and glutathione inhibit salt responses, which show a post-inhibitory rebound, and do not excite water responses in the blowfly (*Phormia regina*). This inhibition can only partly be attributed to the low pH of the solutions of these substances (Wolbarsht and Hanson, 1967).

In the blowfly *Calliphora vomitoria* substances such as calcium chloride, quinine and acetic acid do not produce negative generator potentials (depolarizations) but instead call forth long-lasting positive potentials (hyperpolarizations) that are not followed by nerve impulses. If chemicals evoking positive potentials are added to stimuli-eliciting negative generator potentials, they will eliminate both

the generator potentials and the ensuing nerve impulses, i.e. produce inhibition (Morita and Yamashita, 1959).

Inhibition has also been observed in moth and honeybee olfactory receptors (Boeckh, Kaissling and Schneider, 1965), in the olfactory receptor neurons of the caterpillar of *Protoparce sexta* (Schoonhoven and Dethier, 1966), and in olfactory receptors of the toad *Bufo vulgaris Japonicus* (Takagi and Omura, 1963).

Neurons of the subesophagial ganglia of *Helix pomatia* have been exposed by the removal of a connective tissue covering and then were directly stimulated with odors (Arvanitaki et al., 1967). Benzene, xylene, benzaldehyde, acetone and butyl alcohol caused 20 to 30 per cent of the tested neurons to show hyperpolarization of their cell membranes, akin to inhibition. Thus neurons can undergo changes in response to odor stimulation which resemble those shown by olfactory receptors.

Inhibition appears to be of real significance to arthropods, since they meet inhibitory substances in their environment and react appropriately to them. Inhibitory substances can cause a fly to retract its partly extended proboscis or show avoidance behavior (Hodgson and Steinhardt, 1967).

A natural material may affect an arthropod by the combination of the excitatory and inhibitory compounds it contains.

Seeming inhibitory effects apparently based on mechanisms other than the hyperpolarization of the receptor membrane have been described.

The reversible inhibitory action of straight-chain lower alcohols and long-chain amines on the salt and water receptors of flies resembles the anesthetic effect of hydrocarbons on nerve. On the other hand, these substances seem to inhibit sugar receptors by still different mechanisms, perhaps by denaturation of the receptive membrane molecules or by a more stable combination with them (Hodgson and Steinhardt, 1967). Alcohols of a longer chain length than propanol affected the fly salt receptors to a greater extent than the sugar receptors.

At higher concentrations the mentioned hydrocarbons produced injury discharges.

Results similar to the above were obtained by exposing the amino acid receptors of the spiny lobster (*Panulirus argus*) to pentanol and octylamine.

Dethier (1967b) reports that flies reject various nonelectrolytes because their water and sugar receptors are reversibly inactivated. If alcohol is added to sugar, the latter does not stimulate an insect, indicating narcotization of the sugar receptors (Eisner, 1967).

On the other hand, the salt neuron of the blowfly often gives a considerable response to the anesthetics cocaine, procaine, xylocaine and tetrodotoxin, although these anesthetics also block dendritic conduction (Wolbarsht and Hanson, 1965).

Procaine and other anesthetics have been reported to act on nerve membranes by reducing their ion permeability (Taylor, 1959). Beidler (1967) states that cocaine and iron chloride reduce the potential difference across the plasma membranes of rat and hamster taste cells and may even reverse the polarity.

Andersen *et al.* (1963), using dogs, recorded from single fibers of the chorda tympani nerve which carried impulses after the application of either sucrose or sodium chloride to the tongue. One group of these fibers transmitted a large response to sucrose and only a small one to sodium chloride, but previous application of the latter noticeably reduced the response to sucrose. The same phenomenon was even more apparent in fibers carrying equally large responses to both sucrose and sodium chloride. The authors raise the possibility that in this case previous attachment of the salt to the receptor surface may mechanically prevent the sugar molecules from reaching their proper sites for stimulation.

In insects a good number of compounds— sodium chloride, calcium chloride, ferrous chloride, acetic acid, quinine-HCl and octylamine—may, if they are mixed with sucrose solution, inhibit the response to sucrose.

Similarly, a number of salts, octylamine, mannose and sucrose can, if mixed with sodium chloride solution, inhibit the response to this salt. Wolbarsht (1958) has indicated that sucrose may inhibit the sodium chloride response in the blowfly chemoreceptive hair not only by competitive inhibition at the receptor sites, but also by affecting the thermodynamic properties and the diffusion coefficient of the dissolved sodium chloride.

In the rat 1 molar alanine and also 2 molar glycine irreversibly inhibit the excitatory action of sodium chloride and of potassium chloride. This inhibition often becomes more marked with time (Halpern, Bernard and Kare, 1962). The excitation of the frog's glossopharyngeal nerve by calcium chloride is also inhibited by a number of amino acids (Rapuzzi *et al.*, 1963).

A competitive interaction between alcohol and quinine has been postulated for the depression by alcohol of the response to quinine given by a group of chorda tympani fibers in the cat (Hellekant, 1967).

Beidler (1961) reported that if the tongue is stimulated with both sodium chloride and sodium butyrate, competitive interaction occurs between the chloride and butyrate anions. Rubin *et al.* (1962), using human subjects, found competitive interaction between quinine sulfate and 6-n-propylthiouracil.

Another significant way in which a receptor may be able to discriminate between qualitatively different effective stimuli is by producing differing patterns of impulse firing.

A good example of such a phenomenon can be observed with the blowfly's salt receptor, which could be said to show an intermediate degree of nonspecificity. Although the taste receptors of *Phormia regina's* labella are each specific for a certain modality, the salt receptor will respond to organic sodium salts of up to four carbons (Na butyrate) as it does to sodium chloride (Dethier, 1967a).

However, if one stimulates with aliphatic sodium salts containing a still higher number of carbon atoms, the pattern of firing changes. In such a response there at first occurs that firing of nerve impulses which is the normal response to sodium chloride, but it is followed by a barrage of firing. Then the number of impulses returns to normal, and recovery is complete. Stimulation with aliphatic sodium salts having still longer carbon chains produces one barrage-type burst of firing after another.

The above results indicate that the transmission of two qualitatively different kinds of messages over a single axon is possible, and that some receptors can produce more than one kind of message.

Of course, receptors excited with different stimuli of the same concentration will respond with different impulse frequencies. That different frequencies could be centrally translated into different effects is indicated by the work of Fessard (MacKay, 1968). He found that in *Aplysia*, a marine slug, the same nerve fiber can either excite or inhibit a neuron with which it synapses, depending on its transmitted impulse frequency.

Dethier (1967a) indicates that amplitude modulation may also provide a means of differentiating stimuli. The impulse spikes called forth by various stimuli can differ in height, and spikes of different amplitude could differ in their effectiveness at synapses.

The size of nerve impulses may change with both impulse frequency and amplitude of the generator potential. This was observed by Wolbarsht (1960) in insect mechanoreceptors, such as those of the grasshopper's (*Melanoplus*) antennae. In certain receptors the impulse spike may reach a particular final size, irrespective of its starting height, while in others this is not true. The spike size in the latter, however, varies directly with the amplitude of the generator potential (*Melanoplus*).

It should not be forgotten that there can be differences in the temporal patterns of responses to differing stimuli. Characteristic forms of response, such as peaks of nerve activity followed by plateaus, are evoked by certain stimulating compounds and may provide vital information for central identification of the stimulus.

Thus in the rabbit's chorda tympani nerve the time course of a single salt fiber's response to sodium chloride was noticeably different from the time course of its response to other salts (Beidler, Fishman and Hardiman, 1955).

The temporal patterns of the potentials produced in the *Necrophorus* carrion receptor cell by carrion and fatty acid molecules differ noticeably from the patterns evoked by mercaptans and amines (Boeckh, Kaissling and Schneider, 1965). This is reflected in the resultant impulse frequencies.

The pattern of response has also been reported to vary according to stimulating compound and concentration in the single tarsal chemoreceptors of a butterfly (Takeda, 1961) and in labellar water and salt receptors of *Phormia regina* (Evans and Mellon, 1962a, b).

The potentials developed by individual subesophagial neurons of *Helix pomatia* on odor stimulation had shapes each of which was characteristic of the response to a specific compound (Arvanitaki *et al.*, 1967). The time courses of these potentials were translated into specific impulse frequencies.

The sensitivity of receptors to stimuli, which is provided by their membrane receptor sites, is not a unique capacity. This is evidenced not only by the responses of *Helix* neurons to odors (Arvanitaki *et al.*, 1967) but also by work done on cockroach and on mammalian neurons.

When a series of acidic amino acids were microinjected near the central nervous system neurons of mammals, these neurons responded by discharging groups of impulses. It is believed that in this experiment the acidic amino acids stimulated receptor sites in the surface membrane of the neurons (Eccles, 1964).

Schneider (1969), in the review paper "Insect Olfaction: Deciphering System for Chemical Messages," describes the structure and function of insect olfactory receptors. He deals with both odor specialist and odor generalist receptor cells, and discusses excitatory and inhibitory responses.

REFERENCES

Abrahamson, E.W., and S.E. Ostroy: The photochemical and macromolecular aspects of vision. *Progr. Biophys.*, 17:179-215, 1967.

Adler, J.: Chemoreceptors in bacteria. *Science,* 166:1588-1597, 1969.

Adolph, A.R.: Spontaneous slow potential fluctuations in the *Limulus* photoreceptor. *J. Gen. Physiol.,* 48:297-322, 1964.

Amoore, J.E., G. Palmieri, E. Wanke, and M.S. Blum: Ant pheromone activity: correlation with molecular shape by scanning computer. *Science, 165*:1266-1269, 1969.

Andersen, H.T., M. Funakoshi, and Y. Zotterman: Electrophysiological Responses to Sugars and Their Depression by Salt. In Zotterman, Y. (Ed.): *Olfaction and Taste, Proceedings of the First International Symposium.* Oxford, Pergamon, 1963, pp. 177-192.

Andres, K.H.: Über die Feinstruktur der Rezeptoren an Sinushaaren. *Z. Zellforsch.,* 75:339-365, 1966a.

Andres, K.H.: Der Feinbau der Regio Olfactoria von Makrosmatikern. *Z. Zellforsch.,* 69:140-154, 1966b.

Arduini, A., and L.R. Pinneo: Properties of the retina in response to steady illumination. *Arch. Ital. Biol.,* 100:425-448, 1962.

Arvanitaki, A., H. Takluchi, and N. Chalazonitis: Specific Unitary Osmereceptor Potentials and Spiking Patterns From Giant Nerve Cells. In Hayashi, T. (Ed.): *Olfaction and Taste, Proceedings of the Second International Symposium.* Oxford, Pergamon, 1967, pp. 573-598.

Autrum, H.: Nonphotic Receptors in Lower Forms. In Field, J. (Ed.): *Handbook of Physiology.* Washington, American Physiological Society, 1959, vol. 1, sect. 1, pp. 369-385.

Bannister, L.H.: The fine structure of the olfactory surface of teleostean fishes. *Quart. J. Micr. Sci.,* 106:333-342, 1965.

Bardach, J.E., and J. Case: Sensory capabilities of the modified fins of squirrel hake (*Urophycis chuss*) and searobins (*Prionotus carolinus* and *P. evolans*). *Copeia,* 2:194-206, 1965.

Barlow, H.B., and D.P. Andrews: Sensitivity of receptors and receptor "pools." *J. Opt. Soc. Amer.,* 57:837-838, 1967.

Barlow, H.B., and J.M.B. Sparrock: The role of afterimages in dark adaptation. *Science, 144*:1309-1314, 1964.

Bartoshuk, L.M., D.H. McBurney, and C. Pfaffmann: Taste of sodium chloride solutions after adaptation to sodium chloride: Implications for the "water taste." *Science, 143*:967-968, 1964.

Beidler, L.M.: Taste receptor stimulation. *Progr. Biophys. Biophys. Chem., 12*:107-151, 1961.

Beidler, L.M.: Anion Influences on Taste Receptor Response. In Hayashi, T. (Ed.): *Olfaction and Taste, Proceedings of the Second International Symposium.* Oxford, Pergamon, 1967, pp. 509-534.

Beidler, L.M., I.Y. Fishman, and C.W. Hardiman: Species differences in taste responses. *Amer. J. Physiol., 181*:235-239, 1955.

Békésy, G. von: A new audiometer. *Acta Otolaryng., 34*:411-422, 1947.

Békésy, G. von: *Experiments in Hearing.* New York, McGraw-Hill, 1960.

Békésy, G. von: The effect of adaptation on the taste threshold observed with a semiautomatic gustometer. *J. Gen. Physiol., 48*:481-488, 1965.

Benjamin, R.M.: Some Thalamic and Cortical Mechanisms of Taste. In Zotterman, Y. (Ed.): *Olfaction and Taste, Proceedings of the First International Symposium.* New York, Macmillan, 1963, pp. 309-329.

Bennett, M.V.L.: Mechanisms of Electroreception. In Cahn, P.H. (Ed.): *Lateral Line Detectors.* Bloomington, Indiana U. Pr., 1967, pp. 313-393.

Blümcke, S., and H. R. Niedorf: Electronenmikroskopische Untersuchungen an Lamellenkörpern im regenerierenden peripheren Nerven. *Beitr. Path. Anat., 131*:38-62, 1965.

Blümcke, S., H.R. Niedorf, and J. Rode: Axoplasmic alterations in the proximal and distal stumps of transsected nerves. *Acta Neuropath.,* 7:44-61, 1966.

Boeckh, J.: Elektrophysiologische Untersuchungen an einzelnen Geruchsrezeptoren auf der Antenne des Totengräbers (*Necrophorus, Coleoptera*). Dissertation der Naturwiss. Fak., Univ. München, 1962.

Boeckh, J.: Inhibition and Excitation of Single Insect Olfactory Receptors, and Their Role as a Primary Sensory Code. In Hayashi, T. (Ed.): *Olfaction and Taste, Proceedings of the Second International Symposium.* Oxford, Pergamon, 1967, pp. 721-735.

Boeckh, J., K.E. Kaissling, and D. Schneider: Insect olfactory receptors. In *Sensory Receptors. Cold Spring Harbor Symposia on Quantitative Biology, 30*:263-280, 1965.

Borg, G., H. Diamant, B. Oakley, L. Ström, and Y. Zotterman: A Comparative Study of Neural and Psychophysical Responses to Gustatory

Stimuli. In Hayashi, T. (Ed.): *Olfaction and Taste, Proceedings of the Second International Symposium.* Oxford, Pergamon, 1967, pp. 253-264.

Brammer, J.D., and R. H. White: Vitamin A deficiency: Effect on mosquito eye ultrastructure. *Science, 163*:821-823, 1969.

Bronshtein, A.A., and V.P. Ivanov: Electron optical study of the olfactory organ in the lamprey. *Zh. Evolyuts Biokhim. Fiziol., 1*:251-261, 1965.

Brown, K.T., and K. Watanabe: Neural stage of adaptation between the receptors and inner nuclear layer of monkey retina. *Science, 148*: 1113-1115, 1965.

Bujas, Z.: L'adaptation gustative et son mécanisme. *Acta Inst. Psychol. Univ. Zagreb, 17*: 1-10, 1953.

Bullock, T.H., and F.P. Diecke: Properties of an infra-red receptor. *J. Physiol. (London), 134*: 47-87, 1956.

Bullock, T.H., and D.A. Faulstick: Some properties of unit warm receptors. *Fed. Proc., 12*: 22, 1953.

Burkhardt, D.: Die Eigenschaften und Funktionstypen der Sinnesorgane. *Ergebn. Biol., 22*: 226-267, 1960.

Burkhardt, D.: Allgemeine Sinnesphysiologie und Elektrophysiologie der Receptoren. *Fortschr. Zool., 13*:146-189, 1961.

Burtt, E.T., W.T. Catton, and D.J. Cosens: Electrical Potential Field in Eye and Optic Lobe of Locust: Potential Variations and Changes in Visual Threshold During Light- and Dark-Adaptation. In Bernhard, C.G. (Ed.): *The Functional Organization of the Compound Eye.* Oxford, Pergamon, 1966, pp. 219-230.

Catton, W.T., and N. Petoe: A visco-elastic theory of mechanoreceptor adaptation. *J. Physiol. (London), 187*:35-49, 1966.

Creutzfeldt, O., and B. Sakmann: Neurophysiology of vision. *Ann. Rev. Physiol., 31*:499-544, 1969.

De Lorenzo, A.J.D.: Studies on the Ultrastructure and Histophysiology of Cell Membranes, Nerve Fibers and Synaptic Junctions in Chemoreceptors. In Zotterman, Y. (Ed.): *Olfaction and Taste, Proceedings of the First International Symposium.* Oxford, Pergamon, 1963, pp. 5-17.

Dethier, V.G.: Chemoreceptor mechanisms in insects. *Soc. Exp. Biol. Symp., 16*:180-196, 1962.

Dethier, V.G.: Introductory Remarks. Talk given at A.A.A.S. meeting, New York, Dec. 28, 1967a.

Dethier, V.G.: The hungry fly. *Psychology Today, 1*:65-72, 1967b.

Dethier, V.G., and A. Gelperin: Hyperphagia in the blowfly. *J. Exp. Biol., 47*:191-200, 1967.

Dethier, V.G., and F.E. Hanson: Taste papillae of the blowfly. *J. Cell. Comp. Physiol., 65*:93-100, 1965.

De Voe, R.: A Non-linear Model of Sensory Adaptation in the Eye of the Wolf Spider. In Bernhard, C.G. (Ed.): *The Functional Organization of the Compound Eye.* Oxford, Pergamon, 1966, pp. 309-328.

Dodge, Jr., F.A., B.W. Knight, and J. Toyoda: Voltage noise in *Limulus* visual cells. *Science, 160*:88-90, 1968.

Dodson, C.H., R.L. Dressler, H.G. Hills, R.M. Adams, and N.H. Williams: Biologically active compounds in orchid fragrances. *Science, 164*: 1243-1249, 1969.

Donner, K.O., and T. Reuter: Dark adaptation processes in the rhodopsin rods of the frog's retina. *Vision Res., 7*:17-41, 1967.

Dowling, J.E.: The site of visual adaptation. *Science, 155*:273-279, 1967a.

Dowling, J.E.: The Organization of Vertebrate Visual Receptors. In Allen, J.M. (Ed.): *Molecular Organization and Biological Function.* New York, Harper and Row, 1967b, pp. 186-210.

Dowling, J.E., and B.B. Boycott: Neural connections of the retina: Fine structure of the inner plexiform layer. In *Sensory Receptors. Cold Spring Harbor Symposia on Quantitative Biology, 30*:393-402, 1965.

Duncan, C.J.: The transducer mechanism of sense organs. *Naturwissenschaften, 51*:172-173, 1964.

Easter, S.S.: Adaptation in the goldfish retina. *J. Physiol. (London), 195*:273-281, 1968.

Eccles, J.C.: *The Physiology of Synapses.* Berlin, Springer-Verlag, 1964.

Echandia, E.L.R.: An electron microscopic study on the cochlear innervation. I. The receptoneural junctions at the outer hair cells. *Z. Zellforsch., 78*:30-46, 1967.

Egan, J.P.: Independence of the masking audiogram from the perstimulatory fatigue of an auditory stimulus. *J. Acoust. Soc. Amer., 27*: 737-740, 1955.

Eisner, T.: Cross-specific Chemical Communication. Talk given at A.A.A.S. meeting, New York, Dec. 28, 1967.

Emmers, R.: Modulation of the thalamic relay of taste by stimulation of the tongue with ice water. *Exp. Neurol.*, 16:50-56, 1966.

Engström, H.: The morphology of the normal sensory cells. In Collegium O.R.L.A.S. Lyon. *Acta Otolaryng.*, 63, Suppl. 5-19, 1967a.

Engström, H.: The ultrastructure of the sensory cells of the cochlea. *J. Laryng.*, 81:687-715, 1967b.

Erickson, R.P.: Sensory Neural Patterns and Gustation. In Zotterman, Y. (Ed.): *Olfaction and Taste, Proceedings of the First International Symposium*. Oxford, Pergamon, 1963, pp. 205-213.

Evans, D.R.: Chemical Structure and Stimulation by Carbohydrates. In Zotterman, Y. (Ed.): *Olfaction and Taste, Proceedings of the First International Symposium*. Oxford, Pergamon, 1963, pp. 165-176.

Evans, D.R., and D. Mellon, Jr.: Electrophysiological studies of a water receptor associated with the taste sensilla of the blowfly. *J. Gen. Physiol.*, 45:487-500, 1962a.

Evans, D.R., and D. Mellon, Jr.: Stimulation of a primary taste receptor by salts. *J. Gen. Physiol.*, 45:651-661, 1962b.

Farbman, A.I.: Fine structure of the taste bud. *J. Ultrastruct. Res.*, 12:328-350, 1965.

Flock, Å.: Ultrastructure and Function in the Lateral Line Organs. In Cahn, P.H. (Ed.): *Lateral Line Detectors*. Bloomington, Indiana U. Pr., 1967, pp. 163-197.

Florey, E.: Chemical transmission and adaptation. *J. Gen. Physiol.*, 40:533-545, 1957a.

Florey, E.: Further evidence for the transmitter function of Factor I. *Naturwissenschaften*, 44:424-429, 1957b.

Frisch, D.: Ultrastructure of mouse olfactory mucosa. *Amer. J. Anat.*, 121:87-120, 1967.

Fuortes, M.G.F.: Initiation of impulses in the visual cells of *Limulus*. *J. Physiol. (London)*, 148:14-28, 1959.

Fuortes, M.G.F., and A.L. Hodgkin: Changes in time scale and sensitivity in the ommatidia of *Limulus*. *J. Physiol. (London)*, 172:239-263, 1964.

Fuortes, M.G.F., and S. Yeandle: Probability of occurrence of discrete potential waves in the eye of *Limulus*. *J. Gen. Physiol.*, 47:443-463, 1964.

Gesteland, R.C., J. Y. Lettvin, W.H. Pitts, and A. Rojas: Odor specificities of the frog's olfactory receptors. In Zotterman, Y. (Ed.): *Olfaction and Taste, Proceedings of the First International Symposium*. Oxford, Pergamon, 1963, pp. 19-34.

Granit, R.: *Receptors and Sensory Perception*. New Haven, Yale U. Pr., 1955.

Granit, R.: *Sensory Mechanisms of the Retina*. New York, Hafner, 1963.

Gray, E.G., and K.C. Watkins: Electron microscopy of taste buds of the rat. *Z. Zellforsch.*, 66:583-595, 1965.

Graziadei, P.: Electron microscopic observations of the olfactory mucosa of the mole. *J. Zool. (London)*, 149:89-94, 1966.

Grignolo, A., N. Orzalesi, and G.A. Calabria: Studies on the fine structure and the rhodopsin cycle of the rabbit retina in experimental degeneration induced by sodium iodate. *Exp. Eye Res.*, 5:86-97, 1966.

Hahn, H.: Beiträge zur Reizphysiologie. Heidelberg, Scherer Verlag, 1949.

Hahn, J.F.: Tactile Adaptation. In Kenshalo, D.R. (Ed.): *The Skin Senses*. Proceedings of the First International Symposium. Charles C Thomas, Springfield, 1968a, pp. 322-330.

Hahn, J. F.: Low-frequency vibrotactile adaptation. *J. Exp. Psych.*, 78:655-659, 1968b.

Halpern, B.P.: Some Relationships Between Electrophysiology and Behavior in Taste; Notes. In Kare, M.R., and O. Maller (Eds.): *The Chemical Senses And Nutrition*. Baltimore, Johns Hopkins, 1967, pp. 213-241.

Halpern, B.P., R.A. Bernard, and M.R. Kare: Amino acids as gustatory stimuli in the rat. *J. Gen. Physiol.*, 45:681-701, 1962.

Hartline, H.K.: The dark adaptation of the eye of *Limulus*, as manifested by its electric response to illumination. *J. Gen. Physiol.*, 13:379-389, 1929.

Heist, H.E., B.D. Mulvaney, and D.J. Landis: Odor Sensing Cell Ultrastructure by Electron Microscopy, Final report to Air Force Office of Scientific Research, contract no. AF49 (638)-1618. Presented by Honeywell Inc., Corporate Research Center, Hopkins, Minn, 1967.

Hellekant, G.: Action and Interaction of Ethyl Alcohol and Some Other Substances on the Receptors of the Tongue. In Hayashi, T. (Ed.): *Olfaction and Taste, Proceedings of* the Second International Symposium. Oxford, Pergamon, 1967, pp. 465-479.

Hensel, H., and Y. Zotterman: The response of mechanoreceptors to thermal stimulation. *J. Physiol. (London),* 115:16-24, 1951.

Hodgson, E.S.: Electrophysiological studies of arthropod chemoreception. II. Responses of labellar chemoreceptors of the blowfly to stimulation by carbohydrates. *J. Insect Physiol.,* 1:240-247, 1957.

Hodgson, E.S.: Taste receptors. *Sci. Amer.,* 204: 135-144, 1961.

Hodgson, E.S.: The Chemical Senses and Changing Viewpoints in Sensory Physiology. In Carthy, J.D., and C.L. Duddington, (Eds.): *Viewpoints in Biology.* London, Butterworths, 1965, vol. 4, pp. 83-124.

Hodgson, E.S.: Chemical Senses in the Invertebrates. In Kare, M.R., and O. Maller (Eds.): *The Chemical Senses and Nutrition.* Baltimore, Johns Hopkins, 1967, pp. 7-18.

Hodgson, E.S., and K.D. Roeder: Electrophysiological studies of arthropod chemoreception. I. General properties of the labellar chemoreceptors of diptera. *J. Cell. Comp. Physiol.,* 48: 51-75, 1956.

Hodgson, E.S., and R.A. Steinhardt: Hydrocarbon Inhibition of Primary Chemoreceptor Cells. In Hayashi, T. (Ed.): *Olfaction and Taste, Proceedings of the Second International Symposium.* Oxford, Pergamon, 1967, pp. 737-748.

Hollenberg, M.J., and M.H. Bernstein: Fine structure of the photoreceptor cells of the ground squirrel *(Citellus tridecemlineatus tridecemlineatus). Amer. J. Anat.,* 118:359-374, 1966.

Hood, J.D.: Studies in auditory fatigue and adaptation. *Acta Otolaryng. (Suppl.),* 92:1-57, 1950.

Ishii, K., and T. Oosaki: Electron microscopy of the chemoreceptor cells of the carotid labyrinth of the toad. *Nature,* 212:1499-1500, 1966.

Ishikawa, S.: Responses of maxillary chemoreceptors in the larva of the silkworm, *Bombyx mori,* to stimulation by carbohydrates. *J. Cell. Comp. Physiol.,* 61:99-107, 1963.

Ishiko, N., and W.R. Loewenstein: Effects of temperature on the generator and action potentials of a sense organ. *J. Gen. Phys.,* 45:105-124, 1961.

Katz, B.: Action potentials from a sensory nerve ending. *J. Physiol. (London),* 111:248-260, 1950a.

Katz, B.: Depolarization of sensory terminals and the initiation of impulses in the muscle spindle. *J. Physiol. (London),* 111:261-282, 1950b.

Katz, B.: How cells communicate. *Sci. Amer.,* 205:209-220, 1961.

Kiang, N. Y-S., *et al.: Discharge Patterns of Single Fibers in the Cat's Auditory Nerve.* Res. Monograph 35. Cambridge, M.I.T. Pr., 1965.

Kimura, K., and L.M. Beidler: Microelectrode study of taste receptors of rat and hamster. *J. Cell. Comp. Physiol.,* 58:131-140, 1961.

Kimura, R., H.F. Schuknecht, and I. Sando: Fine morphology of the sensory cells in the organ of Corti of man. *Acta Otolaryng.,* 58:390-408, 1964.

Koitchev, K.A.: Electron-microscopic study of Corti's organ during relative quiet and after sound stimulation. *Arkh. Anat.,* 56:45-53, 1969.

Krnjević, K., and N.M. van Gelder: Tension changes in crayfish stretch receptors. *J. Physiol. (London),* 159:310-325, 1961.

Lacher, V.: Elektrophysiologische Untersuchungen an einzelnen Rezeptoren für Geruch, Kohlendioxyd, Luftfeuchtigkeit und Temperatur auf den Antennen der Arbeitsbiene und der Drohne *(Apis mellifica* L.), *Z. Vergl. Physiol.,* 48:587-623, 1964.

Landgren, S., G. Liljestrand, and Y. Zotterman: Chemical transmission in taste fibre endings. *Acta Physiol. Scand.,* 30:105-114, 1954.

Lenhoff, H.M.: Behavior, hormones and hydra. *Science,* 161:434-442, 1968.

Lippold, O.C.J., J.G. Nicholls, and J.W.T. Redfearn: Electrical and mechanical factors in the adaptation of a mammalian muscle spindle. *J. Physiol. (London),* 153:209-217, 1960.

Lissmann, H.W.: Electric location by fishes. *Sci. Amer.,* 208:50-59, 1963.

Loewenstein, W.R.: Biological transducers. *Sci. Amer.,* 203:98-108, 1960.

Loewenstein, W.R.: On the specificity of a sensory receptor. *J. Neurophysiol.,* 24:150-158, 1961a.

Loewenstein, W.R.: Excitation and inactivation in a receptor membrane. *Ann. N. Y. Acad. Sci.,* 94:510-534, 1961b.

Loewenstein, W.R., and M. Mendelson. Components of receptor adaptation in a Pacinian corpuscle. *J. Physiol. (London),* 177:377-397, 1965.

Loewenstein, W.R., and R. Skalak: Mechanical transmission in a Pacinian corpuscle. An analysis and a theory. *J. Physiol. (London), 182*: 346-378, 1966.

Lowenstein, O.: Functional aspects of vestibular structure. In de Reuck, A.V.S., and J. Knight (Eds.): *Ciba Foundation Symposium on Myotatic, Kinesthetic And Vestibular Mechanisms.* London, Churchill, 1967, pp. 121-128.

MacKay, D.M.: Neural communications: experiment and theory. *Science, 159*:335-353, 1968.

Marimont, R.B.: Numerical studies of the Fuortes-Hodgkin *Limulus* model. *J. Physiol. (London), 179*:489-497, 1965.

Matsnev, E.I., and I.Y. Yakovleva: Threshold adaptation in normal conditions and due to fatigue of the auditory analysor. *Vestn. Otorinolaring., 29*:22-26, 1967.

Matsusaka, T.: Lamellar bodies in the synaptic cytoplasm of the accessory cone from the chick retina as revealed by electron microscopy. *J. Ultrastruct. Res., 18*:55-70, 1967.

McBurney, D.H., and C. Pfaffmann: Gustatory adaptation to saliva and sodium chloride. *J. Exp. Psychol., 65*:523-529, 1963.

Mellon, Jr., D.F.: *The Physiology of Sense Organs.* San Francisco, Freeman, 1968.

Mendelson, M., and W.R. Loewenstein: Mechanisms of receptor adaptation. *Science, 144*: 554-555, 1964.

Missotten, L.: Étude des bâtonnets de la rétine humaine au microscope electronique. *Ophthalmologica, 140*:200-214, 1960.

Morita, H.: Initiation of spike potentials in contact chemosensory hairs of insects. III. D. C. stimulation and generator potential of labellar chemoreceptor of Calliphora. *J. Cell. Comp. Physiol., 54*:189-204, 1959.

Morita, H., and S. Yamashita: Generator potential of insect chemoreceptor. *Science, 130*:922, 1959.

Murray, R.G., and A. Murray: Fine structure of taste buds of rabbit foliate papillae. *J. Ultrastruct. Res., 19*:327-353, 1967.

Nagaki, J., S. Yamashita, and M. Sato: Neural response of cat to taste stimuli of varying temperatures. *Jap. J. Physiol., 14*:67-89, 1964.

Naka, K.I., and K. Kishida: Retinal Action Potentials During Dark and Light Adaptation. In Bernhard, C.G. (Ed.): *The Functional Organization of the Compound Eye.* Oxford, Pergamon, 1966, pp. 251-266.

Nemetschek-Gansler, H., and H. Ferner: Über die Ultrastruktur der Geschmacksknospen. *Z. Zellforsch., 63*:155-178, 1964.

Nicklaus, R.: Die Erregung einzelner Fadenhaare von *Periplaneta americana* in Abhängigkeit der Grösse und Richtung der Auslenkung. *Z. Vergl. Physiol., 50*:331-362, 1965.

Nishi, K., and M. Sato: Depolarizing and hyperpolarizing receptor potentials in the non-myelinated nerve terminal in Pacinian corpuscles. *J. Physiol. (London), 199*:383-396, 1968.

Norberg, Å.: Physical factors in directional hearing in *Aegolius funereus* (Linné) (Strigiformes), with special reference to the significance of the asymmetry of the external ears. *Arkh. Zool., 20*:181-204, 1968.

Oakley, B., and R.M. Benjamin: Neural mechanisms of taste. *Physiol. Rev., 46*:173-211, 1966.

Ogawa, H., M. Sato, and S. Yamashita: Multiple sensitivity of chorda tympani fibres of the rat and hamster to gustatory and thermal stimuli. *J. Physiol. (London), 199*:223-240, 1968.

Okano, M., A.F. Weber, and S.P. Frommes: Electron microscopic studies of the distal border of the canine olfactory epithelium. *J. Ultrastruct. Res., 17*:487-502, 1967.

Olney, J.W.: Centripetal sequence of appearance of receptor-bipolar synaptic structures in developing mouse retina. *Nature, 218*:281-282, 1968a.

Olney, J.W.: An electron microscopic study of synapse formation, receptor outer segment development, and other aspects of developing mouse retina. *Invest. Ophthal., 7*:250-268, 1968b.

Ottoson, D., and G.M. Shepherd: Experiments and Concepts in Olfactory Physiology. In Zotterman, Y. (Ed.): *Sensory Mechanisms, Progress In Brain Research.* Amsterdam, Elsevier, 1967, vol. 23, pp. 83-138.

Ozeki, M., and M. Sato: Changes in the membrane potential and the membrane conductance associated with a sustained compression of the non-myelinated nerve terminal in Pacinian corpuscles. *J. Physiol. (London), 180*: 186-208, 1965.

Pfaffmann, C.: De Gustibus. *Amer. Psychol., 20*: 21-33, 1965a.

Pfaffmann, C.: L'adaptation gustative. *Actualities Neurophysiol., 6*:85-97, 1965b.

Pinter, R.B.: Sinusoidal and delta function responses of visual cells in *Limulus* eye. *J. Gen. Physiol., 49*:563-593, 1966.

Rapuzzi, G., and A. Pedrini: Importanza dell' 'acetilcolina sull' attivazione dei ricettori linguali di Rana. *Boll. Soc. Ital. Biol. Sper., 39:* 1851-1853, 1963.

Rapuzzi, G., G. Ricagno, and U. Ventura: Influenza di alcuni aminoacidi sulla sensibilita dei ricettori gustativi di *Rana. Boll. Soc. Ital. Biol. Sper.,* 39:1853-1855, 1963.

Rose, J.E., and V.B. Mountcastle: Touch and Kinesthesis. In Field, J. (Ed.): *Handbook Of Physiology,* Washington, American Physiological Society, 1959, Vol. I, Sect. I, pp. 387-429.

Rubin, T.R., F. Griffin, and R. Fischer: A physicochemical treatment of taste thresholds. *Nature,* 195:362-364, 1962.

Ruck, P.: Retinal structure and photoreception. *Amer. Rev. Ent.,* 9:83-102, 1964.

Rushton, W.A.H.: The Ferrier Lecture: Visual adaptation. *Proc. Roy. Soc. [Biol.],* 162:20-46, 1965.

Sakai, K.: Studies on chemical transmission in taste fibre endings. I. The action of acetylcholinesterase on bitter taste. *Chem. Pharm. Bull. (Tokyo),* 12:1159-1163, 1964.

Sakmann, B., O. Creutzfeldt, and H. Scheich: An experimental comparison between the ganglion cell receptive field and the receptive field of the adaptation pool in the cat retina. *Pflügers Arch.,* 307:133-137, 1969.

Sato, M.: The Effect of Temperature Change on the Response of Taste Receptors. In Zotterman, Y. (Ed.): *Olfaction and Taste, Proceedings of the First International Symposium.* Oxford, Pergamon, 1963, pp. 151-164.

Schneider, D.: Insect olfaction: deciphering system for chemical messages. *Science, 163:* 1031-1037, 1969.

Schneider, D., G. Kasang, and K.E. Kaissling: Bestimmung der Riechschwelle von *Bombyx mori* mit Tritium-markiertem Bombykol. *Naturwissenschaften,* 55:395, 1968.

Schneider, D., V. Lacher, and K.E. Kaissling: Die Reaktionsweise und das Reaktionsspektrum von Riechzellen bei *Antheraea pernyi* (Lepidoptera, Saturniidae). *Z. Vergl. Physiol., 48:* 632-662, 1964.

Scholes, J.H.: Discrete subthreshold potentials from the dimly lit insect eye. *Nature, 202:* 572-573, 1964.

Schoonhoven, L.M., and V.G. Dethier: Sensory aspects of host-plant discrimination by lepidopterous larvae. *Arch. Néerland. Zool., 16:* 497-530, 1966.

Schwartzkopff, J.: Die Verarbeitung von Sinnes-

nachrichten im Organismus. *Naturw. Rdsch., 19:*401-407, 1966.

Shibuya, T., and S. Shibuya: Olfactory epithelium: Unitary responses in the tortoise. *Science,* 140:495-496, 1963.

Sjöstrand, F.: The ultrastructure of the retinal rod synapses of the guinea pig eye as revealed by three-dimensional reconstructions from serial sections. *J. Ultrastruct. Res.,* 2:122-170, 1958.

Smith, T.G., W.K. Stell, J.E. Brown, J.A. Freeman, and G.C. Murray: A role for the sodium pump in photoreception in *Limulus. Science,* 162:456-458, 1968.

Smith, T.G., W.K. Stell, and J.E. Brown: Conductance changes associated with receptor potentials in *Limulus* photoreceptors. *Science,* 162:454-456, 1968.

Spoendlin, H.: Submikroskopische Organisation der Sinneselemente im Cortischen Organ des Meerschweinchens. *Pract. Otorhinolaryng. (Basel),* 21:34-48, 1959.

Spoendlin, H.: The Organization of the Cochlear Receptor. In Rüedi (Ed.): *Advances In Oto-Rhino-Laryngology.* Basel, Karger, 1966, vol. 13.

Steinhardt, R.A.: Physiology of labellar electrolyte receptors of the blowfly, *Phormia regina.* New York, Columbia University, unpublished thesis, 1966.

Stürckow, B.: Über den Geschmackssinn und den Tastsinn von *Leptinotarsa decemlineata* Say (*Chrysomelidae*). *Z. Vergl. Physiol.,* 42:255-302, 1959.

Takagi, S.F., and K. Omura: Responses of the olfactory receptor cells to odours. *Proc. Japan Acad.,* 39:253-255, 1963.

Takeda, K.: The nature of impulses of single tarsal chemoreceptors in the butterfly, *Vanessa indica. J. Cell. Comp. Physiol.,* 58:233-245, 1961.

Taylor, R.E.: Effect of procaine on electrical properties of squid axon membrane. *Amer. J. Physiol.,* 196:1071-1078, 1959.

Tsuiki, T.: Studies on the perstimulatory loudness adaptation. *Intern. Audiol.,* 4:138-140, 1965.

Vries, H. de, and M. Stuiver: The Absolute Sensitivity of the Human Sense of Smell. In Rosenblith, W.A. (Ed.): *Sensory Communication.* New York, M.I.T. Pr. and John Wiley, 1961, pp. 159-167.

Wendler, L.: Über die Wirkungskette zwischen Reiz und Erregung. Versuche an den abdominalen Streckreceptoren des Flusskrebses. *Z. Vergl. Physiol.*, *47*:279-315, 1963.

Wersäll, J., Å. Flock, and P.-G. Lundquist: Structural basis for directional sensitivity in cochlear and vestibular sensory receptors. In *Sensory Receptors. Cold Spring Harbor Symposia on Quantitative Biology*, *30*:115-132, 1965.

Westheimer, G.: Spatial interaction in human cone vision. *J. Physiol. (London)*, *190*:139-154, 1967.

Wittich, B.A.: Experimental studies on auditory adaptation. *Intern. Audiol.*, 5:5-47, 1966.

Wolbarsht, M.L.: Electrical activity in the chemoreceptors of the blowfly. II. Responses to electrical stimulation. *J. Gen. Physiol.*, *42*:413-428, 1958.

Wolbarsht, M.L.: Electrical characteristics of insect mechanoreceptors. *J. Gen. Physiol.*, *44*: 105-122, 1960.

Wolbarsht, M.L.: Receptor sites in insect chemoreceptors. In *Sensory Receptors. Cold Spring Harbor Symposia on Quantitative Biology*, *30*: 281-288, 1965.

Wolbarsht, M.L., and F.E. Hanson: Electrical activity in the chemoreceptors of the blowfly. III. Dendritic action potentials. *Gen. Physiol.*, *48*:673-683, 1965.

Wolbarsht, M.L., and F.E. Hanson: Electrical and Behavioral Responses to Amino Acid Stimulation in the Blowfly. In Hayashi, I. (Ed.): *Olfaction and Taste, Proceedings of the Second International Symposium*. Oxford, Pergamon, 1967, pp. 749-760.

Wolbarsht, M.L., and S.S. Yeandle: Visual processes in the *Limulus* eye. *Ann. Rev. Physiol.*, *29*:513-542, 1967.

Yamashita, S., H. Ogawa, and M. Sato: Multimodal sensitivity of taste units in the rat. *Kumamoto Med. J.*, *20*:67-70,1967a.

Yamashita, S., H. Ogawa, and M. Sato: Analysis of responses of hamster taste units to gustatory and thermal stimuli. *Kumamoto Med. J.*, *20*:159-162, 1967b.

Yur'eva, G. Yu.: Role of macroenergetic compounds in the functioning of the taste receptors (Effect of substances altering energy metabolism on the functional activity of the taste receptors). *Vestn. Mosk. Univ. Ser. 6 Biol. Pochvoved.*, *22*:21-26, 1967.

Yur'eva, G. Yu.: Study of the adaptation mechanism of taste receptors. *Vestn. Mosk. Univ. Ser. 6 Biol. Pochv.*, *23*:45-52, 1968.

SUGGESTED READING

Békésy, G. von: *Sensory Inhibition*. Princeton, Princeton U. Pr., 1967.

Case, J.: *Sensory Mechanisms*. New York, Macmillan, 1966.

Florey, E.: *Nervous Inhibition*. Oxford, Pergamon, 1961.

Granit, R.: *Receptors and Sensory Perception*. New Haven, Yale U. Pr., 1955.

Mc Cashland, B.W.: *Animal Coordinating Mechanisms*. Dubuque, Wm. C. Brown, 1968.

Mellon, Jr. D.: *The Physiology of Sense Organs*. San Francisco, W.H. Freeman, 1968.

Schneider, D.: Insect olfaction: deciphering system for chemical messages. *Science, 163*: 1031-1037, 1969.

Schoonhoven, L.M., and V.G. Dethier: Sensory aspects of host-plant discrimination by lepidopterous larvae. *Arch. Néerland. Zool., 16*: 497-530, 1966.

Chapter IV

Inhibition

Inhibition through the action of other sense receptor cells, centrifugal nerve fibers or central inhibitory neurons is a significant phenomenon in sensory physiology.

Inhibition involving sense cells, or neurons in their proximity, is referred to as peripheral. Such peripheral inhibition may be due to action on the sense cells themselves or may be produced later at synapses.

Inhibition caused by nervous elements originating from the higher nuclei of sensory pathways (which elements may act at various levels) and by portions of the brain is known as central. Specialized neurons within parts of the brain also produce central inhibition.

The type of peripheral inhibition resulting from interaction between receptor cells (and between neurons) lying in more or less one layer is known as lateral inhibition. Lateral inhibition occurs between visual receptors (and neurons) in the vertebrate retina or between neighboring ommatidia to result in greater brightness contrast and more clear-cut contours. In the cochlea of the ear lateral inhibition between hair cells may produce sharper discrimination of pitch. In the skin lateral inhibition may be significant in permitting the perceptual localization of vibratory stimuli to their area of application.

It seems that generally a great deal of stimulus localization is dependent on lateral inhibition.

Lateral nerve fibers connecting neighboring receptors have been demonstrated in the retina, cochlea and skin. There are also interconnecting fibers between the nerve cells of almost all the neuron layers in the vertebrate retina, and there is lateral interaction at several afferent neuron levels in the skin.

Centrifugal control by efferent nerve fibers originating from a higher center and innervating a peripheral sense organ is a form of central inhibition. Centrifugal control is significant in the function of the retina, the cochlea and the gustatory receptors. Efferent (centrifugal) fibers have also been found in the peripheral vestibular and olfactory systems.

The activity of slowly adapting receptors is particularly inhibited by efferent impulses from the reticular substance of the brain stem.

Such centrifugal inhibition of the peripheral portions of sensory systems may play an important role in sensation and increase the capacity of sensory systems to respond delicately. This is true because the efferent nerve fibers which transmit centrifugal impulses represent a potential means of bringing feedback into many sensory systems.

Central inhibition can also be exerted by a higher center on an intermediate level of a sensory pathway. Thus higher brain centers may inhibit the contralateral olfactory bulb.

Inhibition in the brain is essential for the selection of the stimuli to be perceived among an excess of information impinging from the environment. If a cat's attention is directed from an acoustic to a visual, olfactory or tactile stimulus, the afferent potentials evoked in its cochlear nucleus by the acoustic stimulus are inhibited. Similar phenomena have been observed in the visual and tactile pathways and in the cerebral cortex. Thus, when attention shifts to a certain sensory stimulus, the impulses in the other sensory pathways are inhibited.

Habituation to stimuli results in a reduction of the afferent responses evoked by them in secondary neurons, at the thalamic level and in the cortex. Such habituation can be called forth by acoustic stimuli in the cochlear nucleus, by olfactory stimuli in the olfactory bulb, by visual stimuli in the retina and the higher levels of the visual pathway, and by tactile stimuli in the spinal cutaneous pathways.

Von Békésy (1967a) has proposed that at various levels of the sensory pathways inhibition and summation act to funnel excitation, which would otherwise spread laterally, into narrow neural routes. Such a funneling process, consisting of both a filtering of the total induced excitation by inhibition and its amplification by summation, should raise the signal-to-noise ratio.

According to von Békésy, funneling acts to produce localization and a low threshold. It also tends to reduce the level of the perception of differences between stimuli and decreases the rate at which the magnitude of sensation rises with increasing stimulus amplitude. The last effect should broaden the range over which a sensory system is differentially sensitive to include greater stimulus intensities.

Funneling may have both temporal and spatial attributes. Thus the proper timing of two sounds produces a funneling effect in directional hearing, and tactile, gustatory or olfactory sensation is localized to the area at which one of two stimuli was directed if the other stimulus is applied 1 msec later. Spatial funneling results in the summation of adjacent excitation and the inhibition of excitation which is further removed.

Von Békésy considers all stimuli to give rise to a central zone of sensation with a periphery of inhibition. He defines such a functional pattern as a neural unit.

Von Békésy (1967a), on the basis of psychological studies, believes only the beginning of a neural discharge to function in localization. He suggests that the inhibitory neural activity responsible for such localization is transmitted more rapidly than the impulses which produce an increase in sensation magnitude.

Funneling can be observed at the cortical level when information is gathered in a temporally discontinuous manner. A process similar to funneling seems to occur when sensations are projected beyond the body.

The term *funneling* is particularly fitting when vibrations applied to the skin on either side of a middle vibration are not perceived separately, but contribute to the magnitude of the sensation apparently emanating from the middle vibration. Similarly, in binaural hearing a sufficient time lag will localize a sound in one ear, but the sound stimulus to the other ear contributes to the total perceived loudness (von Békésy, 1959).

Beck (1967) clearly expresses von Békésy's concepts in a superior review of von Békésy's book, *Sensory Inhibition*.

Inhibition of receptor cells may take place through the action of stimulating substances themselves. These may act to hyperpolarize the receptor membrane, may inactivate the receptor, or may compete with other substances. Such inhibition through reactive substances is described in Sensitivities.

THE VISUAL SYSTEM

Peripheral Inhibition in Invertebrates

Lateral inhibition in a visual organ has been most successfully investigated in the compound lateral eye of the horseshoe crab (*Xiphosura* or *Limulus*). In this organism's eye the lateral interactions do not have the complexity of those in vertebrate retinas.

There are approximately 1,000 ommatidia in the compound lateral eye of *Limulus*. Each ommatidium is composed of about twelve retinular cells and the eccentric cell, a bipolar neuron whose dendrite is surrounded by the retinular cells (Fig. 4-1). The visual pigment of the horseshoe crab, a rhodopsin, is concentrated at the inner surfaces of the retinular cells, in their rhabdoms, adjacent to the eccentric cell dendrite. The eccentric cell and the retinular cells proximally give rise to axons which join those from other ommatidia to form the optic nerve.

Internal to the layer of ommatidia the eccentric cell axons and retinular cell axons give off small lateral branches which form a plexus of interconnecting nerve fibers (Fig. 4-1). This fiber plexus is the basis of the inhibitory interactions between ommatidia. The lateral axonal branches contain vesicles, indicating that transmission between ommatidia requires the crossing of a synapse by a chemical agent. The synapses are located in clumps of neuropile, and have the appearance of two-way synapses.

In the horseshoe crab the response of each ommatidium to light is reduced by the activity of the surrounding ommatidia. As the intensity of the light stimulus acting on its neighboring ommatidia is increased, the discharge frequency of an ommatidium falls (Fig. 4-2). This decrease in impulse frequency is only determined by the extent of surrounding impulse activity; it is independent of the degree to

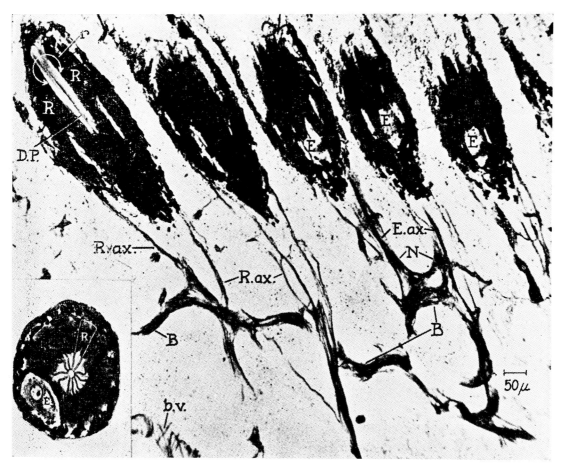

FIGURE 4-1. Photomicrograph of a section through a *Limulus* eye, showing several ommatidia and their connections. (*E*) Unstained eccentric cells, (*R*) retinular cells, (*r*) rhabdom, (*DP*) dendritic process of an eccentric cell, (*R. ax.*) retinular cell axons, (*E. ax.*) two of the thicker eccentric cell axons, (*B*) small axonal branches forming a plexus of lateral interconnections, (*N*) neuropile, in which synapses are located; (*b. v.*) blood vessel.

INSET. Cross-section of an ommatidium through the soma (E) of the eccentric cell. One of the retinular cells (R) is outlined, and the rhabdom has the appearance of the spokes of a wheel. (From Ratliff, F.: Inhibitory Interaction and the Detection and Enhancement of Contours. In Rosenblith, W.A. [Ed.]: *Sensory Communication.* Copyright 1961 by Massachusetts Institute of Technology.)

which the subject ommatidium has been excited and of its resulting discharge level. In turn, the absolute reduction in impulse frequency, irrespective of the level of discharge, is the best indicator of the inhibitory influences acting on an ommatidium.

Antidromic stimulation of *Limulus* optic nerve fibers has shown inhibition to be an S-shaped function of the frequency of the impulses giving rise to it (Lange, Hartline and Ratliff, 1966). This indicates that a sufficient rate of impulses can raise the degree of inhibition to a saturation level.

Antidromic stimulation of optic nerve fibers, rather than photic stimulation of nearby receptors, is used to call forth lateral inhibition when complete control of the temporal aspects of inhibition is needed.

An after discharge, a dark discharge provoked by the addition of ions to the medium in which the eye is bathed, and spontaneous activity are as effectively inhibited by neighboring ommatidia as is a normal response discharge. The same holds true for an impulse discharge produced by stimulating the eccentric cell with an intracellularly applied electric current.

It has been determined that inhibitory action ceases if the interommatidial nerve plexus is interrupted. The site of inhibition has seemed to lie distal to the nerve plexus in the ommatidium itself. However, an electrical model based on the changes in potential and resistance which occur during inhibition suggests that the last is accomplished in the branches of the eccentric cell axon (Purple and Dodge, 1965). This might actually put the site of inhibition as close to the point of presumed impulse generation, in the eccentric cell's axon near its origin from the soma, as if inhibition acted within the soma. In any case, inhibition acts in a visual unit at a level from which it can affect the unit's impulse generation.

The inhibition of an ommatidium gives rise to an inhibitory postsynaptic potential (IPSP) which hyperpolarizes the cell plasma membrane of its eccentric cell (see the action of inhibitory substances on insect olfactory receptors, in Sensitivities). The eccentric cell's membrane also undergoes a reduction in electrical resistance. Further, inhibition brings the membrane potential of weakly depolarized cells toward the normal resting potential (Hartline, Ratliff and Miller, 1961). A similar action has been described for inhibitory impulses in the section on the crustacean stretch receptor (Chap. II).

Concentrations of ethyl alcohol which do not abolish impulses in the axons of eccentric cells block lateral inhibition (MacNichol, Jr. and Benolken, 1956). Thus the synapses or axonal branches forming the lateral plexus have a higher sensitivity to ethyl alcohol than the eccentric cell axons.

Picrotoxin, a GABA (γ-aminobutyric acid) antagonist, also preferentially ends lateral inhibition (Adolph, 1966). However, if picrotoxin is applied in combination with GABA, inhibition is not prevented. These and other findings suggest that GABA is the transmitter substance released into the synapses of the lateral plexus.

The extent of an ommatidium's inhibition increases with the size of the area illuminated around it. Thus spatial summation of the impinging inhibitory actions takes place.

The inhibitory effect exerted by other ommatidia on the average increases with their proximity. Ommatidia which are further than 5 mm away from another have little or no interaction with it. Nevertheless, a few relatively distant ommatidia may show a stronger inhibitory action on an ommatidium than some of the closer units. The inhibitory effects on a *Limulus* ommatidium decrease more rapidly with distance in a dorsoventral direction than in an anteroposterior direction.

If each synaptic ending of the lateral plexus produces a definite amount of an inhibitory transmitter substance, such as GABA, the magnitude of lateral inhibition should be proportional to the number of endings acting on a subject visual unit. Greater distance could then on the average be associated with lower inhibitory action because it may result in a lower number of synaptic endings making con-

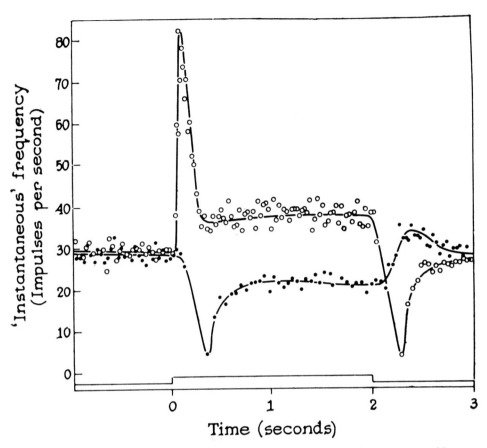

FIGURE 4-2. Simultaneous excitatory and inhibitory transients from two neighboring ommatidia (lateral eye, *Limulus*). The responses recorded from the eccentric cell axon of one ommatidium, which was illuminated steadily, are indicated by black dots. The other ommatidium (empty circles) was subjected to unvarying illumination until time 0, when the light intensity was suddenly raised to a higher level that was maintained for the indicated 2 seconds. Then the illumination was quickly reduced to the original level. The increase in light intensity caused the impulse rate to reach a marked peak. Then, because of adaptation, the frequency fell to a steady level above that of the original discharge rate. Reduction of the illumination to the original intensity was followed by a sizeable transient decrement in discharge frequency, whereupon the frequency rose to the level observed before time 0. The described excitatory transients were mirrored by inhibitory changes in the activity of the first ommatidium (black dots). When there was a precipitous drop in the impulse rate of the second ommatidium (empty circles) at time 2, the first showed a release from inhibition. Some mutual inhibition must be assumed. (From Ratliff, F.: Inhibitory Interaction and the Detection and Enhancement of Contours. In Rosenblith, W.A. [Ed.]: *Sensory Communication.* Cambridge, M.I.T. Pr., 1961, pp. 183-203.)

tact with the subject unit (Lange, Hartline and Ratliff, 1966).

A postinhibitory rebound in impulse rate (a true "off" response which is always present—

see Fig. 4-2) varies with distance as does the exerted inhibition.

The decrease in inhibitory effect with distance is also associated with a greater time delay in the exertion of this inhibition. However, a few preliminary experiments suggest that the impulse rate of the inhibiting ommatidia has a greater effect on the latent period of the inhibition than the distance (Ratliff, Hartline and Lange, 1966).

The latent periods for inhibition following antidromic stimulation may be several hundred milliseconds in length. Higher initial antidromic stimulation or a greater change in the level of such stimulation results in a shorter latent period.

Using antidromic stimulation, Lange, Hartline and Ratliff (1966) showed that the inhibition produced by a high rate of impulses was often followed by a long-lasting postinhibitory rebound. At medium impulse frequencies inhibition was not complete; instead, often the output of the subject ommatidium at first fell below a steady state level in a phenomenon named *undershoot*. On termination of inhibition a rapidly developing postinhibitory rebound was observed. At a rate of only 5 antidromic pulses per second, inhibition developed very slowly and no undershoot was present. However, inhibition ended quickly and was followed by a clear-cut postinhibitory rebound.

The fact that an undershoot at the onset of inhibition does not always balance an equivalent rebound at its end indicates that the inhibition system is not linear. Nonlinearity is also evidenced by the change in shape of the start of inhibition as the magnitude of the antidromic stimulation is varied. Although the steady state levels of inhibition can be described by n linear equations, the time-dependent responses to changes in stimulation have nonlinear components.

During another experiment a strong single antidromic volley produced an inhibition lasting for close to 200 msec in a test fiber bundle. This inhibition was followed by a postinhibitory rebound having approximately the same length.

Since very low antidromic stimulation (1-2 impulses/sec or 2 consecutive volleys) produces no inhibition, it is evident that there is a threshold for inhibition. The latent period preceding inhibition probably is partially due to the time required for passing the inhibitory threshold. A barrier which must be overcome, perhaps located in the synaptic cleft, the presynaptic ending or the site of action of the inhibitory transmitter agent in the postsynaptic membrane, may account for the inhibitory threshold (Lange, Hartline and Ratliff, 1966).

Thresholds for inhibition generally rise with the distance between the interacting ommatidia (Hartline, 1969).

The interaction between ommatidia is mutual. The inhibitory action of one ommatidium on nearby others depends on its level of impulse activity. This level is determined by the magnitude of the light stimulus received by the ommatidium and the extent of inhibition exerted on it by the other ommatidia. The extent of inhibition received from the other ommatidia in turn depends on their impulse frequencies, which are themselves affected by the influence of the first ommatidium.

Inhibitory actions are not only reciprocal but also appear to be recurrent (Hartline, Ratliff and Miller, 1961). Such recurrent inhibition is known from spinal reflexes.

When two widely separated groups of ommatidia both inhibit one ommatidium, their combined effect is greater than the sum of their separate effects. This is true because the greater reduction of the inhibited ommatidium's impulse frequency results in a lower reciprocal inhibitory action by it on the response discharges of the two groups, allowing each of them to in turn exert a greater inhibitory influence.

With the exception of the effects produced by reciprocal inhibition, the inhibitory influences originating from a variety of sources simply sum to reduce a receptor's discharge.

The inhibitory action of two ommatidia on each other, when they are subjected to an identical level of illumination, is often unequal and sometimes clearly one-sided. Yet in all cases, even when the two ommatidia are stimulated with different light intensities, the decrease in the impulse frequency of one ommatidium is directly related only to the response level of the other. The drop in impulse frequency is not a function of the stimulus intensity used on the inhibiting ommatidium.

The combined inhibitory actions between compact, moderately large groups of ommatidia show much more regularity.

The reciprocal inhibitory influences in the *Limulus* eye are complicated by the adaptation of the ommatidia to illumination. Also, a period of time must elapse before inhibition is initiated, inhibitory interactions must reach a mutual equilibrium, and inhibitory effects may show fluctuations in magnitude. In one experiment the discharge rate of an illuminated ommatidium fell 0.13 seconds after a burst of impulses was evoked in an inhibiting ommatidium, and 0.20 seconds after the last was stimulated with a flash of light.

When a test ommatidium and a large area surrounding it are illuminated, the test ommatidium's response shows a burst of impulses, followed by a precipitous drop in discharge frequency. Then the impulse rate returns to a higher level, but remains below the response shown at this time by an ommatidium illuminated by itself. The steep drop in frequency (silent period) is interpreted to reflect the original, preadaptation peak in the responses of the surrounding receptors which, after a latent period, gives rise to a transient, high inhibitory effect on the test ommatidium's response (Hartline, Ratliff and Miller, 1961).

Hartline, Ratliff and Miller (1961) developed a theoretical formulation, consisting of n simultaneous, linear equations, which describes the lateral inhibitory interaction in the *Limulus* (xiphosuran) eye. The equations have the form

$$M_s = r_s - \Sigma_c K_{s,c} (M_c - M^o_{s,c})$$

in which M_s is the response of a selected ommatidium, r_s is the response of this ommatidium in the absence of inhibition, and the subtracted term represents the summed inhibitory effects emanating from the close-by ommatidia c. Every one of the individual inhibitory effects is the product of the portion of

the response M_c that is above the threshold for inhibitory action $M^o_{s,c}$, times its respective inhibitory coefficient $K_{s,c}$.

The steady state equations were later modified to incorporate the temporal changes taking place in the system (Ratliff, Hartline and Lange, 1966). The set of modified, dynamic equations reads

$$M_s(t) = r_s(t) - \sum_{c=1}^{n} K_{s,c} [r_c(t - T_{s,c}) - M^o_{s,c}].$$

In the above the response M_s of a selected ommatidium at any time t is determined by the degree of excitation r_s shown by that ommatidium at time t, minus the summated inhibitory effects acting on it from the close-by ommatidia c. The mentioned effects emanated from the surrounding ommatidia c at a previous time $t - T_{s,c}$, the term $T_{s,c}$ representing the delay involved before the activity of any of the close-by ommatidia c takes effect on the test ommatidium s.

The values and sites of origin of the inhibitory actions (inhibitory coefficients K) impinging on a group of receptors from numerous locations in the surrounding area have been exactingly mapped by Barlow (1967).

Inhibitory actions, although delayed and reduced by distance, basically reflect a level of impulse-initiating excitation. However, previous inhibition may exert a facilitatory effect on inhibitory action.

If an ommatidium is subjected to a steady, low level of background inhibition by continuous, weak illumination of a nearby group of ommatidia, the inhibitory effect of a neighboring short, high-frequency impulse discharge is markedly enhanced. There is also a significant increase in the postinhibitory rebound. This increase in rebound may, in fact, compensate for the greater previous drop in impulse frequency due to facilitation of the inhibitory action.

If a short impulse discharge closely follows upon a first equivalent burst of impulses and its inhibitory action, the inhibitory effect of the second discharge is greatly heightened (Fig.

4-3). The shorter the time interval between the two bursts, the greater is the facilitation of the second inhibitory effect. If more than 4 seconds elapse between the impulse bursts, no facilitation of inhibition is observed. It is assumed that after the first inhibition some subthreshold inhibitory influence persists for a few seconds in the affected visual unit (Ratliff, Hartline and Lange, 1966).

The inhibitory effect of the second of two closely spaced impulse bursts has a considerably shorter latent period, even if its generating discharge has the lesser magnitude. The second burst's inhibitory effect also has a lower threshold.

Lange, Hartline and Ratliff (1966), on the basis of experiments involving the antidromic stimulation of optic nerve fibers, developed a theoretical, nonlinear model for the inhibitory effects produced by the illumination of *Limulus* ommatidia. The inhibitory effects were studied as complex functions of time, and the undershoot at onset, rebound at termination of inhibition, portions of the latent period, and facilitatory effects were all taken into consideration. The listed features of inhibition are indicative of the probable inadequacy of a linear model.

The mentioned model is expressed as both an integral equation, based on the steady state formulation, and a computer program. It assumes ommatidial activity to result from the summation of excitatory and inhibitory effects. It includes a threshold for the effects of a pool of lateral inhibitory influences, and this makes the model nonlinear. Above the mentioned threshold, inhibition develops in a linear manner (Lange, Hartline and Ratliff, 1966).

The results obtained by antidromic stimulation and with illumination-produced inhibition are sufficiently similar to indicate that the described model is equally applicable to both types of experiment.

By sufficiently strong antidromic stimulation of the optic fibers originating from neighboring receptors, Dodge, Jr., Knight and Toyoda (1969) subjected a test receptor to suprathreshold, sinusoidally modulated inhibition.

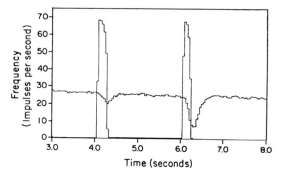

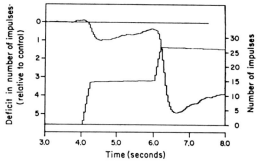

FIGURE 4-3. Facilitation of inhibition (*Limulus*). (Top) The unvarying illumination of an ommatidium gave rise to a relatively steady impulse frequency. Another ommatidium, approximately 0.5 mm away, was partially light adapted and subjected to two consecutive light flashes of unequal duration so as to produce two almost equal, compact bursts of impulses (at 4 and 6 sec). The inhibition exerted on the steadily illuminated ommatidium by the second impulse burst was noticeably augmented if it followed shortly after the first burst. (Bottom) Two consecutive step increases in the impulses produced by an adjacent ommatidium (right-side ordinate) elicited extremely unequal decreases in the impulse discharge of a test ommatidium (left ordinate). (From Ratliff, F., H.K. Hartline, and D. Lange: The Dynamics of Lateral Inhibition in the Compound Eye of *Limulus*. I. In Bernhard, C.G. [Ed.]: *The Functional Organization of the Compound Eye*. Long Island City, Pergamon, 1966, pp. 399-424.)

Since the effects produced by them exceeded threshold levels, they were then able to study their results by linear systems analysis.

Self-inhibition also occurs in the *Limulus* ommatidium (Ratliff, Hartline and Lange, 1966). Each impulse produced by the eccentric cell initiates an inhibitory potential in the same cell.

An impulse gives rise to an inhibitory potential by evoking an action potential which travels a circuitous route to return to, and affect, the impulse-generating portion of the eccentric cell axon. The action potential may be sent out in the eccentric cell's axon collateral (in the lateral plexus) to, in the neuropile, evoke the release of transmitter substance from the synaptic vesicles of the axon collateral's branches. The transmitter agent, after crossing a synapse, may initiate an incoming action potential in another part of the axon collateral or perhaps in other collaterals or in the eccentric cell axon itself. The endings in the lateral plexus are heavily endowed with synaptic vesicles, and a longer circuitous route is also possible (Purple and Dodge, 1966).

The self-inhibitory action potential results in a transient conductance increase in the eccentric cell's membrane, which lasts 400 to 500 msec and hyperpolarizes the membrane. This hyperpolarization can delay the appearance of another eccentric cell impulse.

Some aspects of the membrane conductance increases which take place during self-inhibition are most compatible with a chemical synaptic origin for self-inhibition. For example, the conductance increases, unlike those produced by accommodation, can summate. The change in resistance is a linear function of the change in membrane potential resulting from conductance increases. Further, the decay of the conductance increases has a time course similar to that for the synaptic lateral inhibition.

Also, the equilibrium potential for self-inhibition has a value similar to that of the equilibrium potential for lateral inhibition.

The development of an IPSP (inhibitory postsynaptic potential) following an eccentric cell impulse, to be expected after chemical mediation of an inhibitory potential across a synapse, is not normally discernible. However, in special preparations a slow, IPSP-like component of the spike after-potential can be demonstrated (Purple and Dodge, 1966).

The self-induced inhibitory potentials probably decay exponentially, and, as in the case of lateral inhibition, their sum may persist through a large number of interspike intervals.

Self-inhibition exerts a stronger effect on the eccentric cell than does lateral inhibition. Thus the entire optic nerve had to be stimulated antidromically with 30 pulses/sec to produce the increase in inhibitory conductance called forth by stimulating the eccentric cell directly with 15 short depolarizing pulses per second.

Self-inhibition may well play the primary role in the development of a steady state during light adaptation. The considerable negative feedback supplied to the eccentric cell by self-inhibition may be significant in producing stable responses in the steady state.

When the sudden action of lateral inhibition on a receptor causes its impulse discharge to fall, it will concomitantly produce a drop in the level of self-inhibition. This will partly counteract the effects of the lateral inhibition (Hartline, 1969).

Since lateral inhibition has a shorter time constant than self-inhibition, there is normally an undershoot when lateral inhibition quickly rises, and postinhibitory rebound when it falls. The existence of a threshold for lateral inhibition tends to reduce the undershoot and enhance the postinhibitory rebound (Hartline, 1969).

Self-inhibition, like other forms of synaptic activity, emphasizes a portion of the presynaptic information.

It will be interesting to see whether self-inhibition is present in a variety of animal eyes.

Reciprocal inhibition between visual receptors has the effect of increasing brightness contrast and sharpening contours.

If a brightly lit shape is projected on the retinal mosaic of *Limulus*, the receptors at the edge of the strongly illuminated area will have a much greater response than those adjacent ommatidia receiving considerably less light. Since the inhibitory action exerted by an ommatidium is a linear function of its impulse frequency, the highly stimulated receptors will inhibit their weakly illuminated neighbors much more strongly than vice versa. As a result the high response of the receptors at the illuminated area's periphery will undergo relatively little reduction due to inhibition, while the already low discharge of the nearby poorly illuminated ommatidia will be noticeably reduced by the strong inhibitory action of the neighboring highly illuminated receptors. Thus the inequality of the mutual inhibition across a border between different levels of stimulation increases the brightness contrast between differently illuminated areas in the visual field.

Furthermore, as a consequence of the low inhibition from the weakly stimulated receptors, the receptors at the highly illuminated area's periphery will have a greater response discharge than the receptors deeper within the highly illuminated area. Similarly, because of their proximity to receptors with a large discharge and strong inhibitory action, the receptors at the edge of the region of low illumination will produce impulses at a lower rate than the receptors deeper within this region (Fig. 4-4). The effect of these adjacent zones of, respectively, unusually high and low discharges, one on each side of every border between differently illuminated areas, is to accentuate contours.

Self-inhibition should reduce the enhancement of contrast and contour produced by lateral inhibition.

The mentioned zones of outstandingly high and markedly low discharge flanking the edges of differently illuminated areas result in the appearance to the human eye of bands of higher and lower brightness. Such bordering bands are known as Mach bands.

The increase in contrast and the emphasis of contour, as produced in a visual image at the edges of objects by the inhibitory interaction between visual receptors, should be of considerable value to the organism. These effects represent a first step in the modification of the incoming image by components of the visual pathway.

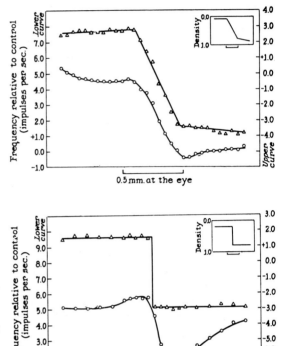

FIGURE 4-4. Counterparts of Mach's bands from the *Limulus* eye. (Top) Relative discharge rate of a receptor as a pattern composed of two areas of unlike brightness and an intermediate transitional zone (inset, upper right) was shifted past the receptor by degrees. The higher (rectilinear) graph indicates the impulse frequency when all the other receptors were masked. This graph directly reflects the intensity distributions in the pattern. When there was no masking (lower graph), maximum and minimum discharge rates were called forth by the zones at which Mach's bands appear to man. (Bottom) A pattern having no transitional zone between its bright and dark areas was also employed (inset, upper right). Again, masking of the other units caused a receptor's impulse rate to mirror the distribution of light intensities (higher graph). In the absence of masking (lower graph), the border zones of the bright and dark areas produced highly accentuated maxima and minima of impulse frequency, apparently equivalent to Mach's bands in human vision. (From Ratliff, F., and H.K. Hartline: The responses of *Limulus* optic nerve fibers to patterns of illumination on the receptor mosaic. *J. Gen. Physiol.*, 42:1241-1255, 1959.)

The fact that the degree of inhibitory interaction is dependent on the distance between groups of ommatidia may play an important role in pattern vision. Also, lateral and self-inhibition, by heightening the effect of light transients, might considerably increase the organism's sensitivity to movement in the visual field. Further, both forms of inhibition should raise the range of differential response of *Limulus* ommatidia to higher intensities of illumination. The intensity of the maximum, saturating stimulus should be greater as a consequence of inhibition, since the last can reduce the frequency of an impulse response to below the physiological limit of an axon.

In the *Limulus* eye lateral inhibition also has the following effects: It causes an increase in the illuminated area to be accompanied by a reduction in the size of the flicker response to low-frequency modulation of the light. At medium frequencies of modulation it causes enlargement of the illuminated area to produce an increase in the size of the flicker response (Ratliff *et al.*, 1967). When the illuminated area is enlarged, more inhibitory influences act on a test ommatidium.

The second amplification effect can be understood on the basis of the delay between the response of ommatidia and their inhibitory action on other ommatidia. The responses and inhibitory effects may be out of phase to varying degrees. At the medium frequencies the inhibitory action is greatest and the response smallest for a large area, and this results in the largest amplitude of the flicker response.

Thus lateral inhibition not only magnifies spatial differences in illumination, as discussed previously, but also emphasizes variations in the temporal pattern of a light stimulus.

Lateral inhibition can be said to sharpen spatial and temporal resolution, and it provides for greater versatility of response. It has an integrative action on the spatial and temporal aspects of the receptor response.

Therefore, the interaction between visual receptors gives rise to new and important functional properties of the eye.

In *Limulus* lateral interactions are only inhibitory in nature.

Hartline, Ratliff and Miller (1961), Ratliff (1961) and Hartline (1969) have written outstanding articles on lateral visual inhibition in *Xiphosura* (*Limulus*), and Wolbarsht and Yeandle (1967) review all aspects of Xiphosuran visual reception.

Retinal inhibition also has the significant function of making possible "off" discharges.

The retinas of most animals, including lower invertebrates, respond with nerve impulse activity to shadows or the termination of a light stimulus. It appears that in at least a number of cases illumination inhibits an impulse discharge, which subsequently occurs when the exposure of the retina to light ceases.

During a photic stimulus inhibitory potentials transmitted across synapses to retinal neurons reduce the elicited impulse frequency. When the illumination is terminated, inhibition ceases, permitting the development of a ganglion cell "off" discharge. Such "off" discharges are important in the perception of movement and in lower animals are frequently followed by escape or protective responses.

"Off" or "on-off" responses do not occur naturally in the *Limulus* eye, but may be artificially produced by providing a proper combination of carefully selected excitatory and inhibitory influences (Hartline, Ratliff and Miller, 1961). These influences include time delays and postinhibitory rebounds.

On the other hand, recordings made from the optic lobe of the *Limulus* brain, sufficiently posterior to the point of entrance of the optic nerve, show clear "off" and "on-off" responses (Wilska and Hartline, 1941). Apparently neural interactions similar to those which produce "off" and "on-off" discharges in the vertebrate retina take place in the horseshoe crab's brain.

In certain Mollusca responses to the cessation of a light stimulus are produced via a different mechanism.

In clams the pallial nerve circles along the edge of the mantle and then enters the visceral ganglion. In the surf clam *Spisula* a single fiber of the pallial nerve shows a spontaneous discharge of 5 impulses/sec in darkness. On illumination this discharge ends, and a burst of impulses follows the termination of illumination.

The described "off" response of *Spisula* originates from a single pallial nerve neuron. It seems that the total light reaction of this neuron consists of an excitatory component dependent on a primarily red-sensitive pigment, and an inhibitory component mediated by a pigment most sensitive to blue light. During a white light stimulus the inhibitory component prevents a response. On cessation of stimulation the inhibitory component falls faster than the excitatory component, permitting the development of the "off" burst of impulses (Kennedy, 1963).

Thus in *Spisula* inhibition is a primary event, as it takes place within the receptor neuron. Primary inhibition also occurs in the receptor cells of the outer layer of the retina of the scallop *Pecten*.

Toyoda and Shapley (1967), recording intracellularly, found that when certain retinal cells of the scallop were illuminated, they underwent hyperpolarization. The last had an estimated equilibrium potential of −70 to −80 mV. The resting potential of the cells was −30 to −40 mV.

Gorman and McReynolds (1969) conducted a more complete investigation of the "off" and also the "on" responses in the retina of the scallop (*Aequipecten irradians*, previously known as *Pecten irradians*). By means of intracellular and extracellular recording, they essentially confirmed earlier evidence that the photoreceptors of the outer, distal layer of the retina respond to a decrease of illumination, while the photoreceptors of the proximal retinal layer fire upon being illuminated or are the source of the "on" response.

The cells in the distal layer responded to a light flash with a hyperpolarizing potential (Fig. 4-5C), which developed 15 to 25 msec after the start of the light flash. In the distal cells which continued to discharge after electrode penetration, the hyperpolarizing potential was associated with an absence of firing.

However, when these last cells were exposed to long flashes, they produced a burst of spikes as the hyperpolarizing potential dissipated. The termination of a light stimulus also resulted in a transient discharge.

Gorman and McReynolds (1969), as well as Toyoda and Shapley (1967), discount a synaptic origin of the hyperpolarization.

The photoreceptors in the proximal layer of the retina underwent depolarization on illumination (Fig. 4-5B). The depolarizing potential had a longer latency (30-80 msec), and also a greater rise time (Fig. 4-5B, C), than the hyperpolarizing potential.

Both the distal and proximal layer cells, which differ in structure, had similar resting potential levels.

Thus the scallop possesses two types of photoreceptors which have opposing responses to light. The potentials recorded extracellularly from two depths of the scallop's retina on light stimulation can be seen in Figure 4-5D. Both traces were recorded simultaneously, the upper one stemming from the more proximal electrode.

Vertebrate cones have also been noted to respond to illumination with hyperpolarization.

In the sea hare *Aplysia* some central ganglion neurons exhibit a reduced spontaneous discharge on exposure to light, while others are excited. The sea urchin *Diadema* shows its "off" response when a shadow falls on particular peripheral nerves.

Certain species of worms and mollusks are especially prone to hide or flee from contoured shadows which have the size, speed and type of movement characteristic of an enemy organism. Thus particularly the scallop (*Pecten*) swims off when a starfish casts its shadow on a group of invertebrates (Boernstein, 1967). Von Buddenbrock (1958) refers to the "biological alarm signal" of the shadow phenomenon.

The Structure and Functional Organization of the Vertebrate Retina

In order to deal with the inhibitory mechanisms which are operative in the vertebrate

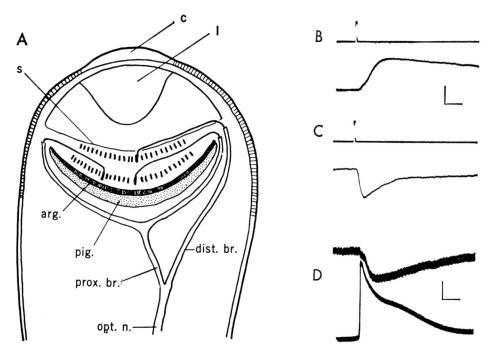

Figure 4-5. Potentials from the retinal receptors of the scallop (*Aequipecten*). A. Diagrammatic section of the eye. One receptor in the distal layer of the retina and two in the proximal layer are magnified, and the courses of their axons to the appropriate branches of the optic nerve are shown. The cornea (*c*), lens (*l*) and septum (*s*) are peripheral to the double-layered retina. Central to it lie the reflecting argentea (*arg.*) and the pigment layer (*pig.*). The distal and proximal layers of the retina are respectively the origins of the distal (*dist. br.*) and proximal (*prox. br.*) branches of the optic nerve (*opt. n.*). B. Intracellular, proximal-layer recording of depolarizing potential. C. Intracellular, distal-layer recording of hyperpolarizing potential. Upper traces of B and C record the light flash. Calibration—B and C: 10 mV, 100 msec. D. Simultaneous extracellular recording of proximal (upper) and distal (lower) retinal responses. Calibration for upper trace 0.5 mV, 100 msec; lower trace 1 mV, 100 msec. (From Gorman, A.L.F. and J.S. McReynolds: Hyperpolarizing and depolarizing receptor potentials in the scallop eye. *Science, 165*:3890, 309-310, 1969 [Copyright 1969 by the American Association for the Advancement of Science].)

retina, it is first necessary to review the structure and functional organization of this organ.

The visual receptors form the outermost or receptor layer of the vertebrate retina. Because of retinal inversion, light has to pass through the retina's neural layers to reach the receptors, and these face the "wrong way." The receptors form axo-axonic contacts with each other, and these may be electrotonic junctions (Dowling and Boycott, 1966). Interior to the receptors, toward the posterior chamber of the eye, are found two types of laterally oriented neurons,

the more externally located horizontal cells and the inner amacrine cells. Vertically oriented neurons, the bipolar cells, connect visual receptors with the innermost element of the retina, the retinal ganglion cells (Fig. 4-6). The last give rise to the axons which form the optic nerve.

The vertebrate retina can be divided into three main layers of cellular elements—the subdivided receptor layer (this includes the outer nuclear layer), the inner nuclear layer, and the ganglion cell layer. Interposed be-

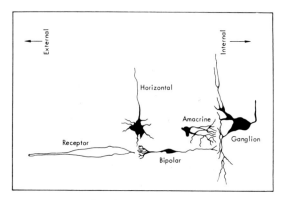

FIGURE 4-6. The five primary types of retinal neurons. (From MacGregor, R.J.: Neural organization in the primate retina. RM-4912-ARPA, The Rand Corp., Santa Monica, 1967.)

tween the receptors and the inner nuclear layer lies a layer of synaptic connections, the outer plexiform layer. An inner plexiform layer contains synaptic connections between the elements of the inner nuclear layer and the retinal ganglion cells (Fig. 4-7).

The horizontal cells, amacrine cells and bipolar cells are all found in the inner nuclear layer of the retina. The horizontal cells are in the external edge of this layer, while the amacrine cells lie close to its inner border (Fig. 4-7).

Horizontal cells have a lateral orientation, and their branches may spread over a distance of 1 mm. Typically their dendrites terminate in small baskets, each of which has been said to synapse with one cone. Along the periphery of the retina a horizontal cell's dendrites are described as synapsing with a few dozen cones, while in the central fovea they are reported to make contact with six or fewer cones (Polyak, 1957). The long axons (a few hundred microns) of horizontal cells appear to synapse with both cones and rods. The axons end in arborizations which ramify over a wider area than that covered by the dendrites.

Horizontal cell processes have also been found to make contact with each other (Dowling and Boycott, 1966, could not confirm this from the primate retina) and with bipolar cell bodies and their processes. Horizontal cell processes are said to form a lateral plexus.

The bodies of bipolar cells are vertically oriented. These cells lie across the inner nuclear layer. A single dendritic stem extends into the outer plexiform layer, where it ramifies, perhaps over a distance of 50μ, close to the synaptic terminals of the visual receptors. An axon runs into the inner plexiform layer to make contact with retinal ganglion cells.

Polyak (1957) reports the dendritic arborization of a bipolar cell to synapse with several receptors. A single visual receptor also synapses with a few bipolar cells. The majority of bipolar cells are served by several retinal ganglion cells. Sjöstrand (1965) estimates that each bipolar cell has at least seventy synaptic junctions.

Dowling and Boycott (1965) found bipolar axons to typically synapse with both a ganglion cell dendrite and an amacrine cell process. They called these synapses with two cells dyad synapses. Bipolar axons also formed axosomatic synapses having no visible intercellular space with retinal ganglion cells, suggesting electrotonic transmission. Dowling and Boycott further noted an occasional connection between two bipolar axons.

The dendritic stem of some bipolar cells terminates in a peculiar club-shaped process, Landolt's club, which bears a single cilium. The function of Landolt's club is not yet known (Hendrickson, 1966). Bipolar cells equipped with Landolt's club are very common in the pigeon (Runge, Uemura and Viglione, 1968).

There are seven layers of bipolar cells 3 mm from the fovea of the pigeon retina (Runge, Uemura and Viglione, 1968).

The laterally oriented amacrine cells lack axons. They possess dendrites which enter the inner plexiform layer. The two to several dendrites branch and spread over a diameter of 100μ to 300μ. Their innermost ramifications at times form junctions with the soma of retinal ganglion cells. Synapses between amacrine processes are frequent in the chicken retina (Dowling and Boycott, 1965), but may not be present in the primate retina. It has also been suggested that interactions of a non-

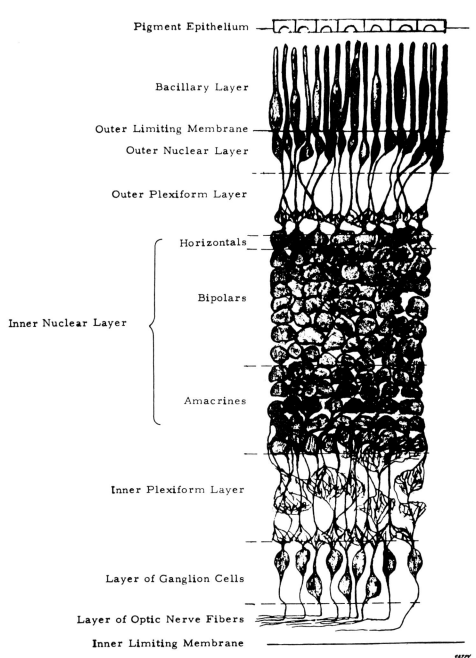

Pigment Epithelium

Bacillary Layer

Outer Limiting Membrane
Outer Nuclear Layer

Outer Plexiform Layer

Horizontals

Bipolars

Inner Nuclear Layer

Amacrines

Inner Plexiform Layer

Layer of Ganglion Cells

Layer of Optic Nerve Fibers

Inner Limiting Membrane

FIGURE 4-7. The neural layers of the vertebrate retina. The rods and cones of the bacillary and outer nuclear layers synapse with horizontal and bipolar cells of the inner nuclear layer in the outer plexiform layer. The inner plexiform layer is the zone of contact between amacrine and bipolar cells of the inner nuclear layer and the retinal ganglion cells. (From Runge, R.G., M. Uemura, and S.S. Viglione: Electronic synthesis of the avian retina. I. E. E. E. Trans. Bio-Med. Engineering, BME-15, pp. 138-151.)

synaptic nature occur between neighboring amacrine cells (Negishi and Svaetichin, 1966).

Beyond bipolar axon-amacrine dendrite synapses, the amacrine dendrite connects with an additional cell process, so that the first-mentioned contact can be considered presynaptic. Amacrine processes also form presynaptic contacts with bipolar axons that then synapse with ganglion dendrites. In at least most cases the amacrine dendrite of a bipolar-amacrine-retinal ganglion synapse makes another connection (reciprocal synapse) with the bipolar axon. An amacrine-bipolar synapse is also frequently next to a bipolar-amacrine junction (Dowling and Boycott, 1966). It thus seems that bipolar axons may synapse on amacrine dendrites, and vice versa. The amacrine dendrites exhibit a cluster of vesicles at the points of synaptic contact (Dowling and Boycott, 1965).

The many instances of apparent presynaptic contacts on the part of amacrine dendrites suggest an inhibitory role for the amacrine cell (presynaptic inhibition). Presynaptic facilitation is also possible.

Birds possess more amacrine cells than primates. There are five layers of amacrine cells 3 mm from the pigeon's fovea (Runge, Uemura and Viglione, 1968).

Castro (1966) has obtained excellent photographs of three kinds of amacrine cells in the retinas of embryonic and young chickens.

The innermost layer of the retina, adjacent to the posterior chamber of the eye, is composed of retinal ganglion cells. The dendrites of these cells run into the inner plexiform layer, and their ramifications may extend over a length of up to 700μ. Ganglion cells with very extensive dendritic fields typically give rise to three to five major dendrites, while those with very restricted fields, cells which are usually near the fovea, have but one main dendrite (Leicester and Stone, 1967). Over most of the chimpanzee retina the retinal ganglion cells form a single layer, but the number of layers increases toward the margin of the fovea, where there are eight to ten cell layers (Carpenter, 1967). The ganglion cells' axons

cross the inner surface of the retina to converge at the optic disc (blind spot) and become the optic nerve.

The four described types of neurons which make up the vertebrate retina interior to the receptor layer have been divided into a number of subgroups. Many of these subtypes could have functional specializations.

The functions of the horizontal and amacrine cells, beyond the fact that they form a feltwork of lateral interconnections, are particularly poorly understood at present.

Dowling and Boycott (1965) hypothesize that the horizontal and amacrine cells may provide for lateral interaction in the vertebrate eye, producing Mach bands (border contrast).

Since there are reciprocal synapses between bipolar and amacrine cells, it may be possible for nearby bipolar cells to act on each other reciprocally through amacrine cells. Bipolar cells could thus modulate each other's activities. Feedback (negative or positive) to bipolar or amacrine cells may therefore have the role of making lateral and reciprocal interactions between bipolar cells possible. These interactions would be presynaptic (Dowling and Boycott, 1966).

If the transmission of impulses from a bipolar cell to an amacrine cell in turn gives rise to inhibitory feedbacks from the amacrine cell to the same bipolar cell, the sensitivity or gain of the bipolar cell could be reduced in proportion to its degree of excitation. The adaptation of bipolar cells might result from this mechanism (Dowling, 1967).

The horizontal cells could be the basis of lateral and reciprocal presynaptic interaction between the visual receptors. They may also permit feedback to occur.

On the basis of experimental hyperpolarization of turtle retina horizontal cells, Byzov (1967) believes the horizontal cells to regulate transmission across the synapses between the photoreceptors and the bipolar cells. He suggests that this regulation takes place through currents generated in the horizontal cells' post-synaptic membranes.

The circular area of the retina which transmits its excitatory potentials to a single retinal ganglion cell comprises the receptive field of that cell. In mammals such receptive fields most commonly consist of a circular central portion and an antagonistic concentric peripheral zone. Separate stimulation of these two portions of a characteristic receptive field gives rise to opposite responses by the ganglion cell.

The areas of these two parts of typical receptive fields vary in different regions of the retina; as the fovea is approached, the central portions of the fields become smaller. Also, there is a lower number of receptors and connecting neurons per retinal ganglion cell within the central region of the primate retina (Rohen and Castenholz, 1967). In this region the ganglion cell dendrites and bipolar cell terminals do not spread over as large an area.

There is reason to believe that the receptors of the central portion of each receptive field transmit their responses to the field's ganglion cell "vertically," by way of bipolar cells. On the other hand, the peripheral zone's receptor responses may travel laterally from the bipolar cells through amacrine cells to the ganglion cell. The amacrine cells, by synapses with the retinal ganglion cell, could evoke an opposed response in the ganglion cell when the peripheral field is stimulated (Dowling and Boycott, 1966). A similar scheme is espoused by Brown and Major (1966).

The amacrine cells, and also perhaps the horizontal cells, may thus commonly have the function of transmitting antagonistic, often inhibitory, potentials to the ganglion cell.

It has been possible to identify a chromatic response, the result of two antagonistic potentials, with the bipolar cell layer (inner nuclear layer) of the goldfish (Mac Nichol, Jr., 1966).

Hiwatashi, Yasuda and Nagata (1967), and Yasuda and Hiwatashi (1968), have developed a model for the information-processing mechanism operative in vertebrate vision. They assume that the retinal neurons are connected in series (temporally) and in parallel (spatially), so that overlapping circular receptive fields are organized. The neural networks are

regarded as composed of excitatory and inhibitory neurons. The inhibitory neurons are considered to be horizontal cells or amacrine cells, and it is supposed that they have a higher response time and threshold than the excitatory neurons. The inhibitory neurons also are assumed to be more easily saturated than their excitatory counterparts. The results from the model agree well with data for the Mach phenomenon, and with the temporal and spatial frequency responses reported for human vision.

An electronic model which can, to a significant measure, duplicate the visual data processing of the bird's retina has been constructed by Runge, Uemura and Viglione (1968). All six types of pigeon retinal ganglion cells are represented in the model. The electrical output of a total of 145 cone analogs finally converges on seven ganglion cell analogs. The model represents a postulated mode of operation for cone retinas.

The neural pathways of the retina converge on a relatively small number of retinal ganglion cells, whose axons then make up a similarly restricted number of optic nerve channels. There are also multiple pathways leading from each receptor to the ganglionic dendrites in the inner plexiform layer. This suggests to Sjöstrand (1965) that the inner plexiform layer is the site of the selection and coding of the retinal impulses. Each of a number of circuit groups in the inner plexiform layer could code for one of the basic qualities of the received image.

Pedler (Discussion, Sjöstrand, 1965) would instead place the processes of information selection, coding and integration in the outer plexiform layer. He would only leave a few functions, such as impulse delay to change spatial into temporal resolution, to the inner plexiform layer. This would avoid the mixing of the incoming signals with the large amount of retinal spontaneous activity. However, Sjöstrand (Discussion) feels that the outer plexiform layer, with its bipolar cell branches and horizontal cells (according to one system of retinal layers), lacks the necessary complexity for performing the bulk of information processing.

The inner plexiform layer contains the majority of retinal synapses and thus has the greatest complexity. In the pigeon the inner plexiform layer not only shows much more profuse dendritic branching than the outer plexiform layer but has five times the thickness of the last (Runge, Uemura and Viglione, 1968).

Sjöstrand regards the outer plexiform layer only as the site of short- and medium-range direct lateral interactions between receptors and of long-distance lateral interactions by means of horizontal cells.

The impulses fed into the information-processing layer of the retina are themselves the product of interactions in the lateral plexus of connections between the visual receptors.

The ability of some ganglion cells to respond differentially to various directions of image movement provides evidence that the separation and coding of impulses had taken place previous to the ganglion cell level.

The a-wave of the electroretinogram may develop in the outer plexiform layer of the retina or perhaps in the horizontal cells (Dowling, 1967).

The S-potentials also could well develop from the horizontal cells, and may have the same origin as the a-wave (Dowling, 1967).

It is believed that the b-wave of the electroretinogram originates from cells of the inner nuclear layer (Brown and Watanabe, 1965; Poppele and Maffei, 1967), probably the bipolar cells. The b-wave is the first retinal response to show full adaptation (Dowling, 1967).

The work of Steinberg (1968a) suggests that the changes in the slow, d.c. component of the local electroretinogram, which component probably also emanates from the inner nuclear layer, can be correlated with ganglion cell activity.

Mac Gregor (1967) has written an excellent review of the present state of our knowledge of the structure of the retina. He points out that there are contradictions in the available literature and that it must be used with caution. Much is still to be learned of the interconnections within the retina, and considerable research with the electron microscope is in progress.

Peripheral Inhibition in Vertebrates

Receptors, Mach Bands and Potentials

As in the case of the ommatidia of *Limulus,* interactions also occur in the vertebrate retina. These interactions bear some resemblance to those in *Limulus* in probably being chiefly inhibitory. However, because of the interposition of several layers of neurons between the visual receptors and the optic nerve in the highly complex vertebrate retina, vertebrate retinal interactions take place at several levels.

In the outer plexiform layer there are direct axo-axonal junctions between visual receptors, permitting lateral interaction at the receptor level. Sjöstrand (1965) observed two kinds of connections between the visual receptors of the guinea pig. Short processes link adjacent receptors, while long processes connect photoreceptors that are 7μ to 10μ apart.

According to Missoten (1960), in man processes originating in cone peduncles synapse with rod endings by entering their terminal invaginations. Richards (1967), using perceptual brightness matching tests, found that at higher suprathreshold light intensities, cones can inhibit rods. However, at lower suprathreshold intensities the differences in the latent periods of response between rods and cones (up to 100 msec), and between different kinds of cones (perhaps 30 msec), should be sufficient to introduce receptor specificity into certain kinds of contrast interactions. Such specificity can be advantageous. When, on the other hand, high stimulus intensities are used, the excitation of the receptors should last for a sufficient time to eliminate that interaction specificity which is based on the length of the latent period.

Alpern and Rushton (1965), working with perceptual thresholds for light increment detection, observed that only receptors of the same type, such as rods, or cones with the same spectral sensitivity, could inhibit each other. It must be remembered that Alpern and Rushton used threshold-strength stimuli. Dowling and Boycott (1966) cite several papers as evidence that retinal receptors interact chiefly with other receptors of the same kind.

Dowling and Boycott (1966) suggest that specific receptor interactions are mediated by the horizontal and amacrine cells. In such a case these interneurons would have to be receptor and color coded. While each horizontal cell would connect with only a specific receptor type, each amacrine cell would contact only rod bipolar cells or bipolar cells connecting with one kind of cone. Rod bipolar cells having a unique structure have been described, and midget as well as flat bipolars are reported to serve the cones.

The interaction between receptors in the light-adapted state differs from that after dark adaptation. Receptor interaction is further highly sensitive to barbiturate anesthesia.

The late receptor potential of vertebrate visual receptors can be modified by interaction between the receptors (Brown and Murakami, 1964) and therefore is also affected by adaptation.

Direct lateral interactions between receptors may be significant in the enhancement of contrast and the delineation of contours. In conjunction with long-range interactions involving the lateral horizontal cells, direct vertebrate visual receptor interactions may also play a role in the perception of shapes as well as of movement (Sjöstrand, 1965).

In the vertebrate retina there are not only direct contacts between retinal receptors, but also the lateral interconnections formed by the horizontal cells and the amacrine cells which were described in the previous section. All these lateral connections may make possible in the vertebrate retina the lateral, reciprocal interactions which have been observed in the compound eye of *Limulus* (*Xiphosura*).

Rall and Shepherd (1968), who postulate that the granule cells of the olfactory bulb form part of an inhibitory dendrodendritic pathway (see p. 209), suggest that the amacrine cells of the retina may also function in this manner. In this way the amacrine cells could bring about lateral inhibition in the retina and contribute to adaptation.

Rall and Shepherd point out that the amacrine cells in the optic lobe of the octopus are suspected of functioning as inhibitory interneurons and possess synapses of opposite polarities.

The existence of reciprocal synapses has been established at the periphery of a visual system. In the spider *Lycosa* there are reciprocal synaptic connections between photoreceptors and second-order visual neurons (Trujillo-Cenoz, 1965).

The amacrine cells of the retina, like the granule cells of the olfactory bulb, are innervated by centrifugal fibers.

Papers by Westheimer (1967, 1968) deal with lateral excitation and inhibition in the cone (central) retina, and with lateral inhibition in the rod (peripheral) retina of man, as indicated by changes in perceptual increment threshold. Westheimer observed that in the cone retina illumination of immediately adjacent areas has an excitatory effect, while illuminated areas beyond a zone 5 minutes of arc in diameter exert an inhibitory action. Westheimer also found that lateral excitation in the cone retina is not related to the presence of a border.

In man lateral interaction plays a more significant role in cone vision than in rod vision.

It has also been observed that metarhodopsin II, formed by the bleaching of rhodopsin, can start a negative feedback that reduces rod sensitivity (Donner and Reuter, 1967).

Evidence has been obtained that in the human retina the transmission of inhibitory effects to their points of action is slower than that of excitatory effects. An asynchrony of these two types of influences could produce a duration-dependent low-frequency decline of perceptual contrast sensitivity (Nachmias, 1967).

Lateral inhibition in the vertebrate retina may be different from that in *Limulus*. It has been reported that in the vertebrate retina inhibition does not appear to be mutual, although mutual inhibition is present at other levels of the vertebrate visual system (Wolbarsht in Discussion, Sjöstrand, 1965).

The function of the vertebrate retina is not yet as well understood as that of the *Limulus* eye.

As explained in the section on peripheral inhibition in invertebrates, mutual inhibition in the visual system results in the appearance of Mach bands. If there is a gradual increase in brightness across a contour, a zone of reduced brightness is seen on the darker side of the contour line, and vice versa. If the transition in luminance is more abrupt, as in the case of a step function, the dark Mach band is visualized in the area of lower illumination, and the light Mach band beyond the border of greater illumination. In order to determine the brightness (L) of his light and dark bands, Mach developed the formula

$$L = f\,(\,U, d^2U/dx^2\,)$$

in which U is the local luminance and d^2U/dx^2 is a term describing the curve of distribution of the luminance over a distance x at and perpendicular to a contour. The second derivative of the luminance distribution (d^2U/dx^2) here is employed to denote the approached limits when the span of the mentioned curve is reduced to infinite minuteness. When the second derivative of U has a positive value, the Mach band in question is light, whereas if d^2U is negative, the Mach band is dark.

Although Van der Horst and Bouman (1967) conclude that no Mach band phenomena occur in color vision, Jacobson and Mac Kinnon (1969) demonstrated a colored Mach band.

Von Békésy (1968) has obtained evidence suggesting that in man Mach bands result from lateral inhibition at a level of the visual system beyond the receptor cells.

A book dealing with the formation of Mach bands and with various types of visual inhibition has been written by Ratliff (1965).

The potentials which develop in the retina show depolarizing or exciting and hyperpolarizing or inhibiting components.

The slow- and long-lasting S-potentials arise between the receptors and the ganglion cell layer, perhaps from horizontal cells. In the carp there are three types of S-potentials—monophasic, biphasic and triphasic. The common form of the biphasic S-potential has a hyperpolarizing component evoked by the green wavelengths of the spectrum, and a depolarizing component elicited by the red wavelengths. The triphasic S-potentials have a depolarizing component in the green part of the spectrum, and hyperpolarizing components in blue and red light. The functional significance of the S-potentials, which show full summation over their whole receptive fields, is not yet known (Norton *et al.*, 1968).

A chromatic response, Svaetichin's "C" response, which can be recorded from the inner nuclear layer of the fish retina, is the product of two antagonistic potentials. One of these potentials is hyperpolarizing and is depressed by short wavelengths, while the other is depolarizing and is sensitive to long wavelengths. The so-called "C" response represents the algebraic sum of the two aforementioned potentials and is negative when provoked by the short wavelengths of the spectrum, and positive if initiated by any of the long wavelengths. It is marked at the middle wavelengths by brief transients at its start and termination, because of the faster rise and drop of the hyperpolarizing potential. At one intermediate wavelength the two opposed potentials are of equal magnitude and neutralize each other, so that there is no "C" response (Mac Nichol, Jr., 1966).

It could be expected that the opposed potentials giving rise to the "C" response would be transmitted to the retinal ganglion cells, at the next higher level of the visual pathway. The records obtained from ganglion cell axons, at the optic nerve or the tectum, show that this is indeed the case.

Retinal Ganglion Cells and Their Fields

Inhibitory actions of the greatest significance occur in the vertebrate retina at the level of the retinal ganglion cells. As indicated in the preceding section of the chapter, it is possible that one group of impulses reaches many retinal ganglion cells from the central portions of their receptive fields directly by way of bipolar cells, whereas amacrine cells might transmit opposed responses from the peripheral portions of the receptive fields.

The above concept is supported by the fact that responses from the peripheral zone seem not to appear as quickly as responses from the central core of a receptive field (Barlow, Hill and Levick, 1964; Gouras, 1967). Lateral inhibition has been said to spread through the retina at only a rate of 80 to 100 mm·sec^{-1} (Wuttke and Grüsser, 1966). However, it has also been surmised that in the case of cat "on" center retinal ganglion cells, the inhibitory impulses from the field periphery may have a latent period which exceeds the latent period of the central excitatory responses by 5 to 10 msec (Grüsser and Snigula, 1968).

Each optic nerve fiber, the axon of a retinal ganglion cell, serves a usually circular retinal surface, its receptive field, which is composed of some thousands of visual receptors. In mammals such receptive fields are approximately 1 mm in diameter.

In the area centralis of the cat most receptive fields are more than 1.5 mm across, but 40 per cent range from 0.80 mm to 1.50 mm in diameter. As determined by an area-threshold technique, most central portions of receptive fields measure about 0.33 mm in diameter, and centers vary from 0.125 mm to 0.80 mm (Steinberg, 1968a).

The double-responsive color receptive fields of the goldfish (*Carassius auratus*) are 5.5 mm or more in diameter, or measure 40 to 60 degrees. Their red central cores cover 10 to 15 degrees and their green central cores 15 to 20 degrees (Daw, 1968).

The impulses emanating from the visual receptors converge, through several layers of neural cells, unto the retinal ganglion cells.

Thus information from thousands of receptor cells is primarily channeled to one retinal ganglion cell.

The middle of many receptive fields gives off impulses on being specifically illuminated, while the periphery responds only to the cessation of a light stimulus. Other receptive fields show the reverse functional arrangement. Such receptive fields are known as "on-off" fields.

The illumination with white light of the entirety of normal "on-off" fields results in retinal ganglion discharges both on initiation and cessation of a light stimulus. However, discharges provoked by or following general illumination are of lower frequency.

The area of the central "on" region of an "on" center field varies with the intensity of illumination. During a low-intensity photic stimulus, or in a dark-adapted state, almost all of the receptive field shows the "on" response, but as the light intensity is raised, there is a gradual increase in the peripheral "off" region. Now the receptive field develops concentric zones (Yasuda and Hiwatashi, 1968).

The described functional change in "on" center receptive fields with light intensity is explained on the basis of a higher threshold level for the inhibitory actions. During the application of a weak photic stimulus the inhibitory activities do not reach threshold, but in stronger light they exceed the threshold level.

Yasuda and Hiwatashi (1968) consider the height of the gaussian curve for the inhibitory effect to vary, over a range, in proportion to input light intensity. The input-output relation for the inhibitory action should then be a quadratic function.

Enroth-Cugell and Robson (1966) found the relative influence of the peripheral zones of various receptive fields to rise with increasing intensity of illumination.

At the same time, Steinberg (1968a) corroborates that the response produced by the central portion of the field is dominant at very high light intensities. He hypothesizes that close to 1.0 log units above threshold the peripheral response mechanism becomes saturated, whereas the central response continues to increase in magnitude. The central core of a receptive field has a larger, comparative-excess number of receptors, and its dominance at higher light intensities may perhaps be ascribed to this fact.

The size of the total receptive field as well is affected by stimulus intensity and the state of adaptation, and also by spectral composition (Mac Gregor, 1966). Higher light intensity is accompanied by a reduction in the diameters of both zones of a receptive field (Enroth-Cugell and Robson, 1966).

"On-off" and purely "on" or "off" discharge ganglion cells all are found in vertebrates. In primates the response type of 3 per cent of the ganglion cells changes with wavelength (Mac Gregor, 1966).

In mammals most retinal ganglion cells have receptive fields consisting of two portions which produce antagonistic effects. Receptive fields of this kind do not seem to be as predominant in reptiles and birds.

The discharge evoked by illumination of a point is a triphasic function of its location on any diameter of its receptive field. Rodieck and Stone (1965) and Rodieck (1965) attempt to describe this function by adding a gaussian function for the response of the middle of the receptive field to one of the opposite sign representing the peripheral discharge.

Butenandt and Grüsser (1968) interpret their results on the response-stimulus area relationship shown by frog ganglion cells in terms of spatial gaussian distributions. An inhibitory gaussian distribution is assumed to overlie an excitatory gaussian distribution of lesser width. The lateral inhibition is considered to be multiplicative.

Imazawa (1966) found cat retinal ganglion cells to give responses of different latency to transretinal electrical currents of opposed polarity. "On" and "off" units showed reverse latency-current direction relations. All responses were increased by maintained illumination, and their latencies were generally reduced by a rise in light intensity.

Enroth-Cugell and Robson (1966) obtained evidence that the impulses from the central photoreceptors of a receptive field are not additive with those from the peripheral receptors before excitation of the field's ganglion cell. Instead, the two zones of each receptive field, which have forms described by gaussian functions, produce discharges which summate independently before acting on the ganglion cell. This is corroborated by Kostelyanets (1965), who synchronously and separately applied dark stimuli to the peripheral and central zones of "off" receptive fields in the frog retina. He found that the response of a field's ganglion cell to synchronous stimulation was equal to the sum of its responses to each of the stimuli. This observation precludes direct inhibitory interaction between the zones. In one experiment Kostelyanets even noted an interstimulatory phenomenon between the two "off" field zones.

On the other hand, the sum of the responses to two dark stimuli applied separately to the center region of a frog "off" receptive field exceeded the single ganglion cell response to the two stimuli when they were applied at the same time to the central region. Perhaps activity from the central core of the field can inhibit other central activity.

An experimental result indicates that the discharge from a receptive field may be inhibited by responses elicited in adjacent regions. If a dark stimulus was projected beyond the limits of an "off" receptive field in the frog retina, the latent period of the ganglion cell response was lengthened. However, the magnitude of the response remained unchanged (Kostelyanets, 1965).

Wolbarsht, Wagner and Mac Nichol, Jr. (1961), have offered a tentative explanation for the "on" and the "off" responses of many retinal ganglion cells, and for the frequent inhibitory effect of the activity of one part of the receptive field on the response called forth by another. First, they suggest that the "on" response is produced when a ganglion cell is

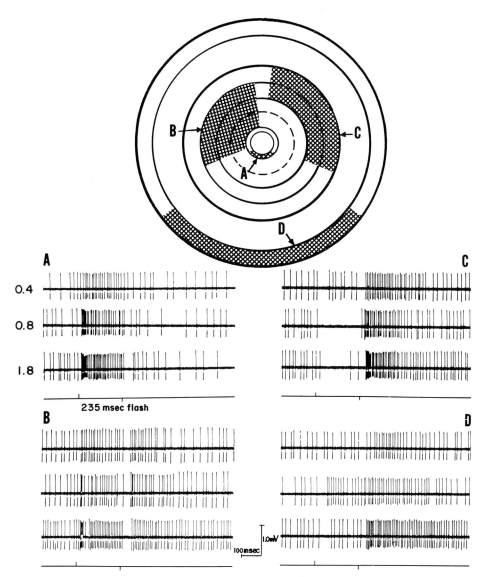

FIGURE 4-8. Responses of a cat retinal ganglion cell to annular flashes of three intensities directed at various portions of its receptive field. (Top) Receptive field diagram, scale of 1:100. The dotted line represents the limit of the 0.33 mm diameter optimal center stimulus. The solid lines outline the annular zones exposed to the flashes; each such annular area is partially crosshatched. The outer diameter of the optimal surround stimulus (also the outer diameter of *D*) was 1.34 mm. The retinal ganglion cell had an "on" excitation center mechanism. (Bottom) The responses obtained by stimulating each indicated area of the illustrated receptive field with flashes at 0.4, 0.8 and 1.8 $\log_{10}$ units above threshold. Negative responses are displayed upward. The flash duration (235 msec) is indicated by the marks below each group of responses. Area *A* gave "on" excitation, "off" inhibition responses which increased with intensity. At *B* both "on" and "off" excitation responses were evoked, but the center "on" excitation response became dominant with higher intensities. At *C* the surround "off" excitation mechanism was activated by all intensities. However, the "on" center mechanism expressed itself at 0.8 log units when *D* was stimulated, whereas the surround mechanism became dominant at 1.8 log units. All areas were preadapted with 45 lumens/meter². (From Steinberg, R.H.: Ganglion cell response characteristics from the area centralis in the intact eye of the cat. NAMI-1031, Naval Aerospace Med. Inst. and U. S. Army Aeromed. Res. Unit, Pensacola, 1968.)

excited by impulses emanating from a portion of its receptive field upon photic stimulation. Illumination can also cause another group of receptors to transmit an inhibitory input. The last acts to hyperpolarize the ganglion cell so that it no longer responds to an excitatory input. The hyperpolarization of the ganglion cell membrane, as effected by an inhibitory input, dissipates upon the cessation of illumination. This termination of the hyperpolarizing potential is followed by a postinhibitory rebound, the "off" response.

The "on" response, just like the "off" response, is said to be associated with inhibition. At the time of the "on" response, normal spontaneous activity is inhibited (Mac Nichol, Jr., 1966).

The investigations of Hughes and Maffei (1966) on the retinal ganglion cell responses evoked by sinusoidal light stimulation in the decerebrate cat provide further information on the function of "on," "off" and "on-off" cells. It was found, contrary to earlier opinion, that both "on" and "off" cells transmit evidence of any light intensity change to the brain, although by opposite signals. A rise in intensity produces a drop in the impulse frequency of an "off" cell and elicits a higher rate of discharge in an "on" cell. A reduction in light intensity gives rise to the reverse changes in impulse rate. The collected data indicate that more than the linear addition of antagonistic effects is involved in the observed functioning of the "on-off" cells.

The responses during variations in the rate of light intensity change bring out the largest differences among the several ganglion cell types; then the magnitude, phase, form, and so on, of the responses are dissimilar for various cells.

The results of Hughes and Maffei show that complex nonlinear nervous or receptor mechanisms exist in the retina and modify the parameters of its responses.

If it is assumed that the inhibitory input to an "off" cell may only reduce its spontaneous discharge, the findings of Hughes and Maffei (1966) can be integrated with the concept of "on-off" cell operation proposed by Wolbarsht, Wagner and Mac Nichol, Jr. (1961).

Grüsser and Snigula (1968) found the in-

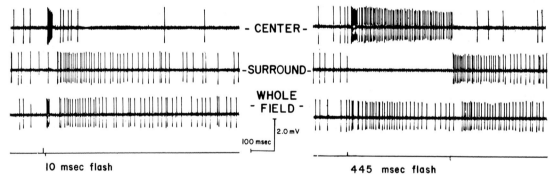

FIGURE 4-9. Retinal ganglion cell responses to optimal center, optimal surround and total receptive field stimulation with two flash durations. Both the center and surround responses can be recognized in the total field response. Thus there is no marked inhibitory interaction between the center and the surround. However, some response decrement can be noted. Negative responses are displayed upward. Intensities—10 msec flashes, 1.2 $\log_{10}$ units above optimal center-response threshold; 445 msec flashes, 1.4 $\log_{10}$ units over this threshold. Adapted with 45 lumens/m². Optimal center stimulus— 0.33 mm diameter; optimal surround stimulus—between diameters of 0.33 mm and 1.50 mm. (From Steinberg, R.H.: Ganglion cell response characteristics from the area centralis in the intact eye of the cat. NAMI-1031, Naval Aerospace Med. Inst. and U. S. Army Aeromed. Res. Unit, Pensacola, 1968.)

fluences from the peripheral zones of cat "on" center retinal ganglion cells and "off" center cells to reach their peak between 100 and 200 msec after the initiation of light stimulation.

Cat "off" center cells are completely inhibited when their central zones are subjected to photic stimuli with luminances between 0.5 and 80 asb (Snigula and Grüsser, 1968).

In primates cone and rod discharges are apparently transmitted to the same ganglion cell in the retinal zone around the fovea. However, the two groups of discharges exert a mutually antagonistic action, each making the ganglion cell unresponsive to the other. The antagonistic effect takes place beyond the bipolar cell level (Gouras, 1966).

The rod and the cone receptive fields of a rhesus perifoveal ganglion cell are superimposed, but the rod field shows a higher level of spatial summation than the cone field (Gouras, 1967).

Cone threshold activity reaches the ganglion cell within less than 50 msec after stimulation, while rod threshold activity arrives after this time (Gouras, 1967). When both cones and rods are stimulated at the same moment, the cone signals, which are generally faster, reach the ganglion cell first. The cone signals are then followed by a temporary refractory state on the part of the ganglion cell (Gouras and Link, 1966).

Either rod impulses or cone impulses can evoke activity in a ganglion cell when the retina is at least primarily dark adapted. However, in the light-adapted retina, ganglion cell activity is only called forth by cone discharges (Gouras, 1967).

In a marine fish, the plaice (*Pleuronectes platessa*), most ganglion cells responding differentially to colors also receive both a cone and a rod input. In the case of these fish ganglion cells as well, the cone signals initiate a discharge after a shorter latent period, or reach the ganglion cells sooner, than the rod signals (Hammond, 1968).

Grüsser, Finkelstein and Grüsser-Cornehls (1968) have developed a model of a retinal receptor unit in which, at the bipolar cells,

a bandpass RC-filter mechanism is operative. The bipolar cells of receptive units terminating in different kinds of retinal ganglion cells would have differently functioning filter mechanisms with different time constants.

The model is based on the finding that the exponent of the power function relating frog ganglion cell responses to the angular velocity of stimuli varies for different types of ganglion cells. The unlike values of the mentioned exponent appear to reflect the existence of different time constants of decay for the responses of each of three kinds of ganglion cells. It has been shown that these differences originate neither at the receptor cell level or the retinal ganglion cell level. However, it is possible that they may arise not only at the bipolar cells, but also at the bipolar-ganglion cell synapses or at the horizontal cells and perhaps the amacrine cells.

Mammalian retinal ganglion cells may discriminate between directions, as is the case in the cat, rabbit and ground squirrel. In the last (*Citellus mexicanus*) movement across the receptive field of such a ganglion cell calls forth a high response only if it is in a particular, preferred direction. Movement in the opposite, the null, direction elicits no response; it only evokes inhibition. When an area within the middle portion of such a receptive field is excited, critical retinal elements on its null-direction side are inhibited. A photic stimulus moving in the null direction is therefore always preceded by a wave of inhibition which prevents a response. The direction of "preferred" movement appears to vary randomly among the movement-sensitive fields, which are scattered over the retina (Michael, 1966a).

Barlow and Levick (1965) offer a hypothesis for the operation of directionally sensitive receptive units. According to these authors, horizontal cells could conduct impulses laterally in the null direction from the excited area of the receptive field. This horizontal cell activity would inhibit the bipolar cells on the null-direction side of the excited area, so that they could not transmit impulses from excited receptors in that direction. Only bipolars serving receptors in the preferred direction from the excited area would convey impulses to their retinal ganglion cells.

It is significant that an inhibited zone of the central receptive field, although not transmitting impulses to the ganglion cell, can on stimulation inhibit the neighboring area on the null-direction side. This indicates that the receptor cells themselves are not inhibited, but that inhibition takes place at a higher level in the receptive unit.

The pigeon retina also contains directionally sensitive ganglion cells.

In receptive fields of the above type, the periphery exerts an inhibitory effect on the center. Inhibitory impulses from the peripheral zones of such "on-off" fields might be carried by amacrine cells (Barlow and Levick, 1965).

In the rabbit retina's visual streak there are not only retinal ganglion cells differentially responsive to direction of movement, but also others that are respectively most reactive to rapid movement, quick variations in light intensity, uniformity of the visual image, contrasting borders projected on the receptive field, and so on (Levick, 1967).

Spinelli (1967) found that in the cat concentric receptive fields with antagonistic central cores and peripheral surrounds were divisible into two kinds. In one type the center is always clearly ringed by an opposed zone, sometimes consisting of two components. In the other type of field the opposed periphery is often demonstrable only when leaving the central core with the scan. The last group of fields can exhibit strong and long-maintained interactions between the central core and the periphery. Central-peripheral interactions may apparently differ between unlike fields.

The cat retina, in addition to having ganglion cells with the typical antagonistic central-peripheral receptive field organization, also has ganglion cells with diffuse receptive fields and ganglion cells whose fields do not seem to have an opposed peripheral zone. Bar-shaped and edge-shaped receptive fields were also found in the cat retina (Spinelli,

1967). Rodieck (1967) discovered two cat retinal ganglion cells with still another type of receptive field organization. The spontaneous impulse firing of these ganglion cells was suppressed by the presence of any type of contrast and by a change in contrast. Although inhibition of the discharge was weaker when a small area of contrast was thrown on the receptive field's periphery, all parts of the receptive field gave the same kind of response. None of the employed stimuli evoked an excitatory discharge from these ganglion cells with unique "suppressed-by-contrast" receptive fields.

Büttner and Grüsser (1968) have reported the response of cat retinal ganglion cells with "on" center and "off" center receptive fields to be a logarithmic function of stimulus area.

Six classes of retinal ganglion cells have been observed in the pigeon retina by Maturana (1962). These consist of verticality detectors, horizontality detectors, general edge detectors, directional moving edge detectors, convex edge detectors and luminosity detectors. Directional moving edge detectors, which possess unusually small receptive fields ($\frac{1}{2}$ of a degree to 1 degree, or 55μ-110μ), made up about 30 per cent of the ganglion cells investigated by Maturana and Frenk (1963).

In general, the magnitude of pigeon ganglion cells' responses can be said to be determined by the direction and degree of contrast and by the rate of movement (Maturana and Frenk, 1963).

By means of optic nerve recordings, four classes of retinal ganglion cells in a frog (*Rana esculenta*) have been discovered to all respond to angular velocity, angular size of entities in motion, the location of objects in the receptive field and the contrast between a moving object and its background. The time interval elapsing between consecutive stimulations of the same receptive field locus by the images of two moving objects was a factor in the excitation of two types of ganglion cells. The discharge of another kind of ganglion cell was affected by the brightness of moving objects (Grüsser and Grüsser-Cornehls, 1968). Thus

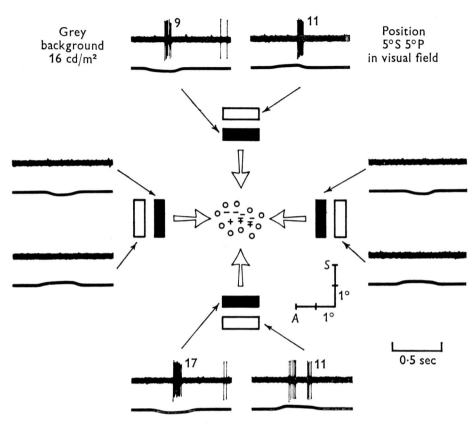

FIGURE 4-10. Responses of a rabbit retinal ganglion cell selective for target orientation. Discharges were evoked by vertical movements of horizontally oriented rectangles but not by vertical rectangles passing across the receptive field horizontally. The rectangle's position and not the direction of movement was most significant. The receptive field is mapped in the center (+ indicates response to stationary spot at on; —, at off; ∓, at both on and off, especially at off; O, no response). The visual field's anterior (A) and superior (S) meridians are indicated, and 1 degree calibration marks are provided. The records read from left to right. Upper trace, response with negativity upward, number of spikes given; lower trace, output of a photomultiplier focused on receptive field (upward deflection, increased light). (From Levick, W.R.: Receptive fields and trigger features of ganglion cells in the visual streak of the rabbit's retina. *J. Physiol. [London]*, 188:285-307, 1967.)

in the frog retina visual stimulation is coded into the discharge patterns of at least four types of ganglion cells. Most of the frog retina's ganglion cells show little or no response to steady illumination.

It can be said that a great deal of the activity of vertebrate retinal ganglion cells is phasic (Lange, Hartline and Ratliff, 1966).

Grüsser, Finkelstein and Grüsser-Cornehls (1968) described the relationship between the angular velocity of a stimulus and the average impulse frequency it elicits from the central excitatory zones of frog (*Rana esculenta*) retinal ganglion cells by the equation

$$R = k \cdot v^c \text{ (impulses} \cdot \text{sec}^{-1})$$

where R is the response, k is a constant, and v represents the angular velocity. The exponent c was found to vary between different classes of retinal ganglion cells, having a value of 0.5 for class I, 0.7 for class II, and 0.95 for

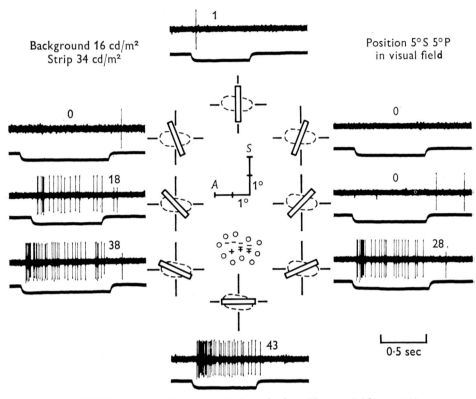

FIGURE 4-11. "Off" responses by the unit described in Figure 4-10 to stationary rectangles oriented in different directions. A thin, rectangular strip of light was focused on the receptive field and its orientation varied. As the strip of light was turned on and off, strong "off" responses appeared only when the strip approached a horizontal orientation. Same signs and conventions as in Figure 4-10. In addition, the strip of light is drawn over an outline of the receptive field at each record. Most of the orientation-selective cells had an "off" core receptive field, and nearly half responded to horizontal targets. (From Levick, W.R.: *J. Physiol. [London]*, 188:285-307, 1967.)

class III cells. The authors suggest that the unlike values of c for different types of ganglion cells may be based on the operation of unlike filter mechanisms, perhaps with different time constants, at each group of bipolar cells serving a different class of ganglion cells.

In the case of class IV ganglion cells no relation could be discovered between R and v for moving stimuli covering less than 5 degrees. The response evoked in class IV cells by large stimuli varied linearly with the angular velocity of the stimulus.

The value of the exponent c is unaffected by any irregularity or nonlinearity in stimulus movement and by the direction of motion. The value of c also does not vary with contrast or the size of the stimulus. On the other hand, k changes with contrast, stimulus size and the direction of the contrast against the background.

The response-velocity equation is not applicable if the image of the stimulus covers much more than the central excitatory zone of a retinal ganglion cell's receptive field.

Grüsser, Finkelstein and Grüsser-Cornehls (1968) found that the frog retina can differentiate angular velocities between 0.5 and 100 degrees · sec^{-1} or more. While class I neurons are most sensitive to movement of only approximately 2 degrees · sec^{-1}, at the other extreme class III neurons are most responsive to movement at 40 to 80 degrees · sec^{-1}.

The relations between stimulus area and cell discharge and between contrast and cell discharge also differ for class I, II, and III ganglion cells.

By virtue of its various parameters one stimulus may excite all classes of frog retinal ganglion cells. A class of retinal ganglion cells is not specialized for the reception of any one stimulus parameter.

The impulse frequency elicited from a class II or a class III frog retinal ganglion cell by the passage of a stimulus across the central excitatory zone of its receptive field is a logarithmic function of the stimulus area (Butenandt and Grüsser, 1968). However, if the image of the stimulus projects beyond the central excitatory zone, the involvement of the inhibitory peripheral surround results once again in a reduction of ganglion cell activity. This drop in activity also is logarithmically related to the area of the stimulus.

The class I retinal ganglion cells of the frog *Rana esculenta* discharge when sharp edges move over their receptive field. However, they also give a sustained discharge to a stationary edge. Pickering and Varjú (1967), using non-moving stimuli, observed the latency of the response to be a power function of the light intensity. At their highest intensity the latent period was 13 seconds.

Crescitelli (1968) studied a slow potential wave in the frog retina which was increasingly delayed with rising photic stimulus intensity. He found this potential, which was accompanied by impulse discharges, to emanate from the rhodopsin-containing rods. Crescitelli hypothesizes that the increase in latent period with intensity is associated with an inhibition (a negativity appeared after the b-wave).

A contrast presented to the central portion of the class I receptive field evoked excitation, while a contrast presented to the concentric peripheral receptive field produced inhibition. If sufficient contrasts were thrown on the peripheral receptive field the activity of the ganglion cell elicited by a 5-degree black disc

could be totally suppressed (Pickering and Varjú, 1967).

Grüsser *et al.* (1967) corroborate the existence of outer concentric inhibitory zones in the receptive fields of frog moving-edge detectors (class I ganglion cells).

The receptive field of the frog's class II retinal ganglion cells is also divided into a central excitatory field (2.5-4 degrees in diameter) and a concentric peripheral inhibitory zone (at least 6-8 degrees in diameter). The same is true of class III frog ganglion cells when the applied stimuli are close to threshold. Class III neurons have an average field of 6 degrees diameter and a peripheral inhibitory zone at least 10 degrees in diameter.

Class III ganglion cells are characterized by responses to alterations in background illumination. Their discharges have a long latent period, which rises with the degree of dark adaptation to a maximum of over 10 seconds (Pickering, 1968). The effect of dark adaptation may be based on the regeneration of rhodopsin.

In the frog *Rana catesbeiana* the three groups of optic nerve fibers, which are distinguished by conduction speeds, can be related to different retinal ganglion cells and receptive fields (Kyoji Tasaki, personal communication).

It has been known for a long time that in the frog the retinal receptive fields of diverse ganglion cells may overlap to a considerable degree (Hartline, 1969).

In his discussion Maturana (1962) develops the idea that while the retinal ganglion cells of mammals transmit a relatively unspecific and ambiguous output to the brain, the information conveyed by the retinal ganglion cells of amphibians, reptiles and birds is more specific. In the retinas of the last, lower groups of animals, visual processing reaches the point where the essential characteristics of the form and shape (edges, corners, etc.), color, intensity and movement of a visual image are defined. In mammals, on the other hand, basic information on shape and color reaches the brain in the form of a combined output from a group of ganglion cells. The mammalian mechanism has the advantages that more information can be communicated to the brain and that the combined output can be subjected to more complex processing in the brain.

In the retina of birds, reptiles and amphibians, there is a greater reduction of the visual data supplied by the receptors, as the large amount of specific processing selects from this data the content of the impulse-coded output of the comparatively specialized ganglion cells.

Pantle and Sekuler (1968) dealt with the question of whether man's ability to discriminate the size of an object is partially based on the transmission of direct information about the retineal area occupied by an image. In their experiments Pantle and Sekuler determined if adaptation to selected patterns of alternating light and dark bars, which differed in frequency or bar diameter, had an effect on the visibility of a test pattern. This was done on the supposition that a transfer of effect from one pattern to another is indicative of the operation of a single mechanism of response, or the existence of a common detector type, for both patterns. The results suggest that a limited number of different size detector unit types, each maximally responsive to a different stimulus size range, operate in the visual system. Similar results have been reported by Campbell and Robson (1968). The shapes and sizes of their receptive field components could determine the responses given by size detectors.

The size detectors may be retinal ganglion cells and their receptive fields, neurons higher in the visual pathway, or both. Cells in the lateral geniculate nucleus have been shown to have receptive fields similar to those of retinal ganglion cells, and simple visual cortex cells also have "on-off" receptive fields, although these are not concentric. Complex visual cortex cells have nonconcentric receptive fields without an "on-off" organization, and the receptive fields of hypercomplex visual cortex cells exhibit antagonistic regions

(Hubel, 1963; Hubel and Wiesel, 1968).

The phenomenon of size constancy might be based on the existence of different groups of size detectors. There could be shifts between such detector groups.

The various size detector units may further be differentially involved in the perception of objects moving at unlike speeds. Units most responsive to bars of large size also seem to be highly reactive to rapidly moving targets, while small-area detectors appear to be very significant in the perception of slow targets (Pantle and Sekuler, 1968).

Research on the ganglion cells serving the cone receptive fields of the ground squirrel (*Citellus mexicanus*) has revealed some to be stimulated by green light and inhibited by blue light, while others showed the reverse responses. The responses to yellow or red light were always similar to the responses to green light. The opposed responses to different colors may involve the entire receptive field, or they may respectively be observable only in the central and peripheral portions of the field. Work on the last type of receptive field has shown the peripheral response to be distributed throughout the field and has vindicated Rodieck and Stone's concept of the relations of the receptive field discharge (Michael, 1966b).

Primates as well possess ganglion cells whose receptive fields are divided into opposed zones most responsive to different colors (Hubel and Wiesel, 1964).

Ganglion cell receptive fields with antagonistic responses to different wavelengths have also been found in fish.

The marine plaice (*Pleuronectes platessa*) possesses color-sensitive "on-off" receptive fields in which, instead of there being opposed central-peripheral zones, every point in the field produces both "on" and "off" responses at normal stimulus intensities. Nevertheless, at the center of the field either the "on" or the "off" component is dominant, and this dominant component's sensitivity drops more quickly than that of the other component with distance from the center. In these fields (type 1) the colors of light eliciting opposed responses may be orange and green, green and blue, and so on. The ganglion cells having the above fields adapt rapidly.

Another kind of plaice color-responsive receptive field (type 2) has the antagonistic central-peripheral zone organization. In such fields one of the zones gives rise only to "off" responses while the other produces both "on" and "off" responses to strong photic stimuli, and perhaps only "on" responses to low levels of illumination. A single color provokes both the "on" and the "off" responses of the zone showing the combination of responses. Thus in one such field green elicited both the "on" and "off" responses of the central core, while the "off" response of the peripheral zone was called forth by blue. The opposed responses of the center and the peripheral surround ("on" of the center and "off" from the periphery, or vice versa), if evoked at the same time, generally strongly inhibit each other's effect on the ganglion cell discharge. An exception to this is that the "off" responses of the "on-off" zone are subjected to but little inhibition. The ganglion cells of these fields adapt slowly (Hammond, 1968).

It has been suggested (Dowling and Boycott, 1966) that the "off" response of the "on-off" zone is due to stimulation by this zone's "on" activity of amacrine cells which extend laterally into the "off" portion of the receptive unit. This explanation would jibe with the absence of such a mixed-in "off" response at low stimulus intensities, and with the identical spectral sensitivity of the mixed "on-off" responses (Hammond, 1968).

Type 1 fields are considered to function in color coding. The mutually antagonistic effects of the "on" and "off" activities at the ganglion cell level could make the retina more sensitive to color contrast. Type 2 fields, because they are divided into two zones of unlike reactivities, are thought to play a role in discrimination of shape and size. Since the type 2 fields include both rods and cones, they should function over a large range of wavelengths and light intensities.

Receptive fields similar to those dealt with above have been described from the goldfish (*Carassius auratus*) by Jacobson and Gaze (1964).

A later paper, by Daw (1968), indicates that 49 per cent of the color-responsive receptive fields of the goldfish may have either a central core giving both an "on" response to red and an "off" response to green light, while the periphery is "on green" and "off red," or the reverse.

Daw points out that there may be no peripheral responses to a small spot of light because the peripheral zone reacts better to a stimulus when it is spread over a large area, even though this reduces its intensity per unit of surface. With small spots of light the color receptive fields described above may appear to simply be either "on red" or "on green" in the center and "off" for the opposite color in the periphery.

However, some 5 per cent of all color-responsive ganglion cells seem really to have receptive fields with centers which are either "on" or "off" to one color and whose peripheries show the opposite response to the other color.

Daw further determined that when the stimulus applied to the first-mentioned, more complex fields consists of both red and green spots, the response is equivalent to the sum of the responses to the two color components. The organization of the complex fields with double-responsive cores and surrounds is suited for the perception of simultaneous color contrast, while the simpler opponent color fields are structured to instead transmit successive color contrast.

In 14 per cent of the double-responsive fields the activity originating from the red-sensitive cones overrides or masks the response component emanating from the green cones.

The discovery in fish of double color-sensitive receptive fields, in which each locus gives rise to "on" as well as "off" responses, adds additional interest to the conceptualizations of Enroth-Cugell and Robson (1966). These investigators interpreted the spatial frequency response of cat retinal ganglion cells in terms of two superimposed, antagonistic receptive fields.

In the cat a sufficiently bright background fully inhibited the inner nuclear layer's b-wave response to a flash of light, but only reduced the magnitude of the late RP (receptor potential) of the visual receptors. These results indicate that visual responses can be suppressed within the neural networks of the retina by strong background illumination (Poppele and Maffei, 1967).

A study of the simultaneous discharges of numbers of retinal ganglion cells in the cat has shown that such discharges have periodic patterns. It is hypothesized that these periodic discharge patterns contribute to mechanisms which in turn affect the spatial distribution of retinal excitation and inhibition (Laufer and Verzeano, 1967). Thus the periodic discharge patterns may help to set the degree of responsiveness of the retina.

In darkness retinal activity oscillates at a slower rate. Nevertheless, a synchronous oscillatory discharge is maintained in the dark, and many investigators consider the dark discharge of ganglion cells to have a sensory function. Jung (1964) deals with the activity of a separate "dark-sensitive" system of retinal neurons.

The periodic patterns of discharge which emanate from the retina, and are highly affected by its responses, appear to inhibit the spontaneous periodic activity of the lateral geniculate body at a higher level of the visual pathway.

Oscillatory and synchronized retinal ganglion cell activity has also been noted after flash stimulation in rabbits (Crapper and Noell, 1963) and cats (Steinberg, 1966). In the rabbit the ganglion cells' responses to a flash are massed into 30 msec bursts alternating with 30 msec periods of inactivity. In the cat a flash elicits 10 msec discharges. Pacheco, Bear and Ervin (1968) also observed that in monkeys the termination of a period of visual stimulation with subdued light is followed by a synchronized ganglion cell afterdischarge.

The last has a frequency of 50-60/sec and lasts for as much as 1 minute. The ganglion cell afterdischarge appears to result from cone excitation which is linked with a suppression of rod impulses.

Oscillatory activity is most pronounced at the level of the bipolar cells (inner nuclear layer), suggesting that cells of this zone of the retina are basically involved in the oscillatory phenomenon.

When an eye-optic nerve preparation from the sea hare *Aplysia californica* (Mollusca) is maintained in complete darkness, the impulses recorded from the optic nerve show a circadian rhythm. Thus eyes from animals previously subjected to 12-hour periods of light and darkness, when kept totally dark in culture medium, give rise to peaks of optic nerve activity at approximately 27-hour intervals (Jacklet, 1969).

The considerable variety of receptive fields and ganglion cell types observed in each investigated group of vertebrates indicates that an important part of visual processing occurs in the retina. The shape of a ganglion cell's receptive field, for instance, determines which image configurations will stimulate it most effectively. Summation over the receptive fields of different cells may be linear or nonlinear.

The combination of excitatory and inhibitory activities characteristic of "on-off" retinal ganglion cells can be employed, as has been shown in the preceding material, both for the discrimination of color and of pattern. In both cases the pairing of the excitatory with the inhibitory effects may act to accentuate contrasts (Mac Nichol, Jr., 1966).

The discharge bursts produced by most ganglion cells in response to transient variations in illumination may emphasize temporal contrasts (Mac Nichol, Jr., 1966).

It has been established that visual images which are stabilized on the retina soon fade (Pritchard, 1961). Therefore, while images move over the retina in normal vision, a constant barrage of "on" and "off" responses must emanate from the retina.

Hartline (1969) has stated that vision is a dynamic process, and that the visual system is to a very high degree structured to respond to change and movement.

Maturana (1962) suggests that retinal ganglion cells are not adequately stimulated by just a sufficiently large input, but to be excited, the cells must receive a certain spatial and temporal distribution of impulses. Thus in the case of pigeon horizontal edge detector ganglion cells, a horizontal edge must be projected on the peripheral zone of the receptive field if the cells are to give a response. However, the casting of a horizontal edge on the peripheral zone by itself is insufficient to produce a discharge, indicating that such stimulation is only an essential part of a total stimulus configuration which is required for excitation. The stimulus configurations necessary for excitation are presumably determined by the connections the ganglion cell makes with afferent processes. When a proper visual image falls on the receptive field, these connections cause such a combination of excitatory and inhibitory inputs to reach the ganglion cell as will result in its excitation.

Maturana and Frenk (1963) reiterate that particular retinal ganglion cells appear to be selectively responsive to certain spatiotemporal afferent impulse configurations, and they also indicate that no specific pathways exist for such afferent influences. Ganglion cells which differ in function have connections with the same bipolar cells.

An excellent review of sensory mechanisms by Goldberg and Lavine (1968) includes a valuable section on the organization and function of retinal receptive fields. Creutzfeldt and Sakmann (1969) also deal with the organization of the retina and the function of the retinal ganglion cells in an extensive review of the neurophysiology of the visual system.

Centrifugal Inhibition

Retinal ganglion cells may also be indirectly inhibited by centrifugal impulses transmitted from the brain through efferent optic nerve fibers. An extensive literature deals with this subject, and it appears that numerous vertebrates have efferent optic nerve fibers.

Maturana and Frenk (1965), verifying earlier studies, found that in the pigeon efferent fibers end in the inner nuclear layer of the retina. They traced these efferent (centrifugal) fibers to the inner portion of the inner nuclear layer, where they synapse with two types of amacrine cells and also with displaced ganglion cells. The terminal branchings of the efferent fibers may converge on primarily one cell, or these branchings may be fanlike and contact several cells. Convergent endings form synaptic nests on the small parasol amacrine cells, while divergent endings make synaptic junctions with the flat amacrine cells.

The displaced ganglion cells, each of which has a centrifugal synapse, are all of one morphological type. This, the differing kinds of complex centrifugal synapses on respectively unlike types of amacrines, and the high number and apparently even distribution of centrifugal terminals ($1/1{,}500\mu^2$) suggest to Maturana and Frenk that in the pigeon centrifugal influences may have multiple effects on retinal output. There may also be different, localized centrifugal effects on various areas of the retina.

Branston and Fleming (1968) are inclined to consider amacrine cells the connecting link between centrifugal optic fibers and retinal ganglion cells in the frog.

Cowan and Powell (1963) traced the efferent optic fibers of the pigeon centrally to the contralateral isthmo-optic nucleus of the midbrain. By counting the cells in the isthmo-optic nucleus, they were able to offer the approximate number of 10,000 for the pigeon's efferent fibers, which they observed to terminate at amacrine cells. This would make the efferent fibers about 1 per cent of the total fibers in the optic nerve. In the pigeon the efferent fibers form a distinct bundle between the isthmo-optic nucleus and the optic chiasma.

McGill (1964) has traced the orderly representation, through afferent fibers, of the pigeon's retina on the tectum of its brain, the representation of the tectum on the isthmo-optic nucleus, and the organized projection of the isthmo-optic nucleus on the retina by means of centrifugal fibers. McGill has thus followed the complete circuit from the retina to parts of the brain, and back again by efferent fibers. This circuit of fiber connections suggests that the efferent fibers are part of a feedback mechanism.

The topographically ordered projection from the pigeon's tectum to its isthmo-optic nucleus was clearly demonstrated by McGill, Powell and Cowan (1966).

Holden (1966b, 1968a) has been able to confirm the origin of the pigeon's efferent optic fibers from the isthmo-optic nucleus by use of antidromic stimulation of the retina, and by blocking antidromic spikes from the retina through orthodromic electrical stimulation of the tectum. It was also established that orthodromic impulses from the isthmo-optic nucleus are transmitted centrifugally to the retina.

Holden (1968b) recorded the responses of the pigeon's isthmo-optic nucleus to electrical stimulation of the lateral tectum. An early response is produced through monosynaptic impulses traveling down the tecto-isthmo-optic tract, and a later discharge is evoked by way of more complex pathways. While most of the output cells of the isthmo-optic nucleus emit impulses on tectal stimulation, about one tenth of these cells can be excited synaptically from the retina. The output cells of the isthmo-optic nucleus receive impulses by both excitatory and inhibitory synapses.

A peak of centrifugal activity reaches the pigeon retina 5 msec after electrical stimulation is applied to the lateral tectum.

Two extremely favorable human preparations resulting from the removal of eyes, and showing complete degeneration of the afferent optic fibers, made it possible for Wolter (1965) to study the nature and course of the efferent optic fibers in man. Wolter estimated that 10 per cent of the optic nerve fibers in man are efferent (centrifugal). The efferent fibers differ greatly in diameter, and some are unmyelinated. Previous studies have shown one group of human efferent fibers to serve blood vessels in the optic nerve and the retina. Another group of efferent fibers, which are thin and unmyelinated, enter into the optic chiasma from the direction of the pituitary stalk. All the myelinated efferent fibers could be traced up the optic tracts to the level of the lateral geniculate bodies. There seem to be several types of efferent fibers.

Some myelinated efferent fibers were seen to remain uncrossed in the optic chiasma, a finding which does not have a counterpart in the studies on the pigeon.

Branston and Fleming (1968) observed that in the frog retina the activity of "off" and "on-off" ganglion cells was inhibited by cutaneous and auditory stimulation, irrespective of whether this activity was spontaneous or in response to visual stimuli. Furthermore, extravisual stimulation was followed by a decrease in sensitivity of moving-edge detector receptive fields. These receptive fields underwent an apparent reduction in size because of their lowered sensitivity. Also, the response, but not the peak response, of an "off" ganglion cell appeared some milliseconds earlier after single auditory clicks. These results generally indicate that efferent optic nerve activity leads to the inhibition of "off," "on-off" and moving-edge detector retinal ganglion cells.

Weingarten and Spinelli (1966) as well reported that auditory and somatic stimulation gives rise to changes in retinal receptive fields. In their experiments on the cat, such stimulation caused the majority of receptive fields to expand. The impulse activity of the stimulated units was affected too, but it did not vary as a simple function of receptive field changes.

Sympathetic activity has been found to reduce retinal sensitivity to the long wavelengths of the spectrum (Kravkov and Galochkina, 1947).

Ogden and Brown (1964) recorded from the retina of the cynomolgus monkey while electrically stimulating the optic nerve (and retina). They identified a positive response, the P-wave, which they found to emanate from the parafoveal ganglion cells. Ogden and

Brown believed their P-wave to be evoked by efferent activity from centrifugal fibers synapsing with amacrine cells.

A number of features of the P-wave indicate that it is postsynaptic. Also, Ogden (1966) followed the P-wave fibers centrally to the lateral geniculate bodies. This origin of the P-wave fibers appears to integrate well with the anatomical results of Wolter (1965).

On the other hand, the pigeon, with its well-established centrifugal optic fiber tract, does not, in its retina, give rise to a P-wave. Furthermore, Ogden (1966) has postulated that the P-wave originates from a recurrent collateral system. Retinal ganglion cells, by means of electrotonic junctions, could excite bipolar cells which would in turn transmit potentials to amacrine cells to produce the postsynaptic P-wave.

In the rabbit the application of strychnine to the right retina results in the appearance of rhythmic spontaneous impulselike activity in the left retina and left optic nerve. If the right eye is stimulated with flashes, a response in the right optic nerve is followed in a few milliseconds by a response in the left optic nerve. It is possible to conclude from the last observation that afferent impulses in the right visual pathway lead to the release of efferent impulses in the left visual pathway. If the right retina is stimulated with flashes after strychnine has been applied to it, the efferent response is increased, and occasionally doubled (Vatter, 1967).

Vatter was also able to demonstrate the effects of centrifugal activity on the a- and b-waves of the electroretinogram. The efferent potentials tend to reduce the a-wave components. If an eye is stimulated by flash simultaneously with the action of efferent impulses on its retina, the resulting a-wave and the ascending portion of the b-wave are both enhanced.

Ogden (1968) recorded the local electroretinogram of the pigeon after denervation of the retina. Denervation produced no changes in the a- and b-waves. However, 3 hours after the cutting of the optic tract, maintained oscillations in retinal potential (30-40 cps) appeared on illumination of the retina. The light-evoked oscillations later declined, and ended when ganglion cell activity terminated. If, instead of interrupting the optic tract, the retina was blocked with procaine, photic stimulation also gave rise to oscillations.

In another experiment Ogden attempted to produce efferent discharges to the retina through electrical stimulation of the tectum. This resulted in a decrease in amplitude of the oscillatory potentials which sometimes follow illumination of the normal retina.

Ogden concludes that in the pigeon the efferent pathway to the retina permits central control of a photically-induced oscillatory mechanism which seems to function in the inner plexiform layer. Perhaps higher centers modulate inhibition in the retina by means of the centrifugal fibers.

It is possible that degenerative changes in the retinal ganglion cells may have produced effects contributing to the light oscillations. Functional ganglion cells may also be necessary for the development of the oscillatory mechanism. During the effort to initiate efferent discharges, tectal stimulation could well have resulted in the antidromic activation of ganglion cells. However, it was found unlikely that such activation affected the oscillatory potentials.

It has been reported that after sectioning of one optic nerve in each of two human patients, the affected eye showed electroretinographic responses of greater amplitude than the other eye. Also, the ERG flicker responses were larger than normal in the eye with the cut nerve (Gills, Jr., 1966). The author considers these results to indicate an inhibitory action by centrifugal fibers in the normal condition. However, he also refers to numerous previous similar as well as contradictory findings and points out that further research must be performed.

Haft and Harman (1967) observed an evoked response in the optic chiasma which resulted from weak photic stimulation of the right eye and which was of small amplitude and was marked by a long latent period, to be suppressed by synchronous strong light stimulation of the left eye. The investigators concluded from this result that the response from the right retina had been inhibited by some central influence.

On the other hand, Brindley and Hamasaki (1962, 1966) were unable to find either centrifugal optic nerve fibers or indications of efferent activity in the cat. Steinberg (1968b) has published a letter expressing doubt about Haft and Harman's (1967) interpretation of their findings, pointing out a number of pitfalls which can be encountered in such research. The weaknesses of the methods used in seeking evidence of centrifugal fibers are also dealt with by Granit (1962).

Gliozzi (1966) recorded S-potentials from the retina of the goldfish (*Carassius auratus*) while electrically stimulating the optic nerve. He was unable to observe any changes in the S-potentials. Gliozzi therefore suggests that optic nerve stimulation does not significantly affect the activity of the visual receptor cells.

Spinelli and Weingarten (1966), using the cat, were the first to obtain recordings of activity from purported efferent fibers of the optic nerve.

Branston and Fleming (1968) found that in the frog most efferent optic nerve activity was near noise level, as had also been reported for the cat by Spinelli and Weingarten (1966). The estimated 1 per cent of the optic nerve fibers which were efferent produced impulses at lower frequencies than did afferent optic fibers during their spontaneous activity.

Efferent optic fibers showed adaptation and forms of "off" responses upon extravisual stimulation of the frog (Branston and Fleming, 1968).

Ogden (1968), in a paper presented in 1966, reviews the anatomical and physiological literature pertaining to the existence of centrifugal optic fibers in various animal groups. He considers the morphological evidence for the presence of efferent optic fibers in cephalopods, insects and birds conclusive but cannot say the same for vertebrates other than Aves.

Ogden also views the results of physiological investigations as inconclusive.

Holden (1966a) has offered a few possible functions for optic efferent activity. It may serve to suppress the retinal discharge from one eye if the two eyes have totally different (chameleon, pigeon) or partially different (man) visual fields. It may also suppress diplopic images of objects falling beyond the horopter in binocular vision. The last function would demand a spatially highly organized centrifugal system, which would quickly produce activity changes in various retinal regions with eye movement. Further, efferent activity may be involved in several of the phenomena of saccadic suppression and in various spatial suppressions linked with head and eye movements.

Piggins (1966) restates the likelihood of central control of retinal activity through centrifugal fibers. He also suggests that the fragmentation of a geometric figure, when it is visible as a long-lasting afterimage or as a partly stabilized retinal image, is due to centrifugal activity. Perhaps fluctuations in attention, possibly produced by nonvisual stimuli, may be responsible for the fading and return of sections of a geometric figure (fragmentation).

The possibility has been raised that feedback from the brain to the eye may occur by two mechanisms—centrifugal nerve impulses to the retina, and the more indirect mechanism of eye movements, particularly the minute eye movements of fixation. By these two means the brain could constantly affect the function of the retinal receptor units. The brain could slow or stop visual reception on receiving an excess of data or when a shift in attention is taking place. The brain might also cause the visual system to "lock" onto a visual field in which change would be significant, and it could initiate a search for some lacking element. Such central manipulation of visual receptor activity might in addition play a role in illusions and hallucinations (Gaarder, 1963).

Inhibition at Higher Levels of the Visual System

The optic nerves from both eyes, composed of the axons of the retinal ganglion cells, form the optic chiasma at the base of the brain. Here the medial optic nerve fibers cross over to the contralateral side, while the lateral fibers do not (Fig. 4-12). On each side, beyond the optic chiasma, the crossed medial fibers and the uncrossed lateral fibers compose the optic tract. Most fibers of the last end in the lateral geniculate body of the same side, but some go to the thalamus and to the superior colliculus. The neurons of the lateral geniculate body, and neurons in the thalamus, give rise to ascending fibers which form the optic radiation. The fibers of the optic radiation then terminate in the visual cortex, which occupies the surface of the medial part of the occipital lobe and the gyri at the sides of, and near to, the calcarine fissure.

A second human visual system, concerned with orientational and general spatial adjustments, is reported to operate through centers in the brain stem. In this newly discovered, subconscious system, both eyes are represented in each cerebral hemisphere.

Much evidence has also accumulated for inhibition in the higher portions of the visual pathway. A sample of this material is given below.

Evidence for inhibitory connections within the central visual system of the toad was obtained in a behavioral study performed by Ewert and Härter (1968).

Suzuki and Ichijo (1967) found that in the cat retinal spontaneous activity gives rise to a postsynaptic inhibition in the lateral geniculate nucleus. The inhibitory influence emanating from the optic nerves produces maintained suppression of the activity of the geniculate neurons.

When two light flashes are separated by a suitable time interval, the first exerts an inhibitory effect on the second at the geniculate level in the cat. This inhibitory action, which reaches its peak after about 30 msec, also involves postsynaptic hyperpolarization (Bremer, 1967). Kuman and Skrebitskii (1968) as well observed a long inhibitory period in the lateral

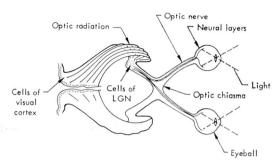

FIGURE 4-12. Simplified schematic drawing of the visual pathway. Each of the optic tracts, which lie beyond the optic chiasma, sends some of its nerve fibers to the pulvinar of the thalamus and some to the superior colliculus. The thalami and superior colliculi are not shown. A few optic tract fibers also run to the hypothalamus and the mesencephalon. (From MacGregor, R.J.: Pulse trains in lateral geniculate and retinal ganglion nerve cells. RM-4870-ARPA, The Rand Corp., Santa Monica, 1966.)

geniculate body subsequent to flash stimulation. An inhibitory interval of 140 to 300 msec was preceded and often followed by impulse discharges.

Approximately half of the lateral geniculate neurons investigated by Kuman and Skrebitskii (1968) also responded to auditory stimuli, most being excited but some showing inhibition. In the neurons activated by auditory stimulation, the last affected the photic response by inducing either a reduction of the inhibitory period or causing the postinhibitory discharge to increase in magnitude. Auditory stimuli primarily facilitated the lateral geniculate body's transmission of photically excited discharges.

Somatic stimulation exerts similar effects on lateral geniculate body photic responses (Hotta and Kameda, 1963).

It has been reported that in the auditory system interference by stimuli of a different modality, as well as habituation and conditioning, affect impulse activity at the receptor level by way of centrifugal fibers (Buño *et al.*, 1966, see p. 177).

Vastola (1967) studied the effects of striate cortical polarization (inhibition) on the neurons of the cat's lateral geniculate body. Many experiments included optic nerve stimulation in the hope of discovering any unusual feedback phenomena by their absence during cortical inhibition. Vastola found the inferred normal corticofugal influence to be facilitatory in most cases and did not observe optic nerve stimulation to initiate any strikingly new mechanisms. Meulders and Colle (1966) used removal of the striate cortex to show that a corticofugal influence is exerted on the lateral geniculate body. Widén and Ajmone-Marsan (1960) determined that cortical stimulation could facilitate or suppress the response of lateral geniculate body neurons to subsequent stimulation of the optic tract. Hull (1968) showed that while the excitatory and inhibitory responses of some cells of the macaque's (*Macaca irus*) lateral geniculate nucleus are facilitated by impulses from the striate visual cortex, the excitatory responses of other cells are inhibited.

Evidence that the cortex exerts presynaptic inhibition at the level of the lateral geniculate body was provided by Suzuki and Kato (1965). The experiments of Kahn, Magni and Pillai (1967) indicate that presynaptic inhibition of optic fiber impulses at the level of the lateral geniculate body also emanates from the mesencephalic reticular formation.

Montero and Guillery (1968) trace the route of corticogeniculate fibers in the rat.

Suzuki and Kato (1966) and Sefton and Burke (1966) have provided evidence that inhibitory interneurons exist in the lateral geniculate body. Saavedra and Vaccarezza (1968) described the glomerular synaptic complex in the neuropil of the lateral geniculate nucleus of the Cebus monkey. They determined the giant central axon terminal of this complex to be of retinal origin and suggest that the peripheral axon terminals of the complex have an inhibitory function.

When Shevelev (1968) applied diffuse stimulation to the contralateral retina, he found the cat lateral geniculate neurons having average latencies of response to inhibit the beginning reactions and responses of the other neurons. Shevelev also observed the system of inhibitory neurons to function primarily in the day range (at high thresholds).

Some possible roles of inhibition in the lateral geniculate body are given by Creutzfeldt (1968). It may be advantageous for the proper stimuli, visual ones, to produce inhibition because this could, during a visual input, prevent a general discharge in response to impulses called forth by other stimuli. Inhibitory interaction akin to and with the same function as lateral inhibition in the retina may occur in the lateral geniculate body. Postexcitatory IPSP's may act to dampen rapidly developing, strong responses to light. Also, stimulation of the entire receptive field with a diffuse photic stimulus results in only a small degree of lateral geniculate activity, perhaps due to collateral inhibition of the excited neurons.

In the squirrel monkey (*Saimiri sciureus*) the receptive fields of lateral geniculate neurons have been found to exhibit antagonistic center and surround mechanisms (excitatory and inhibitory zones) which to a high degree overlap spatially (Jacobs and Yolton, 1968). On the other hand, Wiesel and Hubel (1966) reported that in *Macaca* the antagonistic center and peripheral receptive field mechanisms of the neurons in the lateral geniculate nucleus are to a considerable extent spatially distinct.

Montero and Brugge (1969) describe directionally selective lateral geniculate neurons in the rat. While movement across their visual receptive field in one direction evokes a maximum response, movement in the opposite direction produces no impulses, gives rise to a preceding wave of inhibition, and often results in the cessation of spontaneous activity. There was a spread of facilitation in the preferred direction. Such neurons probably reflect the properties of directionally selective retinal ganglion cells.

Levick, Oyster and Takahashi (1969) found directionally selective neurons in the lateral geniculate nucleus of the rabbit to generally function like directionally selective rabbit retinal ganglion cells of the "on-off" type. However, the geniculate neurons respond to only a smaller range of directions, or signal direction more precisely. Thus, while the retinal ganglion cells are quite reactive (25% of the maximum) to movements at right angles to their preferred direction-null direction axis, the geniculate cells show no response to such stimulation. In fact, geniculate cell activity falls beneath the maintained rate on stimulation at ± 80 degrees from the preferred direction, while retinal ganglion cell responses never drop below the maintained rate. These results also show that a strong inhibitory input acts on each directionally sensitive geniculate neuron.

Further, movement in the null direction gives rise to a much greater inhibition in the case of the geniculate cells, and they do not discharge at the initiation of null-direction movements.

Levick, Oyster and Takahashi postulate that each directionally sensitive geniculate cell receives inputs from two (or perhaps two groups of) retinal ganglion cells, one excitatory and the other inhibitory. The preferred directions of movement of the two retinal ganglion cells are directly opposed, or are divergent by 180 degrees. Of course, the preferred direction for response of the geniculate cell is identical with the preferred direction of the excitatory retinal ganglion cell.

The responses of the geniculate cells are less repetitive than those of the retinal ganglion cells. This possibly reflects activities occurring at the lateral geniculate nucleus level.

In the optic tectum (superior colliculus) of the frog, adjacent "on" neurons, which fail to exhibit spontaneous activity, inhibit each other following photic stimuli. This interaction between tectal neurons may lead to considerable differences in neural visual thresholds and sensitivities at later points in the visual pathway (Samsonova, 1967).

McIlwain and Buser (1968) observed a transitory, quickly habituating inhibition to appear in the periphery of the receptive fields of some neurons located in two laminae of the superior colliculus.

Neuronal activity in the cat's superior colliculus is depressed, presumably by discharges passing down corticotectal paths, when hypothermia is induced in the cerebral cortex. The experimental procedure appears to result in presynaptic inhibition within the superior colliculus (Marchiafava, Rizzolatti and Sprague, 1968).

Ablation of visual areas 17, 18 and 19 and surrounding cortical regions had no effect on collicular responses. However, Wickelgren and Sterling (1967) found that removal of the cat's visual cortices resulted in a loss of directional specificity and other symptoms in certain laminae of the superior colliculi.

Silakov (1968) reported that elimination of the neocortex produces a stable increase in all facets of the response activity of the superior colliculi and the exterior geniculate bodies. There is also an increase in response duration. In a few cases elimination of the neocortex results in a decrease in the amplitude of the evoked potentials. The normal inhibitory actions of the cortex are presumably transmitted by corticocollicular and corticogenicular tracts.

According to Sprague (1966), the two superior colliculi also seem to exert inhibition on each other.

While certain frequencies of light or auditory stimulation evoke discharges in the hippocampus (an olfactory center invaginated from the cortex), higher frequencies of such stimuli result in depression of hippocampal activity (Ungiadze, 1966).

Cortical responses to light appear to be associated with inhibitory postsynaptic potentials (IPSP's) in the cortical neurons (Skrebitskii, 1966; Kondratjeva and Polyansky, 1968). IPSP's are also evoked in the cat's visual cortex by electrical shocks to the optic tract and optic radiation (Creutzfeldt and Ito, 1968a). These IPSP's had latencies exceeding those of the frequently preceding excitatory postsynaptic potentials (EPSP's) by 1.0 msec.

Toyama and Matsunami (1968) recorded the effects of visual afferents on the parastriate portion of the visual cortex of the cat. They observed IPSP's to follow the EPSP's after a time lag of approximately 0.8 msec, and consider the IPSP's to have a disynaptic origin. The duration of the IPSP's exceeded 100 msec.

In the recovery cycle of the visual cortex of the tortoise (*Emys orbicularis*) as well, the return of facilitation precedes that of depression (Belekhova, 1968).

Creutzfeldt and Ito (1968b) found the cat's primary visual cortex to show spontaneous EPSP's and IPSP's. The former had a frequency of 150-300/sec, and outnumbered the latter by 10 to 1.

Armstrong (1968) applied two successive electrical stimuli to the optic radiation. He observed that a response in the visual cortex to the second stimulus was inhibited between 0.4 to 300 msec after the first stimulus, even if the latter was quite weak. An optimum inhibition could be obtained during a period of approximately 1 msec.

The inhibitory effect of the first electrical stimulus could be prevented by applying strychnine sulfate to the surface of the cortex. This and other features of the system indicate that the inhibition is postsynaptic.

Armstrong concludes that optic radiation fibers synapse with inhibitory interneurons which act on pyramidal cells in layer 3 or 4. Impulses from the optic radiation (geniculocortical) fibers excite the cortical cells before inhibition sets in because an excitatory pathway to the pyramidal cells is more quickly traversed than is the inhibitory pathway. It also appears that optic radiation fibers have more inhibitory than excitatory contacts.

Using only records obtained from rabbit visual cortex neurons responding to both light and sound, Skrebitskii (1967) determined that the amplitudes of the IPSP's produced in response to photic stimuli are reduced by irrelevant (auditory) stimuli. It is postulated that this reduction of the inhibitory responses is due to inhibition of inhibitory internuncial neurons or is a consequence of presynaptic inhibition.

Spinelli, Starr and Barrett (1968) corrobo-

rate that a fraction of the neurons in the primary visual cortex are responsive to both photic and acoustic stimuli. Several multisensitive neurons were not all excited by the same parameters of sound stimulation. Their visual receptive fields were generally more diffuse than those of purely visually responsive neurons.

No inhibition is observed in the primary visual cortex (area 17) of cats during stimulation of the skin and the labyrinth. Further, such stimulation only enhances the response to flashes of light (Gorgiladze and Smirnov, 1967).

Long inhibitory postsynaptic potentials produced in cat cortical neurons by electrical shocks to the caudate nucleus can be shortened by similar stimulation of the lateral geniculate body. Such disinhibition again appears to be presynaptic (Hull, Buchwald and Vieth, 1967). Like results are obtained by electrical stimulation of the auditory or the somatic sensory pathway and by the presentation of auditory, somatic and visual stimuli.

In addition to the inhibitory actions described earlier, recurrent inhibition appears to occur in the cerebral cortex.

If in the rabbit two or three stimuli with intervals of 3 to 5 msec are applied to the reticular formation of the midbrain, the activity of the majority of cortical neurons is facilitated. This facilitation has a latent period of about 20 to 35 msec, and reaches its peak after 35 to 50 msec. The rise in neuronal activity is attributed to the suppression of the recurrent inhibition of the cortex (Supin, 1968).

A superficial slow negative oscillation is elicited in the rabbit's visual cortex by afferent or direct stimulation. This negative oscillation can also be suppressed by stimulation of the reticular formation, and this effect is linked by Supin with the abolition of the cortex's recurrent inhibition.

The late "off" component of the response of the visual cortex to multiple flashes is known to be depressed by stimulation of the mesencephalic reticular formation. The same phenomenon can be observed by, instead of using visual flashes, stimulating the optic tract or lateral geniculate body with trains of electrical pulses (Steriade and Demetrescu, 1967).

Sukhov (1968) found that direct and antidromic electrical stimulation of the rat's sensorimotor cortex produced inhibition in the vast majority of cortical neurons. However, 3 per cent of the neurons responded with a high rate of impulses (maximum at onset 300-1,000/sec). Their discharge coincided with the initiation of inhibition of the other neurons and also resembled the inhibitory response in duration. Sukhov believes this 3 per cent of the cortical neurons to be inhibitory neurons which are at least partly responsible for the inhibition of the other cortical neurons.

A stabilization of the responses of visual cortex neurons to repetitive light stimulation was noted in unanesthetized rabbits by Sokolov, Polyanskii and Bagdonas (1968). They tentatively ascribed this stabilization to a postactivation potentiation of excitatory and inhibitory synapses and to lateral inhibition.

Shevelev and Hicks (1968), using anesthetized cats, observed an increasing reduction in summation at successively higher levels of the visual pathway. They considered the decrease in summation to result from horizontal inhibition in the consecutive stations of the visual pathway, particularly in the higher visual centers.

The primary visual area of the cat cortex was observed to contain neurons showing only inhibitory responses or having only inhibitory receptive fields. Other neurons had receptive fields composed of both excitatory and inhibitory areas, and a third group of neurons

showed excitation alone on photic stimulation of the retina (Creutzfeldt and Ito, 1968a).

By means of averaged records Creutzfeldt and Ito (1968b) determined that each neuron of the cat's primary visual cortex has two to four receptive-field areas of "on" or "off" excitation or inhibition. These areas overlap to different degrees. They show the properties of single geniculocortical "on" or "off" center fibers, and the differing responses of the cortical neurons can be explained on the basis of synapses with varying combinations of such fibers. The last can be either excitatory or inhibitory, but inhibitory effects may be indirectly transmitted by way of another cortical pyramidal neuron.

Movement sensitivity appears to be conveyed by excitatory "off" center fibers.

The experimental results given in this section indicate significant functional parallels between the inhibitory mechanisms of the lateral geniculate nucleus and the visual cortex. In both cases impulses which have been transmitted orthodromically along the visual pathway produce postsynaptic inhibition. Inhibitory interneurons appear to play a role in this inhibitory phenomenon. Also, in the case of both visual centers impulses of other origins than the preceding station of the visual pathway act to reduce the level of inhibition.

Goldberg and Lavine (1968) review recent work dealing with inhibitory phenomena in the higher portions of the visual pathway.

The structure and physiology of the lateral geniculate nucleus, the superior colliculi and the visual cortex are covered in a review by Creutzfeldt and Sakmann (1969).

THE AUDITORY SYSTEM

Structure and Functional Organization of the Peripheral Auditory Pathway

In higher vertebrates the auditory system's sense cells, the hair cells, are located in the cochlea. Within the cochlea the hair cells form rows in the organ of Corti, a structure which overlies the basilar membrane. While birds

possess approximately thirty rows of hair cells, mammals have four or five rows. In mammals the hair cells are structurally and topographically differentiated into outer rows of outer hair cells and an inner row of inner hair cells.

While the outer hair cells are cylindrical and have a flat free surface, the inner hair cells are of a lopsided flask shape that culminates in a small upper surface.

The free surface of both outer and inner hair cells is divided into a larger cuticular area and a noncuticular cytoplasmic region. Usually about a hundred stereocilia are borne by the cuticular portion of the free surface. They are longest at the periphery. The stereocilia of inner hair cells are also thicker and longer than those of outer hair cells.

In the noncuticular region a single kinocilium is represented in the adult by only a type of basal body, the kinetosome. This kinetosome may be of importance, according to one view, in transduction (Engström, 1967).

The stereocilia project from the free surface of each of the hair cells to embed themselves into the surface grooves of the gelatinous tectorial membrane, which lies parallel to and above the organ of Corti and the supporting basilar membrane (Fig. 4-13). The basilar membrane is set into vibration by the action of sound waves. Then the movements of the basilar membrane (and of the organ of Corti and thus the hair cells) in relation to the tectorial membrane subject the hair cells' stereocilia to shearing forces. These shearing forces are believed to initiate excitation of the hair cells.

The inner hair cells are considered more primitive and less sensitive than the outer hair cells. They appear to be more resistant to injury by noise and ototoxic drugs (Engström, 1967).

The fibers of the auditory nerve form the afferent innervation of the hair cells. These fibers are divided into radial fibers serving at least primarily the inner hair cells and spiral fibers innervating the outer hair cells. Most of the auditory fibers synapse with inner hair cells, and each of the last is innervated by a good number of neurons. The sensory innervation of the outer hair cells is less extensive (Spoendlin, 1966).

The portions of the outer hair cells adjacent to synapses with the afferent auditory fibers lack synaptic vesicles but contain large numbers of canaliculi of the smooth endoplasmic reticulum. These canaliculi appear to be involved in synaptic function (Echandia, 1967).

The bipolar cell bodies of the auditory nerve fibers are located in the spiral ganglion. The axons originating from these cell bodies run centrally to form the main portion of the auditory (eighth) nerve. These axons then terminate in the cochlear nuclei of the medulla oblongata. Each auditory nerve fiber (axon) divides centrally to send a branch to the dorsal cochlear nucleus and a branch to the ventral cochlear nucleus (Fig. 4-14).

It has been estimated that after a branch of an auditory fiber enters a cochlear nucleus, it ramifies to contact several hundred neurons (Lorente de Nó, 1933). Also, each cochlear nucleus neuron has synapses with hundreds of auditory fibers (Whitfield, 1967a).

The inner and outer hair cells are also innervated by efferent fibers, which form the olivocochlear bundle. These efferent fibers originate in or near the left and right superior olivary nuclei of the medulla oblongata (Fig. 4-14), most from a periolivary cell group, and show considerable branching at various levels. Close to the internal auditory meatus they travel in the vestibular portion of the auditory nerve but can be recognized by their characteristic ultrastructure. The efferent fibers have been reported to synapse with the hair cells and with the afferent fibers (dendrites which are axonal in structure) of the auditory nerve (Spoendlin, 1966).

Nerve tracts run, mainly contralaterally, from the ventral cochlear nucleus to the superior olivary nuclei (Fig. 4-14). The distribution of these fiber tracts to the superior olivary complex of both sides forms the basis for the lowest level of binaural interaction.

Recordings from individual auditory nerve fibers have shown that each is most sensitive to a certain, characteristic frequency. Fibers innervating the basal turn of the cochlea, near the foramen ovale, have high characteristic frequencies, while fibers coming from the apical portion of the cochlea exhibit low characteristic frequencies.

The response area of an auditory unit might

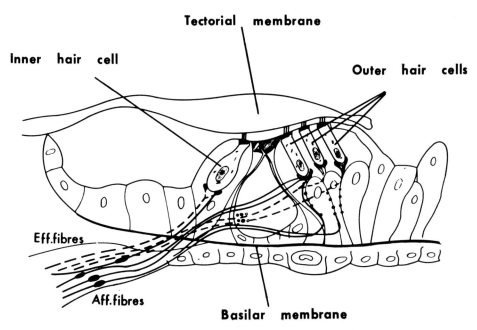

FIGURE 4-13. Diagrammatic cross-section through a mammal's organ of Corti. The supporting basilar membrane lies beneath the organ of Corti. Afferent and efferent nerve fibers innervate the hair cells. (Adapted from Wersäll, J., Å. Flock, and P.-G. Lundquist: Structural basis for directional sensitivity in cochlear and vestibular sensory receptors. In *Sensory Receptors. Cold Spring Harbor Symposia on Quantitative Biology*, *30*:115-132, 1965.)

be defined as an area on an intensity versus frequency graph which includes all combinations of intensities and frequencies to which the auditory unit is reactive (Galambos and Davis, 1943).

A good treatment of the structure and function of all parts of the auditory pathway, including the centrifugal pathways, can be found in the book *The Auditory Pathway*, by Whitfield (1967a). Spoendlin (1966), in his volume *The Organization of the Cochlear Receptor*, makes a detailed study of the cochlea. He emphasizes the hair sense cells and their afferent and efferent innervations and includes material on the physiology of the olivocochlear bundle. A detailed examination of the organ of Corti—the hair cells, supporting cells and nervous innervations—is made in *Structural Pattern of the Organ of Corti*, by Engström, Ades and Andersson (1966). The ultrastructure of the sensory cells of the cochlea is treated in a paper by that name written by Engström (1967).

Peripheral Inhibition
Primary-order Neurons

A number of research papers point to the existence of inhibition, other than that produced by efferent fibers, in the peripheral portion of the auditory system at the level of the auditory nerve neurons or earlier.

Several investigators have observed that if an auditory fiber is transmitting a discharge in response to a stimulus, the application of a second, less effective stimulus (a stimulus acting on the periphery of the fiber's receptive area, for example) may be followed by a drop in impulse frequency.

Thus Nomoto, Suga and Katsuki (1964) and Frishkopf (1964), respectively using the monkey and the bat, reported that a combination of two tones may elicit a lower impulse frequency than that called forth by either tone

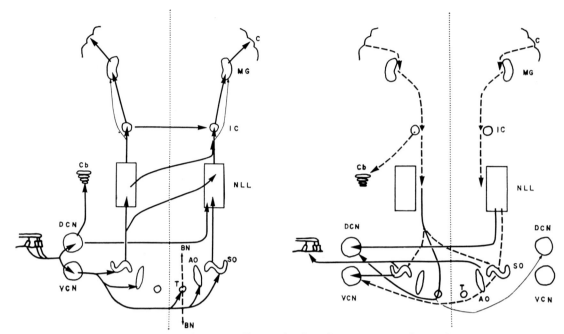

FIGURE 4-14. Afferent (left) and efferent (right) fiber tracts of the auditory system. Connections whose existence is still open to question are indicated by dashed lines. (*DCN*) dorsal cochlear nucleus, (*VCN*) ventral cochlear nucleus, (*Cb*) cerebellum, (*AO*) accessory olivary nucleus, (*SO*) lateral olivary nucleus, (*T*) nucleus of the trapezoid body, (*BN*) brain stem motor nuclei, (*NLL*) nuclei of the lateral lemniscus, (*IC*) inferior colliculus, (*MG*) medial geniculate body, (C) cortex. The accessory olivary nucleus, lateral olivary nucleus (S-shaped segment) and nucleus of the trapezoid body belong to the superior olivary complex, and the nuclei of the lateral lemniscus are considered to be extensions of this complex. (From Whitfield, I.C.: *The Auditory Pathway.* London, Edward Arnold, 1967.)

alone. The intense tone burst used by Nomoto, Suga and Katsuki (1964) to inhibit a continuous background tone generally was most effective if its frequency was below the characteristic frequency of the auditory nerve fiber. However, in the case of some fibers, inhibition was called forth by tone bursts having frequencies either below or above the characteristic frequency. In still other fibers inhibition was best produced by frequencies above the characteristic frequency. Frishkopf (1964) observed that in over 80 per cent of the bat's primary auditory neurons elicited activity was inhibited by frequencies just beyond the higher limits of the neuron's excitatory range. Fewer units were inhibited by frequencies at either side of their excitatory range.

In both the experiments of Nomoto, Suga and Katsuki (1964) and of Frishkopf (1964), the inhibition produced by the addition of the second tone stimulus to the first had but a short latent period. The possibility of an efferent effect is further reduced by such inhibitory results being obtained after sectioning of the auditory nerve (Kiang *et al.*, 1965). A role by efferent fibers in the preparations of Nomoto, Suga and Katsuki (1964) is contraindicated by the lack of an effect on the part of strychnine. The stimulation of olivocochlear efferent impulses also produced no results.

Nomoto, Suga and Katsuki further report that the inhibition they evoked was followed by a postinhibitory rebound.

Hind *et al.* (1967) determined that the response to two tones applied together is usually less than the discharge elicited by the more stimulating tone when it is used by itself.

One cannot ignore the chance that in these experiments the movements of the basilar membrane elicited by one stimulus interfered with the oscillations provoked by the other. The likelihood that such mechanical interaction between basilar membrane oscillations accounts for the phenomena of afferent inhibition is increased by the fact that inhibiting tone bursts have had to be of relatively high intensity. Nomoto, Suga and Katsuki (1964) take cognizance of the possibility that their findings are the result of such mechanical interaction. They also observed that summation between two nonexciting tones can take place. Sometimes two tones, which separately produced no discharge because they lay beyond the response area of the tested auditory unit, in combination called forth impulses.

Adaptation also exerts an effect in inhibition experiments (Kiang *et al.*, 1965).

Two groups of investigators (Katsuki, Suga and Kanno, 1962; Rupert, Moushegian and Galambos, 1963) have published results which seem to satisfy the objections given above. They observed single tones to depress spontaneous activity being transmitted by the auditory nerve. The second group of investigators noted an immediate inhibition with a latent period of less than 20 msec. This last finding reduces the likelihood of efferent fiber involvement.

Kiang *et al.* (1965), in spite of strenuous efforts, failed to obtain inhibition of spontaneous activity by means of a single tone. This group of investigators regards the results of the earlier single-tone experiments with some reservations.

Thus in regard to the experiment by Katsuki, Suga and Kanno (1962), it is pointed out by Kiang *et al.* (1965) that inhibition appeared in association with "on" and "on-off" discharges to tone bursts. Sound frequencies other than that of the selected single tone are produced when a tone burst starts and ceases. Therefore, Kiang *et al.* (1965) suggest that the termination of the responses, by several auditory units,

to the initial, transient, extra sound frequencies may have been misconstrued by Katsuki, Suga and Kanno as a reduction in activity due to inhibition.

Kiang *et al.* (1965) also remark that the unanesthetized cats used in the research of Rupert, Moushegian and Galambos (1963) may themselves have produced a noisy environment. In such a case the inhibition observed by these investigators could have been due to the interaction of the effects evoked by two tones. Although both unanesthetized and anesthetized cats were employed by Rupert, Moushegian and Galambos, their results for inhibition by one tone were obtained with the former.

Kiang *et al.* (1965) determined one auditory unit in the cat to produce a relatively high level of spontaneous activity (100 impulses/ sec). They then subjected this unit to a continuous tone at the characteristic frequency of the unit's auditory nerve fiber. This elicited a higher impulse rate. If now tone bursts clearly capable of exciting the auditory unit were superimposed on stimulation with the aforementioned continuous tone, the unit's impulse frequency fell beneath the spontaneous level (Fig. 4-15). This drop in activity below the spontaneous level is not very likely to be due to interference between two sets of basilar membrane oscillations.

Kiang *et al.* provide adequate evidence that the described inhibitory phenomenon did not involve centrifugal fiber activity.

The condensation phase of clicks, which results in an inward motion of the tympanic membrane, produces a decrease in baseline auditory nerve activity. Kiang *et al.* (1965) cite this as a rapidly appearing inhibitory phenomenon.

If true afferent inhibition indeed occurs below the level of the brain's cochlear nuclei, its structural basis is yet unknown. Perhaps inhibitory action takes place at the layers of cochlear hair sense cells.

Spoendlin (1966) writes that a noticeable increase in sound contrast (presumably by some inhibition) can already be noted in recordings from the auditory nerve fibers. He suggests that this original sharpening of the auditory response may occur in the peripheral nerve plexus beneath the bases of the sense cells, since no other significant connections between nerve fibers have been found up to the level of the cochlear nuclei. The hair cells in the organ of Corti receive a multiple innervation from nerve fibers which form a nerve plexus.

A comparatively ineffective stimulus, if it has sufficiently high intensity, can also mask a stimulus which normally elicits a much greater discharge. This typically results in a lowered impulse frequency, and sometimes the drop in discharge rate is great (Kiang *et al.*, 1965; Hind *et al.*, 1967). However, the masking effect cannot truly be considered an inhibitory phenomenon. Hind *et al.* state that the masking tone acts by causing the auditory nerve fiber to "phase-lock" its activity to the sinusoidal cycle of the masker. The phase-locked response to the masked tone, which the last normally elicits, is thus prevented.

Goldberg and Lavine (1968), as well as Bishop (1967), discuss inhibition in primary auditory neurons.

Second-order Neurons (Cochlear Nuclei)

The first-order auditory nerve neurons synapse with the second-order cochlear nucleus neurons.

Just as retinal ganglion cells typically have an inhibitory zone in their visual receptive field, most cochlear nucleus neurons have response areas partly composed of inhibitory portions. The majority of cat and monkey cochlear nucleus neurons possess a central excitatory response area which is flanked at lower and higher frequencies by inhibitory areas. Suga (1964) was able to observe only one inhibitory area and one excitatory area in bat (*Myotis lucifugus*) cochlear units, and the inhibitory area always had higher frequencies than its neighboring excitatory area. In the bat, however, the cochlear nuclei play a special role in echolocation and are hypertrophied.

In the little brown bat the higher frequency

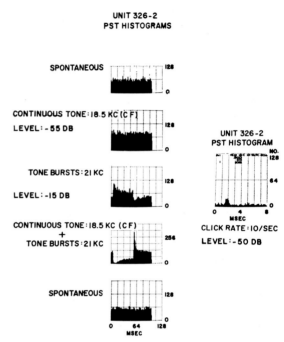

FIGURE 4-15. Responses of a cat auditory unit to a continuous tone, tone bursts, and a combination of both. The top histogram demonstrates the unit's level of spontaneous activity (100 spikes/ sec). Impulse activity was augmented by a continuous tone at the unit's characteristic frequency (second histogram) and also by 21-kc tone bursts (third histogram). If tone-burst stimulation was added to a continuous-tone background (fourth histogram), there was a large transient decrease in discharge, followed by a plateau considerably below the level of spontaneous activity. Termination of the tone bursts resulted in a sizeable transient increase in activity and a subsequent return to the baseline level. Bottom histogram, control record of spontaneous activity. Zero time for all histograms, 2.5 msec preceding the electrical input to the earphone; continuous tone, 55 dB; tone bursts, duration of 50 msec, 2.5 msec rise-fall time, 10 bursts/sec, 15 dB. Histogram on right pictures short latency of click response, identifying unit as an auditory nerve fiber (50 dB clicks, 10/sec). (From Kiang, N. Y-S., *et al.*: *Discharge Patterns of Single Fibers in the Cat's Auditory Nerve*. Cambridge, M.I.T. Pr., 1965.)

inhibitory area begins close to the excitatory area's best frequency, and the boundary between these excitatory and inhibitory areas is narrow and sharp (Suga, 1964).

The widths of response areas, and presumably their excitatory and inhibitory components, vary among cochlear neurons.

Greenwood and Maruyama (1965) determined that a cochlear neuron's near-peak response to a band of sound around the neuron's most stimulating frequency could usually be suppressed by a band of noise at any frequencies of the inhibitory areas. As the intensity of an effective noise band is heightened, the response to an unchanging tone is increasingly inhibited.

Sound frequencies at the inhibitory areas can also suppress spontaneous activity (Rose, Galambos and Hughes, 1959).

Inhibition at the level of the cochlear nucleus has a typical latent period of 1 to 2 msec, and is not affected by strychnine, even when the last is directly applied to the neuron under investigation (Whitfield and Comis, 1967).

Stopp and Whitfield (1961) determined the proportions of cells exhibiting inhibitory phenomena in the nucleus magnocellularis of the pigeon, which is homologous to the ventral cochlear nucleus of mammals. In almost half of the one hundred investigated neurons, a response to one tone could be suppressed with another, while one fifth of the units exhibited inhibition of their spontaneous activity by a tone but gave no responses to the employed stimuli. The other recorded neurons were successfully excited by tones but showed no inhibition. Since in some of the first group of neurons only a small degree of inhibition was called forth by intense tones, Whitfield (1967a) suggests that cochlear neurons may show a spectrum of variation in the proportions of their excitatory and inhibitory connections.

Unlike previous workers, Gerstein, Butler and Erulkar (1968) recorded intracellularly from cochlear nucleus neurons. They simultaneously stimulated the ears of their anesthetized cats with sequences of brief tone bursts at different frequencies and with fixed tones.

Gerstein, Butler and Erulkar (1968) found that the impulse discharges maintained in most neurons for the length of an exciting tone stimulus were accompanied by sustained membrane depolarizations of the same duration. In many neurons the long-lasting impulse discharges were interrupted or the firing rate temporarily dropped for some reason. Such disturbances were frequently systematic functions of the stimulating frequency and the time interval since initial application of the stimulus.

In some neurons the period during which there was a suppression of the impulse discharge was a linear function of the logarithm of the stimulus (tone) frequency. Upon comparing subjective responses of humans with the recorded suppressions of firing in the cat, the authors also hazard the suggestion that the period of impulse inhibition is linearly related to the subjective tone frequency. It thus appears quite possible that in certain neurons information about an exciting sound frequency may be coded in terms of the period of inhibition of impulses.

In the discharges of other neurons highly complex changes were noted.

Since a hyperpolarizing potential was only rarely seen during the inhibition of an impulse discharge, even if depolarization had earlier been recorded from the same neuron, Gerstein, Butler and Erulkar believe that inhibitory potentials act at some distance from the cell soma, the presumed location of the recording electrode. This finding also suggests that the site of impulse generation lies beyond the cell body.

Erulkar, Butler and Gerstein (1968) assume that auditory (primary) fibers may form both inhibitory and excitatory synapses with a cochlear nucleus neuron.

The impulse discharge of some cochlear nucleus units did not vary synchronously with the course of the associated membrane depolarization. This indicates that the time courses of excitatory and inhibitory synaptic inflows are unlike. The occasionally seen long latent period of response may be the result of an inhibitory process which not only appears earlier but also dissipates more rapidly than excitation. The suppression of spontaneous activity after the termination of excitation at the characteristic or surrounding frequencies may be due to an inhibitory influence outlasting excitation. The virtual absence of "off" responses in the cochlear nucleus may indicate that the excitatory synaptic inflow is not maintained beyond either the inhibitory inflow or the period of stimulation.

Both the "on" discharges and the periods of lowered impulse activity which are sometimes observed are also believed to be consequent to interactions between excitatory and inhibitory influences.

In the little brown bat (*Myotis lucifugus*) some cochlear nucleus neurons produce marked afterdischarges (Suga, 1964). In a number of cases these afterdischarges could be identified as postinhibitory rebounds. The afterdischarges may serve to increase the contrast between the excitatory and the inhibitory responses of the said neurons.

In most cochlear nucleus neurons the responses to slow frequency modulation of tones resembled those to tones of unchanging frequency (Erulkar, Butler and Gerstein, 1968). However, three main kinds of firing pattern in response to slow linear frequency modulation could be identified. One firing pattern, named "mirror symmetry," indicated sensitivity to only the momentary tonal frequency. Another firing pattern, "translation symmetry," was purely a function of the time of stimulation. It included no element of response to frequency or the order of frequency stimulation. Perhaps neurons reacting with "translation symmetry" only code timing information. The third type of firing pattern, "asymmetry," reflected momentary frequency, the direction of frequency change, and the rate of frequency change.

The presence of excitatory and inhibitory areas in the response area of a cochlear nucleus neuron may derive some of its significance from the accentuation of temporal contrast. An increase in temporal contrast may be called forth as sound frequencies shift from the excitatory area of a neuron to its inhibitory area (Evans and Nelson, 1966). Certain sound stimuli have been found to alternately produce excitatory and inhibitory effects during the period of their presentation (Greenwood and Maruyama, 1965; Kiang, 1965).

Suga (1964) points out that in the little brown bat (*Myotis lucifugus*) the adjacent, sharply separated inhibitory and excitatory areas of some cochlear units could produce a temporal effect during echolocation. The echolocating sound pulses of *Myotis lucifugus* start at high frequencies and then drop one octave. This should first evoke inhibitory responses and then excitatory responses, the point and thus the timing of transition varying among neurons.

Greenwood and Maruyama (1965) suggest that the relationship between excitatory and inhibitory areas may vary with time. They base themselves on the complex manner in which the impulse frequency of some cochlear nucleus cells changes with sound intensity.

An inhibition of firing can be elicited in neurons of the cat's cochlear nucleus by triangular or trapezoidal modulating waveforms. This inhibition is affected by the direction of change of frequency with time. It is not associated with hyperpolarization of the neuron membrane. The duration of the inhibition depends on the frequency (Butler, Gerstein and Erulkar, 1967).

A good number of cochlear nucleus neurons show the expected increase in impulse frequency with a rise in sound intensity, but then, as the stimulus intensity is raised farther, their impulse rate falls again. In addition, such nonmonotonic cochlear units may not maintain a regular asymptotic decrease in impulse frequency during long-continued stimulation. Goldberg and Greenwood (1966) report that most cochlear nucleus neurons are not observed to be nonmonotonic units when stimulated with prolonged pure tones. When discovered nonmonotonic neurons were subjected to increasingly intense pure tones, an earlier portion of their response was markedly depressed, but the later part of the response showed relatively little effect.

The depressive effect obtained with non-monotonic cochlear nucleus neurons by increasing the intensity of an inhibiting noise band during monotonal stimulation at a fixed intensity resembles the effect produced by raising the stimulus intensity above the maximum response level. This appears to indicate that inhibitory influences are called forth at the response area frequencies when the intensity is raised above that provoking a maximum discharge. There seems to be an overlap between excitatory and inhibitory actions at the intensities exceeding the maximum response intensity and perhaps even at somewhat lower intensities.

Radionova (1968) has made a detailed analysis of several diverse types of inhibitory processes which she observed in the cochlear nucleus of the cat.

Starr and Wernick (1968) observed that stimulation of the cat's olivocochlear bundle, while depressing the activity in the cochlear nucleus called forth by tones of threshold intensity, increased the activity produced by tones at higher intensities. This may be correlated with the described fact that at supra-optimal intensities tones may give rise to inhibitory influences in cochlear nucleus neurons.

Whitfield (1967a) raises the possibility that inhibitory internuncial neurons are present in the cochlear nuclei.

After ablation of the ipsilateral cochlea, stimulation of the crossed olivocochlear bundle in unanesthetized cats still modified the spontaneous discharge in the dorsal and postero-ventral subdivisions of the cochlear nucleus (Starr and Wernick, 1968). This indicates that the olivocochlear bundle exerts a direct effect on these portions of the cochlear nucleus, presumably through those of its fibers which innervate the cochlear nucleus.

Koerber *et al.* (1966) state that while spontaneous activity in the ventral cochlear nucleus is probably dependent on an afferent input from the cochlea, this is not true of the spontaneous discharge in the dorsal and postero-ventral subdivision of the cochlear nucleus.

The results of Starr and Wernick (1968) corroborate this conclusion.

Olivocochlear stimulation resulted in more complex changes in cochlear nucleus activity than had been observed after such stimulation in the discharge of auditory nerve fibers. Spontaneous activity, as well as responses to tones, were decreased, increased or not affected in different cochlear nucleus neurons (Starr and Wernick, 1968).

The division of the response areas of cochlear nucleus neurons into excitatory and inhibitory areas indicates that an important stage in the processing of sound information occurs in the cochlear nuclei.

Goldberg and Lavine (1968) devote a section of their review paper to the cochlear nuclei, and Bishop (1967) also deals extensively with this subject. Whitfield (1967a) treats the cochlear nuclei in a separate chapter.

Centrifugal Inhibition

The hair sense cells and endings of the auditory nerve in the organ of Corti are subject to inhibition through efferent impulses transmitted by the olivocochlear fibers.

Uncrossed reticulocochlear fibers are also said to innervate the cochlea in rodents and rabbits (Rasmussen, 1965; Rossi and Cortesina, 1965).

In mammals the olivocochlear fibers consist on each side of a larger crossed group and less than one quarter as many uncrossed fibers.

The crossed fibers originate from a mass of minute multipolar cells which lies dorsomedially from the accessory olive nucleus and dorsally to the nucleus of the trapezoid body (Fig. 4-14). This mass of cells is known as the retrolateral olivary cell group. Morest (1968) describes this origin of the crossed olivocochlear fibers, and hypothesizes about its function.

The uncrossed fibers are the processes of cell bodies in the S-segment of the superior olive nucleus (Fig. 4-14) or may also originate from the dorsolateral periolivary cell group (Rasmussen, 1967).

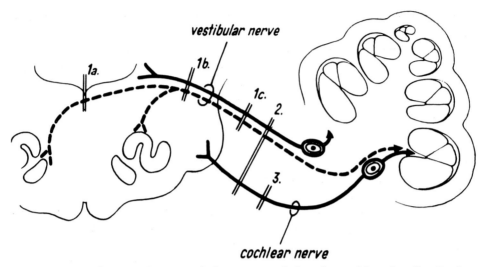

vestibular nerve

cochlear nerve

FIGURE 4-16. Schematic drawing of the courses of the olivocochlear bundle (broken line) and related nerves. The contralateral portion of the olivocochlear bundle may be selectively sectioned (*1a*), or the whole bundle can be interrupted in the vestibular root (*1b*) or in the vestibular nerve (*1c*). In the internal acoustic meatus the entire VIII nerve (*2*) or only the cochlear (auditory) nerve (*3*) may be transected. (From Spoendlin, H.: *The Organization of the Cochlear Receptor. Advances Otorhinolaryng.*, vol. 13 [S. Karger, Basel/New York], 1966.)

The cells of the uncrossed efferent fibers are said to be capable of receiving impulses from only the ipsilateral cochlear nucleus, while the cell mass of the crossed olivocochlear fibers has connections at least primarily with the contralateral cochlear nucleus (Rasmussen, 1960).

Warr (1969), using degeneration methods, found that while the anteroventral cochlear nucleus sends fibers to the lateral and medial superior olivary nuclei, the posteroventral cochlear nucleus projects to the periolivary cell groups located close to the lateral superior olivary nucleus. At least some of these destinations of cochlear nucleus fibers act as origins of olivocochlear fibers.

Soon after the crossed fibers join the uncrossed fibers of the opposite side, most of each now mixed olivocochlear bundle passes out of the medulla oblongata together with the vestibular nerve. The olivocochlear fibers then shift from the vestibular nerve to the cochlear portion of the auditory nerve, and travel to the cochlea in company with the afferent auditory fibers. In the cochlea the efferent fibers

form the intraganglionic (spiral ganglion) spiral bundles (3-6) which course toward the apex and as well in the opposite direction toward the round window.

However, a few fibers of the olivocochlear bundle leave it before it emerges from the medulla oblongata. These fibers pass through the vestibular nerve to the ventral cochlear nucleus (Rasmussen, 1960).

The olivocochlear fibers are myelinated up to the basilar membrane.

The terminations of the olivocochlear fibers in the organ of Corti have diameters of less than 1μ, and are thus differentiated from the bigger (2μ-5μ) endings of the afferent auditory fibers. The terminal branches of the efferent fibers also have a unique beaded structure.

The large endings of the olivocochlear fibers contain high numbers of synaptic vesicles, granulated vesicles and mitochondria (Kimura and Wersäll, 1962; Spoendlin, 1966; Echandia, 1967). Echandia (1967) did not see any granulated vesicles directly beneath the synaptic membrane; they probably are not involved in synaptic transmission. Adjacent to their efferent synapses the outer hair cells possess a uniquely clear-cut reticulum of subsurface cisternae (Echandia, 1967).

Sectioning of the olivocochlear fibers has clearly shown that they innervate the outer hair cells of the organ of Corti by means of most of their large vesiculated endings (Spoendlin, 1966). There are fewer large vesiculated endings in the region of the inner hair cells. Spoendlin also mentions efferent terminal fibers which appear to end beneath the inner hair cells. These fibers make up the majority of the numerous, typically quite small inner spiral fibers and also are a part of the olivocochlear system.

The inner hair cells have less sensitivity than the outer hair cells.

The outer hair cells of the basal coil of the cochlea seem to have the richest efferent innervation (Smith and Sjöstrand, 1961). Spoendlin (1966) estimates that in the cochlea's basal turn there are six to ten efferent nerve endings and five to eight afferent endings per outer hair cell. Thus in this region there seem to be a majority of efferent terminals. At the end of the cochlea's first coil, however, there is already a diminution in the number of efferent endings serving the first two rows of outer hair cells, and only a few efferent endings still innervate the outer hair cells of the third row. At the cochlea's apex generally only the outer hair cells of the first row have any efferent innervation.

According to Spoendlin (1966) the approximately 500 fibers of the olivocochlear bundle ramify to give rise to at least 40,000 efferent endings in the cochlea.

More afferent than efferent endings serve the total of outer hair cells in the cochlea.

Smith and Rasmussen (1963) postulate that the repetitive widenings of the efferent fibers seen in certain species may represent points of synaptic contact with afferent dendrites. Smith (1968), who is quite positive in regarding contacts between efferent-fiber enlargements and afferent dendrites as synaptic, points out

that the efferent bulbous widenings contain numerous vesicles and some mitochondria.

Membrane thickenings and clusters of vesicles are also present in efferent terminals which supposedly make synaptic contact with afferent fibers just beyond the hair cell synapse.

Since over most of their course to the cochlea the efferent fibers run separately from the afferent auditory fibers in the cochlear nerve, it is possible to section only the olivocochlear fibers alone (Fig. 4-16).

Efferent fibers have also been described from the pigeon and caiman (Boord, 1961), and from the auditory nerve of the bullfrog (Robbins, Bauknight and Honrubia, 1967).

The efferent olivocochlear impulses bring about a reduction in the afferent activity transmitted along the auditory nerve. They also produce an enhancement of the cochlear microphonic, which is the hair cell receptor potential (Desmedt, 1962; Fex, 1962). These effects have been considered to be due to postsynaptic inhibition of, respectively, the auditory nerve endings and the hair cells (Desmedt and Monaco, 1961).

Fex (1967) believes the decrease in afferent auditory impulses to directly result from the inhibitory action on the hair cells, which are hyperpolarized. He rests his conviction on the histological findings of other investigators and on the following facts: Electrical stimulation of the crossed efferents elicits postsynaptic potentials reaching 3 mV in the cat's scala media. Intracochlear potentials of such large amplitude are most likely to arise from the membranes of rows of parallel cells. Also, the centrifugally provoked potentials are positive in the organ of Corti and negative in the scala media. This change in sign resembles the 180 degree phase shift undergone by the cochlear microphonics, and again implicates the hair cell membranes (Fex, 1968).

Spoendlin (1966) contends that the fibers of the olivocochlear bundle which innervate the outer hair cells probably act chiefly on these sense cells. He bases his view on the greater areas of contact between efferent endings and outer hair cells than between these efferent endings and nearby afferent dendrites. In fact, Spoendlin found numerous efferent endings in the cochlea's basal coil to have no demonstrable direct contact with afferent dendrites. Also, concentrations of synaptic vesicles, and so on, are much more commonly present in efferent endings where they come into the proximity of outer hair cells.

At the same time, Spoendlin notes that there are synapses between efferent endings and afferent dendrites, particularly in the apical coils of the cochlea. Echandia (1967) observed efferent and afferent endings to be apposed. However, he saw no synaptic structural differentiations and assumes the absence of a true synaptic relationship at the points of afferent-efferent proximity which were examined by him.

The efferent endings of the internal spiral plexus, beneath the inner hair cells, on the other hand, form synapses almost entirely with afferent dendrites, according to Spoendlin (1966).

Fex (1967) and Iurato (1964) assume at least a portion of the cat's uncrossed olivocochlear fibers to terminate below the inner hair cells, and there synapse with afferent dendrites. Fex (1967) tentatively suggests that the uncrossed olivocochlear fibers of the cat may only act on the afferent dendrites beneath the inner hair cells.

Desmedt and Monaco (1962) were proponents of the hypothesis that efferent endings in general act primarily on the afferent dendrites. Smith (1968) suggests that both the efferent ending–hair cell synapses and efferent axon–afferent dendrite synapses contribute to inhibition.

The application of strychnine prevents the effects of centrifugal fiber activity (Desmedt and Monaco, 1961; Desmedt and La Grutta, 1963; Desmedt and Delwaide, 1965).

It has been possible to clearly demonstrate with electrical stimuli that efferent fiber discharges can lead to the inhibition of afferent auditory nerve responses in the cat. Galambos (1956) and Desmedt (1962) obtained such

results after the removal of the middle ear muscles. Also, if the olivocochlear bundle was transected peripherally to the region of stimulus application, a change in afferent activity no longer occurred.

Fex (1962), by recording from single afferent auditory nerve fibers, determined that the application of electric shocks to the efferent fibers suppressed both resting activity and sound-evoked impulse discharges in the great majority of auditory fibers. There were no instances of facilitation.

Electrical stimulation of the uncrossed olivocochlear fibers also brings about reduced afferent auditory responses, but the action of the uncrossed fibers is markedly weaker than that of the crossed fibers (Desmedt and La Grutta, 1963).

Dewson (1967) reduced the amplitudes of click-evoked cat auditory nerve discharges by electrically stimulating the crossed olivocochlear fibers. He found that such reduction is not significantly additive with that produced by broad-band noise if both methods are applied simultaneously.

The results of efferent stimulation have been reported to depend on the attributes of the auditory stimulus (Sohmer, 1965; Wiederhold and Peake, 1966). The last authors found efferent activity in anesthetized cats to produce no noticeable inhibition when a click exceeded its intensity at the lowest observable response level by 60 to 70 dB. Further, at intensities producing discharges of equal amplitude, the responses evoked by high-frequency (10,000 Hz) stimuli were inhibited more than those provoked by low-frequency (400 Hz) stimuli. Wiederhold and Peake suggest that this greater inhibition of responses to high frequencies may be related to the much more extensive efferent innervation of the cochlea's basal coil. Sohmer (1965) reported that electrical shocking of the crossed centrifugal fibers in the anesthetized cat resulted in the greatest inhibition when auditory stimulation was of low intensity or of low frequency. Sohmer did not equalize the amplitudes of the responses to different frequencies of sound. The effects produced by efferent discharges appear to also differ among individual auditory nerve fibers (Wiederhold and Swift, 1967).

The efferent fibers themselves apparently also each preferentially discharge following contralateral auditory stimulation with a characteristic range of frequencies.

Fex (1965) stimulated uncrossed efferent fibers in the cat with electrical shocks to the ipsilateral auditory nerve and with sound directed to the contralateral ear. Higher frequencies to this ear particularly excited the uncrossed efferents innervating the basal portion of the cochlea, while the fibers to the apical portion preferentially reacted to lower frequencies. It thus appears that excitation of the basal or apical portion of one cochlea produces impulses in the uncrossed olivocochlear fibers respectively serving the basal or the apical turns of the other cochlea. On this basis Fex postulates that the cochleas are projected on each other and that afferent auditory fibers from one cochlea are indirectly connected with uncrossed efferents innervating the corresponding points in the other cochlea. These indirect afferent-efferent connections probably involve third-order auditory neurons.

A few crossed fibers investigated by Fex (1962) also showed a differential distribution according to the sound frequencies of their activation. Apparently a similar arrangement of afferent-efferent projections applies to the crossed fibers.

Fex (1965) notes that the uncrossed efferents are affected by both cochlear nerves. He then states the belief that both the uncrossed and crossed olivocochlear fibers are part of an auditory feedback system. Such a system is probably under central control. This is evidenced by the finding of Buño *et al.* (1966) that habituation can affect the cochlear microphonic and the primary auditory discharge by way of the efferent system (see page 177). Veselý and Faltýnek (1964) observed that during spreading cortical depression, the guinea pig's cochlea shows increased sensitivity to a wide range of tones (500-2000 Hz), as

seen by amplitude changes in the cochlear microphonics.

Fex (1965) puts much emphasis on the fact that the uncrossed efferent fibers are subject to inhibition (their spontaneous activity can at least typically be suppressed by stimulating the contralateral ear with sound). He suggests that this may refine the function of the described orderly arrangement of the uncrossed fibers and permit a more effective or delicate control of the total efferent output. Inhibition could supplement control through the level of excitation.

The crossed fibers do not undergo such inhibition.

There is some evidence that the cat's crossed efferents are more successfully influenced through the cochlea that they innervate than through the opposite cochlea (Fex, 1963). On this score the observations on the uncrossed efferents are insufficient.

The inhibitory actions of the crossed as well as the uncrossed olivocochlear fibers show long latencies at auditory thresholds. Fex (1962) noted that stimulation of the efferent fibers reduced the afferent discharge following a barely exciting click only if it preceded the click by over 15 msec. It took 75 msec for inhibition of the response to a tone to reach its peak. This inhibition was also maintained for close to 70 msec after the cessation of olivocochlear stimulation. Desmedt (1962) found efferent inhibition to undergo decay according to an exponential curve having a time constant of approximately 150 msec.

The long latent periods of action, and the regular, low-rate discharge of efferent fibers, mean that an input fed into the efferents is probably integrated over a lengthy time period.

Whitfield (1967a) states that the long latencies of efferent action are indicative of a slow peripheral process. He further points out that this peripheral process is probably also responsible for the fact that continuous electrical stimulation is not accompanied by continued inhibition. Instead, groups of 40 to 100 electrical pulses are most effective.

High-frequency stimulation must be applied in the case of both the crossed and the uncrossed olivocochlear fibers to bring about a noticeable drop in afferent neural activity. Trains of shocks with a frequency of 250-400/sec give the best results, while a frequency of 50/sec produces little effect (Desmedt, 1962; Fex, 1962). The maximum reduction of afferent auditory nerve activity achieved by efferent fiber stimulation was equivalent to a drop of 25 dB in the intensity of a sound stimulus. This decrease was obtained by stimulating the crossed olivocochlear tract of the cat at a high rate. In most tested species peak inhibitions equivalent to 14 dB or more could be produced (Desmedt, 1962). The highest inhibition obtained by stimulating the less numerous uncrossed efferent fibers in the cat corresponded to an intensity drop of 6 or 7 dB (Desmedt and La Grutta, 1963).

In contrast, the maximal obtainable increase in amplitude of the cochlear microphonics by means of efferent stimulation is equivalent to but 3 to 4 dB (Desmedt, 1962; Desmedt and Monaco, 1962).

Desmedt and Delwaide (1965) compared their results with the efferent cochlear bundle of the pigeon to those gained by the other investigators with the olivocochlear bundle of the cat. By recording, from the round window, the responses to clicks and tone pips, they determined the effects of electrically stimulating the pigeon's efferent fibers. Desmedt and Delwaide observed such stimulation to enhance the cochlear microphonics and inhibit the afferent auditory discharges, and they consider the bird's efferent cochlear bundle to be essentially physiologically homologous with the olivocochlear bundle of the mammal.

However, there are also significant differences between the efferent effects in the pigeon and the cat. In the pigeon the auditory nerve action potentials are never totally inhibited, and the greatest suppression of auditory nerve activity is equivalent to only a drop of 7 dB in sound intensity. On the other hand, the cochlear microphonics are augmented to an unusual extent. These receptor potentials may be increased by as much as the equivalent of 7 dB. Furthermore, in the pigeon the augmentation of the cochlear microphonics is maintained for a longer period than the partial inhibition of the auditory response, while both effects decay at the same rate in the cat.

If the cochlear microphonics are really receptor potentials that give rise to auditory nerve action potentials, then the maintenance of enhanced cochlear microphonics beyond the period of nerve inhibition should result in an increased afferent auditory discharge. Desmedt and Delwaide indeed report a temporary increase in the nerve discharge after the inhibition of nerve activity has dissipated.

Smith (1968) attributes the lesser inhibition of the auditory nerve action potential in the pigeon to a far lower number or absence of efferent-afferent fiber synapses in this bird.

Over 10 per cent of the cat's efferent fibers exhibit resting activity. The last consists of a regular, low impulse frequency of 1-10/sec (Fex, 1962).

A similar type of spontaneous activity was obtained by Rupert, Moushegian and Whitcomb (1968) on recording from olivocochlear neurons in the superior olivary complex of the cat. This spontaneous activity could be modified by central and peripheral influences. Whether an auditory stimulus would raise, depress or not affect the olivocochlear discharge depended on the existing spontaneous activity of the neurons.

One type of olivocochlear neuron was found to have only a net excitatory output, another kind only a net inhibitory output, and a third showed both.

Fex (1962, 1965) determined that in the cat the initiation of contralateral afferent fiber stimulation did not evoke an "on" burst of activity in either group of efferent fibers. Fex rarely noted impulse rates of more than 50/sec in crossed or uncrossed fibers after sound stimulation of the contralateral ear. He surmises that the decrease in afferent activity produced by the centrifugal fibers may be little in terms of an equivalent drop in sound stimulus intensity. Fex suggests that the centrifugal fibers might, however, be significant in controlling afferent fiber activity.

It is still within the realm of possibility that the dendrites of the afferent auditory fibers exert an electrical action on the final branchings of the efferent fibers (Spoendlin, 1966).

The afferent auditory fibers from the basal coil of the cochlea have been found to have one-sided, quickly rising threshold frequency curves which drop off suddenly at frequencies above the characteristic frequencies. In contrast to this the afferent fibers coming from the apical coil have symmetrical threshold frequency curves which fall gradually on the higher frequency side as well. The cochlea's basal coil also receives a much more extensive efferent innervation. These observations suggest that efferent inhibition, perhaps by olivocochlear fibers discharging particularly after certain higher sound frequencies, might produce the sharp cutoff in the threshold frequency curves of the basal coil's afferent fibers. In addition, the cochlea's basal coil has noticeably narrower fields of excitation.

Capps and Ades (1968) used four squirrel monkeys (*Saimiri sciureus*) to investigate the effects of interrupting the olivocochlear bundle on the acuity of auditory frequency discrimination. The crossed fibers of the olivocochlear bundle were lesioned by means of focused ultrasonic energy.

A clear-cut loss in ability to discriminate between frequencies lying within the same range was noticed after the elimination of the efferent influence. The postoperative animals required larger frequency differences than those successfully recognized preoperatively to make a correct (rewarded) response. This suggests that the efferent innervation acts to refine the cochlea's ability to resolve frequencies.

Fex (1962) postulated that the efferent fibers may play the part of a gating mechanism. They would permit the transmission of that sensory activity which is of prime importance in a situation and inhibit discharges of less significance.

Fex's hypothesis appears to gain some support from the findings of Buño *et al.* (1966).

These researchers looked for an effect of acoustic habituation on afferent auditory nerve potentials and on cochlear microphonics. They recorded from 45 awake guinea pigs by means of electrodes which had been permanently implanted in the middle ear, close to the round window. Click and pure tone pip stimuli were piped into the middle ear by an implanted polyethylene tube connected to an earphone. Acoustic habituation was produced by repeating a stimulus for long periods.

Buño *et al.* found that acoustic habituation to a certain sound frequency caused both the afferent discharge and the cochlear microphonics to fall in amplitude. This represents the first instance in which habituation has been shown to have an effect on a receptor potential (the cochlear microphonics). Similar decreases in the magnitudes of response potentials upon habituation have been observed from all later levels of the auditory pathway in the cat and man.

That both the afferent discharge and the cochlear microphonics changed in the same direction is surprising, but Buño *et al.* offer several possible explanations for this phenomenon. It is significant in this connection that the afferent discharge and the cochlear microphonics did not vary in a strictly parallel manner.

The application of another type of sensory stimulation, such as a light flash or an electric shock to the pinna, produced a fall in amplitude of the afferent nerve potentials and the cochlear microphonics if it preceded habituation. However, if such an extraneous stimulus was introduced following habituation, it evoked an increase to about the original level in response amplitudes. It may be correct to explain this last effect in relation to an increase in attention on the part of the organism. A stimulus which distracts preceding habituation "wakes up" a subject following habituation. A change in sound frequency after habituation had a like effect.

Interference by stimuli from other modalities produces similar results at various levels in several sensory pathways.

The effects of conditioning noted for the cochlea also resemble those which occur in the higher nervous system. Association of the auditory stimulus with a conditioning electric shock following habituation resulted in a rise in the amplitudes of the afferent discharge and the cochlear microphonics. Perhaps a rise in attention should also be considered here.

When the crossed olivocochlear fibers were sectioned, the described changes in amplitude either did not occur or were insignificant. In view of the several precautions taken by Buño *et al.*, it appears correct to assume that habituation, interference and conditioning affect the hair cells and possibly the afferent dendrites by way of appropriate changes in centrifugal inhibitory influences.

Wiederhold and Peake (1966) also suggest that the olivocochlear bundle can have specific effects on certain frequency ranges.

Spoendlin (1966) expresses the viewpoint that the long latencies involved in inhibitory actions by the efferent fibers preclude a specialized function on the part of these fibers in any peripheral integration of auditory responses. Nevertheless, Spoendlin feels that the extensive efferent innervation of the cochlea must play some significant role. Perhaps the efferent fibers play a part in the primary coding of auditory responses, or some unknown process of short latencies exists.

It is possible that olivocochlear inhibitory impulses act on local potentials in the afferent dendrites. In that case the extent of depolarization of the dendrites would be determined by the sum of the excitatory and inhibitory influences acting on them. The degree of hair cell depolarization might also be under olivocochlear control. Inhibitory effects on such easily influenced graded potentials (no threshold or all-or-none characteristics) might permit peripheral integration before propagated impulses develop. A protozoan cell has been found to apparently differ in its responses with the degree of depolarization (Tamar, 1967).

In this connection it is interesting that Echandia (1967) found canaliculi of the smooth endoplasmic reticulum, rather than synaptic vesicles, in outer hair cells at the synapses with afferent dendrites. This suggested to him that either no significant quantities of transmitter are stored at these afferent synapses, or that the canaliculi are the source of a transmitter substance. The subsurface reticulum at afferent synapses is highly developed, and it seems possible that it plays a role in the function of these synapses. Acanthous vesicles, presumably micropinocytic, are also present.

Leibbrand's (1965) findings suggest that the olivocochlear system contributes to adaptation to auditory stimulation.

There is a thorough description of the efferent innervation of the organ of Corti in Spoendlin (1966), and this is followed by a discussion of the physiology of efferent inhibition. Whitfield (1967a) includes a chapter on the centrifugal pathways in his book, and Goldberg and Lavine (1968) have a short section on efferent inhibition in their review. Wersäll (1968), in a 1966 report, summarizes findings on the afferent and efferent innervations of the inner ear.

The functions of the centrifugal pathways connecting the higher centers of the auditory system are examined in the next section on inhibition at higher levels of the auditory system.

Inhibition at Higher Levels of the Auditory System

As in the case of the visual system, inhibitory influences play an important role in the functioning of the higher portions of the auditory system. Some of the more significant of these inhibitory actions will be briefly described.

The superior olivary complex, one on each side of the brain, is the next "relay" station of the auditory pathway beyond the cochlear nucleus (Fig. 4-14). The cells of the nuclei of this complex are the lowest in the auditory system to receive ascending fibers originating from both ears. The superior olivary complex may play an important role in binaural hearing and sound localization.

About a quarter of the cells in the medial superior olive nucleus of the dog are excited when one ear, in over 80 per cent of the cases the contralateral ear, is stimulated, and they are inhibited when the other ear is stimulated (Goldberg and Brown, 1966). Monaural neurons of this kind have been reported to respond (or show inhibition) according to the time interval between impulses engendered by separate click stimulation of each ear. The responses of these neurons are also affected by intensity differences between the stimuli presented to each ear, and they are a product of the interplay between the effects of intensity and of length of the time interval (Hall, 1965).

Allowing for species differences, the above findings have been confirmed by Watanabe, Liao and Katsuki (1968) on the cat. These investigators found the inhibition produced in monaurally responding superior olivary neurons by stimulation of the "nonexciting" ear to be very short. Three of a large number of contralaterally activated monaural neurons were facilitated if the ipsilateral ear was stimulated simultaneously with the contralateral one.

Watanabe and his co-workers suggest that monaurally responding neurons may be innervated by an "excitatory" axon coming from one cochlear nucleus and an "inhibitory" axon originating from the opposite cochlear nucleus. The monaural units, consisting of two primary types of opposite functional orientation, probably play a significant role in localization of sound.

Contralaterally responding monaural neurons were localized in the accessory nucleus of the superior olivary complex, and ipsilaterally activated ones were chiefly identified in the trapezoid and S-segment nuclei. In agreement with the last observation, Tsuchitani and Boudreau (1966) found a number of the cells of the S-segment (lateral superior olivary) nucleus to be inhibited upon stimulation of the contralateral ear.

According to Moushegian, Rupert and Langford (1967), varied intensity differences between stimuli of the same frequency presented binaurally call forth inhibitory interactive effects over larger or smaller ranges of phase differences. If, for example, the excitatory signal is intensified relative to the inhibitory signal, the time range of interaction is reduced. In the reverse case the time range of interaction is extended.

The interaction of the exciting impulses from one ear and the inhibitory impulses from the other ear can further in a systematic manner determine the latent period of response of these neurons (Rupert, Moushegian and Whitcomb, 1966).

In medial superior olivary neurons inhibitory interactions cluster around a zero interaural time difference for binaurally applied click stimuli. This raises the possibility that the contralateral input to these neurons is transmitted more rapidly than the ipsilateral input (Moushegian, Rupert and Langford, 1967).

In the case of superior olivary cells stimulated by excitatory impulses from both ears, impulses from one ear generally reduced the response to later impulses originating in the other ear, even when the time interval between the two groups of impulses was about 10 msec.

Watanabe, Liao and Katsuki (1968) also found binaurally responding units of the superior olivary complex to show an exceedingly long inhibition upon binaural interaction. The significance of this lasting inhibition, which may be produced by interneurons that give burst discharges to clicks, is not yet known.

Binaurally responsive olivary neurons have similar response areas and latencies to clicks for the two ears. However, the thresholds of the response areas differ.

Some neurons of the cat's superior olivary complex show sensitivity to the direction of FM stimuli (Watanabe, Liao and Katsuki, 1968; Watanabe and Ohgushi, 1968) whereas no such neurons could be discovered in the cat's cochlear nucleus.

The afferent fibers from the superior olivary complex seem to generally synapse with neurons in the next highest cell masses of the auditory pathway on each side, the nuclei of the lateral lemniscus. The ventral nucleus of the lateral lemniscus also receives afferent fibers from the cochlear nucleus (Warr, 1969). From here fibers pass up to the inferior colliculi, mostly to the one on the same side.

The neurons of the inferior colliculus, just as those of lower auditory centers, respond according to a product of excitatory and inhibitory influences. Again the response to stimulation of both ears depends on such excitatory-inhibitory interaction.

The inferior colliculus, like the superior olivary complex, is involved in the location of sound sources and is important in echolocation by bats. In fact, the inferior colliculus is considered to be the chief center for the spatial analysis of sounds.

The interplay of excitatory and inhibitory influences appears to cause many neurons in the inferior colliculus to show an initial depolarization and resultant short burst discharge which are suddenly terminated by a sizeable hyperpolarizing potential. Such cessation of discharges before the termination of a stimulus is also found in other higher auditory centers and contrasts sharply with the sustained response of cochlear nucleus neurons (Gerstein, Butler and Erulkar, 1968).

Rose *et al.* (1966) provide evidence that in the anesthetized cat a stimulus presented to either ear may give rise to a cycle of excitatory and inhibitory events in neurons of the inferior colliculus. When both ears are stimulated at once, the response of neurons reactive to an interaural time lag depends upon the time gap between the stimuli and the intensity of each stimulus. The interstimulus time lag determines how the excitatory and inhibitory cycles of the two stimuli will sum. The amplitude, duration and perhaps rise time of these periodic excitatory and inhibitory events are in turn dependent on the intensity of the evoking stimulus. Two stimuli that each have an overall excitatory effect when employed alone may, when presented binaurally, produce a deep inhibition if there is a proper time lag between them.

Rose *et al.* (1966) also found neurons which responded to small intensity differences in binaurally-presented stimuli. Some of these neurons showed no discharge when the two stimuli were of equal strength or if the assumed inhibitory stimulus had greater intensity. However, as the excitatory stimulus became the more intense one, the discharge increased rapidly. Other such neurons showed a minimal impulse rate when the inhibitory stimulus was more intense and a maximum discharge when the excitatory stimulus was stronger.

The neurons which are sensitive to minor interaural intensity differences are normally excited by stimulation of the contralateral ear and inhibited by stimuli directed to the ipsilateral ear.

If a neuron of the inferior colliculus which has been responding uninterruptedly to a monaural stimulus for a sufficient period is then also stimulated by way of the other ear, an "on" inhibitory effect can be obtained. This effect is always sharp and transitory, and could inform the higher brain of the appearance of a new sound source (Rose *et al.*, 1966).

Vasil'ev and Matyushkin (1967) recorded from single neurons of the inferior colliculus of the bat *Myotis oxygnathus*. As in previous studies, some neurons exhibited inhibition when the stimulus intensity was excessively raised. The frequency-threshold response curves of these neurons, whether wide or narrow, were partially or totally cut off by a line marking the threshold of inhibition. In the case of two neurons the frequency-threshold curves for inhibition had a complex form and at certain frequencies resembled the frequency-threshold curves for excitation. Vasil'ev and Matyushkin consider their results to be evidence for a special inhibitory mechanism.

Suppression on raising the intensity of tones has also been reported from the bat (*Myotis lucifugus*) by Suga (1965), and from the cat's inferior colliculus by Rose *et al.* (1963).

Potter (1965) recorded from neurons in the torus semicircularis (mesencephalon) of the bullfrog (*Rana catesbeiana*). In a large percentage of these neurons he observed similar inhibition when the intensity of previously exciting frequencies was raised, and he also considered the phenomenon as due to a neural mechanism. Potter states that this inhibition phenomenon should reduce the response area of a neuron to certain intensity-frequency combinations, and should sharpen tuning. Such high-intensity inhibition may also cause the best frequency to change as the stimulus intensity is varied.

In the case of other neurons an increase in intensity eliminated the early discharge and caused it to be replaced by discharges of much greater latency.

Neurons in the inferior colliculus of the bat (*Myotis lucifugus*) were found to exhibit differing kinds of inhibition during their recovery cycles by Friend, Suga and Suthers (1966). While 4 per cent of the neurons showed short suppression, 11 per cent underwent a delayed inhibition, and 78 per cent had an undelayed inhibition lasting from 4 to 26 msec. It is postulated that these differences in recovery rates could provide a means for discriminating between echoes reflected at varying distances during echolocation.

The inferior colliculus is also probably significant in simple frequency discrimination. In the inferior colliculus a discharge to a click can frequently be inhibited by a band of tonal stimuli.

Suga (1964) observed that in the inferior colliculus of the bat (*Myotis lucifugus*) neurons had either wide or narrow response areas, with some possessing extremely narrow response areas. The neurons with narrow response areas normally had inhibitory areas at one or both edges of the excitatory area (Suga, 1965). Such arrangements could be correlated with differences in responses to various tone pulses. The responses of the neurons were normally extremely phasic "on" types, with but a few impulses being produced at the start of a stimulus (Suga, 1964).

Some neurons showed different response thresholds when frequency-modulated tone pulses passed over their best frequency from different directions. Such sensitivity to the dynamic aspects of a stimulus is most common in the higher auditory centers. Other neurons did not respond to frequency-modulated tone pulses (Suga, 1965). Neurons differentially responsive to the direction of FM stimuli have also been described from the cat's superior olivary complex and inferior colliculus (Watanabe and Ohgushi, 1968).

David *et al.* (1967) report observations indicating the presence of temporal inhibition and facilitation in the inferior colliculus and the medial geniculate body. There was inhibition and facilitation of both individual impulse responses (or changes in impulse intervals) and impulse (interval) combinations. Certain neurons could be inhibited for a period of one, two or more spike intervals but nevertheless maintained their basic rhythm. These units were particularly excitable through tones whose frequencies are whole multiples of the neuron's basic frequency. Such neurons should be able to discriminate harmonies. The neurons of the inferior colliculus exhibited directionality, and there were differences in threshold to contralateral and ipsilateral stimuli presented at the best angle of 40 degrees (Suga, 1964).

The lateral mesencephalic nucleus of the barbary dove (*Streptopelia risoria*) has been shown to be physiologically homologous to the inferior colliculus of mammals by Biederman-Thorson (1967), corroborating earlier histological studies. The lateral mesencephalic nucleus neurons are either only inhibitory, excitatory for a central range of frequencies and inhibitory for surrounding frequencies, or mainly inhibitory with one or several small excitatory zones. The dove differs from the cat in having neurons with exclusively or primarily inhibitory responses. Even the neurons with excitatory responses exhibit more inhibitory reactions than is the case in the cat.

Fibers arising from the inferior colliculus form the majority of the afferent fibers which terminate in the ipsilateral medial geniculate body (Fig. 4-14). From the last fibers project to the true auditory portions (AI and AII) of the temporal cortex and the insulotemporal cortex on the same side (Figs. 4-17, 4-18).

Some auditory neurons of both the medial geniculate body and the temporal cortex show binaural sensitivities much like those observed in the lower centers of the auditory pathway. These neurons, like many at lower levels, seem to be significant in localizing sounds.

In the cat 15.5 per cent of the medial geniculate neurons are excited by stimulation of the contralateral ear and inhibited by tones directed to the ipsilateral ear, while binaural units with contralateral inhibition make up only 2.4 per cent of the neurons (Adrian *et al.*, 1966). The described neurons are sensitive to time lags and differences in intensity between the binaurally applied stimuli. Such binaurally responsive neurons may play a role in fusion interval discrimination, laterality discrimination, and in organizing the input to the auditory cortex which indicates sound direction.

The inhibitory effect on binaural units generally lasts between 3 to 5 msec. In most of these units inhibition from one ear has the same maximal frequency as excitation through the other ear.

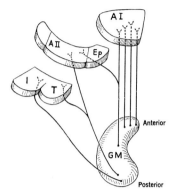

FIGURE 4-18. Projection of the medial geniculate body (*GM*) on auditory areas of the cat's cerebral cortex. Designations same as in Figure 4-17. (From Neff, W.D.: Neural Mechanisms of Auditory Discrimination. In Rosenblith, W.A. [Ed.]: *Sensory Communication.* Cambridge, M.I.T. Pr., 1961, pp. 259-278.)

In some other neurons continuous sound inhibits spontaneous activity.

The medial geniculate body is not held to be vital for the discrimination of sound frequencies. Nevertheless, its response to a click may be suppressed by a band of frequencies presented to the same ear. Since no such binaural inhibition can be obtained, this inhibition may well be passed up from a lower center.

Recovery from the effects of a click is relatively slow in the medial geniculate body of unanesthetized cats and may only be completed after several seconds. The refractory period thus evidenced may well involve inhibition, possibly of a recurrent postsynaptic nature. In cats anesthetized with barbiturates, recovery is marked by cycles of excitation and inhibition (Webster, 1969).

Hyperpolarizing potentials, possibly associated with inhibition, have been noted in inferior colliculus and medial geniculate neurons by Nelson and Erulkar (1963). The neurons from these brain centers often responded to transient stimuli with a short excitatory postsynaptic potential followed by a more lasting inhibitory postsynaptic potential.

Studies on cortical neurons have generally

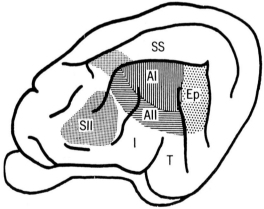

FIGURE 4-17. Diagram of the auditory areas of the cat's cerebral cortex. (*AI*) auditory area I, (*AII*) auditory area II, (*Ep*) posterior ectosylvian area, (*I*) insular area, (*T*) temporal area, (*SII*) somatic area II, (*SS*) suprasylvian area. (From Neff, W.D.: Neural Mechanisms of Auditory Discrimination. In Rosenblith, W.A. [Ed.]: *Sensory Communication.* Cambridge, M.I.T. Pr., 1961, pp. 259-278.)

had ambiguous results. Cortical cells often do not respond in a consistent and sustained manner and many show no impulse discharge at all.

A considerable variety of responses are observed in the auditory cortex. Hall II and Goldstein, Jr. (1968) noted monaural and binaural stimulation to evoke in different neurons an increased or a reduced discharge at the initiation, cessation or throughout the application of a stimulus. A fraction of the neurons showing binaural interaction are inhibited through one ear, and some binaural units exhibit a complex interplay of summation and inhibition. In the case of certain neurons of the last group, tone-burst stimuli give rise to summation at particular frequencies and to inhibition at different frequencies. In other neurons binaural stimulation augments some portions of the response and weakens other components. Sometimes the application of a stimulus to the inhibiting ear totally suppresses only one component of the discharge.

Parker and Mundie (1967) differentiated five types of sensitivity patterns in neurons of the guinea pig's auditory cortex which responded to paired sound stimuli. They suggested that these patterns resulted from an interplay of excitatory and inhibitory synaptic input.

There are neurons in the cat's auditory cortex, in which, as in neurons of the cochlear nucleus and of the inferior colliculus, excitation is supplanted by suppression as the stimulus intensity is raised (Goldstein, Jr., Hall II and Butterfield, 1968).

The classes of neurons in the cat's auditory cortex described by Hall II and Goldstein, Jr. (1968) resemble the classes into which Adrian *et al.* (1966) divided the neurons of the cat's medial geniculate body.

It should be noted in connection with the above findings that the properties of the responses of neurons in higher auditory centers may in many cases simply reflect the nature of the responses taking place in lower level neurons.

Bogdanski and Galambos (1960), and Kat-

suki, Suga and Kanno (1962) noticed sustained inhibition, and "on-off" responses based on inhibition, in the auditory cortex. The last investigators also observed most of the responses to be phasic and in one neuron found suppression of spontaneous activity by a continuous pure tone.

In the auditory cortex recovery from the effects of a click may take a number of seconds.

A loud tone has been reported to produce an initial period of facilitation in the spinal cord, lasting for approximately 33 msec. This is followed by a period of inhibition which is about 58 msec long. The described effect is believed to originate in the reticular formation of the brain stem (Barnes and Thomas, 1968).

Centrifugal Inhibition at Higher Levels

In addition to its ascending fiber tracts, the auditory system seems to include equivalent centrifugal pathways which parallel the sets of afferent tracts. The centrifugal fibers are not mixed with the afferent fibers but form discrete bundles close to them (Desmedt, 1960). The olivocochlear bundle of centrifugal fibers has already been discussed in the last section.

The activity of each "relay" station of the auditory system may thus be a product of both afferent influences arriving from a more peripheral site and efferent influences emanating from a more central location.

A number of studies have dealt with the effects of habituation to sound on various centers of the auditory system. These investigations were based on the supposition that such habituation acts on the auditory cortex and causes the cortex to initiate impulse activity in the centrifugal pathways. The different studies produced largely contradictory results, however, and such research is said to be hampered by many variables that are difficult to control. Whitfield (1967a) suggests that only more delicate experiments at the unit level can yield really meaningful results. This may be especially true because of the considerable number of smaller and less known efferent fiber bundles, some of which have complex connections.

Watanabe *et al.* (1966) investigated the effect of corticofugal fibers originating in the left auditory cortex of cats on neurons in the principal division of the left medial geniculate body. They observed that in the small, affected fraction of neurons auditory responses were chiefly inhibited upon stimulation of auditory area AI in the cortex. Stimulation of auditory area AII instead primarily enhanced the auditory responses of the small number of affected cells.

Electrical stimulation of the AI auditory cortex and the posterior ectosylvian gyrus (Fig. 4-17) raised the threshold of response to sound in affected units. A neuron with a high characteristic frequency showed parallel threshold elevation over all of its response area, and the greatest effect was produced when stimulation was focused on the anterior ectosylvian gyrus (in AI). In the case of a neuron with a low characteristic frequency, the threshold was not equally elevated over the entire response area. While stimulation of the anterior ectosylvian gyrus raised thresholds primarily in the high-frequency portion of this neuron's response area, stimulation of the posterior ectosylvian gyrus produced some effect in the low-frequency range of the response area.

Watanabe *et al.* (1966) conclude that only a limited number of corticofugal fibers make contact with neurons of the ipsilateral medial geniculate body. They suggest that these fibers transmit a cortical feedback, perhaps frequency-specific for each fiber and both inhibitory and facilitatory, which could make an important contribution to the frequency-specific "gating" mechanism of the higher auditory pathway. The gating mechanism may function in the discrimination of a certain sound from a background of other sounds.

It was also corroborated by Watanabe *et al.* (1966) that many neurons of the inferior colliculus are innervated by efferent fibers from both the ipsilateral and the contralateral

auditory cortex. These efferent fibers exert patterns of inhibition and facilitation on inferior colliculus neurons which resemble those modifying the activity of medial geniculate neurons. However, the latent period elapsing between cortical stimulation and an efferent effect is considerably longer in the case of the inferior colliculus, where it lasts 30 to 40 msec.

About 1.7 times as high a percentage of inferior colliculus neurons as medial geniculate neurons are acted on by corticofugal fibers. In the inferior colliculus the threshold for an ipsilateral cortical inhibitory effect may be lower than that for a contralateral one.

In addition to efferent pathways to the ipsilateral medial geniculate body and the bilateral inferior colliculi, each auditory cortex also originates fibers running to the ipsilateral dorsal nucleus of the lateral lemniscus (Otani and Hiura, 1962).

Granstrem (1968) performed an anatomical study, supplemented by electrical stimulation and subsequent Nissl staining of synapses, on the fiber tracts descending from areas Al and Al y of the cat's auditory cortex. Direct corticofugal pathways were found to end not only in the medial geniculate body, the superior and inferior colliculi and the nucleus of the lateral lemniscus, but they were also seen to terminate in the nuclei of the superior olivary complex and in the trapezoid body. The contralateral trapezoid body was innervated only by descending fibers from area Al y. The corticofugal fibers did not follow the course of the afferent fibers between the medial geniculate body and the inferior colliculi.

Teramoto and Snider (1966) report results indicating that the auditory area of the cerebellum gives rise to two ascending pathways to the auditory cortex of the cerebrum. One of these pathways could well involve the reticular formation. There also appears to be an efferent connection between the auditory area of the cerebellum and the inferior colliculus.

The cerebellar-cerebral tracts may significantly affect the second and third waves of the cortical response.

According to Rasmussen (1953, 1955), centrifugal fiber tracts extend from the dorsal nucleus of the lateral lemniscus and from the nucleus of the inferior colliculus to the superior olivary complex.

Each cochlear nucleus is innervated by three major groups of centrifugal fibers. One of these bundles of centrifugal fibers originates in part from the ventral nucleus of the contralateral lateral lemniscus. Another bundle comes from the S-shaped segment of the ipsilateral superior olivary complex (Fig. 4-19). A third bundle of efferent fibers takes its origin in the ipsilateral inferior colliculus and in the dorsal nucleus of the ipsilateral lateral lemniscus. Some of these fibers pass to the contralateral cochlear nucleus.

A few fibers of the olivocochlear bundle also end in the cochlear nucleus (Fig. 4-19), as was indicated in the section on centrifugal inhibition.

Of the three important centrifugal bundles terminating in the cochlear nucleus, only the one originating in the superior olivary complex has been extensively investigated. Whitfield and Comis (1967) determined that stimulation with direct current near the medial portion of the S-segment of the superior olivary complex gives rise to a higher discharge by cells in the anteroventral cochlear nucleus. The augmented discharge of the responding cochlear nucleus neurons appears with a latency of at least 30 msec. The direct current stimulation must therefore exert its effect by exciting centrifugal neurons in the superior olivary complex.

The researches of Whitfield and Comis (1967) and Whitfield (1966) have shown this olivary complex–ventral cochlear nucleus efferent pathway to be cholinergic and excitatory.

It is likely that at least one of the other efferent pathways to the cochlear nucleus has the inhibitory action usually attributed to centrifugal fibers. The threshold of cochlear nucleus neurons to acoustic stimuli is not only

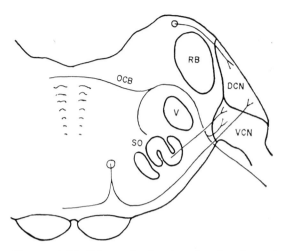

FIGURE 4-19. Schematic drawing showing four of the centrifugal fiber tracts which innervate the cochlear nucleus. The olivocochlear bundle (*OCB*) sends some fibers into the ventral cochlear nucleus (*VCN*). Fibers originating mainly in the contralateral ventral nucleus of the lateral lemniscus (represented by upper small circle) run laterally past the restiform body (*RB*) to end in the dorsal cochlear nucleus (*DCN*). Fibers from the S-shaped segment (lateral olivary nucleus) of the superior olivary complex (*SO*) course around the ventrolateral limit of the descending root of the fifth nerve (*V*) and later terminate in the anteroventral cochlear nucleus. Fibers from the inferior colliculus and the dorsal nucleus of the lateral lemniscus (represented by lower small circle) reach the dorsal cochlear nucleus. (From Whitfield, I.C.: *The Auditory Pathway*. London, Edward Arnold, 1967.)

lowered by acetylcholine, but approximately 75 per cent of these neurons are inhibited, and show a higher threshold, on local application of adrenalin or noradrenalin (Whitfield, 1967b). This suggests that an adrenergic group of fibers is inhibitory. Comis and Whitfield (1967) observed that stimulation with direct current of an area in the dorsal nucleus of the lateral lemniscus can cause the inhibition of a unit in the dorsal cochlear nucleus of the opposite side. Whitfield (1967a) reports that in preliminary work the administration of reserpine to the organism has prevented the inhibitory effect of stimulating the lemniscus.

If, instead of the dorsal nucleus, the ventral nucleus of the lateral lemniscus is stimulated, either excitation of the contralateral ventral cochlear nucleus or inhibition of the contralateral dorsal cochlear nucleus results, depending on the placement of the electrodes (Comis and Whitfield, 1968). Several efferent pathways terminating in these nuclei have not yet been studied.

Desmedt (1960) showed that stimulating a small region of the lateral lemniscus reduced the response to a click in the cochlear nucleus. This effect could not have been called forth more peripherally by the olivocochlear bundle. Similar results have been obtained by stimulating an area just anterior to the inferior colliculus, one near the entry of the lateral lemniscus or an area on the medial surface of the medial geniculate body. Dewson, Nobel and Pribram (1966) provide evidence that the cortex exerts an inhibitory action on the cochlear nucleus.

The above research indicates that there exists a reciprocal efferent gating mechanism at the cochlear nucleus which controls the response to different impulses.

Auditory stimulation of the contralateral ear has been found to reduce elicited compound action potentials in the guinea pig cochlear nucleus by up to 89 per cent (Pfalz and Pirsig, 1966). Preceding these experiments, the homolateral cochlea was destroyed. Activity in probably crossed centrifugal fibers was thus shown to affect large numbers of neurons in the cochlear nucleus. The threshold for the observed efferent inhibition lay at a broad-band noise or pure-tone intensity of 60 dB, and the latency of inhibition was 8 to 12 msec. The inhibition reached its peak between 60 to 100 msec after the start of acoustic stimulation.

In a further study (Pirsig and Pfalz, 1967) action potentials were initiated in a small, high-frequency fraction of the examined neurons of the ventral cochlear nucleus by, as in the previous investigation, electrically stimulating the lamina spiralis (auditory nerve) on the same side. About half of the excited secondary neurons were inhibited by sinus-tone stimulation of the contralateral ear, and inhibition was dependent on intensity and frequency. The normally phasic-tonic course of excitation in these ventral cochlear nucleus neurons was converted into a purely phasic process by inhibition, and the period required for transmission of afferent impulses through the second afferent synapse was approximately doubled.

It was found that in the mentioned inhibited neurons afferent excitation and spontaneous activity were suppressed to an equal degree. Koerber *et al.* (1966) have made observations indicating that most of the spontaneous activity in the ventral cochlear nucleus originates from the auditory nerve running into it. This is not true of neurons in the dorsal cochlear nucleus.

Pirsig, Pfalz and Sadanaga (1968) showed crossed efferent inhibition of the ventral cochlear nucleus to be blocked by strychnine. Thus the assumption that this inhibition is postsynaptic is supported. Evidence is also offered that the strychnine acted on the inhibitory synapses in the ventral cochlear nucleus.

A spontaneous discharge can be recorded from deafferented neurons of the dorsal cochlear nucleus. If now the contralateral ear is subjected to auditory stimulation, an efferent inhibitory effect again appears. This effect normally rises with greater stimulus intensity. In cats intensities of 15 to 40 dB or more over the threshold of 60 dB are required to obtain maximum inhibition. In the case of some neurons a rise in stimulus intensity beyond an optimum value leads to a decrease in inhibition (Grubel, Dunker and Rehren, 1964).

In dogs a mediosagittal section of the pons varolii up to the trapezoid nucleus reduces the induced efferent inhibitory effect by at least 61 per cent. If in addition a sagittal section is made of the caudal or rostral half of the trapezoid body, efferent inhibition is reduced by a minimum of 81 per cent. The threshold curves for inhibition are essentially unaffected by this procedure. Total section of the trapezoid body results in the cessation of any inhibitory effect on resting activity (Dunker and Grubel, 1965).

On the basis of their results Dunker and Grubel believe contralateral auditory stimulation to exert its inhibitory effect on the dorsal cochlear nucleus not only by way of tracts passing through the trapezoid body but also by crossed pathways running outside this nucleus. The comparatively long latent periods of the observed efferent effects indicate that the involved neurons have extensive functional connections at various stations of the pons.

The spontaneous impulse frequency of deafferented neurons of the dorsal cochlear nucleus of dogs and cats has a gaussian distribution both at rest and during contralateral acoustic stimulation. The variation in the intervals between impulses is increased by efferent inhibition (Dunker and Wachsmuth, 1965) and is reduced by brain sections. This suggests that the spontaneous discharge of the deafferented dorsal cochlear nucleus is entirely initiated by efferent impulses (Dunker and Grubel, 1965).

Webster *et al.* (1965), using unanesthetized cats, determined that at the cochlear nucleus auditory habituation develops rapidly, dissipates more slowly and is a direct function of the stimulus frequency. The reticular formation is apparently not involved, as barbiturates do not eliminate habituation at the cochlear nucleus.

Barbiturates do appear to eliminate habituation decrements in the medial geniculate body, but they also produce similar increased activity in this structure in the absence of habituation (Webster, 1969).

On the other hand, Hernandez-Peon *et al.* (1956) provide partial evidence that the pathway for central inhibition of the cochlear nuclei may pass through the reticular formation. When these investigators subjected the reticular formation in the midbrain of cats to electrical stimulation, afferent activity in the cochlear nuclei was greatly suppressed.

Visual, olfactory or somatic stimulation of unanesthetized cats had a similar result.

The inhibitory mechanism appears to favor attention to an outstanding stimulus. The same principle is illustrated by the effect of distraction on the activity of the human optic radiations and on the discharge of the posterior ventrolateral nucleus of the human thalamus.

Inhibition has been found to be the basis for the enhancement of contours and the sharpening of contrast in vision. The difference in the degree of lateral inhibition at both sides of the edges of differently illumined object images is responsible for Mach bands. Inhibition also plays a role in the localization of cutaneous sensations (von Békésy, 1959). The interactions between excitatory and inhibitory influences at various levels of the auditory system seem to have similar functions, although more research is needed along these lines.

Temporal discrimination may also be significant in the auditory system.

During sound localization the inhibition of binaurally excitable neurons through impulses originating from one ear is accompanied in the auditory system by a summation of the impulse activity called forth by the sound intensities acting on both ears. Von Békésy (1967) considers such synchronous inhibition and summation as part of a sensory funneling process. The inhibition of some neural activity, and the summation of other discharges in the channels of the auditory system, results in improved signal-to-noise ratios.

Kudryavtseva (1968) believes changes in the EEG of dogs during lasting acoustic stimuli to be produced by an inhibitory process with a protective function. This inhibitory process is said to appear on strong (80-90 dB) auditory stimulation.

What is known of the functions of the higher centers of the auditory system is reviewed in Goldberg and Lavine (1968) and in Whitfield (1967a). The last provides descriptions of the traced fiber tracts connecting various nuclei. The sensory processes which occur in the central auditory pathway, especially those pertinent to the development of

models, are discussed in a review by Erulkar, Nelson and Bryan (1968).

THE LATERAL LINE SYSTEM

The function of the lateral line sense organs of fish and amphibians also involves inhibition.

Flock (1967) observed nerve endings containing numerous synaptic vesicles to lie adjacent to lateral line hair cells. He considered such nerve endings to be the terminations of efferent fibers (Fig. 4-20). Aronova (1967) reported efferent nerve endings to make contact with receptor hair cells in the lateral line system of the pike (*Esox lucius*).

Görner (1967) showed that the thin myelinated fibers innervating the lateral line hair cells of the South African clawed toad (*Xenopus laevis*) transmit efferent impulses. However, he could not demonstrate an effect of this efferent activity on the impulse discharge of the thicker afferent fibers which serve the hair cells. When the toad was about to move, groups of efferent impulses passed down the lateral line nerve.

Harris and Flock (1967) antidromically stimulated nerves serving the lateral line organs of *Xenopus laevis*. They obtained inhibition of spontaneous activity in these nerves after a latent period of 30 msec.

Katsuki, Hashimoto and Yanagisawa (1968) recorded spontaneous discharges from efferent and afferent fibers of the lateral line nerve of the Japanese sea eel (*Lyncozymba nystromi*). The spontaneous activity was found to undergo cyclical changes in relation to heart beat, lymph heart beat and respiratory gill movement.

When a bundle of the peripheral cut end of the lateral line nerve was repetitively stimulated electrically, both the total spontaneous activity and the response discharges evoked in the lateral line nerve by vibration were partially inhibited.

The Japanese common eel (*Anguilla japonica*) has not been found to possess a similar efferent innervation of its lateral line.

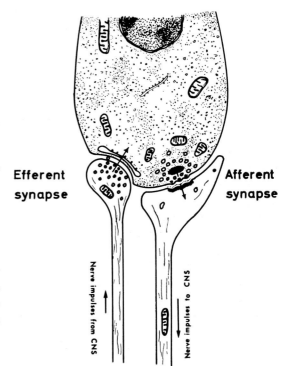

FIGURE 4-20. The double innervation of canal neuromast hair cells. Adjacent to one synapse the cytoplasm of the hair cell contains a concentration of synaptic vesicles around a synaptic body (or rod). The nerve ending beyond is therefore presumably afferent. At the other synapse vesicles are instead concentrated within the synaptic region of the nerve ending, suggesting that the last is efferent and influences the hair cell's activity. (From Flock, Å.: Electron microscopic and electrophysiologic studies on the lateral line canal organ. *Acta Oto-Laryngol., Suppl. 199*:1-90, 1965.)

THE VESTIBULAR SYSTEM

The hair cells of each labyrinth are innervated by dendrites of nerve cell bodies in the vestibular ganglion of the same side. The

axons of these neurons then form the respective vestibular nerve. In the brain stem the vestibular nerves terminate in the vestibular nuclei, which have extensive connections in the brain and spinal cord. An anatomical description of the vestibular system can be found in Sarkisov (1966).

Work with the electron microscope has shown two types of nerve fibers to be present in the vicinity of the vestibular hair cells. These receptors are described as being dually innervated, like the other sense cells of the acousticolateralis system.

Rossi (1968) described two efferent bundles serving exclusively the vestibular receptors and one bundle innervating both the vestibular receptors and the cochlea from rabbits and rodents. The "direct ventral efferent vestibular bundle" originates from a nucleus in the proximity of the inferior and lateral vestibular nuclei. The "direct dorsal efferent vestibular bundle" arises from the ventrocaudal part of the lateral vestibular nucleus, passes around the dorsal side of the descending root of the fifth nerve, and then joins the "direct ventral efferent vestibular bundle." A mixed "direct reticulocochlear and vestibular bundle" originates from lateral cells of the median raphe of the reticular formation and joins the crossed olivocochlear bundle. All these fiber tracts combine into a single bundle on the lateral edge of the descending root of the fifth nerve. The combined bundle then leaves the brain stem together with the vestibular nerve (Fig. 4-21).

Although the efferent vestibular fibers are greatly outnumbered by afferent fibers, they show extensive terminal branching. This apparently permits considerable synaptic contact between the efferent and afferent fibers. Further, many efferent fiber terminals form synapses with vestibular hair cells. In the mammalian labyrinth there seem to be direct synaptic contacts between efferent fibers and type II hair cells. On the other hand, efferent fibers only synapse with the nerve chalices surrounding the type I hair cells (Wersäll, 1968).

The efferent terminals of examined vertebrates have a characteristic synaptic structure and contain concentrations of round and oval vesicles (Wersäll, 1968).

A large number of papers supply information on aspects of the role of inhibition in the operation of the vestibular system. There are also reports dealing with the inhibitory effects exerted by various brain centers or by other sensory systems on the function of the vestibular system. The last has in turn been found to inhibit the activities of certain sensory and motor neurons.

A brief résumé is given below of portions of the literature which cast light on inhibitory actions related to the vestibular system.

In order to investigate the actions of the reported efferent vestibular system in adult cats, Sala (1968) electrically stimulated the floor of the fourth ventricle, at the level of the lateral vestibular nucleus, and recorded from the contralateral vestibular nerve.

Sala observed electrical stimulation of the efferent vestibular fibers to variously produce either an increase or a diminution of spontaneous activity in the vestibular nerve. This suggested that the efferent fibers can give rise to both excitatory and inhibitory effects, the elicited effect being determined by the functional condition of the vestibular receptors. The efferent vestibular system seems to modulate the vestibular discharges.

Sala (1968) showed that the efferent vestibular system forms part of a closed feedback loop between the labyrinthine receptors and the vestibular nuclei, with the excited efferent fibers of the two sides diverging to act on the ipsilateral and contralateral receptors.

Intravenous injection of strychnine blocks the effect of the efferent vestibular system.

Markham, Precht and Shimazu (1966) studied the effects of impinging impulse discharges on neurons in the vestibular nuclei. In the course of their research they classified vestibular neurons as type I if they showed an increased resting discharge on ipsilateral rotation and a reduced discharge on contralateral rotation. Neurons exhibiting the converse responses were labeled type II.

Type I vestibular nucleus neurons whose

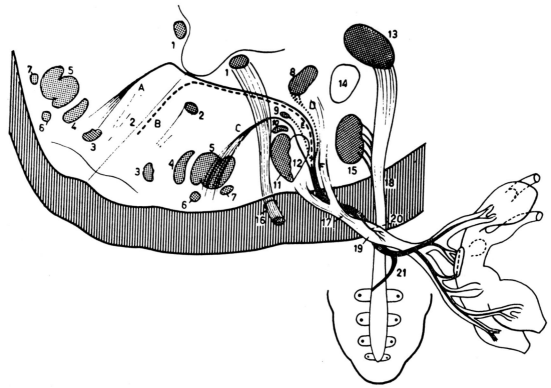

FIGURE 4-21. The efferent cochlear and vestibular fiber tracts of rodents. (*1*) Geniculum of the facial nerve, (*2*) nucleus and root fibers of the abducent nerve, (*3*) nucleus of the trapezoid body, (*4*) accessory olivary nucleus, (*5*) superior lateral olivary nucleus, (*6*) medial preolivary nucleus, (*7*) lateral preolivary nucleus, (*8*) lateral vestibular nucleus, (*9*) interposed vestibular nucleus, (*10*) inferior vestibular nucleus, (*11*) nucleus of the descending root of the trigeminal nerve, (*12*) descending root of the trigeminal nerve, (*13*) dorsal cochlear nucleus, (*14*) restiform body, (*15*) ventral cochlear nucleus, (*16*) facial nerve, (*17*) vestibular branch of the eighth nerve and its superior and inferior roots, (*18*) cochlear branch of the eighth nerve, (*19*) Scarpa's ganglion, (*20*) a small bundle of efferent fibers ending at the level of Scarpa's ganglion, (*21*) Oort's anastomosis. (*A*) Crossed efferent cochlear bundle (——), (*B*) direct reticulocochlear and vestibular bundle (- - - - -), (*C*) direct efferent cochlear bundle (——), (*D*) direct dorsal efferent vestibular bundle (. . . . . . .), (*E*) direct ventral efferent vestibular bundle (. . . . . .), (*F*) bundle resulting from the confluence of the different tracts of efferent fibers. (From Rossi, G., and G. Cortesina: The "efferent cochlear and vestibular system" in *Lepus cuniculus* L. *Acta Anat.*, *60*:362-381, 1965 [Karger, Basel/New York].)

activity is affected by fluid motion in the horizontal canal can be strongly inhibited by either stimulation of the contralateral vestibular nerve or stimulation of the ipsilateral interstitial nucleus of Cajal (midbrain). Type I neurons serving the anterior canal show weaker inhibitory responses on such stimulation (Markham, 1968).

Type II neurons of the horizontal canal are transsynaptically facilitated by the above stimulation, and the activity of type II neurons of the anterior canal is also enhanced by stimulation of the contralateral vestibular nerve.

About half of the type II neurons can further be transsynaptically excited through the ipsilateral vestibular nerve. Normal ipsilateral excitation of these neurons probably stems from some other source than the horizontal canal (Shimazu and Precht, 1966).

The greater inhibition shown by those type I units serving the horizontal canal may indicate a greater need for exact coordination and control in horizontal eye movements.

Precht, Shimazu and Markham (1966) observed that when the vestibular nuclei were chronically deafferented, there was a significant drop in the threshold of electrical stimulation which had to be applied to the contralateral vestibular nerve in order to inhibit type I neurons. Evidence was also obtained that the contralateral labyrinth exerts a strong inhibitory effect on the type I neurons of the vestibular nucleus.

It has been hypothesized that following stimulation of the contralateral vestibular nerve, certain type II neurons are excited by way of transcommissural fibers, and that these type II neurons then inhibit type I neurons, probably of the tonic kind, on the same side (Shimazu and Precht, 1966; Markham, Precht and Shimazu, 1966; Kasahara *et al.*, 1968). It is postulated by Wilson, Wylie and Marco (1968) that the inhibitory pathway is normally composed of an excitatory commissural neuron and an inhibitory neuron ipsilateral to the inhibited target cell. Sometimes the pathway may be made up of only an inhibitory commissural neuron. Such inhibition of type I (tonic) neurons has been found to have an average latent period of 4 msec (Wilson, Wylie and Marco, 1968, report latencies of 1.6 to 3.7 msec).

Kasahara *et al.* (1968) suggest that a comparatively direct commissural pathway transmits the impulses leading to the inhibition of kinetic type I neurons, since the latency of the contralateral inhibition of these cells is only 2.0 to 2.4 msec.

Stimulation of the ascending or the descending medial longitudinal fasciculus results in the transsynaptic excitation of numerous neurons. These frequently receive discharges from the ipsilateral and the contralateral labyrinth. Wilson, Wylie and Marco (1968) believe some of these neurons to be excitatory and inhibitory interneurons which transmit impulses to the ipsilateral and contralateral vestibular nuclei.

Some vestibular neurons of the guinea pig are excited by stimulation of one labyrinth and inhibited by stimulation of the other. When stimulation of a labyrinth with warm water is replaced by treatment with cold water, the response of a number of vestibular neurons also changes. In some instances there is a shift from excitation to inhibition, or the opposite (Manni and Giretti, 1968).

It has been shown that each vestibular apparatus acts to suppress the enhancing effect of the other labyrinth on the extensor tonus of the homolateral limbs (Moruzzi and Pompeiano, 1956).

Among the investigations concerned with the influence of various brain centers on the vestibular system are those of which the results are given below.

Manni and Giretti (1968) deal with the action of the cerebral nystagmogenic center on vestibular nucleus neurons affected by stimulation of the labyrinth. They describe patterns of excitation and inhibition and indicate that labyrinthine and cerebral nystagmogenic discharges converge on the vestibular nuclei.

The relationship between the cerebral nystagmogenic area and the mesodiencephalic nystagmogenic center was investigated by Manni, Azzena and Atzori (1965). The nystagmus-producing action of the mesodiencephalic nystagmogenic center was found to not require transmission by corticofugal fibers. Relay neurons connected to the mesodiencephalic center are present in the pathways linking the cortical nystagmogenic area with the oculomotor nuclei.

Stimulation of the anterior lobe of the cerebellum produces inhibitory postsynaptic potentials in most neurons of the ipsilateral lateral vestibular nucleus (Ito and Yoshida, 1966). The latency of such inhibition may be only 1.06 msec when lobule III or the anterior of lobule IV of the cerebellum are stimulated.

IPSP's produced in this manner are normally followed by a slow and long-lasting depolarization.

Cerebellar discharges can also call forth excitatory postsynaptic potentials in the lateral vestibular nucleus.

The long corticofugal fibers extending from parts of the cerebellum into the lateral vestibular nucleus are the axons of Purkinje cells.

Llinàs, Precht and Kitai (1967) postulate a cerebellovestibular efferent system, presumably inhibitory, on the basis of research on the frog. In this organism section of the eighth nerve produces Purkinje cell degeneration in the auricular lobe of the cerebellar cortex, showing that these Purkinje cells extend axonal elements to the vestibular organ. Further, removal of the cerebellar cortex results in the degeneration of synaptic boutons which lie on the surface of vestibular receptor cells.

The previously mentioned Purkinje cells can be antidromically excited by threshold stimulation of the eighth cranial nerve. This provides strong evidence for a cerebellovestibular pathway.

Blomstrand *et al.* (1968a) found that cerebellectomy reduces the level of RNA and raises the amount of succinoxidase activity in the Deiters' giant cells of the rabbit lateral vestibular nucleus. Blomstrand *et al.* (1968b) determined the effect of cold and warm water irrigation of the outer ear on the levels of RNA and succinoxidase activity in the Deiters' cells of cerebellectomized rabbits. They discuss the inhibitory action of the cerebellum on the lateral vestibular (Deiters') nuclei, and also deal with the function of the fibers connecting the lateral vestibular nuclei.

Hypnosis may produce a suppression of caloric induced nystagmus, which then returns on the termination of hypnosis (Johner and Perlman, 1968). Nystagmus is also inhibited by reverie and may be restored by making the patient attentive. The above observations show that higher nervous centers and mental states can affect the vestibular system. Thus the reticular system seems to exert an influence on nystagmus.

There may be some inhibition of nystagmus during nerve stimulation, possibly by way of reticulocortical tracts.

Somatosensory and optic nerve activity may indirectly affect the function of the vestibular system.

Fredrickson *et al.* (1966) report that the primary cortical vestibular area and the first somatic area (SI) of the cortex overlap. There is thus convergence and interaction between vestibular and somatosensory discharges in the cortex. Gernandt (1968) studied convergence and interaction between extraocular myotatic and afferent vestibular discharges by recording from the oculomotor nerves and the reticular formation. Vestibular discharges were noticeably suppressed by preceding volleys of stretch-receptor impulses, and the last more successfully excited neurons in the reticular formation during competition between the two types of discharges. While vestibular impulses passing through the vestibular nuclei and to the oculomotor nuclei were unaffected by extraocular muscle stretch discharges, these inhibited vestibulo-ocular impulses being transmitted through the reticular formation.

Azzena and Davini (1967) discovered that optic nerve discharges inhibit the ipsilateral cerebral nystagmogenic area. The ocular nystagmus provoked through the optic nerve is in turn inhibited by the ipsilateral cerebral nystagmogenic center and facilitated by the contralateral center. The action of optic nerve discharges on a cerebrally initiated nystagmus and the effect of the cerebral nystagmogenic center on a simultaneous optic nerve–induced nystagmus are both facilitatory when the rapid phases of the mentioned nystagmi have the same direction. These influences are suppressive when the rapid phases of the two nystagmi are opposed in direction.

When the ventral fourth of the spinal cord is stimulated, inhibitory postsynaptic potentials are initiated in a low percentage of the neurons of the lateral vestibular nucleus and the descending vestibular nucleus on the same side (Ito, 1968).

Pompeiano (1967), after describing the excitatory action of the medial and descending vestibular nuclei on ocular and spinal motor neurons, states that these vestibular nuclei give rise to descending inhibitory influences. The last produce presynaptic depolarization of primary (group Ia) afferent neurons (resulting in inhibition) when bursts of rapid eye movements take place. Group Ib afferents, as well as cutaneous and high threshold muscle afferents, are also believed to be subject to such influences. The vestibular nuclei appear to produce inhibition both directly and by way of the sensory-motor cortex and may further act on the lateral geniculate nucleus.

Upon high-frequency stimulation of the labyrinth, a sustained inhibition of spinal reflexes is noted. The vestibular influence on spinal motor neurons can be excitatory, inhibitory or both in parallel (Gernandt, 1967).

The anatomical structure and fiber connections of the vestibular nuclei have been extensively studied by Brodal and his co-workers (Brodal, 1964, 1967; Angaut and Brodal, 1967; Ladpli and Brodal, 1968). Electron microscopical investigations of fiber terminations in the lateral vestibular nucleus have been performed by Mugnaini, Walberg and Brodal (1967) and by Mugnaini and Walberg (1967).

THE GUSTATORY SYSTEM

Structure and Functional Organization

In mammals the taste receptor cells are collected in taste buds which are primarily located in papillae on the tongue—the fungiform papillae on the dorsal surface of the anterior portion of the tongue, the foliate papillae on both sides of the posterior tongue, and the vallate papillae on the dorsal surface near the base of the tongue. Taste buds are also found in the mucous membrane of the posterior buccal cavity, the posterior pharyngeal wall, the tonsils, the epiglottis and the larynx.

Beneath each taste bud there is a plexus of myelinated and unmyelinated nerve fibers. Further, in the center of a taste bud, as observed in the rabbit, there is a second, considerable mixing of nerve fibers. These can be traced back to many loci in the underlying nerve plexus.

Some of the thinner fibers may be branches of larger ones; there appears to be profuse branching before the fibers reach the papillae, and there is branching within papillae. The thinner fibers (.05μ-.5μ), after passing through the taste bud, terminate in one taste cell. The larger diameter fibers (.5μ-1μ) may be associated with several receptor cells and end between two or more taste cells (De Lorenzo, 1963).

Rapuzzi and Casella (1965), working with the frog tongue, have found some but not all of the papillae bearing taste buds to be electrically connected. Typically four to five interconnecting axons innervate such papillae.

The taste buds in the anterior two thirds of the mammalian tongue are innervated by nerve fibers whose most distal portions run in the lingual nerve. As these fibers are followed centrally, they are seen to leave the lingual nerve to form the bulk of the chorda tympani nerve (Fig. 4-22). The last consists primarily of taste fibers but also contains preganglionic efferent nerve fibers to the submaxillary and sublingual salivary glands, sympathetic postganglionic fibers, and groups of a few fibers each respectively sensitive to temperature, touch and pain. Because it is preponderantly composed of taste fibers, the chorda tympani offers an excellent opportunity to record the taste responses of the anterior portion of the mammalian tongue.

The chorda tympani runs centrally through a bone canal into the middle ear cavity, and thereupon crosses the tympanic membrane. It then joins the facial (VII) nerve, of which it is considered a branch. At the genu of the facial nerve lies the geniculate ganglion, which contains the cell bodies of the peripheral gustatory neurons serving the anterior two thirds of the mammalian tongue. The central processes of these neurons, after passing into the brain stem in the nervus intermedius of Wrisberg, terminate close to neurons of the rostral

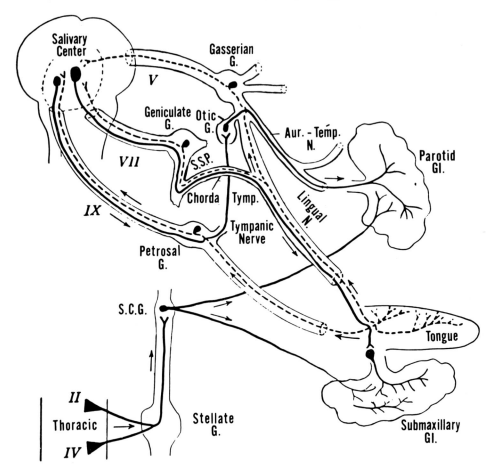

FIGURE 4-22. Schematic drawing of the peripheral gustatory pathway (broken lines) in mammals. Most taste fibers from the anterior two thirds of the tongue leave the lingual nerve with the chorda tympani. The taste fibers from the posterior third of the tongue pass centrally in the glossopharyngeal (IX) nerve (broken line on left). (From Zotterman, Y.: The Neural Mechanism of Taste. In Zotterman, Y. [Ed.]: *Sensory Mechanisms, Progress in Brain Research, 23.* Amsterdam, Elsevier, 1967, pp. 139-154.)

portion of the ipsilateral nucleus of the tractus solitarius.

The chorda tympani's route in tetrapods, and the evolutionary origins of this route, are dealt with by Fox (1965).

A few taste fibers may also pass centrally from the lingual nerve via the trigeminal (V) nerve, since the lingual nerve is a branch of the third division of the trigeminal nerve.

The taste buds of the posterior third of the tongue, the posterior buccal cavity and the tonsils, and some taste buds in the pharynx are

innervated by way of the lingual branches of the glossopharyngeal (IX) nerve (Fig. 4-22). The cell bodies of the neurons serving these taste buds are located in the ganglion petrosum (ganglion inferius in man) of the glossopharyngeal nerve. From the petrosal ganglion the axons of this group of peripheral neurons run with the glossopharyngeal nerve into the brain stem to end close to neurons of the midsection of the ipsilateral nucleus of the tractus solitarius.

Frewein (1965) describes a superior ganglion which is present next to the petrosal ganglion in a series of domestic mammals.

In addition, taste buds in the pharynx, epiglottis and larynx are subserved by branches of the vagus (X) nerve, probably the pharyngeal branches and the internal superior laryngeal nerve. The gustatory nerve fibers in the branches of the vagus nerve join cell bodies in the ganglion jugulare and the ganglion nodosum of the vagus. From these ganglia the central processes of the mentioned peripheral gustatory neurons pass as part of the vagus nerve into the medulla oblongata, to terminate in the proximity of neurons of the caudal portion of the nucleus of the tractus solitarius, including the nucleus commissuralis. Most of the peripheral gustatory neurons in the vagus run to the ipsilateral nucleus, but some cross to reach the contralateral nucleus.

The picture given above of the courses and connections of the peripheral gustatory neurons should be basically correct but may be subject to some modification. Thus Bernard (1964) recorded taste impulses from the chorda tympani of the calf on stimulation of the posterior part of the tongue. It has also been observed that after transection of the glossopharyngeal nerve in man, taste stimulation of the posterior tongue was still effective (Bohm and Strang, 1962).

In the nucleus of the tractus solitarius, the second-order neurons of the gustatory pathway give rise to central fibers, some of which quickly cross over. The decussation of these fibers takes place in the reticular formation. The crossed fibers then enter the medial lemniscus and pass to the thalamus. They seem to end in the medial and ventral nuclei of the thalamus. The thalamic relay station for taste has been localized by electrical recording to the medial tip of the ventromedial complex of the thalamus. Other fibers have been reported to terminate in the mammillary body, and in fishes and amphibians there are fiber connections between the tractus solitarius and the region of the hypothalamus.

From the thalamus nerve fibers run to a presumed cortical taste center, but its location

has not been definitely determined. The cortical taste center has been variously placed near the hippocampus and hippocampal gyrus in the temporal lobe and in the inferior pre- and post-central gyri in the cortex of the operculum Rolandi.

Wolf (1968) has used lesions and the staining of the subsequently degenerated axons to study the courses and terminations of the corticopetal and corticofugal gustatory tracts in the rat. He found the rat's ascending gustatory pathway to terminate in its insular and inferior parietal cortex.

Benjamin and Burton (1968) performed a similar study on the squirrel monkey (*Saimiri sciureus*), employing electrical stimulation of the taste nerves and lesioning of the presumed cortical taste areas. They cite results showing the existence of two separate gustatory areas in the monkey's cortex (the opercular-insular area and somatic sensory area I) and suggest that other mammals, with the possible exception of the rat, may have two distinct cortical taste areas as well. At the same time, Benjamin and Burton indicate that only the opercular-insular area could be devoted purely to taste.

If the chorda tympani and glossopharyngeal nerves of the squirrel monkey are electrically stimulated, the response recorded from the opercular-insular area is of 2 to 3 msec longer duration than the response recorded in the SI area. There is no contralateral effect.

Sanides (1968) makes an attempt to delimit the cortical gustatory areas in the squirrel monkey (*Saimiri sciureus*).

Oakley and Benjamin (1966) deal extensively with the anatomy and physiology of the mammalian gustatory pathway. The anatomy of the human gustatory system is covered by Sarkisov (1966).

Unlike mammals, fish not only have taste buds in their mouths but also have a distribution of taste buds over the surface of their body. Bodrova (1965) describes the taste buds of three freshwater fish (bream, burbot, zander). She reports these fish to have taste buds not only on the head, body and lips, and in the buccal cavity, but also in the gills and the pharynx and on various fins. In catfish taste buds are found in high number on the barbels. In the sea robin (*Prionotus carolinus*) many chemosensitive free nerve endings are located on a portion of the pectoral fins, and in the squirrel hake (*Urophycis chuss*) there are taste buds and possibly also chemosensitive free nerve endings on the pelvic fins.

The taste buds of fish are subserved by the seventh, ninth and tenth cranial nerves. The chemosensitive nerve fibers of the sea robin belong to the third spinal nerve.

In insects taste hairs and taste pegs are located externally, primarily on the maxillary and labial palpi and on the tarsi. Taste receptors have also been reported from antennae (blowfly, bees, ants), ovipositors (blowfly, ichneumon flies, crickets) and wings (blowfly).

The central process of an insect chemoreceptive neuron generally extends directly into the central nervous system. Labellar receptors enter the subesophageal ganglion, while tarsal receptors extend into the thoracic ganglion. Only the chemoreceptors of some Neuroptera are known to synapse distal to the central nervous system.

Although some observations have been made which point to the existence of efferent taste fibers, indisputable proof of an efferent innervation of the taste cells has not been obtained.

In mammals numerous synaptic vesicles have been noted in the endings of large intragemmal taste fibers. Vesicles have also been observed in taste fibers of a fish (*Corydoras paleatus*). However, synaptic vesicles are similarly present in a number of different nerve endings which seem to be sensory in function (Oakley and Benjamin, 1966).

Gray and Watkins (1965) cast doubt on the nature of the vesicles on both sides of taste cell–nerve fiber synapses in the rat. They point to the absence of a clear-cut concentration of these vesicles at the synaptic membranes. Furthermore, while in the taste cell and the nerve fiber terminal there are vesicles falling within the size range of normal synaptic vesicles,

other vesicles are twice or three times this diameter.

Gray and Watkins also give reasons for believing that some structures interpreted as axon terminals may in fact have been portions of taste cells.

Esakov (1963b) reported recording efferent discharges from the glossopharyngeal nerve after stimulating the frog's tongue with sodium chloride.

Taste impulses from both the anterior and posterior portions of the tongue are transmitted to the rostral part of the nucleus of the tractus solitarius. Recordings made from this region of the rat's nucleus showed an augmentation of the activity produced by stimulation of the posterior tongue when transmission through the chorda tympani nerve (subserving the anterior tongue) was blocked. Discharges from the chorda tympani may therefore exert some inhibitory effect in the rostral part of the nucleus of the tractus solitarius (Halpern and Nelson, 1965).

Inhibition can normally be produced in the cat's thalamus (in or near the nucleus ventralis posteromedialis) by stimulating its tongue with sodium chloride. The magnitude of such thalamic inhibition varies more or less linearly with concentration. Occasionally the application of quinine hydrochloride or hydrochloric acid to the tongue also calls forth inhibitory effects in the thalamus (Ishiko, Amatsu and Sato, 1967).

There is evidence for centrifugal tracts at higher levels of the gustatory analyzer.

Wolf (1968) traced the course of corticofugal fibers originating in an apparently gustatory region of the rat's cortex. Lesions in the insular and inferior parietal cortex produced degeneration along a route through the globus pallidus and striatum which was parallel to that of the ascending gustatory pathway. One group of the degenerating, apparently efferent fibers then passed into the ipsilateral thalamus to end just dorsal to the medial subnucleus. A second group curved caudally into the cerebral peduncle and terminated in the ipsilateral substantia nigra. Both some corticofugal and afferent thalamic fibers appeared to end in the striatum.

Wolf also found a group of fibers to connect the cortical gustatory areas of the two sides of the brain.

Benjamin and Burton (1968) ablated the apparently gustatory opercular-insular and SI projection areas of the cortex of a squirrel monkey (*Saimiri sciureus*). This resulted in the degeneration of nearly all of the ventromedial complex (gustatory region) of the thalamus. If either of the above responsive cortical areas is removed alone, no degeneration is produced in the thalamus.

Evidence has been presented that taste substances are directly absorbed from the oral cavity and then, within a matter of tens of seconds, reach the brain, where they especially concentrate in the region of the olfactory lobes (see page 265, Gustatory Reception). Kare (1968) has suggested that absorbed taste stimuli could provoke activity which is transmitted to cerebral structures associated with the mediation of consumption. The possibility that such absorbed taste stimuli may evoke efferent activity in the brain should also be considered.

Gustatory activity is apparently subject to centrifugal effects mediated by way of sympathetic, parasympathetic and vagal nerves. Some ideas have been formed of the routes which are traversed by these centrifugal influences.

Sympathetic action potentials producing a general increase in gustatory response probably pass in the frog from the first sympathetic ganglion to the pneumogastric (jugular) ganglion, and then into the glossopharyngeal nerve. There are two connecting tracts between the first sympathetic ganglion and the pneumogastric ganglion of the frog, and the glossopharyngeal and vagal nerves take origin from the latter ganglion (Chcrnctski, 1964). Activity has been successfully produced in the frog's glossopharyngeal nerve by electrically stimulating the first sympathetic ganglion.

It is believed that in the rat and in man efferent sympathetic fibers from the cervical sympathetic ganglion could reach the tongue by running alongside the lingual artery.

The efferent impulses which call forth increases or reductions in the taste discharges of the frog's glossopharyngeal nerve upon gastric stimulation appear to be transmitted from the stomach to the nucleus of the tractus solitarius in afferent vagal fibers. Removal of the medulla oblongata, in which the nucleus of the tractus solitarius is located, interrupts the pathway from the gastric receptors to the glossopharyngeal taste fibers (Esakov, 1961).

The taste fibers in the glossopharyngeal nerve are known to terminate near the ipsilateral nucleus of the tractus solitarius. Esakov (1961) observed in the frog that if a glossopharyngeal nerve was cut and its central portion stimulated, the contralateral glossopharyngeal nerve showed a reduced discharge to sodium chloride and water. Halpern (1967) suggests that parasympathetic fibers in the glossopharyngeal nerve may propagate inhibitory impulses to the peripheral subgemmal plexus of this nerve. Findings have been published showing that the glossopharyngeal nerve contains not only sensory fibers but also parasympathetic postganglionic fibers and their more central solitary terminal ganglion cells (Chu, 1968).

If the peripheral portion of a transected glossopharyngeal nerve is electrically stimulated, the taste discharge of the contralateral glossopharyngeal nerve is again reduced, indicating transmission in this case of efferent impulses through connections between the subgemmal taste fiber plexi. Rapuzzi and Casella (1965) found fiber connections between different papillae in the frog tongue.

Peripheral Afferent Inhibition

Snyakin (1965) reported the existence of a stable reflex connection between taste receptors. The large number of nerve axons which are often found to be enveloped by the membrane of a single taste cell also caused Beidler (1965) to raise the question of interaction between taste cells. The concept that there is interaction between the taste receptors during adequate stimulation has been espoused by Filin and Esakov (1968). These investigators showed that in the frog an antidromic spread of action potentials takes place along the branchings of the afferent fibers of the lingual nerve.

Beidler (1965) has further suggested that some processing of the gustatory input may already occur in the nerve plexus beneath the taste cells. It has been observed that the responses of taste cells to divalent ions differ in some respects from the responses recorded from single chorda tympani fibers.

Electrophysiological recording from the cat's chorda tympani has been used by Hellekant (1969) to study the effects of taste solutions on the responses to subsequent taste stimuli administered following a water rinse. He found that in the case of some taste solutions (hydrochloric acid, quinine hydrochloride, sodium chloride, potassium chloride, potassium sulfate and ammonium chloride) the response to a different subsequent solution was depressed more than the response to a second volume of the same solution. Hellekant considers it possible that such results may be due to reciprocal inhibition between the neural elements at the periphery of the gustatory system.

Hellekant (1969) also states that lateral inhibition between peripheral gustatory neurons, by enhancing differences between the responses of similarly sensitive neurons, could facilitate stimulus identification.

Von Békésy (1967b) has described a psychophysical experiment proving the existence of peripheral lateral inhibition in the gustatory system. Hydrochloric acid, sugar or quinine solutions, and so on, were flown over an observer's tongue by means of an apparatus designed to maintain the same concentration over a small length of the tongue and then produce a continuous increase in concentration in a posterior direction (Fig. 4-23). When the tongue was stimulated in this manner, a posterior localized area of strong taste sensation was bordered anteriorly by an area of no taste

sensation, followed further anteriorly by another region of taste sensation. This result shows that lateral inhibition like that producing visual Mach bands operates in gustation.

Centrifugal Inhibition

Centrifugal influences on gustation tend to fall into two major groups according to the results which they have been observed to produce. Activity mediated by sympathetic nerve fibers gives rise to a general augmentation of gustatory responses. On the other hand, increases or reductions in taste responses can be respectively evoked by different specific nongustatory stimuli which do not act through the sympathetic system. These changes in gustatory response appear to follow afferent vagal discharges which presumably lead to efferent parasympathetic impulses that are transmitted to the peripheral taste fiber plexus.

A number of investigators have noted sympathetic activity to enhance gustatory re-

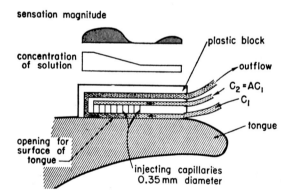

FIGURE 4-23. Apparatus for demonstrating lateral inhibition on the tongue. Tube C_1 carries a taste solution into a plastic block. The block has a 3 mm x 27 mm opening by which the solution reaches the tongue's surface before flowing upward and out (outflow). A higher concentration of the solution flows through tube $C_2=AC_1$ and into capillaries connecting to the opening. These capillaries serve to produce a continuous increase in concentration along the posterior portion of the opening. Middle, distribution of concentrations, top, distribution of sensation magnitudes. (From Békésy, G. von: Mach band type lateral inhibition in different sense organs. *J. Gen. Physiol.*, 50:519-532, 1967.)

sponses. Kimura (1961) recorded larger taste responses from the cut chorda tympani nerve of the rat after he directly stimulated the preganglionic nerve of the cervical sympathetic plexus. The magnitudes of the responses to sodium chloride, hydrochloric acid, sucrose and quinine hydrochloride increased somewhat, and there also resulted a higher level of spontaneous activity. Kimura obtained similar but lesser effects with epinephrine, which is closely related to the sympathetic transmitter.

Chernetski (1964) found that in the frog electrical stimulation of the first sympathetic ganglion moderately increased the afferent discharge elicited in the glossopharyngeal nerve by flowing taste substances over the tongue. Both the number of active nerve fibers and the impulse frequency in individual fibers was higher for 10 seconds after stimulating the sympathetic ganglion. There was an inverse relationship between the unmodified impulse frequency of the gustatory response and the latency of effect of sympathetic stimulation. Any chance of visceral or central nervous system effects was excluded.

A more thorough study of the mode of action of sympathetic activity on taste responses was performed by Esakov, Margolis and Yur'eva (1966), using the frog tongue. It was learned that under certain experimental conditions stimulation of the sympathetic trunk actually leads to the inhibition of receptor activity but that this inhibition is followed by the enhancement of receptor responses during the subsequent recovery phase. Under other experimental conditions only the augmentation of receptor responses is obtained. Esakov and his co-workers state that the sympathetic system can change the functional condition of the taste receptor.

The sympathetic system was also found to interact in a complex manner with other efferent influences. Such interaction results in both reinforcement of the efferent effect and a faster receptor recovery.

Esakov, Margolis and Yur'eva (1966) consider the sympathetic system's action to be of a damping nature, in keeping with the general trophic function of the sympathetic system. They point to the considerably greater duration of lingual nerve inhibition of receptor activity in sympathectomized frogs and, conversely, to the shortening of the inhibitory period in such frogs by epinephrine. Epinephrine also hastens the termination of lingual inhibition in normal organisms.

Epinephrine, unlike sympathetic system stimulation, only enhances receptor responses.

The central nervous system can affect taste receptor activity by way of the lingual nerve and also through the sympathetic system.

Taste discharges in both lingual nerves of the frog can be reduced for a period of 12 to 25 minutes by electrically stimulating one lingual nerve.

Several studies have been made of the actions on taste responses of impulses which seem to be mediated by way of afferent vagal fibers and efferent parasympathetic fibers. Esakov (1961) stimulated the stomach of the frog while flowing taste solutions over its tongue and recording from a glossopharyngeal nerve. Stretching of the stomach with water, which presumably provokes afferent vagal discharges, resulted in a 50 per cent rise in the impulse frequency of the gustatory response to water. When sodium chloride was flown over the tongue, there was a 25 per cent rise in impulse rate following stomach distension. However, during taste stimulation with quinine hydrochloride, a 17 per cent drop in impulse frequency appeared upon gastric distension. Stimulation of the stomach wall with 0.5 ml of peptone produced still other effects —the response to water fell by a third, the response to sodium chloride underwent a slight reduction and the taste response to quinine remained unchanged.

Halpern and Postles (1967) performed an experiment similar to the above on *Rana pipiens*. They distended the stomach with an intragastric balloon to produce a significant increase in the average taste response to 0.5M sodium chloride. The effect on the response to 0.2M potassium chloride was not as clear-cut. Like results were obtained by flowing protein hydrolyzate through the stomach.

Psychophysical experiments on man (Zaiko and Lokshina, 1963) and behavioral experiments on dogs (Kassil, Ugolev and Chernigovskii, 1959) also show the effect of gastric stimulation on gustation. In man the introduction of a meal into the stomach through a gastric fistula resulted in a decrease in the number of taste papillae responding to suprathreshold solutions of sodium chloride and sucrose. In the dog the placement of a solution of hypertonic sodium chloride into the stomach by a fistula was followed by the rejection of previously acceptable concentrations of sodium chloride in milk. These concentrations were once more consumed after the stomach was washed out.

Gastric distension and osmotic pressure were eliminated as factors in the dog. The sensitivity of the response to gastric sodium chloride concentration, irrespective of the total amount of sodium chloride introduced into the stomach, makes it likely that gastric or duodenal chemoreceptors initiated the centrifugal effect in the dog. Sudakov and Rogacheva (1963) have found indications of gastric chemoreceptors sensitive to sodium chloride.

Snyakin (1965) stimulated the interoceptors of the stomach and of the intestine to produce an inhibitory action on the taste papillae of the tongue and on the lingual nerve discharge. He also confirmed the existence, in the reverse direction, of a tongue-stomach reflex.

It can thus be seen that the efferent effects initiated through stomach stimulation are dependent on both the nature of the gastric stimulation and the particular taste stimulant applied to the tongue. Efferent influences could modulate gustatory responses in relation to the condition of lower portions of the digestive tract.

Esakov (1963a), recording from the frog's glossopharyngeal nerve, found that gastric distension caused the frequency of the spontaneous activity of the taste receptors to more than double. When the frog's stomach was rhythmically inflated fifteen to twenty times over a period of 30 to 45 seconds, the increase

in the rate of spontaneous impulses was maintained for over 10 minutes.

On introducing peptone into the stomach, and on stimulating the sympathetic chain, Esakov observed a sizable inhibition of the spontaneous discharge of the taste receptors. The inhibition following sympathetic stimulation, which resulted in a halving of spontaneous activity, had a latent period of 5 to 10 seconds.

However, Esakov (1963a) reported stimulation of the sympathetic chain to also produce a considerable and long-lasting inhibition of the taste responses to water and sodium chloride solution. This finding is not in agreement with the results obtained in other studies of efferent sympathetic effects.

The adaptation of taste receptors on the frog tongue to a stimulus can lead to the inhibition of a response to the same stimulus on the part of other such receptors. This effect operates by way of an arc of afferent and efferent fibers which passes through the medulla oblongata. Esakov (1967) used a chronically split frog tongue to demonstrate the above centrifugal interaction of taste receptors. He found the magnitude and duration of the evoked receptor inhibition to be dependent on the level and nature of the afferent discharge emanating from the adapted receptors.

In another investigation Esakov (1963b) studied centrifugal activity evoked in a tongue motor nerve by taste stimulation of the frog's tongue. He recorded from the central end of the sublingual nerve, whose fibers carry impulses to the tongue muscles. An increase was noted in the frequency of efferent impulses when water on the tongue was replaced by sodium chloride solution or when a saline solution was applied to the tongue for an extended period.

Further studies of a most exacting nature are needed to establish the manner in which the different centrifugal influences modify taste responses, and to determine the degree of the effect.

The significance of different centrifugal actions on the taste receptors is also not yet fully understood. Snyakin and his collaborators postulated that the functional level of the receptors can vary and that efferent discharges act to bring receptor activity to a suitable level for each existing combination of a series of changing internal and external conditions. Esakov (1967) instead suggested that centrifugal impulses act to maintain the taste receptors at a definite basic level of activity. In this way centrifugal influences would play a role in making the analysis of taste stimuli possible.

Halpern (1967) gives a good review of neural effects on the operation of the vertebrate gustatory analyzer.

Inhibition, probably acting in the brain, functions to terminate feeding in flies. Dethier and Gelperin (1967) have shown that feeding in the blowfly *Phormia regina* is regulated by the interaction of excitatory activity transmitted from the chemoreceptors and inhibitory potentials originating from gut and body wall stretch receptors.

Both of these inputs undergo fluctuation. The excitatory input varies as chemoreceptors adapt and new ones come into play. The inhibitory input changes as food moves discontinuously into the foregut and the crop undergoes periods of churning and distension. The fluctuating nature of the excitatory and inhibitory inputs is hypothesized to result in the normal discontinuous feeding of the fly.

The inhibitory input terminating feeding reaches the fly's brain from two chief sources. Stretch receptors in the foregut, which are responsive to the magnitude and rate of peristaltic movements in the foregut, send impulses to the brain by way of the recurrent nerve. Stretch receptors located in the body wall are stimulated by distension produced through filling of the crop. The discharges from these receptors reach the brain by way of the thoracic ganglion and the ventral nerve cord.

Transection of either the recurrent nerve or the ventral nerve cord results in continuous feeding, or hyperphagia. Transection of only the nerves innervating the abdominal body wall also results in hyperphagia.

The input of the oral chemoreceptors is more effectively counterbalanced by the inhibitory input from the ventral nerve cord than by that transmitted via the recurrent nerve. The body wall stretch receptors seem to exert a stronger inhibitory action than the foregut receptors.

Another inhibitory input appears to reach the brain via the ventral nerve cord from a locomotor center in the thoracic ganglion. Flies cannot walk and feed at the same time.

The extent of inhibition acting on the brain shows itself behaviorally as the apparent level of the taste threshold (Gelperin and Dethier, 1967).

Studies of sugar consumption by the blowfly (*Phormia regina*) have shown that there also is a negative feedback relationship between the osmotic pressure of the blood and the rate of food movement out of the crop into the foregut and then the midgut. A rise in blood osmotic pressure beyond a critical value slows the movement of food, and a drop in osmotic pressure below this value speeds up food transport (Gelperin and Dethier, 1967).

Central excitatory and inhibitory states of considerable relative duration can be produced in the blowfly (*Phormia regina*). Thus the stimulation of a salt receptor, which usually prevents or reverses the positive proboscis response, increases the threshold for release of proboscis extension by subsequent stimulation of a sugar receptor. Dethier, Solomon and Turner (1965) postulate a central salt center whose activity can inhibit a motor center for proboscis extension.

The long-lasting central excitatory state called forth by sucrose stimulation can be quickly reduced by stimulation with salt or water.

When *Hydra littoralis* is exposed to the brine shrimp *Artemia* or to reduced glutathione (which initiates a powerful feeding response), column contractions are inhibited.

The electrical pulses associated with this movement are then also absent. The previously mentioned stimuli further lead to the inhibition of contractions and of the related electrical pulses in excised tentacles (Rushforth and Hofman, 1966).

THE OLFACTORY SYSTEM

Structure and Functional Organization

The olfactory receptors of vertebrates are primitive bipolar neurons whose cell bodies lie in the nasal mucosa.

The sensory neurons terminate peripherally in long olfactory cilia. Reese (1965) observed that in the frog a dendrite projects distally from the neuron soma for 40μ to 120μ through the olfactory mucosa. It then gives rise, from a slight enlargement (the olfactory vesicle), to approximately six olfactory cilia. The last may be over 200μ long. While the pike's (*Esox*) and the burbot's (*Lota*) olfactory receptors each have only one cilium, as is also usually the case in the mole (*Talpa*), some mammalian receptors may have as many as fifteen olfactory cilia.

In air-breathing vertebrates the olfactory cilia lie for most of their length close to the surface of the fluid mucous layer which covers the nasal epithelium.

It has been shown, by destroying the olfactory cilia with detergents, that the cilia are not essential for the development of sizeable olfactory potentials (Tucker, 1967).

The sensory neurons of Jacobson's (vomeronasal) organ, which resemble olfactory receptors, have been found to be devoid of cilia in the slow worm (Bannister, 1968), the box turtle and the gopher tortoise (Graziadei and Tucker, 1968). However, these receptors possess complex microvilli.

Centrally the olfactory receptor neurons give rise to very fine, unmyelinated axons which run to the ipsilateral olfactory bulb.

In mammals the olfactory axons, after collecting into bundles each enveloped by a Schwann cell (the fila olfactoria), pass through holes in the cribriform plate of the ethmoid bone to enter into the cranial cavity and reach the olfactory bulb (Fig. 4-25). In amphibians and most actinopterygii, however, the distance between the olfactory neurons on each side and the olfactory bulbs is greater, and in these groups the olfactory axons join together to form a pair of olfactory nerves.

The envelopment of twenty to over one hundred olfactory axons by one Schwann cell is a unique feature of the peripheral olfactory pathway.

When the olfactory axons reach the brain (olfactory bulb), they interlace in a complex manner.

The olfactory axons terminate in the superficial zone of the olfactory bulb. Here they branch to form palisades of endings which synapse with the dendritic processes of the secondary olfactory neurons, chief among which are the mitral cells. As a consequence, spherical plexi of complexly interwoven terminal branchings, known as glomeruli, are formed.

There may be a great deal of summation of afferent olfactory impulses in the glomeruli. Allison and Warwick (1949) report that in a glomerulus of the rabbit 26,000 olfactory axons synapse with only some 100 dendrites of secondary olfactory neurons.

In mammals each of the olfactory axons runs into only a single glomerulus. This is also true of the olfactory nerve fibers in certain fish. However, in some fish and amphibians, individual olfactory axons have been observed to ramify into two or more glomeruli.

Nearby astrocytes send branches into the glomeruli and the more peripheral fiber network to enclose bundles of axons.

In the rabbit and the turtle the terminations of the olfactory nerve fibers have been reported to be spatially localized in the olfactory bulb according to their site of origin in the olfactory epithelium (Le Gros Clark, 1957; Orrego, 1961). Thus the spatial distribution of activity in the surface layer of the olfactory bulb would reflect the distribution of excita-

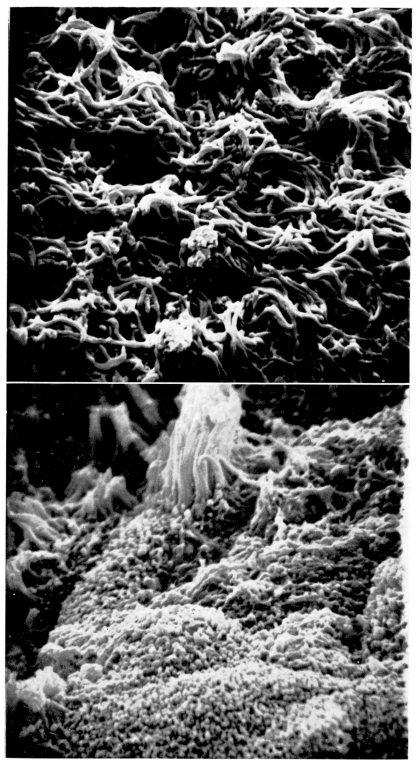

FIGURE 4-24. Electron micrographs of the olfactory mucosa of the box turtle (*Terrapene carolina*) in the absence of (top) and after (bottom) nerve section. Numerous olfactory cilia are present in normal olfactory mucosa. Interruption of the fila olfactoria results in metaplasia, and only respiratory cilia and microvilli are visible. ×5,500. (Courtesy of Dr. Don Tucker, Florida State University, Tallahassee.)

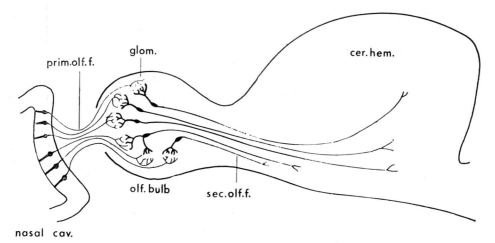

prim.olf. f.　　　glom.　　　　　　　cer. hem.

olf. bulb　　　　sec.olf.f.

nasal cav.

FIGURE 4-25. Diagram illustrating the general organization of the vertebrate olfactory system. The olfactory receptors, which are bipolar sensory neurons, give rise to axons, the primary olfactory fibers (*prim. olf. f.*), which are collected into fila olfactoria. In the olfactory bulb (*olf. bulb*) these axons synapse in glomeruli (*glom.*), chiefly with mitral cells. The axons (*sec. olf. f.*) of the last course to the ipsilateral cerebral hemisphere (*cer. hem.*). Nasal cavity (*nasal cav.*). (From Nieuwenhuys, R.: Comparative anatomy of olfactory centres and tracts. In Zotterman, Y. [Ed.]: *Sensory Mechanisms, Progress in Brain Research, 23.* Amsterdam, Elsevier, 1967, pp. 1-64.)

tion in the olfactory epithelium. However, according to the findings of Herrick (1924), this does not seem to hold for the amphibian *Ambystoma*.

The largest and predominant secondary olfactory neurons, the mitral cells, make up a separate olfactory bulb layer in most vertebrates. In mammals, birds and reptiles, plexiform layers which contain few cells are found on either side of the mitral cell layer, whereas in amphibians, with the exception of caecilians, the internal plexiform layer is either poorly differentiated or absent. In cyclostomes and the majority of other fish, the mitral cells lie mostly directly internal to but also in part between the glomeruli.

The various cell types of the main olfactory bulb are relatively clearly segregated into different cell layers. The six chief cell layers, starting from the surface of the bulb and moving internally, are (1) the fibrous layer, a layer consisting of a plexus of the olfactory axons, (2) the glomerular layer, which contains the glomeruli, (3) the external plexiform layer of some fish and all higher vertebrates, the site of numerous synaptic connections between cell processes (Fig. 4-28) and the location of tufted cells, (4) the mitral body layer, containing the somas of the mitral cells, (5) the granular layer, or internal granular layer of birds and mammals, in which are located the somas and short processes of the numerous granular cells, and (6) the periventricular gray matter, located immediately above the ventricle of the olfactory bulb. The external granular layer of birds and mammals, composed of cells lying central to the glomerular layer, and the internal plexiform layer of some amphibians and of amniotes, beneath the bodies of the mitral cells, are less commonly referred to.

From each mammalian mitral cell one primary dendrite (400μ-600μ long in the rabbit) extends peripherally and enters a glomerulus. In birds, reptiles, amphibians and fish a mitral cell typically gives rise to several main dendrites, each of which may serve more than one glomerulus.

The axons of the mitral cells pass centrally to leave the olfactory bulb in the secondary olfactory pathway, which runs to the ipsilateral cerebral hemisphere (Fig. 4-25).

In mammals the smaller tufted cells of Cajal also contribute dendrites to the olfactory bulb glomeruli and, probably, axons to the secondary olfactory pathway. The tufted cells of Cajal are distributed through the external plexiform layer of the mammalian bulb. Lower vertebrates as well possess smaller cellular elements which add their processes to the glomeruli and the secondary olfactory pathway. However, the bodies of these cells are located centrally to the mitral cells in the periventricular gray matter of the olfactory bulb.

In vertebrates an accessory bulbar formation is associated with the main formation of the olfactory bulb. This accessory olfactory bulb area is entered by the vomeronasal nerve fibers from Jacobson's (vomeronasal) organ, and its size is reported to be proportional to the extent of development of Jacobson's organ. The cellular structure of the accessory bulbar formation resembles that of the main formation but is less highly organized. In the accessory formation of mammals the mitral cells, like those of the main bulb of reptiles, give rise to several dendrites which run to glomeruli.

Lakomy (1966) found tufted cells to be absent from the accessory bulbar formation of the goat.

The secondary olfactory pathways, composed of the axons of secondary olfactory neurons, may vary in length. In cartilaginous fishes, numerous teleosts, and most Reptilia, the cerebral hemispheres lie at some distance from the olfactory bulbs. In these organisms the secondary olfactory pathways form long crura between the olfactory bulbs and the cerebral hemispheres. (Fig. 4-26). On the other hand, in mammals cell groups of the anterior olfactory nucleus may already be found in the caudal olfactory bulb and in the accessory olfactory formation.

In the majority of vertebrates each secondary olfactory pathway consists of a medial tract and a lateral tract. The medial tract of tetrapods is considerably smaller than the lateral tract.

Westerman and Wilson (1968) examined the structure of the medial and lateral olfactory tracts of the carp (*Carassius carassius* L.). Both tracts contain an excess of unmyelinated fibers over myelinated fibers, but the proportion of the first is much higher in the medial tract.

The axons of the tufted cells of the accessory bulbar formation seem to contribute to the lateral olfactory tract, as does the rostral portion of the pars lateralis of the anterior olfactory nucleus in the guinea pig.

Groups of neurons, as well as synapses, have been reported to lie in the human olfactory tracts. The largest bundle of the medial olfac-

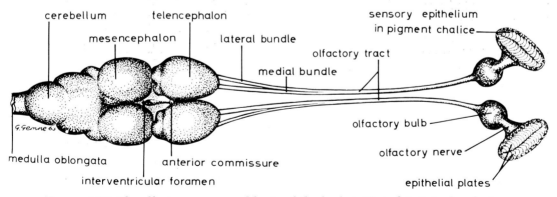

FIGURE 4-26. The olfactory organs and brain of the burbot (*Lota lota* L.), dorsal view. The tracts (crura) are 20 to 30 mm long. (From Döving, K.B., and G. Gemne: Electrophysiological and histological properties of the olfactory tract of the burbot [*Lota lota* L.]. *J. Neurophysiol.*, 28:139-153, 1965.)

tory tract of the carp (*Carassius carassius* L.) contains synapses along its entire length (Westerman and Wilson, 1968).

The many mitral cell axons in the lateral olfactory tract send out numerous collaterals to the cortex of the olfactory peduncle and to the prepyriform cortex, which lie beneath the tract. The axon collaterals form a thick plexus and then make synaptic contact with pyramidal and polymorphic cells. The axons of these two types of cells in turn pass into the internal capsule and give off branches which run into the anterior commissure.

The axons of the secondary olfactory pathways terminate in various secondary olfactory centers of the rhinencephalic portions of the telencephalon. The olfactory system is unique among sensory systems in initially projecting to these rhinencephalic centers rather than to the thalamus.

Lesioning and degeneration experiments to trace the courses of the olfactory pathway fibers have been performed only on the frog, reptiles and mammals, and the identity of the secondary olfactory areas innervated by the olfactory pathway fibers still remains somewhat obscure.

Scalia *et al.* (1968) ablated one olfactory bulb of the frog (*Rana pipiens*) to determine that its medial olfactory tract projects to the anterior border of the hippocampal and septal primordia. The frog's lateral olfactory tract instead appears to innervate the lateral pallium, the amygdala and the dorsal paleostriatum. The ventral habenular region also seems to receive lateral olfactory tract fibers.

The observed olfactory connections in the frog basically resemble those traced in the turtle by Gamble (1956).

In reptiles one group of medial olfactory tract fibers ends in the olfactory tubercle, while another group runs to the contralateral anterior olfactory nucleus (Gamble, 1952, 1956).

The lateral olfactory tract fibers of reptiles and mammals course to the prepyriform cortex, to certain amygdaloid nuclei, and to the lateral portion of the olfactory tubercle (Fig. 4-27). Mammalian lateral tract fibers have also been found to terminate in the periamygdaloid cortex, the pars externa and the caudal pars lateralis of the anterior olfactory nucleus and in the nucleus of the lateral olfactory tract (Mascitti and Ortega, 1966; Lohman and Lammers, 1967). Heimer (1968) further observed the rat's olfactory bulb to give rise to afferent fiber projections to the olfactory peduncle and the ventrolateral entorhinal area. In the cat the lateral olfactory tract has also been traced, by electrical stimulation, to all portions of the parahippocampal area of the cortex, which lies behind the periamygdaloid cortex (Dennis and Kerr, 1968).

The endings of the rat's lateral olfactory tract afferent fibers synapse chiefly with the peripheral branchings of pyramidal cell dendrites in the external plexiform layers of the secondary olfactory areas (Heimer, 1968). Similar observations were made on the cat by Mascitti and Ortega (1966).

Stevens (1969) studied the structure of the cat's prepyriform cortex, using some specimens in which one olfactory bulb had earlier been ablated. He found the fibers of the lateral olfactory tract to terminate mainly on the distal thirds of the apical dendrites of superficial neurons.

Stevens further commonly noted the prepyriform cortex's superficial neurons to send their axons down to deep neurons. The axons of the last synapse with other deep neurons and also with the apical dendrites of superficial neurons. Thus some impulses may follow a circular pathway. The axons of superficial neurons convey impulses out of the prepyriform cortex.

Northcutt (1967) has performed an anatomical study of the telencephalon of *Iguana iguana* and other reptiles, in which he concentrates on the olfactory system.

In the Cyclostomata and other low fish nearly all of the telencephalon is devoted to olfaction, whereas in birds and some microsmatic mammals only reduced portions of the cerebrum are olfactory.

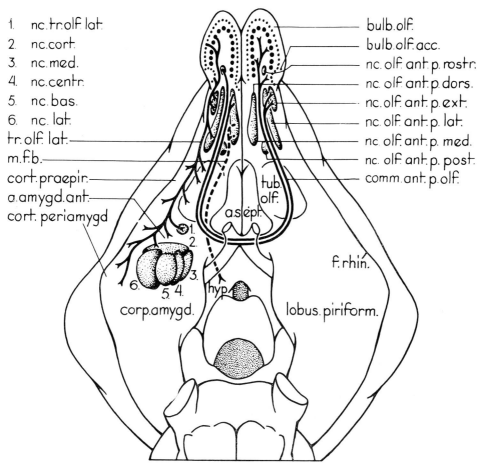

1. nc. tr. olf. lat.
2. nc. cort.
3. nc. med.
4. nc. centr.
5. nc. bas.
6. nc. lat.
tr. olf. lat.
m. f. b.
cort. praepir.
a. amygd. ant.
cort. periamygd

bulb. olf.
bulb. olf. acc.
nc. olf. ant. p. rostr.
nc. olf. ant. p. dors.
nc. olf. ant. p. ext.
nc. olf. ant. p. lat.
nc. olf. ant. p. med.
nc. olf. ant. p. post.
comm. ant. p. olf.

tub. olf.
a. sept.
hyp.
f. rhin.
corp. amygd.
lobus. piriform.

FIGURE 4-27. Diagrammatic representation of the principal connections of the main and accessory olfactory bulbs and of the anterior olfactory nucleus in the guinea pig. Abbreviations, left down: *nc. tr. olf. lat.*, nucleus tractus olfactorius lateralis; *nc. cort.*, corticalis; *nc. med.*, medialis; *nc. centr.*, centralis; *nc. bas.*, basalis; *nc. lat.*, lateralis; *tr. olf. lat.*, tractus olfactorius lateralis; *m. f. b.*, medial forebrain bundle; *cort. praepir.*, cortex prepiriformis; *a. amygd. ant.*, area amygdaloidea anterior; *cort. periamygd.*, cortex periamygdaloidea; *corp. amygd.*, corpus amygdaloideum. Middle: *tub. olf.*, tuberculum olfactorium; *a sept.*, area septalis. Right down: *bulb.* olf., bulbus olfactorius; *bulb. olf. acc.*, bulbus olfactorius accessorius; *nc. olf. ant. p. rostr.*, nucleus olfactorius anterior, pars rostralis; *nc. olf. ant. p. dors.*, pars dorsalis; *nc. olf. ant. p. ext.*, pars externa; *nc. olf. ant. p. lat.*, pars lateralis; *nc. olf. ant. p. med.*, pars medialis; *nc. olf. ant. p. post.*, pars posterior; *comm. ant. p. olf.*, commissura anterior, pars olfactoria; *f. rhin.*, fissura rhinalis; *lobus piriform.*, lobus piriformis. (From Lohman, A.H.M., and H.J. Lammers: On the Structure and Fibre Connections of the Olfactory Centres in Mammals. In Zotterman, Y. [Ed.]: *Sensory Mechanisms, Progress in Brain Research*, 23. Amsterdam, Elsevier, 1967, pp. 65-82.)

The secondary olfactory areas in the cerebral hemispheres have fiber connections with the diencephalon and with brain stem nuclei. Powell, Cowan, and Raisman (1965), and Wolf and Sutin (1966), have traced several connections between olfactory centers and feeding areas in the rat brain. The first authors deal with the olfactory tracts in general.

The terminal olfactory centers may lie in the hippocampus and the hippocampal gyrus (pyriform area of the cortex), but this has not been definitely established.

Yokota *et al.* (1967) recorded from neurons in the hippocampus of the squirrel monkey (*Saimiri sciureus*). Both electrical stimulation of the olfactory bulb and of the septum evoked excitatory postsynaptic potentials in these neurons. However, the EPSP's called forth by olfactory bulb stimulation were subliminal, and only the "septal" EPSP's gave rise to impulses.

The septum has afferent and efferent connections with the hypothalamus, which is significant in positive and negative feeding responses. In addition to other regulatory functions, the hypothalamus influences the activity, by neurosecretion, of the anterior lobe of the pituitary gland.

Insect Olfactory Structures

In insects the olfactory receptor cells, which are bipolar sense neurons, are located in olfactory sensilla that are primarily found on the antennal flagellum.

An olfactory sensillum typically contains one or several sensory neurons within a cuticular hair, peg or plate, and so on. If a number of sensory neurons are present, they may show similar responses or be reactive to different odor qualities and sometimes modalities.

The dendrite of an olfactory neuron passes peripherally toward or into the cuticular specialization of the sensillum and may be branched (Fig. 3-1).

In sensilla of the cuticular hair variety, the dendrite is constricted at the point where it enters the fluid-filled lumen of the hair. A ciliary structure has been seen to extend from this constriction. The portion of the dendrite proximal to and extending into the hair base is surrounded by a cuticular sheath (Schneider and Steinbrecht, 1968).

The axons of the bipolar olfactory neurons of insects always make direct connections with the central nervous system.

The cuticular apparatus of most insect olfactory sensilla has been seen to be penetrated by a large number of complexly structured fine pores (Schneider and Steinbrecht, 1968). These fine pores (of about 150 Å diameter in hairs and pegs) are easily distinguished from the single large opening found on insect taste hairs.

On the grasshopper's antennal flagellum the thin-walled, 16μ long peg of each olfactory sensillum basiconica is pierced by approximately 150 pores. A dendritic branch of one of the 40 to 60 neurons in the sensillum ends at each pore. At its termination adjacent to a pore every branch divides further into twenty-four thin processes (Slifer, Prestage and Beams, 1959).

In the moth *Bombyx* an antennal olfactory hair has about 3,000 pores, each of which is reached by several dendritic branches of 100 to 200 Å diameter. There are two to three sensory neurons in these sensilla (Boeckh *et al.*, 1965).

Electrophysiological recording by means of microelectrodes has made it possible to positively identify sensilla containing olfactory neurons. Sensilla trichodea (large hairs), sensilla basiconica (pegs), sensilla placodea (plates), and sensilla coeloconica and ampullacea (pit-pegs) may all contain olfactory neurons.

In related insect genera the same types of sensilla contain similarly functioning olfactory receptor cells. Thus the sensilla trichodea of male moths contain specialists responsive to the sexual attractant of the species. Generalist cells responding to different combinations of stimulants are found only in sensilla basiconica and sensilla placodea.

Nonafferent Connections

In addition to the afferent pathways described above, the vertebrate olfactory system also contains various intrinsic circuits, associative connections, and centrifugal tracts.

In the mammalian olfactory bulb there are a number of cells and connections which permit intercellular inhibition at the olfactory bulb level. Thus around the glomeruli there are neurons possessing short axons which act as connections between several glomeruli. In the rabbit each glomerulus is reported to contain the dendritic tufts of one or two such periglomerular neurons. Central to the glomerular zone these neurons make up the external granular layer. Also, the mitral cells and tufted cells have, besides their main dendrite which enters into a glomerulus, two or more accessory dendrites (Fig. 4-28). These accessory dendrites run peripherally or laterally into the external plexiform layer of the olfactory bulb, where they may synapse with "recurrent" collateral branches arising from the axons of other mitral and tufted cells and with granular cell processes. The accessory dendrites contribute to a thick fiber plexus in the external plexiform layer. The mitral and tufted cell axons not only give off "recurrent" collateral branches to the external plexiform layer but also give rise to deep collateral branches that make contact with the cells of the internal granular layer, which are described below.

In the internal granular layer of the olfactory bulb, central to the mitral cells, the cells are equipped with one or more long and several short processes. None of these processes is structured like an axon. It is believed that the cell somas and the short processes are contacted by the mitral cells' deep collateral branches, and by centrifugal fibers originating from olfactory centers beyond the olfactory bulb. The one or more long processes of each cell, which extend peripherally to branch in the external plexiform layer, are thought to convey action potentials to the accessory dendrites of the tufted and mitral cells. The granular processes running through the external plexiform layer are supplied with numerous knoblike gemmules, which are connected through short side branches to the main divisions of the processes (Fig. 4-28). The gemmules appear to be the synaptic terminals of the granular processes.

Granule cells are considered by some to be the general inhibitory interneurons of the olfactory bulb.

In the external plexiform layer adjacent synapses have the opposite polarity. The accessory dendrites of mitral cells synapse with the

long processes of granule cells, and the last in turn synapse with the same or other accessory mitral cell dendrites. The accessory dendrites of mitral cells apparently produce excitation in the granule cell processes, and the last act to inhibit the mitral cells. In the neuronal circuits of the external plexiform layer, dendrites appear to transmit potentials to other dendrites; the long processes of the granule cells are essentially dendritic in nature.

Rall and Shepherd (1968) used a computational neuron model to study the origins of the field potentials called forth in the rabbit's olfactory bulb by antidromic volleys evoked in the lateral olfactory tract. Their findings support the hypothesis of dendrodendritic synaptic pathways of the nature described above.

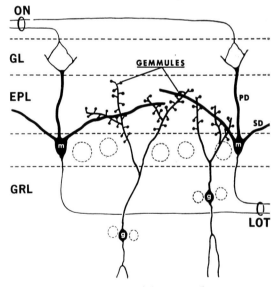

FIGURE 4-28. Diagram of layers and connections in the mammalian olfactory bulb. (*GL*) Glomerular layer, (*EPL*) external plexiform layer, (*GRL*) internal granular layer, (*ON*) olfactory nerve, (*LOT*) lateral olfactory tract, (*g*) granule cell, (*m*) mitral cell, (*PD*) primary (main) mitral dendrite, (*SD*) secondary (accessory) mitral dendrite. The external granular and internal plexiform layers are not shown. (From Rall, W., G.M. Shepherd, T.S. Reese, and M.W. Brightman: Dendrodendritic synaptic pathway for inhibition in the olfactory bulb. *Exp. Neurol., 14:* 44-56, 1966 [Academic].)

Rall's and Shepherd's results are in better agreement with a dendrodendritic inhibitory pathway than with transmission from mitral axon collaterals to accessory mitral dendrites or to granule cells. The hypothesized axon collateral-accessory dendrite route conflicts with the observed long latencies and with the polysynaptic nature of the inhibition. A deep collateral-granule cell route should result in the reverse of the observed potential gradients. The similar time course of orthodromic versus antidromic inhibition weighs against an axon collateral-granule cell long process pathway.

The failure of repetitive lateral olfactory tract stimulation to enhance the inhibitory potentials also points to a dendrodendritic pathway, since the antidromic potentials could only be blocked above the level of the axon collaterals.

The postulated dendrodendritic pathway indicates for the first time the possibility of transmission by dendrites, and thus offers a mechanism for integrative interaction on the part of axonless neurons with other neurons.

Whether interdendritic transmission is based on passive electrotonic spread over the synaptic membrane, whether it requires presynaptic action potentials, or whether both take place at different dendritic synapses, is left a mute point by Rall and Shepherd (1968). However, they report that according to their theoretical calculations the spread of depolarization within the granule cell dendrites may well take a nonpropagating or decrementing form.

By means of the described dendrodendritic pathways, a system of recurrent inhibitions could be established. By this means mitral cells could determine their own impulse rate. The indirect self-inhibition of mitral cells is quite likely.

Because each accessory dendrite and each granular cell process may have multiple synapses, a large number of mitral cells could ultimately be affected by a potential in an original accessory dendrite.

By means of the system of synapses in the external plexiform layer, mitral cells may be able to inhibit other mitral cells receiving a lower olfactory input. This would give rise to lateral inhibition in the olfactory bulb. Because of the spatial arrangement of mitral cell accessory dendrites, a mitral cell exerting such lateral inhibition would be surrounded by an anteroposteriorly elongated zone of inhibition.

Lateral inhibition, as well as self-inhibition, should be significant in the development of adaptation in the olfactory system.

A mitral cell may thus integrate excitatory depolarization, evoked in its primary dendrite through synapses with olfactory axons, with inhibitory potentials passing down its accessory dendrites. The sum of the potential gradients at the mitral cell's axon hillock will determine the frequency of the impulses transmitted through its axon.

Rall and Shepherd (1968) demarcate a greater role for the granule cell as an inhibitory interneuron. The inhibitory function of the granule cell is not only called into play by impulses transmitted from accessory mitral dendrites in the dendrodendritic pathway but also by discharges in the fibers of the anterior commissure. Centrifugal fibers from higher olfactory centers, the stellate cells of the internal granular layer, and the tufted cells represent additional possible sources of input to the granule cells.

Rall and Shepherd (1968) attempt to draw a parallel between the function of the granule cell in the olfactory bulb and the role of the amacrine cell in the retina. They point out that the amacrine cell of the retina also has no axon, and forms synapses of opposite polarities with retinal bipolar cells. Rall and Shepherd suggest that the amacrine cell may also be part of an inhibitory dendrodendritic pathway.

In the internal granular layer of the mammalian olfactory bulb, there are also cell types possessing axonlike processes. Some of these processes run to the external granular layer, while others end within the internal granular layer.

Seifert and Ule (1967) were unable to identify any efferent fibers in the olfactory epithelium of the juvenile white mouse (*Mus*), nor

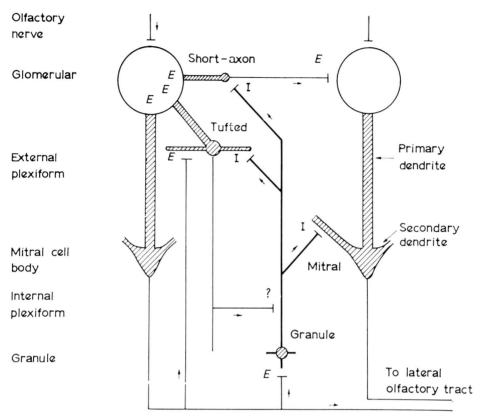

FIGURE 4-29. Diagrammatic representation of the principal hypothesized excitatory and inhibitory pathways in the mammalian olfactory bulb. The cells and excitatory (*E*) and inhibitory (*I*) connections are positioned in reference to the cell layers listed on the left. The term "short axon" refers to short-axon cells (periglomerular neurons), "tufted" to tufted cells. The dendroden-dritic pathway (from mitral cell accessory dendrites to granular cell long processes) postulated by Rall and Shepherd (1968) is not indicated. A possible centrifugal input to the granule cells is also not shown. (From Shepherd, G.M.: Neuronal systems controlling mitral cell excitability. *J. Physiol. [London]*, 168:101-117, 1963.)

have peripheral olfactory centrifugal fibers been reported by other sources.

The likelihood of finding efferent synapses in the olfactory epithelium is diminished by the morphology of the olfactory receptor cells. The olfactory receptors are sensory neurons which are provided with long axons that run centrally into the periphery of the olfactory bulb. Therefore, the impulse output of the receptors could be modified by centrifugal activity within the bulb.

The olfactory bulb appears to be subject to considerable centrifugal influences. Centrifugal fibers course to the main olfactory bulb (and accessory bulb formation) from higher centers, particularly from the olfactory tubercle. Most of these fibers contribute to a thickly interwoven plexus in the internal granular layer. The centrifugal fibers could affect the activity of granule cells by changing the excitability of their synaptic gemmules.

Some of the centrifugal fibers appear to continue toward the periphery of the olfactory bulb and seem to reach the glomeruli. These fibers apparently make contact with periglomerular neurons. This would permit centrifugal activity to act on the primary olfactory neurons (Powell and Cowan, 1963).

Heimer (1968) observed the ipsilateral centrifugal fibers to the rat's olfactory bulb to originate in the anterior prepyriform cortex.

Dennis and Kerr (1968) report that all the telencephalic areas which are terminal destinations of lateral olfactory tract fiber groups also give rise to centrifugal tracts ending in the ipsilateral olfactory bulb. Discharges initiated in these centrifugal systems produce negative potentials in the ipsilateral olfactory bulb even after transection of both the ipsilateral anterior limb of the anterior commissure and the lateral olfactory tract.

Dennis and Kerr suggest that the association of parallel centrifugal systems with the fiber groups of the lateral olfactory tract may be indicative of sensory feedback systems.

The anterior commissure provides significant connections between the two sides of the olfactory system, and the olfactory bulbs also receive fibers by this route. It was observed in the guinea pig by Lohman and Lammers (1967) that a group of fibers originating in the pars dorsalis of the anterior olfactory nucleus runs through the anterior limb of the anterior commissure to innervate the granular cells of both the primary olfactory bulb and the accessory bulb formation on the contralateral side. Such a contralateral olfactory bulb innervation has been noted in the cat as well (Mascitti and Ortega, 1966).

Ablation of the olfactory bulb of the frog (*Rana pipiens*) is followed by degeneration in the contralateral amygdaloid region (Scalia et al., 1968). However, Powell, Cowan and Raisman did not obtain such a result with the rat.

The two olfactory bulbs are also said to be interconnected through the anterior limb of the anterior commissure (Callens, 1967). However, Heimer (1968) and Powell, Cowan and Raisman (1965) were unable to find any such commissural fiber connection between the olfactory bulbs of the rat. Lohman and Lammers (1967) also provide evidence against a direct connection between the olfactory bulbs. It is possible that the axons of neurons in the anterior olfactory nucleus were excited during

stimulation of the cat's contralateral olfactory bulb by Callens (Ottoson and Shepherd, 1967).

Döving and Gemne (1966) discount a commissural connection between the olfactory bulbs of the burbot (*Lota lota* L.).

Induced afferent activity and spontaneous firing in the cat's olfactory bulb have been depressed by exciting the contralateral prepyriform cortex, cortical amygdaloid nucleus and olfactory tubercle. Direct electrical stimulation of the anterior commissure, at a sufficiently high frequency, had a similar result (Kerr and Hagbarth, 1955).

Stimulation of the lateral olfactory tract at the same frequency employed on the anterior commissure (100/sec) produced no depressive effect in the olfactory bulb.

Section of the anterior commissure enhanced olfactory bulb activity evoked by olfactory stimulation, and lesioning of the commissure's anterior limb noticeably lengthened the duration and augmented the synchrony of such activity.

It thus appears that inhibition is exerted on the olfactory bulb by way of centrifugal fibers crossing in the anterior commissure. Kerr and Hagbarth's sectioning and lesioning experiments suggest that this inhibitory action is tonic and regulates the impulse activity of the bulb.

Studies have also been made of the centrifugal and interconnecting fibers terminating in the anterior olfactory nucleus. Thus centrifugal fibers from the median forebrain bundle have been found to course to the pars medialis of the anterior olfactory nucleus. In the guinea pig a group of fibers passes through the anterior limb of the anterior commissure to connect the pars rostralis of one anterior olfactory nucleus with the pars externa of the contralateral nucleus (Lohman and Lammers, 1967). Crossed fibers have been reported to similarly terminate in the pars externa of the cat's anterior olfactory nucleus (Mascitti and Ortega, 1966). However, Scalia (1968) states in a review that there is considerable disagreement among investigators working with mammals as to the destinations in the contralateral anterior olfactory nucleus of crossed fibers originating from one anterior olfactory nucleus.

The anterior olfactory nucleus chiefly contributes to the anterior limb of the anterior commissure.

Heimer (1968) describes a centrifugally conducting olfactory associative system in the rat which involves all of the prepyriform and periamygdaloid cortices, and also the olfactory tubercle and a portion of the olfactory peduncle. The fibers of this system primarily end at proximal segments of pyramidal cells, in the deep portions of the plexiform layers of most of the mentioned brain regions. This suggests a centrifugal effect on pyramidal cell olfactory responses.

The neural circuits and tracts which convey nonafferent impulses in the mammalian olfactory system also seem to be represented for the most part in other vertebrates.

The anatomical studies of the secondary tracts and more central pathways of the olfactory system have brought to light a multiplicity of pathways. Some of these run from olfactory centers to other parts of the brain (to the mammillary bodies in the diencephalon and then to the dorsal tegmental nucleus; or to the habenular nucleus of the epithalamus and then to the interpeduncular nucleus and farther to the dorsal tegmental nucleus, etc.). Additional tracts reenter the olfactory system from various brain nuclei, and many of these may have a modulating function. Neuroanatomists are at present perplexed about the purposes served by many of these tracts.

A good idea of our present knowledge of the anatomy of the peripheral two thirds of the olfactory system may be obtained by reading the excellent reviews by Nieuwenhuys, Lohman and Lammers, and Ottoson and Shepherd in Zotterman (1967). Scalia (1968) reviews the findings on the origins and terminations of the secondary olfactory connections in mammals and cites much valuable literature. Allison's (1953) review, although somewhat outdated in many respects, can be used to gain a good picture of the earlier work on the struc-

ture of the various portions of the vertebrate olfactory system.

Afferent Inhibition

Results confirming the existence of presynaptic inhibition at the level of the olfactory bulb glomeruli were obtained from the frog (*Rana temporaria*) by Voronkov and Gusel'nikova (1968). Afferent impulses transmitted in primary olfactory axons depolarized the endings and probably also a considerable length of other olfactory fibers. This produced a reduction in the amplitudes of presynaptic action potentials in the affected fibers. The observed inhibitory effect showed some latency, suggesting the involvement of an intermediate process or structure, such as an interneuron.

When mitral and tufted cells, the secondary olfactory neurons in the olfactory bulb, are excited by olfactory impulses which reach them through their main dendrites in the glomeruli, their impulses can lead to lateral inhibition and self-inhibition. Such inhibition seems to be accomplished primarily through dendrodendritic pathways. The structural and functional aspects of the dendrodendritic pathways and of other neuronal circuits in the olfactory bulb are treated in the preceding section on olfaction.

Probably as a result of the inhibitory connection within the olfactory bulb, different odor stimuli most commonly cause the majority of secondary olfactory neurons to be inhibited. In the case of many stimulating substances, such as butanol, a low concentration evokes excitation and an impulse discharge in certain olfactory bulb neurons, while a higher concentration brings about the appearance of an inhibitory interval. Inhibition thus often requires a minimal level of stimulation (Döving, 1964).

Many substances simultaneously produce inhibition at certain olfactory bulb loci and excitation at others. This is suggestive of lateral inhibition. Odoriferous compounds may also produce excitation at a certain frequency range of the rhythmical activity shown in olfactory bulb responses and call forth inhibition at the neighboring higher and lower frequencies (Hughes *et al.*, 1968). Both of the mentioned phenomena should produce sharpening or greater contrast, and thus should make the input to higher olfactory centers more definitive.

At threshold a number of odor stimuli may cause some mitral cells of the olfactory bulb to respond with only one action potential. This is followed by a low membrane hyperpolarization of long duration. When stimulus concentrations are increased, the hyperpolarization of the mitral cell membrane rises proportionately in amplitude and duration. Spontaneous mitral cell activity is sometimes inhibited for over 50 msec (Ottoson and Shepherd, 1967).

A variety of responses, including "off" responses, can be obtained in the olfactory bulb by means of odor stimulation.

Callens (1967), using cats, obtained evidence for the existence of two different types of inhibitory circuits in the prepyriform cortex. Both kinds of inhibitory circuits in this secondary olfactory center are triggered by olfactory bulb stimulation.

When either or both olfactory bulbs are stimulated, the first inhibitory mechanism limits the discharge of certain prepyriform neurons to one or a few impulses. This suppression of neuron activity may be indicative of the activation of a recurrent inhibitory pathway.

Other prepyriform neurons display a lasting discharge which after a time progressively increases in frequency. This type of response suggests a release from inhibition, possibly due to the suppression or reduction of activity in a recurrent inhibitory pathway.

The presence of a second type of prepyriform inhibitory circuit can be demonstrated as follows: the impulse discharge evoked in certain neurons by stimulation of one olfactory bulb is recorded, and then this procedure is repeated after stimulating the other olfactory bulb immediately beforehand. Suppression of the impulse discharge by the preceding stimulation of the second olfactory bulb can thus be shown. In some cells ipsilateral bulb stimulation induces impulse activity, and the contralateral bulb has a depressive effect, while for other neurons the reverse is true.

If stimulation of one olfactory bulb facilitates the firing of a group of prepyriform neurons, their normal spontaneous activity is suppressed by action potentials from the other olfactory bulb.

Additional light has been cast on an inhibitory circuit in the prepyriform cortex by the work of Biedenbach and Stevens (1969a, b). These investigators observed that on repetitive stimulation of the cat's lateral olfactory tract, so as to produce synchronous volleys, the prepyriform cortex exhibits compound evoked potentials consisting of a negative wave followed by a positive wave. The first, negative wave is associated with excitation or depolarization of the superficial cells, and the second, positive wave with a sizeable and lasting inhibition or hyperpolarization. Most affected cells showed this depolarization-hyperpolarization sequence. The characteristics of the hyperpolarization identify it as an inhibitory postsynaptic potential (IPSP).

The lateral olfactory tract fibers synapse chiefly on superficial cortex neurons, and the last generally discharge ahead of the neurons which lie deeper in the cortex. Also, while the excitatory postsynaptic potential (EPSP) of the superficial cells shows a latency commensurate with monosynaptic excitation, the latency of the EPSP in the deeper neurons has a longer duration, which would be in keeping with the transmission of excitation from the superficial neurons to the deeper ones. It thus appears that the lateral olfactory tract is excitatory and initiates EPSP's in the superficial cells. These subsequently transmit the excitation to the deeper neurons. Biedenbach and Stevens (1969b) hypothesize that the deeper cells then exert inhibition on or produce IPSP's in other nearby deeper neurons and, by way of the proximal parts of superficial neuron apical dendrites, in superficial cells (Fig. 4-30). The described inhibitory actions of deeper neurons would account for the appearance of hyperpolarization at all cell levels and complete a circuit of impulse propagations.

Evoked potentials resembling those obtained by Biedenbach and Stevens (1969a) have been recorded *in vitro* from the guinea pig olfactory cortex (Richards and Sercombe, 1968). In his studies on the cat prepyriform cortex, Freeman (1968) also found that lateral olfactory tract discharges generally result in excitation and subsequent inhibition and that the superficial neurons mostly have a briefer latency of excitation.

The inhibitory circuits in the prepyriform cortex may well have a function similar to that of the inhibitory dendrodendritic pathways in the olfactory bulb. The prepyriform inhibitory circuits could produce lateral inhibition, which would be most marked in the case of those surrounding neurons receiving relatively few afferent impulses. Thus the "contrast" between more active and less active neurons would be accentuated. This might lead to a more precise identification of odors. The prepyriform cortex acts as an analyzer of the olfactory input.

It is not yet known whether the suppression exerted by an olfactory bulb on a group of prepyriform neurons is direct or whether inhibitory interneurons are involved.

According to Callens (1967) impulses from the contralateral olfactory bulb reach the prepyriform cortex by way of the anterior limb of the anterior commissure.

That the olfactory bulbs exert a tonic inhibitory influence on each prepyriform cortex, perhaps through inhibitory interneurons located in the cortex, is shown by ablation

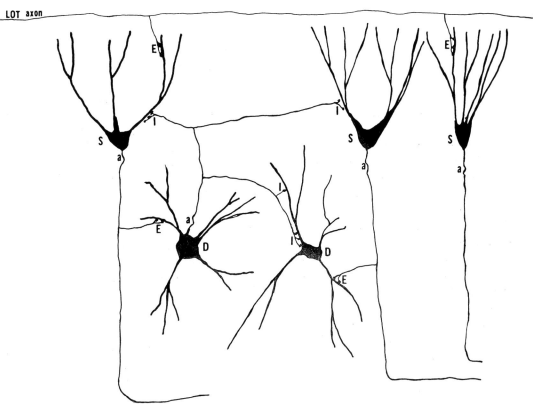

FIGURE 4-30. Schematic diagram of the hypothesized excitatory (*E*) and inhibitory (*I*) connections believed to produce the prepyriform responses to lateral olfactory tract volleys. (*S*) superficial cell, (*D*) deep cell, (*a*) axon. (From Biedenbach, M.A., and C.F. Stevens: Synaptic organization of cat olfactory cortex as revealed by intracellular recording. *J. Neurophysiol.*, 32:204-214, 1969.)

experiments. The excitability of the cat's pre-pyriform cortex is increased (as evidenced by greater response amplitudes) when incoming spontaneous activity is reduced by the removal of either or both olfactory bulbs. Results similar to those on the cat were obtained with the sloth (Callens *et al.*, 1965).

The finding that the spontaneous activity of the olfactory bulbs tonically depresses the excitability of the prepyriform cortex lends a new dimension of significance to olfactory bulb spontaneous activity. Afferent impulses resulting from this spontaneous activity may be responsible for the rapid adaptation of the prepyriform cortex.

The spontaneous activity of the olfactory bulb originates primarily in its glomerular and granular layers. Some glomerular cells show a steady rate of spontaneous firing which is not affected by an impulse input. The spontaneous discharge of other neurons is inhibited by afferent impulses and lateral olfactory tract stimulation.

The presence of strong excitatory connections between the olfactory bulb and the ipsilateral prepyriform cortex has been demonstrated.

It has been determined that olfactory receptor cells continue to show an almost steady level of response during a maintained olfactory stimulus of moderate intensity. Since the receptor potential fails to decline after reaching a plateau, the basis of olfactory adaptation must be sought in the inhibitory mechanisms which operate in the olfactory bulb and in secondary olfactory centers such as the prepyriform cortex.

The finding of Yokota *et al.* (1967) that olfactory bulb stimulation in the squirrel monkey (*Saimiri sciureus*) gives rise to subliminal EPSP's in hippocampal neurons makes neuronal events in the hippocampus of interest.

While the excitatory synapses of the hippocampal pyramidal cells are located on the spines of thin dendrites, comparatively far out on the dendritic tree (Andersen, Blackstad, and Lömo, 1966), inhibitory synapses are found on the somas of the pyramidal cells.

Andersen and Lömo (1968) investigated both inhibitory postsynaptic potentials (IPSP's) and EPSP's in the pyramidal cells of the hippocampal formation. They learned that these cells exhibit very strong IPSP's of long duration. Both forward inhibitions and recurrent inhibitions can be produced. Recurrent inhibitory effects may last for 200 to 600 msec.

Single electric shocks to the fimbria, administered at a rate of 1/sec, as well as tetanic stimulations, evoke recurrent inhibition. Both types of stimulation, and also the tetanic activation of forward inhibition, lead to the same final level of pyramidal cell hyperpolarization. The resultant membrane potential, approximately 85 mV, is thought to be the equilibrium potential for the IPSP, or the most negative intracellular potential which can be achieved. It may take as long as 15 msec from the start of the IPSP to reach this degree of hyperpolarization.

In view of the high strength and duration of the pyramidal cell IPSP's, it is not surprising that afferent impulses generally produce inhibition in these cells. Nevertheless, when the pyramidal cells are very excitable, a high rate of stimulation (10-12/sec) causes the IPSP to be replaced by a very large and lasting EPSP. The EPSP's slowly rise, and this increase is probably due to the accumulation of a greater quantity of a transmitter substance with each succeeding stimulating volley.

The initial portion of the eventually great EPSP appears after a short latent period, indicating it is monosynaptic.

Pyramidal cell IPSP's can be more readily recorded by an intrasomatic electrode than EPSP's, perhaps partly because of the location of the inhibitory synapses on the cell body. Also, the quantity of transmitter released at a dendritic excitatory synapse following a single stimulating volley is probably very small, and the initial low EPSP decrements as it spreads electrotonically along the dendritic tree. Only after a lasting tetanic stimulation is the quantity of released excitatory transmitter sufficient to adequately depolarize the dendritic tree for successful recording (Andersen and Lömo, 1968).

It appears likely that in hippocampal pyramidal cells the impulse rate is dependent both on the frequency of the inhibitory input and the level to which the EPSP is raised by repetitive excitatory stimulation.

It is possible that an olfactory bulb input of sufficient frequency and duration may be necessary to produce superthreshold EPSP's and hence impulses in the hippocampus.

Centrifugal Inhibition

Döving and Hyvärinen (1969) investigated the efferent effects exerted on the secondary olfactory neurons in the olfactory bulb of the burbot (*Lota lota* L.). They found numerous efferent influences to produce complex results, and could not clearly determine the natural role of the efferent system.

In fish efferent fibers may have excitatory or inhibitory actions on neurons in the olfactory bulb (Döving, 1966; Hara, 1967). Electrical stimulation of either the ipsilateral or the contralateral olfactory tract had similar effects. However, while each shock administered to the excitatory efferent fibers of the burbot (*Lota lota* L.) called forth only one action potential in the secondary olfactory neurons, stimulation of the primary olfactory axons elicited a full burst of firing (Döving, 1966).

In the rabbit as well stimulation of the fila olfactoria gives rise to bursts of firing, which emanate from the short-axon periglomerular neurons (Yamamoto *et al.*, 1963).

Inhibition of the spontaneous activity of goldfish (*Carassius auratus* L.) olfactory bulb neurons by antidromic electrical stimulation of the ipsilateral olfactory tract is long lasting (Hara, 1967).

Efferent activity can be evoked in each olfactory tract by electrically stimulating the central portion of a cut bundle of the same or by stimulating the contralateral tract. If contralateral stimulation is followed after suitable intervals of up to 140 msec by ipsilateral stimulation, the effect of the last is inhibited (Döving and Gemne, 1966). The inhibition exerted on one olfactory tract by the other is therefore of long duration.

Since afferent impulses in an olfactory tract can induce efferent activity in it, the efferent tract fibers must form the descending portion of a feedback loop between the olfactory bulb and the telencephalon.

The efferent fibers show spontaneous activity. In some tract fibers the spontaneous activity may be suppressed for a relatively long time by touching the burbot's skin. A similar inhibition is obtained by electrically stimulating the mesencephalon or several telencephalic areas (Döving and Gemne, 1966). Thus the function of other sensory systems may modify olfactory bulb responses.

The lateral olfactory tract of mammals is largely composed of mitral cell axons and probably tufted cell axons.

When the lateral olfactory tract (LOT) of mammals is antidromically stimulated, two negative waves can be consecutively recorded from the ipsilateral olfactory bulb. The first negative deflection is apparently due to the antidromic invasion of the mitral cells. The second negative wave seems to result from the inhibition of numerous tufted and mitral cells by way of synaptic connections.

The LOT mitral and tufted cell axons conduct the antidromic stimuli into the recurrent axon collaterals of the same cells. These collaterals should synapse with granule cells, in addition to mitral and tufted cell accessory dendrites, in the external plexiform layer of the bulb.

Inhibition, probably primarily by way of granule cells, results in the cessation of spontaneous activity on the part of numerous olfactory bulb neurons for 40 to 150 msec. This inhibition, like that produced by afferent olfactory impulses, is accompanied by membrane hyperpolarization of the said neurons, and is sustained.

Antidromic electrical stimulation of the lateral olfactory tract elicits a stronger inhibition of mitral cells than that produced by odor stimulation.

Electrical stimulation of the anterior limb

of the anterior commissure also results in mitral cell hyperpolarization. In addition, anterior commissure activity (probably involving centrifugal fibers) suppresses the hyperpolarization produced by LOT stimulation (Yamamoto et al., 1963).

Trigeminal nerve discharges also seem to initiate a mechanism that inhibits olfactory bulb activity. When Stone et al. (1968) reversibly blocked the trigeminal nerves of rabbits at their ganglia, the sinusoidal wave activity induced in each olfactory bulb by odor stimulation increased markedly in both rate and amplitude. Thus blockage of the trigeminal nerves heightens the excitability of the olfactory bulbs. Stone et al. postulate that trigeminal nerve impulses may induce the reticular formation to exert an inhibitory influence on the olfactory bulbs.

The reticular formation appears to modify the function of the relay stations of the various specific sensory pathways in a facilitatory or inhibitory manner.

The results of Stone et al. (1966, 1968) also suggest that the trigeminal nerve joins with the olfactory neurons in producing some olfactory bulb responses. The endings of the trigeminal nerve can be excited by very low concentrations of some nonirritating chemicals.

Callens (1967) has found that in the cat the removal of one olfactory bulb increases the excitability of the other one. Other investigators as well have noted an effect of one olfactory bulb on the other or, like Döving and Gemne (1966), have obtained evidence for such an action. Impulses may be transmitted between the two olfactory bulbs by way of higher olfactory centers.

Levêteau et al. (1968) have recorded from single glomeruli in the olfactory bulbs of rabbits. They observed the activity of individual glomeruli to be relatively weakly inhibited by electrical stimulation of the contralateral olfactory bulb. However, this weak inhibition may have been due to the localized character of the contralateral electrical stimulation, since contralateral olfactory stimulation had a strong effect.

Stimulation of the anterior commissure gave similar results.

All the demonstrated inhibitory actions showed long latencies.

The work of Levêteau et al. (1968) reinforces the concept that olfactory discrimination may involve interaction between the two olfactory bulbs. Olfactory stimuli presented to different nasal fossae should not produce independent effects.

Yamamoto (1961) reported that the response recorded from mitral cell somas is inhibited by activity from the contralateral bulb.

A considerable number of papers deal with centrifugal actions exerted by secondary olfactory centers on the olfactory bulb. The work of Kerr and Hagbarth (1955) indicates that contralateral secondary olfactory centers have a tonic inhibitory effect on the impulse discharge evoked in the olfactory bulb by odor stimulation. Callens (1967) also concluded that a tonic depressive action is exercised on the olfactory bulb by higher centers. He traced the inhibitory effect to the ipsilateral and contralateral prepyriform cortex and confirmed these centers as the origins of the inhibition by means of stimulation experiments.

Callens (1967) showed that interruption of the connecting tracts heightens the excitability of the olfactory bulb. Section of the anterior commissure raised the amplitude of the responses induced by electrical stimulation of the bulb's external plexiform layer, and the cutting of the ipsilateral olfactory tract or the olfactory peduncle produced a further augmentation. There was also a drop in threshold.

The surgical procedures were performed after ablation of the contralateral olfactory bulb.

Carreras et al. (1967) recorded the slow negative DC changes which take place in the surface of the cat's olfactory bulb after stimulation of various brain regions. They noticed that such changes in DC potential followed the stimulation of midline thalamic structures. The bilateral ablation of the primary olfactory cortices eliminated the thalamically induced negative potentials, suggesting a paleocortical pathway for the thalamic effects. A maintained negative change was also evoked by stimulation of the midbrain reticular formation. However, this DC change was unaffected or augmented by removal of both primary olfactory cortices. The last finding indicates a different pathway for reticular formation influences on the olfactory bulb.

The centrifugal fibers to the olfactory bulb for the most part form synapses with granule cells, which participate in the inhibitory dendrodendritic pathways of the bulb. Therefore, the greater proportion of centrifugal impulses descending from higher olfactory centers should be able to "modulate" the activity of the inhibitory neuronal circuits of the olfactory bulb and enhance or reduce the sensory "contrast" produced by them.

The inhibitory effects of the majority of the centrifugal fibers may also derive from their making contact with granule cells. In this way these centrifugal fibers may "key" into the inhibitory dendrodendritic pathways.

Hughes *et al.* (1968) have presented a scheme for the operation of the olfactory bulb which involves a tonic centrifugal input. A stream of efferent impulses would act on the bulb's cells to continuously desynchronize the background activity emanating from the cells. Afferent activity produced by odor stimulation would "break through" this normally maintained desynchronization to permit the intrinsic rhythms of the responding neuron masses to now show themselves as different frequency components.

The above hypothesis gains interest because of the existence of continuous efferent inputs to sensory receptors such as the muscle spindle.

The olfactory bulb exhibits irregular spontaneous oscillatory activity (EEG waves). The oscillations become enhanced and more regular on stimulation (Kerr and Hagbarth, 1955) and also on section of the peripheral and central connections of the bulb (Gerard and Younge, 1937).

Rall and Shepherd (1968) noted spontane- ous potential oscillations of considerable amplitude in the olfactory bulb of the rabbit. Huggins, Parsons and Peña (1968) found the spontaneous activity of the olfactory bulb of a reptile (*Caiman sclerops*) to consist of a combination of two oscillatory rhythms. Waves having a frequency of 7 to 12 cps and amplitudes of $10\mu V$ to $30\mu V$ appeared simultaneously with oscillations of a frequency of 17 to 27 cps and amplitudes of $5\mu V$ to $10\mu V$. When air was drawn into the nostrils, a sinusoidal wave rhythm of medium rate (12-15 cps) and very large amplitude ($100\mu V$-$200\mu V$) developed. This induced rhythm was abolished by ether.

Rall and Shepherd (1968) and Rall *et al.* (1966) postulate that the circular and often reciprocal dendrodendritic pathways between the mitral cells and the granule cells could well form the basis for the oscillatory activity of the olfactory bulb. As the mitral cells receive a continuous flow of impulses from the glomeruli, they in turn excite the granule cells. The last then inhibit the mitral cells and thus cut off their own source of excitatory input. As a result, the impulse activity of the granule cells falls and the mitral cells receive a lower inhibitory input. Now the mitral cells can once more respond to afferent impulses from the glomeruli and can again excite the granule cells.

Because of the close synaptic coupling between the masses of mitral cells and granule cells, the described neuronal circuit should lend itself to the development of synchronous, repetitive potentials. The amplitude of the extracellular potentials produced in this manner should be augmented by the radial orientation of the neurons' processes.

Gusel'nikova *et al.* (1968) noted that in the frog's olfactory bulb there is a direct correlation between the total inhibitory postsynaptic potentials picked up by intracellular recording and the frequency of the evoked waves. They consider the total inhibitory postsynaptic potentials to be the chief basis of the evoked rhythmic activity.

In the burbot (*Lota lota* L.) the secondary

olfactory neurons exhibit a rhythmical oscillation in the probability of impulse discharge. Since transection or cooling of the olfactory tract does not affect these oscillations in excitability, they may be assumed to have a peripheral source. However, efferent activity may play a role in preventing this rhythm. In a few neurons an afferent input did not permit the oscillations to develop, but only if the centrifugal connections to the bulb were intact (Döving and Hyvärinen, 1969).

Gusel'nikova and Voronkov (1966) determined that in the olfactory bulb of the frog (*Rana temporaria*) oscillatory activity is evoked by a high rate of stimulation of the olfactory nerve even in the absence of the orthodromic potential. Also, the orthodromic potential is fully or partially blocked by evoked rhythmic activity, and reappears upon termination of the oscillations. It seems that evoked oscillatory activity can inhibit the orthodromic potential.

Oscillatory phenomena similar to those in the olfactory bulb have been recorded from various parts of the brain and from the retina and optic tract. Laufer and Verzeano (1967) observed spontaneous oscillatory potentials in the lateral geniculate body to be inhibited by rhythmic activity emanating from the retina.

The retinal neurons were shown to have periodic patterns of discharge. Later Verzeano (1969) found that after light flashes the neurons of the lateral geniculate body show consecutive periods of excitation and inhibition and of the probability of firing. The distribution of these periods changed with the intensity of stimulation. The afferent input modulated the lateral geniculate body's spontaneous activity. In the visual cortex an evoked response is also accompanied by repetitive variations in the probability of neuronal impulse firing (Dill, Vallecalle and Verzeano, 1968).

Rodin and Luby (1966) reported that in human subjects LSD-25 produced progressive desynchronization of the EEG. The effect was most notable for the slower frequencies. It might be interesting to study the effect of LSD-25 on the rhythmic oscillatory activity of the olfactory bulb.

Good descriptions of research findings on the function of the olfactory system can be found in the following reviews: "Problems in the Physiology of Olfaction," by K. B. Döving (1967), "Experiments and Concepts in Olfactory Physiology," by D. Ottoson and G. M. Shepherd (1967), and "The Chemical Senses," by D. Tucker and J. C. Smith (1969).

THE SOMATOSENSORY SYSTEM

Research results obtained on the skin and visceral senses are covered in two important review papers—"Nervous System: Afferent Mechanisms," by Goldberg and Lavine (1968), and "Central Nervous System: Afferent Mechanisms And Perception," by Bishop (1967).

Von Békésy (1968), in a paper concerned with displacement of the sensation maximum by surrounding stimuli, extensively discusses lateral inhibition in the skin.

Mountcastle (1964) indicates that in the somatosensory system afferent inhibition is important for spatial discrimination. A receptor discharge, in addition to exciting central neurons, also produces pre- and post-synaptic inhibition in central cells by way of inter-

neurons. The cells in the middle of the affected central neural field are thought to be primarily excited, while toward the field's periphery there is an increasing inhibitory effect, until at its fringe inhibition greatly exceeds excitation. Such a phenomenon would tend to oppose the central spread of excitation. Despite cumulative divergence at the different levels of the afferent pathway, a localized cortical area of excitation might thus be preserved, making identification of the site of stimulation possible.

Among many interesting papers dealing with inhibition in the cutaneous afferent pathway is one by Sokolov and Dulenko (1968), who worked with the snail *Helix pomatia*.

Four publications which give information on

the inhibition produced by cutaneous afferents in the spinal cord are those by Zimmermann (1968), Jänig, Schmidt and Zimmermann (1967), Schmidt, Senges and Zimmermann (1967), and Mendell (1966). Two efferent systems activated by cutaneous receptors and producing primary afferent depolarization and inhibition in the spinal cord are described by Jänig, Schmidt and Zimmermann (1968), while Schmidt (1968) deals with the organization of the inhibitory input to afferent fibers which originates from skin mechanoreceptors.

Kostyuk (1968) treats the presynaptic and postsynaptic inhibitory phenomena produced in spinal interneurons and spinal motoneurons by impulse activity in visceral afferent fibers.

Kellerth (1968) devotes himself to the roles of the various presynaptic and postsynaptic inhibitions exerted on spinal motoneurons.

Wall (1967) reports that cutaneous responses are inhibited by the brain stem while movement responses are augmented. He also states that action potentials transmitted from the brain stem act to make lamina 6 cells sensitive to proprioceptive rather than to cutaneous inputs.

In a review of the afferent pathway transmitting facial sensation, Darian-Smith (1966) deals with efferent influences acting on this pathway in the brain stem and in the ventrobasal complex of the brain.

Gescheider (1968) found that more inhibition occurs when two different fingers on separate hands are stimulated than when both fingers are on the same hand. He suggests that wide separation of the stimulated skin areas increases the opportunity for inhibitory interaction by way of interneurons.

The organization of the cerebellar efferent system which acts on muscle tone has been described by Ito (1967). The cerebellar areas which are the source of the inhibition of Deiters' neurons were investigated by Ito, Kawai and Udo (1968).

The axons of Deiters' neurons run to motoneurons and inhibitory neurons in the spinal cord.

Inhibition is transmitted from the cerebellum to Deiters' neurons by way of the axons of the cerebellar Purkinje cells. The effects of drugs on the activity of the Purkinje cell axons was studies by Obata *et al.* (1967).

The disinhibition of Deiters' neurons by way of the cerebellum forms the subject of a paper by Ito, Kawai, Udo and Sato (1968).

The corticofugal effects exerted on the pain pathway at the levels of the spinal cord and thalamus are identified, with references, by Melzack and Casey (1968).

REFERENCES

Adolph, A.R.: Excitation and Inhibition of Electrical Activity in the *Limulus* Eye by Neuropharmacological Agents. In Bernhard, C.G. (Ed.): *The Functional Organization of the Compound Eye.* Oxford, Pergamon, 1966, pp. 465-482.

Adrian, H.O., W.M. Lifschitz, R.J. Tavitas, and F.P. Galli: Activity of neural units in medial geniculate body of cat and rabbit. *J. Neurophysiol., 29:*1046-1060, 1966.

Allison, A.C.: The morphology of the olfactory system in the vertebrates. *Biol. Rev., 28:* 195-244, 1953.

Allison, A.C., and R.T.T. Warwick: Quantitative observations on the olfactory system of the rabbit. *Brain, 72:*186-197, 1949.

Alpern, M., and W.A.H. Rushton: The specificity of the cone interaction in the after-flash effect. *J. Physiol. (London), 176:*473-482, 1965.

Andersen, P., and T. Lømo: Counteraction of Powerful Recurrent Inhibition in Hippocampal Pyramidal Cells by Frequency Potentiation of Excitatory Synapses. In von Euler, C., S. Skoglund, and U. Söderberg (Eds.): *Structure and Function of Inhibitory Neuronal Mechanisms.* Oxford, Pergamon, 1968, pp. 335-342.

Andersen, P., T.W. Blackstad, and T. Lømo: Location and identification of excitatory synapses on hippocampal pyramidal cells. *Exp. Brain Res., 1:*236-248, 1966.

Angaut, P., and A. Brodal: The projection of the "vestibulocerebellum" onto the vestibular nuclei in the cat. *Arch. Ital. Biol.*, 105:441-479, 1967.

Armstrong, C.M.: The inhibitory path from the lateral geniculate body to the optic cortex in the cat. *Exp. Neurol.*, 21:429-439, 1968.

Aronova, M.Z.: Electron microscopic study of lateral line organs in pike. *Arkh. Anat.*, 52:30-40, 1967.

Azzena, G.B., and V. Davini: Relationships between cerebral nystagmogenic area and optic nerve. *Arch. Int. Physiol.*, 75:855-858, 1967.

Bannister, L.H.: Fine structure of the sensory endings in the vomeronasal organ of the slow-worm *Anguis fragilis*. *Nature*, 217:275-276, 1968.

Barlow, H.B., R.M. Hill, and W.R. Levick: Retinal ganglion cells responding selectively to direction and speed of image motion in the rabbit. *J. Physiol. (London)*, 173:377-407, 1964.

Barlow, H.B., and W.R. Levick: The mechanism of directionally selective units in rabbit's retina. *J. Physiol. (London)*, 178:477-504, 1965.

Barlow, R.B.: Thesis. New York, Rockefeller University, 1967.

Barnes, C.D., and J.S. Thomas: Effects of acoustic stimulation on the spinal cord. *Brain Res.*, 7:303-305, 1968.

Beck, J.: Man as sensor. *Science*, 158:1296-1298, 1967.

Beidler, L.M.: Comparison of gustatory receptors, olfactory receptors and free nerve endings. In *Sensory Receptors. Cold Spring Harbor Symposia on Quantitative Biology*, 30:191-200, 1965.

Békésy, G. von: Similarities between hearing and skin sensations. *Psych. Rev.*, 66:1-22, 1959.

Békésy, G. von: *Sensory Inhibition*. Princeton, Princeton U. Pr., 1967a.

Békésy, G. von: Mach band type lateral inhibition in different sense organs. *J. Gen. Physiol.*, 50:519-532, 1967b.

Békésy, G. von: Location of maxima and minima in sensation patterns influenced by lateral inhibition. *J. Appl. Physiol.*, 25:200-206, 1968.

Belekhova, M.G.: Electrophysiological characteristics of the visual systems of the tortoise *Emys orbicularis*. *Zh. Evol. Biokhim. Fiziol.*, 4:265-275, 1968.

Benjamin, R.M.: Some Thalamic and Cortical Mechanisms of Taste. In Zotterman, Y. (Ed.): *Olfaction and Taste. Proceedings of the First*

International Symposium. Oxford, Pergamon, 1963, pp. 309-329.

Benjamin, R.M., and H. Burton: Projection of taste nerve afferents to anterior opercular-insular cortex in squirrel monkey *(Saimiri sciureus)*. *Brain Res.*, 7:221-231, 1968.

Bernard, R.A.: An electrophysiological study of taste reception in peripheral nerves of the calf. *Amer. J. Physiol.*, 206:827-835, 1964.

Biedenbach, M.A., and C.F. Stevens: Electrical activity in cat olfactory cortex produced by synchronous orthodromic volleys. *J. Neurophysiol.*, 32:193-203, 1969a.

Biedenbach, M.A., and C.F. Stevens: Synaptic organization of cat olfactory cortex as revealed by intracellular recording. *J. Neurophysiol.*, 32:204-214, 1969b.

Biederman-Thorson, M.: Auditory responses of neurones in the lateral mesencephalic nucleus (inferior colliculus) of the barbary dove. *J. Physiol. (London)*, 193:695-705, 1967.

Bishop, P.O.: Central nervous system: Afferent mechanisms and perception. *Ann. Rev. Physiol.*, 29:427-484, 1967.

Blomstrand, C., O. Hallen, A. Hamberger, and J. Jarlstedt: Effect of cerebellectomy upon the cytochemistry of neurons in the lateral vestibular nucleus. I. Effects on the RNA content and succinoxidase activity in Deiters' neurons at different post-operative intervals. *Brain Res.*, 10:239-244, 1968a.

Blomstrand, C., O. Hallen, A. Hamberger and J. Jarlstedt: Effect of cerebellectomy upon the cytochemistry of neurons in the lateral vestibular nucleus. II. Effects on the RNA content and succinoxidase activity in Deiters' neurons after warm and cold water calorization. *Brain Res.*, 11:648-654, 1968b.

Bodrova, N.V.: Taste and olfactory receptors in fish. *Tr. Inst. Biol. Vnutr. Vod. Akad. Nauk SSSR*, 9:148-162, 1965, and *Ref. Zh. Biol.*, No. 5124, 1966.

Boeckh, J., K.E. Kaissling, and D. Schneider: Insect olfactory receptors. In *Sensory Receptors. Cold Spring Harbor Symposia on Quantitative Biology*, 30:263-280, 1965.

Boernstein, W.S.: Optic perception and optic imageries in man. Their roots and relations studied from the viewpoint of biology. *Int. J. Neurol.*, 6:147-181, 1967.

Bogdanski, D.F., and R. Galambos: Studies of the Auditory System With Implanted Electrodes:

Chronic Microelectrode Studies. In Rasmussen, G.L., and W.F. Windle (Eds.): *Neural Mechanisms of the Auditory and Vestibular Systems.* Springfield, Charles C Thomas, 1960, pp. 143-148.

Bohm, E., and R.R. Strang: Glossopharyngeal neuralgia. *Brain,* 85:371-388, 1962.

Boord, R.L.: The efferent cochlear bundle in the caiman and pigeon. *Exp. Neurol.,* 3:225-239, 1961.

Branston, N.M., and D.G. Fleming: Efferent fibers in the frog optic nerve. *Exp. Neurol.,* 20:611-623, 1968.

Bremer, F.: Interactions binoculaires dans l'aire visuelle corticale et le corps genouillé latéral du chat. *Arch. Int. Physiol.,* 75:835-854, 1967.

Brindley, G.S., and D.I. Hamasaki: Evidence that the cat's electroretinogram is not influenced by impulses passing to the eye along the optic nerve. *J. Physiol. (London),* 163:558-565, 1962.

Brindley, G.S., and D.I. Hamasaki: Histological evidence against the view that the cat's optic nerve contains centrifugal fibers. *J. Physiol. (London),* 184:444-449, 1966.

Brodal, A.: Anatomical Organization and Fiber Connections of the Vestibular Nuclei. In Fields, W.S., and B.R. Alford (Eds.): *Neurological Aspects of Auditory and Vestibular Disorders.* Springfield, Charles C Thomas, 1964.

Brodal, A.: Anatomical Organization of Cerebello-Vestibulo-Spinal Pathways. In de Reuck, A.V.S., and J. Knight (Eds.): *Myotatic, Kinesthetic and Vestibular Mechanisms.* London, Churchill, 1967, pp. 148-166.

Brown, J.E., and D. Major: Cat retinal ganglion cell dendritic fields. *Exp. Neurol.,* 15:70-78, 1966.

Brown, K.T., and M. Murakami: Receptive field organization of S-potentials and receptor potentials in light and dark adapted states. *Fed. Proc.,* 23:517, 1964.

Brown, K.T., and K. Watanabe: Neural stage of adaptation between the receptors and inner nuclear layer of monkey retina. *Science, 148:* 1113-1115, 1965.

Buddenbrock, von, W.J.: *The Senses.* Ann Arbor, U. of Michigan Pr., 1958.

Buño (Jr.), W., R. Velluti, P. Handler, and E. Garcia Austt: Neural control of the cochlear input in the wakeful free guinea-pig. *Physiol. Behav.,* 1:23-35, 1966.

Butenandt, E., and O.-J. Grüsser: The effect of stimulus area on the response of movement detecting neurons in the frog's retina. *Pflügers Arch.,* 298:283-293, 1968.

Butler, R.A., G.L. Gerstein, and S.D. Erulkar: Inhibitory phenomena in cat cochlear nucleus. *Fed. Proc.,* 26:543, 1967.

Büttner, U., and O.-J. Grüsser: Quantitative Untersuchungen der räumlichen Erregungssummation im rezeptiven Feld retinaler Neurone der Katze. I. Reizung mit zwei synchronen Lichtpunkten. *Kybernetik,* 4:81-94, 1968.

Byzov, A.L.: Horizontal cells of the retina as the regulators of synaptic transmission. *Fiziol. Zh. SSSR Sechenov.,* 53:1115-1124, 1967.

Callens, M.: *Peripheral and Central Regulatory Mechanisms of the Excitability in the Olfactory System.* Brussels, Presses Academiques Europeennes S.C., 1967.

Callens, M., J. Colle, M.A. Gerebtzoff, and M. Goffart: Excitatory and depressive phenomena in the olfactory system of the sloth (*Choloepus hoffmanni* P.). *Arch. Int. Physiol.,* 73:748-761, 1965.

Campbell, F.W., and J. Robson: Application of Fourier analysis to the visibility of gratings (human). *J. Physiol. (London),* 197:551-566, 1968.

Capps, M.J., and H. W. Ades: Auditory frequency discrimination after transection of the olivo-cochlear bundle in squirrel monkeys. *Exp. Neurol.,* 21:147-158, 1968.

Carpenter, R.L.: A histological study of the chimpanzee eye. ARL-TR-67-9. Aerospace Med. Div., Holloman A. F. Base, N. M., 1967, pp. 1-72.

Carreras, M., D. Mancia, and M. Mancia: Centrifugal control of the olfactory bulb as revealed by induced DC potential changes. *Brain Res.,* 6:548-560, 1967.

Castro, G.D.O.: Branching pattern of amacrine cell processes. *Nature, 212:*832-834, 1966.

Chernetski, K.E.: Sympathetic enhancement of peripheral sensory input in the frog. *J. Neurophysiol.,* 27:493-515, 1964.

Chu, C.H.U.: Solitary neurons in human tongue. *Anat. Rec.,* 162:505-510, 1968.

Comis, S.D., and I.C. Whitfield: Centrifugal excitation and inhibition in the cochlear nucleus. *J. Physiol. (London),* 188:34-35, 1967.

Comis, S.D., and I.C. Whitfield: Influence of centrifugal pathways on unit activity in the cochlear nucleus. *J. Neurophysiol., 31*:62-68, 1968.

Cowan, W.M., and T.P.S. Powell: Centrifugal fibres in the avian visual system. *Proc. Roy. Soc. [Biol.], 158*:232-252, 1963.

Crapper, D.R., and W.K. Noell: Retinal excitation and inhibition from direct electrical stimulation. *J. Neurophysiol., 26*:924-947, 1963.

Crescitelli, F.: Delayed off-responses recorded from the isolated frog retina. *Vision Res., 8*: 801-816, 1968.

Creutzfeldt, O.D.: Functional Synaptic Organization in the Lateral Geniculate Body and Its Implication for Information Transmission. In von Euler, C., S. Skoglund, and U. Söderberg (Eds.): *Structure and Function of Inhibitory Neuronal Mechanisms.* Proceed. Fourth Int. Meet. Neurobiologists, 1966. New York, Pergamon, 1968, pp. 117-122.

Creutzfeldt, O.D., and M. Ito: Inhibition in the Visual Cortex. In von Euler, C., S. Skoglund, and U. Söderberg (Eds.): *Structure and Function of Inhibitory Neuronal Mechanisms.* Proceed. Fourth Int. Meet. Neurobiologists, 1966. New York, Pergamon, 1968a, pp. 343-349.

Creutzfeldt, O., and M. Ito: Functional synaptic organization of primary visual cortex neurones in the cat. *Exp. Brain Res., 6*:324-352, 1968b.

Creutzfeldt, O., and B. Sakmann: Neurophysiology of vision. *Ann. Rev. Physiol., 31*:499-544, 1969.

Darian-Smith, I.: Neural mechanisms of facial sensation. *Int. Rev. Neurobiol., 9*:301-395, 1966.

David, E., P. Finkenzeller, S. Kallert, and W. D. Keidel: Die Bedeutung der temporalen Hemmung im Bereich der akustischen Informationsverarbeitung. *Pflügers Arch., 298*:322-335, 1967.

Daw, N.W.: Colour-coded ganglion cells in the goldfish retina: Extension of their receptive fields by means of new stimuli. *J. Physiol. (London), 197*:567-592, 1968.

Dennis, B.J., and D.I.B. Kerr: An evoked potential study of centripetal and centrifugal connections of the olfactory bulb in the cat. *Brain Res., 11*:373-396, 1968.

Desmedt, J.E.: Neurophysiological Mechanisms Controlling Acoustic Input. In Rasmussen, G.L., and W.F. Windle (Eds.): *Neural Mechanisms of the Auditory and Vestibular Systems.* Springfield, Charles C Thomas, 1960, Chapter 11.

Desmedt, J.E.: Auditory-evoked potentials from cochlea to cortex as influenced by activation of the efferent olivo-cochlear bundle. *J. Acoust. Soc. Amer., 34*:1478-1496, 1962.

Desmedt, J.E., and P.J. Delwaide: Functional properties of the efferent cochlear bundle of the pigeon revealed by stereotaxic stimulation. *Exp. Neurol., 11*:1-26, 1965.

Desmedt, J.E., and V. La Grutta: Function of the uncrossed efferent olivo-cochlear fibres in the cat. *Nature, 200*:472-474, 1963.

Desmedt, J.E., and P. Monaco: Mode of action of the efferent olivo-cochlear bundle on the inner ear. *Nature, 192*:1263-1265, 1961.

Desmedt, J.E., and P. Monaco: The pharmacology of a centrifugal inhibitory pathway in the cat's acoustic system. *Proc. First Int. Pharmacol. Meeting, 8*:183, 1962.

Dethier, V.G., and A. Gelperin: Hyperphagia in the blowfly. *J. Exp. Biol., 47*:191-200, 1967.

Dethier, V.G., R.L. Solomon, and L.H. Turner: Sensory input and central excitation and inhibition in the blowfly. *J. Comp. Physiol. Psychol., 60*:303-313, 1965.

Dewson, III, J.H.: Efferent olivocochlear bundle: Some relationships to noise masking and to stimulus attenuation. *J. Neurophysiol., 30*:817-832, 1967.

Dewson, III, J.H., K.W. Nobel, and K.H. Pribram: Corticofugal influence at cochlear nucleus of the cat: Some effects of ablation of insular-temporal cortex. *Brain Res., 2*:151-159, 1966.

Dill, R.C., E. Vallecalle, and M. Verzeano: Evoked potentials, neuronal activity and stimulus intensity in the visual system. *Physiol. Behav., 3*:797-801, 1968.

Dodge, Jr., F.A., B.W. Knight, and J. Toyoda: In preparation.

Donner, K.O., and T. Reuter: Dark-adaptation processes in the rhodopsin rods of the frog's retina. *Vision Res., 7*:17-41, 1967.

Döving, K.B.: Studies of the relation between the frog's electro-olfactogram (EOG) and single unit activity in the olfactory bulb. *Acta Physiol. Scand., 60*:150-163, 1964.

Döving, K.B.: Efferent influence upon the activity of single neurons in the olfactory bulb of the burbot. *J. Neurophysiol., 29*:675-683, 1966.

Döving, K.B.: Problems in the physiology of olfaction. In Schultz, H.W., E.A. Day, and L.M. Libbey (Eds.): *Symposium on Foods: The Chemistry and Physiology of Flavors.* Westport, Avi Publ., 1967, pp. 52-94.

Döving, K.B., and G. Gemne: An electrophysiological study of the efferent olfactory system in the burbot. *J. Neurophysiol., 29*:665-674, 1966.

Döving, K.B., and J. Hyvärinen: Afferent and efferent influences on the activity pattern of single olfactory neurons. *Acta Physiol. Scand., 75*:111-123, 1969.

Dowling, J.E.: The site of visual adaptation. *Science, 155*:273-279, 1967.

Dowling, J.E., and B.B. Boycott: Neural connections of the retina: Fine structure of the inner plexiform layer. In *Sensory Receptors. Cold Spring Harbor Symposia on Quantitative Biology, 30*:393-402, 1965.

Dowling, J.E., and B.B. Boycott: Organization of the primate retina: Electron microscopy. *Proc. Roy. Soc. [Biol.], 166*:80-111, 1966.

Dunker, E., and G. Grubel: Zur Funktionsweise des efferenten auditorischen Systems. II. Mitteilung. Änderung von Variabilität der Spike-Intervalle und Hemmungs-Empfindlichkeit deafferentierter Cochlearis-Neuronen nach Durchschneidung ventral im Brückenhirn kreuzender Bahnen (Hund). *Pflügers Arch., 283*: 270-284, 1965.

Dunker, E., and D. Wachsmuth: Zur Funktionsweise des efferenten auditorischen Systems. III. Mitteilung. Analyse der Fluktuation von Spike-Intervallen deafferentierter Einzelneurone des Nucleus cochlearis dorsalis bei hemmend und fördernd beeinflusster Aktivität. *Pflügers Arch., 284*:347-359, 1965.

Echandia, E.L.R.: An electron microscopic study on the cochlear innervation. I. The Receptoneural junctions at the outer hair cells. *Z. Zellforsch., 78*:30-46, 1967.

Engström, H.: The ultrastructure of the sensory cells of the cochlea. *J. Laryng., 81*:687-715, 1967.

Engström, H., H.W. Ades, and A. Andersson: *Structural Pattern of the Organ of Corti.* Baltimore, Williams and Wilkins, 1966.

Enroth-Cugell, C., and J.G. Robson: The contrast sensitivity of retinal ganglion cells of the cat. *J. Physiol. (London), 187*:517-552, 1966.

Erulkar, S.D., R.A. Butler, and G.L. Gerstein:

Excitation and inhibition in cochlear nucleus. II. Frequency-modulated tones. *J. Neurophysiol., 31*:537-548, 1968.

Erulkar, S.D., P.G. Nelson, and J.S. Bryan: Experimental and Theoretical Approaches to Neural Processing in the Central Auditory Pathway. In Neff, W.D. (Ed.): *Contributions to Sensory Physiology.* New York, Academic, 1968, vol. 3, pp. 149-189.

Esakov, A.I.: The efferent control of receptors (on the example of the chemoreceptors of the tongue). *Byul. Eksp. Biol. Med. (USSR), 51*: 283-289, 1961.

Esakov, A.I.: Reflex regulation of the "spontaneous" activity of the chemoreceptors of the tongue. *Byul. Eksp. Biol. Med. (USSR), 55*:7-11, 1963a.

Esakov, A.I.: Efferent reactions in the sublingual nerve. *Byul. Eksp. Biol. Med. (USSR), 56*: 1184-1186, 1963b.

Esakov, A.I.: Role of afferentation from the taste receptors in the regulation of their functional activity. *Fiziol. Zh. SSSR Sechenov., 53*:575-581, 1967.

Esakov, A.I., S.E. Margolis, and G. Yu. Yur'eva: Interaction of somatic and sympathetic influences on activity of taste receptors. *Biol. Nauk, 9*:92-96, 1966.

Evans, E.F., and P.G. Nelson: Responses of neurones in cat cochlear nucleus to modulated tonal stimuli. *J. Acoust. Soc. Amer., 40*:1275, 1966.

Ewert, J.P., and H.A. Härter: Inhibitions-Phänomene im visuellen System der Erdkröte. *Die Naturwissenschaften, 5*:235, 1968.

Fex, J.: Auditory activity in centrifugal and centripetal cochlear fibres in cat, a study of a feedback system. *Acta Physiol. Scand., 55 (Suppl. 189)*:1-68, 1962.

Fex, J.: Crossed cochlear efferents activated by sound through both ears. *Acta Physiol. Scand., 59 (Suppl. 213)*:41, 1963.

Fex, J.: Auditory activity in uncrossed centrifugal cochlear fibres in cat. A study of a feedback system, II. *Acta Physiol. Scand., 64*:43-57, 1965.

Fex, J.: Efferent inhibition in the cochlea related to hair-cell dc activity: Study of postsynaptic activity of the crossed olivo-cochlear fibres in the cat. *J. Acoust. Soc. Amer., 41*:666-675, 1967.

Fex, J.: The Mechanisms of Centrifugal Inhibition in the Organ of Corti in Mammals. In Euler,

C. von, S. Skoglund, and U. Söderberg (Eds.): *Structure and Function of Inhibitory Neuronal Mechanisms.* Oxford, Pergamon, 1968, pp. 147-155.

Filin, V.A., and A.I. Esakov: Interaction of gustatory receptors. *Byul. Eksp. Biol. Med. (USSR),* 65:12-15, 1968.

Flock, Å.: Ultrastructure and Function in the Lateral Line Organs. In Cahn, P.H. (Ed.): *Lateral Line Detectors.* Bloomington, Indiana U. Pr., 1967, pp. 163-197.

Fox, R.C.: Chorda tympani branch of the facial nerve in the middle ear of tetrapods. *U. of Kansas Publ. (Museum Nat. Hist.),* 17:15-21, 1965.

Fredrickson, J.M., U. Figge, P. Scheid, and H.H. Kornhuber: Vestibular nerve projection to the cerebral cortex of the rhesus monkey. *Exp. Brain Res.,* 2:318-327, 1966.

Freeman, W.J.: Relations between unit activity and evoked potentials in prepyriform cortex of cats. *J. Neurophysiol.,* 31:337-348,1968.

Frewein, J.: Ein Beitrag zur Kenntnis der sensiblen Wurzelganglien des N. glossopharyngeus. *Zbl. Veterinaermed. [A],* 12:511-519, 1965.

Friend, J.H., N. Suga, and R.A. Suthers: Neural responses in the inferior colliculus of echolocating bats to artificial orientation sounds and echoes. *J. Cell. Physiol.,* 67:319-332, 1966.

Frishkopf, L.S.: Excitation and inhibition of primary auditory neurons in the little brown bat. *J. Acoust. Soc. Amer.,* 36:1016, 1964.

Gaarder, K.: Alternative physiological mechanisms of information transfer between the retina and the brain in visual perception. *Brit. J. Physiol. Opt.,* 20:1-7, 1963.

Galambos, R.: Suppression of auditory nerve activity by stimulation of efferent fibers to cochlea. *J. Neurophysiol.,* 19:424-437, 1956.

Galambos, R., and H. Davis: The response of single auditory-nerve fibers to acoustic stimulation. *J. Neurophysiol.,* 6:39-57, 1943.

Gamble, H.J.: An experimental study of the secondary olfactory connexions in *Lacerta viridis. J. Anat.,* 86:180-196, 1952.

Gamble, H.J.: An experimental study of the secondary olfactory connexions in *Testudo graeca. J. Anat.,* 90:15-29, 1956.

Gelperin, A., and V.G. Dethier: Long-term regulation of sugar intake by the blowfly. *Physiol. Zool.,* 40:218-228, 1967.

Gerard, R., and J.Z. Younge: Electrical activity of central nervous system in frog. *Proc. Roy. Soc. [Biol],* 122:343-352, 1937.

Gernandt, B.E.: Vestibular Influence Upon Spinal Reflex Activity. In de Reuck, A.V.S., and J. Knight (Eds.): *Myotatic, Kinesthetic and Vestibular Mechanisms.* London, Churchill, 1967, pp. 170-204.

Gernandt, B.E.: Interactions between extraocular myotatic and ascending vestibular activities. *Exp. Neurol.,* 20:120-134, 1968.

Gerstein, G.L., R.A. Butler, and S.D. Erulkar: Excitation and inhibition in cochlear nucleus. I. Tone-burst stimulation. *J. Neurophysiol.,* 31:526-536, 1968.

Gescheider, G.A.: Role of phase-difference cues in the cutaneous analog of auditory sound localization. *J. Acoust. Soc. Amer.,* 43:1249-1254, 1968.

Gills, Jr., J.P.: The electroretinogram after section of the optic nerve in man. *Amer. J. Ophthal.,* 62:287-291, 1966.

Gliozzi, A.: Effect of electrical stimulation of the optic nerve on retinal potentials. *Arch. Ital. Biol.,* 104:511-515, 1966.

Goldberg, J.M., and P.B. Brown: Response of neurons of the superior olivary complex of the dog to dichotic stimuli. *Physiologist,* 9:190, 1966.

Goldberg, J.M., and D.D. Greenwood: Responses of neurons of the dorsal and posteroventral cochlear nuclei of the cat to acoustic stimuli of long duration. *J. Neurophysiol.,* 29:72-93, 1966.

Goldberg, J.M., and R.A. Lavine: Nervous system: Afferent mechanisms. *Ann. Rev. Physiol.,* 30:319-358, 1968.

Goldstein, Jr., M.H., J.L. Hall, II, and B.O. Butterfield: Single-unit activity in the primary auditory cortex of unanesthetized cats. *J. Acoust. Soc. Amer.,* 43:444-455, 1968.

Gorgiladze, G.I., and G.D. Smirnov: Effect of vestibular stimulation on neuronal activity in the visual cortex of the cat. *Zh. Vyssh. Nerv. Deyat. Pavlov.,* 17:345, 1967.

Gorman, A.L.F., and J.S. Mc Reynolds: Hyperpolarizing and depolarizing receptor potentials in the scallop eye. *Science,* 165:309-310, 1969.

Görner, P.: Independence of Afferent Activity from Efferent Activity in the Lateral Line Organ of *Xenopus laevis* Daudin. In Cahn,

P.H. (Ed.): *Lateral Line Detectors*. Bloomington, Indiana U. Pr., 1967, pp. 199-214.

Gouras, P.: Rod and cone independence in the electroretinogram of the dark-adapted monkey's perifovea. *J. Physiol. (London)*, *187*:455-464, 1966.

Gouras, P.: The effects of light-adaptation on rod and cone receptive field organization of monkey ganglion cells. *J. Physiol. (London)*, *192*:747-760, 1967.

Gouras, P., and K. Link: Rod and cone interaction in dark-adapted monkey ganglion cells. *J. Physiol. (London)*, *184*:499-510, 1966.

Granit, R.: Neurophysiology of the Retina. In Davson, H. (Ed.): *The Eye*. New York, Academic, 1962, Vol. II.

Granstrem, E.E.: Topography and ending places of straight corticofugal fibers of the auditory analyzer of the cat. *Arkh. Anat.*, *55*:22-27, 1968.

Gray, E.G., and K.C. Watkins: Electron microscopy of taste buds of the rat. *Z. Zellforsch.*, *66*:583-595, 1965.

Graziadei, P., and D. Tucker: Vomeronasal receptors' ultrastructure. *Fed. Proc.*, *27*:583, 1968.

Greenwood, D.D., and N. Maruyama: Excitatory and inhibitory response areas of auditory neurons in the cochlear nucleus. *J. Neurophysiol.*, *28*:863-892, 1965.

Grüsser, O.-J., U. Grüsser-Cornehls, D. Finkelstein, V. Henn, M. Patutschnik, and E. Butenandt: A quantitative analysis of movement detecting neurons in the frog's retina. *Arch. Ges. Physiol.*, *293*:100-106, 1967.

Grüsser, O.J., and U. Grüsser-Cornehls: Neurophysiologische Grundlagen visueller angeborener Auslosemechanismen beim Frosch. *Z. Vergl. Physiol.*, *59*:1-24, 1968.

Grüsser, O.-J., and F. Snigula: Vergleichende verhaltensphysiologische und neurophysiologische Untersuchungen am visuellen System von Katzen. II. Simultankontrast. *Psychol. Forsch.*, *32*:43-63, 1968.

Grüsser, O.-J., D. Finkelstein, and U. Grüsser-Cornehls: The effect of stimulus velocity on the response of movement sensitive neurons of the frog's retina. *Pflügers Arch.*, *300*:49-66, 1968.

Grubel, G., E. Dunker, and D. von Rehren: Zur Funktionsweise des efferenten auditorischen Systems. I. Mitteilung. Hemmung deafferentierter, sekundärer Cochlearis-Neurone durch Gegenohr-Beschallung nach Durchschneidung

descendierender und dorsal kreuzender Bahnen (Katze). *Pflügers Arch.*, *281*:109-121, 1964.

Gusel'nikova, K.G., and G.S. Voronkov: Orthodromic potential and evoked rhythmic activity of the frog olfactory bulb. *Biol. Nauk.*, *9*:101-105, 1966.

Gusel'nikova, K.G., G.S. Voronkov, L.E. Tsitolovskii and V.V. Engovatov: Intracellular and pharmacological study of evoked waves of the olfactory bulb of the frog. *Biol. Nauk.*, *11*:28-34, 1968.

Haft, J.S., and P.J. Harman: Evidence for central inhibition of retinal function. *Vision Res.*, *7*:499-501, 1967.

Hall, J.L.: Binaural interaction in the accessory superior-olivary nucleus of the cat. *J. Acoust. Soc. Amer.*, *37*:814-823, 1965.

Hall, II, J.L., and M.H. Goldstein, Jr.: Representation of binaural stimuli by single units in primary auditory cortex of unanesthetized cats. *J. Acoust. Soc. Amer.*, *43*:456-461, 1968.

Halpern, B.P.: Some Relationships Between Electrophysiology and Behavior in Taste. In Kare, M.R., and O. Maller (Eds.): *The Chemical Senses and Nutrition*. Baltimore, Johns Hopkins, 1967, pp. 213-241.

Halpern, B.P., and L.M. Nelson: Bulbar gustatory responses to anterior and to posterior tongue stimulation in the rat. *Amer. J. Physiol.*, *209*:105-110, 1965.

Halpern, B.P., and D.H. Postles: Facilitation of gustatory responses in the frog. *Fed. Proc.*, *26*:544, 1967.

Hammond, P.: Spectral properties of dark-adapted retinal ganglion cells in the plaice (*Pleuronectes platessa*, L.). *J. Physiol. (London)*, *195*:535-556, 1968.

Hara, T.J.: Electrophysiological studies of the olfactory system of the goldfish, *Carassius auratus* L.-II. Response patterns of the olfactory bulb neurones to chemical stimulation and their centrifugal control. *Comp. Biochem. Physiol.*, *22*:199-208, 1967.

Harris, G.G., and Å. Flock: Spontaneous and Evoked Activity from the *Xenopus laevis* Lateral Line. In Cahn, P.H. (Ed.): *Lateral Line Detectors*. Bloomington, Indiana U. Pr., 1967, pp. 135-161.

Hartline, H.K.: Visual receptors and retinal interaction. *Science*, *164*:270-278, 1969.

Hartline, H.K., F. Ratliff, and W.H. Miller: Inhibitory Interaction in the Retina and Its Significance in Vision. In Florey, E. (Ed.): *Nervous Inhibition,* Proceedings Second Friday Harbor Symposium. Oxford, Pergamon, 1961, pp. 241-284.

Heimer, L.: Synaptic distribution of centripetal and centrifugal nerve fibres in the olfactory system of the rat. An experimental anatomical study. *J. Anat., 103*:413-432, 1968.

Hellekant, G.: Inhibitory processes in gustation. *Acta Physiol. Scand., 75*:39-48, 1969.

Hendrickson, A.: Landolt's club in the amphibian retina: A Golgi and electron microscope study. *Invest. Ophthal., 5*:484-496, 1966.

Hernandez-Peon, R., H. Scherrer, and M. Jouvet: Modification of electric activity in cochlear nucleus during "attention" in unanesthetized cats. *Science, 123*:331-332, 1956.

Herrick, C.J.: The amphibian forebrain. II. The olfactory bulb of *Ambystoma. J. Comp. Neurol., 37*:373-396, 1924.

Hind, J.E., D.J. Anderson, J.F. Brugge, and J.E. Rose: Coding of information pertaining to paired low-frequency tones in single auditory nerve fibers of the squirrel monkey. *J. Neurophysiol., 30*:794-816, 1967.

Hiwatashi, K., M. Yasuda, and S. Nagata: A model of the receptive fields in the vertebrate visual system. *Digest, 7th Int. Conf. Med. Biol. Eng., Stockholm, 36-5*:478, 1967.

Holden, A.L.: Two possible visual functions for centrifugal fibres to the retina. *Nature, 212*: 837-838, 1966a.

Holden, A.L.: An investigation of the centrifugal pathway to the pigeon retina. *J. Physiol. (London), 186*:133P, 1966b.

Holden, A.L.: Antidromic activation of the isthmo-optic nucleus. *J. Physiol. (London), 197*:183-198, 1968a.

Holden, A.L.: The centrifugal system running to the pigeon retina. *J. Physiol. (London), 197*: 199-219, 1968b.

Hotta, T., and K. Kameda: Interactions between somatic and visual or auditory responses in the thalamus of the cat. *Exp. Neurol., 8*:1, 1963.

Hubel, D.H.: The visual cortex of the brain. *Sci. Amer., 209*:54-62, 1963.

Hubel, D.H., and T.N. Wiesel: Receptive fields, binocular interaction and functional architecture in the cat's visual cortex. *J. Physiol. (London), 160*:106-154, 1962.

Hubel, D.H., and T.N. Wiesel: Responses of monkey geniculate cells to monochromatic and white spots of light. *Physiologist, 7*:162-163, 1964.

Hubel, D.H., and T.N. Wiesel: Receptive fields and functional architecture of monkey striate cortex. *J. Physiol. (London), 195*:215-243, 1968.

Huggins, S.E., L.C. Parsons, and R.V. Peña: Further study of the spontaneous electrical activity of the brain of *Caiman scleraps:* Olfactory lobes. *Physiol. Zool., 41*:371-383, 1968.

Hughes, G.W., and L. Maffei: Retinal ganglion cell response to sinusoidal light stimulation. *J. Neurophysiol., 29*:333-352, 1966.

Hughes, J.R., D.E. Hendrix, and N. Wetzel: Evidence from the Human Olfactory Bulb for the Frequency Component Hypothesis. In Tanyolaç, N.N. (Ed.): *Theories of Odor and Odor Measurement.* N.N. Tanyolaç, Robert College Research Center, Bebek, Istanbul, 1968, pp. 87-111.

Hull, C.D., N.A. Buchwald, and J. Vieth: Cortical intracellular analyses of responses to inhibitory and disinhibitory stimuli. *Brain Res., 6*:12-21, 1967.

Hull, E.M.: Corticofugal influence in the macaque lateral geniculate nucleus. *Vision Res., 8*: 1285-1298, 1968.

Imazawa, Y.: Facilitatory effects of spectral lights upon unit discharge caused by electrical stimulation of the cat's retina. *Tohoku J. Exp. Med., 90*:175-187, 1966.

Ishiko, N., M. Amatsu, and Y. Sato: Thalamic Representation of Taste Qualities and Temperature Change in the Cat. In Hayashi, T. (Ed.): *Olfaction and Taste II, Proceedings of the Second International Symposium.* Oxford, Pergamon, 1967, pp. 563-572.

Ito, M.: Neuronal Circuitry in the Cerebellar Efferent System. In Yahr, M.D., and D.P. Purpura (Eds.): *Neurophysiological Basis Of Normal And Abnormal Motor Activities,* Proc. 3rd Symp., Hewlett, L.I., Raven, 1967, pp. 119-140.

Ito, M.: Two Extensive Inhibitory Systems for Brain Stem Nuclei. In Euler, C. von, S. Skoglund, and U. Söderberg (Eds.): *Structure and Function of Inhibitory Neuronal Mechanisms.* Oxford, Pergamon, 1968, pp. 309-322.

Ito, M., N. Kawai, and M. Udo: The origin of cerebellar-induced inhibition of Deiters' neurones. III. Localization of the inhibitory zone. *Exp. Brain Res.*, *4*:310-320, 1968.

Ito, M., N. Kawai, M. Udo, and N. Sato: Cerebellar-evoked disinhibition in dorsal Deiters' neurones. *Exp. Brain Res.*, *6*:247-264, 1968.

Ito, M., and M. Yoshida: The origin of cerebellar-induced inhibition of Deiters' neurones. I. Monosynaptic initiation of the inhibitory postsynaptic potentials. *Exp. Brain Res.*, *2*:330-349, 1966.

Iurato, S.: Fibre efferenti dirette e crociate alle cellule acustiche dell'organo del Corti. *Atti Soc. Ital. Anat.*, *72*:60(A), 1964.

Jacklet, J.W.: Circadian rhythm of optic nerve impulses recorded in darkness from isolated eye of *Aplysia*. *Science*, *164*:562-563, 1969.

Jacobs, G.H., and R.L. Yolton: Distribution of excitation and inhibition in receptive fields of lateral geniculate neurones. *Nature*, *217*:187-188, 1968.

Jacobson, J.Z., and G.E. MacKinnon: Coloured Mach bands. *Canad. J. Psychol.*, *23*:56-65, 1969.

Jacobson, M., and R.M. Gaze: Types of visual response from single units in the optic tectum and optic nerve of the goldfish. *Quart. J. Exp. Physiol.*, *49*:199-209, 1964.

Janig, W., R.F. Schmidt, and M. Zimmermann: Presynaptic depolarization during activation of tonic mechanoreceptors. *Brain Res.*, *5*:514-516, 1967.

Janig, W., R.F. Schmidt, and M. Zimmermann: Two specific feedback pathways to the central afferent terminals of phasic and tonic mechanoreceptors. *Exp. Brain Res.*, *6*:116-129, 1968.

Johner, C.H., and H.B. Perlman: Hypnosis and vestibular function. *Ann. Otol.*, *77*:126-138, 1968.

Jung, R.: Neuronale Grundlagen des Hell-Dunkelsehens und der Farbwahrnehmung. *Ber. Deutsch. Ophth. Ges.*, *LXVI*:69-111, 1964.

Kahn, N., F. Magni, and R.V. Pillai: Depolarization of optic fiber endings in the lateral geniculate body. *Arch. Ital. Biol.*, *105*:573-582, 1967.

Kare, M.R.: The Functions of the Sense of Taste. Tele-lecture given to the sensory physiology class, Indiana State University, 1968.

Kasahara, M., N. Mano, T. Oshima, S. Ozawa, and H. Shimazu: Contralateral short latency inhibition of central vestibular neurons in the horizontal canal system. *Brain Res.*, *8*:376-378, 1968.

Kassil, V.G., A.M. Ugolev, and V.N. Chernigovskii: Gastric receptors and regulation of feeding behavior in the dog. *Dokl. Akad. Nauk SSSR*, *126*:546-548, 1959.

Katsuki, Y., T. Hashimoto, and K. Yanagisawa: Information processing in fish lateral-line sense organs. *Science*, *160*:439, 1968.

Katsuki, Y., N. Suga, and Y. Kanno: Neural mechanism of the peripheral and central auditory system in monkeys. *J. Acoust. Soc. Amer.*, *34*: 1396-1410, 1962.

Kellerth, J.O.: Aspects on the Relative Significance of Pre- and Postsynaptic Inhibition in the Spinal Cord. In von Euler, C., S. Skoglund, and U. Söderberg (Eds.): *Structure and Function of Inhibitory Neuronal Mechanisms.* Oxford, Pergamon, 1968, pp. 197-212.

Kennedy, D.: Inhibition in visual systems. *Sci. Amer.*, *209*:122-130, 1963.

Kerr, D.I.B., and K.E. Hagbarth: An investigation of olfactory centrifugal fiber system. *J. Neurophysiol.*, *18*:362-374, 1955.

Kiang, N.Y.-s.: Stimulus coding in the auditory nerve and cochlear nucleus. *Acta Otolaryng. (Stockholm)*, *59*:186-200, 1965.

Kiang, N.Y.-s., T. Watanabe, E.C. Thomas, and L.F. Clark: *Discharge Patterns of Single Fibers in the Cat's Auditory Nerve.* Cambridge, M.I.T. Pr., 1965.

Kimura, K.: Factors affecting the response of taste receptors of rat. *Kumamoto Med. J.*, *14*: 95-99, 1961.

Kimura, R., and J. Wersäll: Termination of the olivo-cochlear bundle in relation to the outer hair cells of the organ of Corti in guinea pig. *Acta Otolaryng. (Stockholm)*, *55*:11-32, 1962.

Koerber, K.C., R.R. Pfeiffer, W.B. Warr, and N.Y.-s. Kiang: Spontaneous spike discharges from single units in the cochlear nucleus after destruction of the cochlea. *Exp. Neurol.*, *16*: 119-130, 1966.

Kondratjeva, I.N., and V.B. Polyansky: Inhibition in the neuronal systems of the visual cortex. *Activ. Nerv. Sup. (Praha)*, *10*:1-11, 1968.

Kostelyanets, N.B.: Investigation of the receptive off-fields of the retina of the frog by means of moving darkness stimuli. *Zh. Vyssh. Nerv. Deyat. Pavlov.*, *15*:521-528, 1965.

Kostyuk, P.G.: Presynaptic and Postsynaptic Changes Produced in Spinal Neurons by an Afferent Volley from Visceral Afferents. In von Euler, C., S. Skoglund, and U. Söderberg (Eds.): *Structure and Function of Inhibitory*

Neuronal Mechanisms. Oxford, Pergamon, 1968, pp. 239-248.

Kravkov, S.V., and L.P. Galochkina: Effect of a constant current on vision. *J. Opt. Soc. Amer.*, 37:181-186, 1947.

Kudryavtseva, N.N.: Change of background EEG in dogs under the effect of acoustic stimulation of varying intensity. *Zh. Vyssh. Nerv. Deyat. Pavlov.*, 18:120-125, 1968.

Kuman, E.A., and V.G. Skrebitskii: Visual-acoustic afferent interaction in the lateral geniculate body in rabbits. *Zh. Vyssh. Nerv. Deyat. Pavlov.*, 18:507-513, 1968.

Ladpli, R., and A. Brodal: Experimental studies of commissural and reticular formation projections from the vestibular nuclei in the cat. *Brain Res.*, 8:65-96, 1968.

Lakomy, M.: The structure of the bulbus olfactorius of the goat. *Ann. Univ. Curie Sklodowska [Med]*, 21:219-235, 1966.

Lange, D., H.K. Hartline, and F. Ratliff: The Dynamics of Lateral Inhibition in the Compound Eye of *Limulus.* II. In Bernhard, C.G. (Ed.): *The Functional Organization of the Compound Eye.* Oxford, Pergamon, 1966, pp. 425-449.

Laufer, M., and M. Verzeano: Periodic activity in the visual system of the cat. *Vision Res.*, 7:215-229, 1967.

Le Gros Clark, W.: Inquiries into the anatomical basis of olfactory discrimination. *Proc. Roy. Soc. [Biol.]*, 146:299-319, 1957.

Leibbrandt, C.C.: The significance of the olivocochlear bundle for the adaptation mechanism of the inner ear. *Acta Otolaryng.*, 59:124-132, 1965.

Leicester, J., and J. Stone: Ganglion, amacrine and horizontal cells of the cat's retina. *Vision Res.*, 7:695-705, 1967.

Levêteau, J., S. Fanjat, and G. Daval: Influence de la stimulation électrique contralatérale sur la réponse des glomérules olfactifs du Lapin à une stimulation odorante. *C.R. Soc. Biol. (Paris)*, 162:42, 1968.

Levick, W.R.: Receptive fields and trigger features of ganglion cells in the visual streak of the rabbit's retina. *J. Physiol. (London)*, 188:285-307, 1967.

Levick, W.R., C.W. Oyster, and E. Takahashi: Rabbit lateral geniculate nucleus: Sharpener of directional information. *Science*, 165:712-714, 1969.

Llinàs, R., W. Precht, and S.T. Kitai: Cerebellar Purkinje cell projection to the peripheral vestibular organ in the frog. *Science, 158*:1328-1330, 1967.

Lohman, A.H.M., and H.J. Lammers: On the Structure and Fibre Connections of the Olfactory Centres in Mammals. In Zotterman, Y. (Ed.): *Sensory Mechanisms, Progress in Brain Research.* Amsterdam, Elsevier, 1967, vol. 23, pp. 65-82.

Lorente de Nó, R.: Anatomy of the eighth nerve. I. The central projection of the nerve endings of the internal ear. *Laryngoscope, 43*:1-38, 1933.

Lorenzo, A.J. de: Studies on the Ultrastructure and Histophysiology of Cell Membranes, Nerve Fibers and Synaptic Junctions in Chemoreceptors. In Zotterman, Y. (Ed.): *Olfaction and Taste, Proceedings of the First International Symposium.* New York, Macmillan, 1963, pp. 5-18.

Mac Gregor, R.J.: Pulse trains in lateral geniculate and retinal ganglion nerve cells. Memorandum RM-4870-ARPA, Rand Corp., Santa Monica, Calif., 1966.

Mac Gregor, R.J.: Neural organization in the primate retina. Memorandum RM-4912-ARPA, Rand Corp., Santa Monica, Calif., 1967.

Mac Nichol, Jr., E.F.: Retinal processing of visual data. *Proc. Nat. Acad. Sci. U.S.A., 55*:1331-1344, 1966.

Mac Nichol, Jr., E.F., and R. Benolken: Blocking effect of ethyl alcohol on inhibitory synapses in the eye of *Limulus. Science, 124*:681-682, 1956.

Manni, E., G.B. Azzena, and M.L. Atzori: Relationships between cerebral and mesodiencephalic nystagmogenic centers in the rabbit. *Arch. Ital. Biol., 103*:136-145, 1965.

Manni, E., and M.L. Giretti: Vestibular units influenced by labyrinthine and cerebral nystagmogenic impulses. *Exp. Neurol., 22*:145-157, 1968.

Marchiafava, P.L., G. Rizzolatti, and J.M. Sprague: Studies on corticotectal activity in the unanesthetized mid-pontine cat. Effects of cortical cooling and ablation. *Arch. Ital. Biol., 106*:21-40, 1968.

Markham, C.H.: Midbrain and contralateral labyrinth influences on brain stem vestibular neurons in the cat. *Brain Res., 9*:312-333, 1968.

Markham, C.H., W. Precht, and H. Shimazu:

Effect of stimulation of interstitial nucleus of Cajal on vestibular unit activity in the cat. *J. Neurophysiol.*, 29:493-507, 1966.

Mascitti, T.A., and S.N. Ortega: Efferent connections of the olfactory bulb in the cat. An experimental study with silver impregnation methods. *J. Comp. Neurol.*, 127:121-136, 1966.

Maturana, H.R.: Functional Organization of the Pigeon Retina. In *Information Processing in the Nervous System*. Vol. III, Proc. Intl. Union Physiol. Sc., Netherlands, Excerpta Medica, 1962, Vol. III, pp. 170-178.

Maturana, H.R., and S. Frenk: Directional movement and horizontal edge detection in the pigeon retina. *Science, 142*:977-979, 1963.

Maturana, H.R., and S. Frenk: Synaptic connections of the centrifugal fibers in the pigeon retina. *Science, 150*:359-361, 1965.

Mc Gill, J.I.: Organization within the central and centrifugal fibre pathways in the avian visual system. *Nature, 204*:395-396, 1964.

Mc Gill, J.I., T.P.S. Powell, and W.M. Cowan: The retinal representation upon the optic tectum (mesencephalon, brain) and isthmo-optic nucleus in the pigeon. *J. Anat., 100*: 5-33, 1966.

Mc Ilwain, J.T., and P. Buser: Receptive fields of single cells in the cat's superior colliculus. *Exp. Brain Res.*, 5:314-325, 1968.

Melzack, R., and K.L. Casey: Sensory, Motivational, and Central Control Determinants of Pain. In Kenshalo, D. (Ed.): *The Skin Senses.* Springfield, Charles C Thomas, 1968, Chapter 20.

Mendell, L.M.: Physiological properties of unmyelinated fiber projection to the spinal cord. *Exp. Neurol.*, 16:316-332, 1966.

Meulders, M., and J. Colle: Influence du cortex visuel sur l'activité évoquée dans les voies optiques sous-corticales. *Electroenceph. Clin. Neurophysiol.*, 20:475-484, 1966.

Michael, C.R.: Receptive fields of directionally selective units in the optic nerve of the ground squirrel. *Science, 152*:1092-1095, 1966a.

Michael, C.R.: Receptive fields of opponent color units in the optic nerve of the ground squirrel. *Science, 152*:1095-1097, 1966b.

Missoten, L.: Étude des batonnets de la rétine humaine au microscope electronique. *Ophthalmologica, 140*:200-214, 1960.

Montero, V.M., and J.F. Brugge: Direction of movement as the significant stimulus parameter for some lateral geniculate cells in the rat. *Vision Res.*, 9:71-88, 1969.

Montero, V.M., and R.W. Guillery: Degeneration in the dorsal lateral geniculate nucleus of the rat following interruption of the retinal or cortical connections. *J. Comp. Neurol., 134*: 211-242, 1968.

Morest, D.K.: The collateral system of the medial nucleus of the trapezoid body of the cat, its neuronal architecture and relation to the olivo-cochlear bundle. *Brain Res.*, 9:288-311, 1968.

Moruzzi, G., and O. Pompeiano: Crossed fastigial influence on decerebrate rigidity. *J. Comp. Neurol., 106*:371-392, 1956.

Mountcastle, V.B.: The Neural Replication of Sensory Events in the Somatic Afferent System. In Eccles, J.C. (Ed.): *Brain and Conscious Experience.* New York, Springer-Verlag, 1964, pp. 85-115.

Moushegian, G., A.L. Rupert, and T.L. Langford: Stimulus coding by medial superior olivary neurons. *J. Neurophysiol., 30*:1239-1261, 1967.

Mugnaini, E., and F. Walberg: An experimental electron microscopical study on the mode of termination of cerebellar corticovestibular fibres in the cat lateral vestibular nucleus (Deiters' nucleus). *Exp. Brain Res.*, 4:212-236, 1967.

Mugnaini, E., F. Walberg, and A. Brodal: Mode of termination of primary vestibular fibres in the lateral vestibular nucleus. An experimental electron microscopical study in the cat. *Exp. Brain Res.*, 4:187-211, 1967.

Nachmias, J.: Effect of exposure duration on visual contrast sensitivity with square-wave gratings. *J. Opt. Soc. Amer.*, 57:421-427, 1967.

Negishi, K., and G. Svaetichin: Effects of temperature on S-potential producing cells and on neurons. *Pflügers Arch.*, 292:206-217, 1966.

Nelson, P.G., and S.D. Erulkar: Synaptic mechanisms of excitation and inhibition in the central auditory pathway. *J. Neurophysiol., 26*:908-923, 1963.

Nieuwenhuys, R.: Comparative Anatomy of Olfactory Centres and Tracts. In Zotterman, Y. (Ed.): *Sensory Mechanisms, Progress in Brain Research.* Amsterdam, Elsevier, 1967, vol. 23, pp. 1-64.

Nomoto, M., N. Suga, and Y. Katsuki: Discharge pattern and inhibition of primary auditory nerve fibers in the monkey. *J. Neurophysiol.*, 27:768-787, 1964.

Northcutt, R.G.: Architectonic studies of the telencephalon of *Iguana iguana. J. Comp. Neurol., 130*:109-148, 1967.

Norton, A.L., H. Spekreijse, M.L. Wolbarsht, and H.G. Wagner: Receptive field organization of the S-potential. *Science, 160*:1021-1022, 1968.

Oakley, B., and R.M. Benjamin: Neural mechanisms of taste. *Physiol. Rev., 46*:173-211, 1966.

Obata, K., M. Ito, R. Ochi, and N. Sato: Pharmacological properties of the postsynaptic inhibition by Purkinje cell axons and the action of γ-aminobutyric acid on Deiters' neurones. *Exp. Brain Res., 4*:43-57, 1967.

Ogden, T.E.: Studies of intraretinal slow potentials evoked by brain stimulation in the primate. *J. Neurophysiol., 29*:898-908, 1966.

Ogden, T.E.: On the Function of Efferent Retinal Fibres. In von Euler, C., S. Skoglund, and U. Söderberg (Eds.): *Structure and Function of Inhibitory Neuronal Mechanisms.* Proceed. Fourth Intl. Meet. Neurobiologists, 1966. New York, Pergamon, 1968, pp. 89-109.

Ogden, T.E., and K.T. Brown: Intraretinal response of the cynomolgus monkey to electrical stimulation of the optic nerve and retina. *J. Neurophysiol., 27*:682-705, 1964.

Oreggo, F.: The reptilian forebrain. I. The olfactory pathways and cortical areas in the turtle. *Arch. Ital. Biol., 99*:425-445, 1961.

Otani, K., and M. Hiura: Projection fibers from the auditory cortex of the cat. *Progr. Neurol. Psychiat., 7*:485-494, 1962.

Ottoson, D., and G.M. Shepherd: Experiments and Concepts in Olfactory Physiology. In Zotterman, Y. (Ed.): *Sensory Mechanisms, Progress in Brain Research.* Amsterdam, Elsevier, 1967, vol. 23, pp. 83-138.

Pacheco, P., D. Bear, and F. R. Ervin: Synchronized retinal afterdischarge and neural dark adaptation in the monkey (*Cebus albifrons*). *Exp. Neurol., 20*:635-654, 1968.

Pantle, A., and R. Sekuler: Size-detecting mechanisms in human vision. *Science, 162*:1146-1148, 1968.

Parker, D.E., and J.R. Mundie: Neural sensitivity changes following stimulation with transient sound bursts. *J. Aud. Res., 7*:287-301, 1967.

Pfalz, R.K.J., and W. Pirsig: Compound afferent action potentials of the cochlear nucleus evoked electrically: Inhibition due to acoustic stimulation of the contralateral cochlea (guinea pig). *Ann. Otol., 75*:1077-1088, 1966.

Pickering, S.G.: The extremely long latency response from on-off retinal ganglion cells: Relationship to dark adaptation. *Vision Res., 8*:383-387, 1968.

Pickering, S.G., and D. Varjú: Ganglion cells in the frog retina: Inhibitory receptive field and long-latency response. *Nature, 215*:545-546, 1967.

Piggins, D.J.: A possible function of centrifugal fibres to the human retina. *Brit. J. Physiol. Opt., 23*:258-259, 1966.

Pirsig, W., and R. Pfalz: Neurone im Nucleus cochlearis ventralis, die von homolateral durch elektrischen Reiz an der Schneckenbasiswindung erregt wurden: Zentrifugale Hemmung durch kontralaterale Beschallung (Meerschweinchen). *Arch. Klin. Exp. Ohr., Nas. Kehlk. Heilk., 189*:135-157, 1967.

Pirsig, W., R. Pfalz, and M. Sadanaga: Postsynaptische, auditorische, gekreuzte, efferente Hemmung im Nucleus cochlearis ventralis und ihre Blockade durch Strychninnitrat (Meerschweinchen). *Arch. Klin. Exp. Ohr. Nas. Kehlkopfheilk., 190*:60-68, 1968.

Polyak, S.: *The Vertebrate Visual System.* Chicago, U. of Chicago Pr., 1957.

Pompeiano, O.: Sensory Inhibition During Motor Activity in Sleep. In Yahr, M.D., and D.P. Purpura (Eds.): *Neurophysiological Basis of Normal and Abnormal Motor Activities.* Hewlett, Raven, 1967, pp. 323-375.

Poppele, R.E., and L. Maffei: Retinal responses with different background light and psychophysical correlation. *Arch. Ital. Biol., 105*:189-200, 1967.

Potter, D.: Patterns of acoustically evoked discharges of neurons in the mesencephalon of the bullfrog. *J. Neurophysiol., 28*:1155-1184, 1965.

Powell, T.P.S., and W.M. Cowan: Centrifugal fibres in the lateral olfactory tract. *Nature, 199*:1296-1297, 1963.

Powell, T.P.S., W.M. Cowan, and G. Raisman: The central olfactory connexions. *J. Anat., 99*:791-814, 1965.

Precht, W., H. Shimazu, and C.H. Markham: A mechanism of central compensation of vestibular function following hemilabyrinthectomy. *J. Neurophysiol., 29*:996-1010, 1966.

Pritchard, R.M.: Stabilized images on the retina. *Sci. Amer., 204*:72-78, 1961.

Purple, R.L., and F.A. Dodge: Interaction of excitation and inhibition in the eccentric cell in the eye of *Limulus*. In *Sensory Receptors. Cold Spring Harbor Symposia on Quantitative Biology*, 30:529-538, 1965.

Purple, R.L., and F.A. Dodge: Self-inhibition in the Eye of *Limulus*. In Bernhard, C.G. (Ed.): *The Functional Organization of the Compound Eye*. Oxford, Pergamon, 1966, pp. 451-464.

Radionova, E.A.: Inhibitory phenomena in impulse activity of neurons in the cochlear nucleus of cats. *Zh. Vyssh. Nerv. Deyat. Pavlov.*, 18:133-136, 1968.

Rall, W., and G.M. Shepherd: Theoretical reconstruction of field potentials and dendrodendritic synaptic interactions in olfactory bulb. *J. Neurophysiol.*, 31:884-915, 1968.

Rall, W., G.M. Shepherd, T.S. Reese, and M.W. Brightman: Dendrodendritic synaptic pathway for inhibition in the olfactory bulb. *Exp. Neurol.*, 14: 44-56, 1966.

Rapuzzi, G., and C. Casella: Innervation of the fungiform papillae in the frog tongue. *J. Neurophysiol.*, 28:154-165, 1965.

Rasmussen, G.L.: Recurrent or "feed-back" connections of the auditory system of the cat. *Anat. Rec.*, 115:361, 1953.

Rasmussen, G.L.: Recurrent or "feed-back" connections of the auditory system of the cat. *Amer. J. Physiol.*, 183:653, 1955.

Rasmussen, G.L.: Efferent Fibers of the Cochlear Nerve and Cochlear Nucleus. In Rasmussen, G.L., and W.F. Windle (Eds.): *Neural Mechanisms of the Auditory and Vestibular Systems*. Springfield, Charles C Thomas, 1960, Chapter 8.

Rasmussen, G.L.: Personal communication. In Filogamao, G., L. Candiollo, and G. Rossi: *Le Basi Morfo-Functionali Del Controllo Della Sensazioni Acustiche*. Torino, Soc. Ital. Laringol. Otol. Rhinol., 1965.

Rasmussen, G.L.: Efferent Connections of the Cochlear Nucleus. In Graham, A.B. (Ed.): *Sensorineural Hearing Processes and Disorders*. Boston, Little, Brown, 1967, pp. 61-75.

Ratliff, F.: Inhibitory Interaction and the Detection and Enhancement of Contours. In Rosenblith, W.A. (Ed.): *Sensory Communication*. New York, M.I.T. Pr. and John Wiley, 1961, pp. 183-203.

Ratliff, F.: *Mach Bands: Quantitative Studies on Neural Networks in the Retina*. San Francisco, Holden-Day, 1965.

Ratliff, F., H.K. Hartline, and D. Lange: The Dynamics of Lateral Inhibition in the Compound Eye of *Limulus*. I. In Bernhard, C.G. (Ed.): *The Functional Organization of the Compound Eye*. Oxford, Pergamon, 1966, pp. 399-424.

Ratliff, F., B.W. Knight, J.-I. Toyoda, and H.K. Hartline: Enhancement of flicker by lateral inhibition. *Science*, 158:392-393, 1967.

Reese, T.S.: Olfactory cilia in the frog. *J. Cell. Biol.*, 25:209-230, 1965.

Richards, C.D., and R. Sercombe: Electrical activity observed in guinea-pig olfactory cortex maintained *in vitro*. *J. Physiol. (London)*, 197:667-683, 1968.

Richards, W.: Interacting spectral sensitivity functions obtained in a contrast situation. *Vision Res.*, 7:629-644, 1967.

Robbins, R.G., R.S. Bauknight, and V. Honrubia: Anatomical distribution of efferent fibers in the 8th cranial nerve of the bullfrog (*Rana catesbeiana*). *J. Acoust. Soc. Amer.*, 41:1585, 1967.

Rodieck, R.W.: Quantitative analysis of cat retinal ganglion cell response to visual stimuli. *Vision Res.*, 5:583-601, 1965.

Rodieck, R.W.: Receptive fields in the cat retina: A new type. *Science*, 157:90-92, 1967.

Rodieck, R.W., and J. Stone: Analysis of receptive fields of cat retinal ganglion cells. *J. Neurophysiol.*, 28:833-849, 1965.

Rodin, E., and E. Luby: Effects of LSD-25 on the EEG and photic evoked responses. *Arch. Gen. Psychiat. (Chicago)*, 14:435-441, 1966.

Rohen, J.W., and A. Castenholz: Über die Zentralisation der Retina bei Primaten. *Folia Primat. (Basel)*, 5:92-147, 1967.

Rose, J.E., R. Galambos, and J.R. Hughes: Microelectrode studies of the cochlear nuclei of the cat. *Johns Hopkins Med. J.*, 104:211-251, 1959.

Rose, J.E., D.D. Greenwood, J.M. Goldberg, and J.E. Hind: Some discharge characteristics of single neurons in the inferior colliculus of the cat. I. Tonotopical organization relation of spike-counts to tone intensity, and firing patterns of single elements. *J. Neurophysiol.*, 26: 294-320, 1963.

Rose, J.E., N.B. Gross, C.D. Geisler, and J.E. Hind: Some neural mechanisms in the inferior colliculus of the cat which may be relevant to localization of a sound source. *J. Neurophysiol.*, 29:288-314, 1966.

Rossi, G.: Anatomical Organization of the Efferent Cochlear and Vestibular System. In Euler,

C. von, S. Skoglund, and U. Söderberg (Eds.): *Structure and Function of Inhibitory Neuronal Mechanisms.* Oxford, Pergamon, 1968, pp. 157-168.

Rossi, G., and G. Cortesina: The efferent cochlear and vestibular system in *Lepus cuniculus* L. *Acta Anat. (Basel), 60*:362-381, 1965.

Runge, R.G., M. Uemura, and S.S. Viglione: Electronic synthesis of the avian retina. I.E.E.E. Trans. Bio-Med. Engineer., BME-15, pp. 138-151, 1968.

Rupert, A., G. Moushegian, and R. Galambos: Unit responses to sound from auditory nerve of the cat. *J. Neurophysiol., 26*:449-465, 1963.

Rupert, A., G. Moushegian, and M.A. Whitcomb: Superior-olivary response patterns to monaural and binaural clicks. *J. Acoust. Soc. Amer., 39*: 1069-1076, 1966.

Rupert, A.L., G. Moushegian, and M.A. Whitcomb: Olivocochlear neuronal responses in medulla of cat. *Exp. Neurol., 20*:575-584, 1968.

Rushforth, N.B., and F. Hofman: Behavioral sequences in the feeding response of *Hydra littoralis. Biol. Bull., 131*:403-404, 1966.

Saavedra, J.P., and O.L. Vaccarezza: Synaptic organization of the glomerular complexes in the lateral geniculate nucleus of Cebus monkey. *Brain Res., 8*:389-393, 1968.

Sala, O.: Some Remarks on the Vestibular Efferent System. In Euler, C. von, S. Skoglund, and U. Söderberg (Eds.): *Structure and Function of Inhibitory Neuronal Mechanisms.* Oxford, Pergamon, 1968, pp. 169-179.

Samsonova, V.G.: Inductive inhibition of contiguous neurons of the visual center of the frog following light stimulation. *Dokl. Akad. Nauk. SSSR., 177*:1497-1500, 1967.

Sanides, F.: The architecture of the cortical taste nerve areas in squirrel monkey (*Saimiri sciureus*) and their relationships to insular, sensorimotor and prefrontal regions. *Brain Res., 8*:97-124, 1968.

Sarkisov, S.A.: *The Structure and Functions of the Brain.* Transl. Scripta Technica, Inc., Bloomington, Indiana U. Pr., 1966.

Scalia, F.: A review of recent experimental studies on the distribution of the olfactory tracts in mammals. *Brain Behav. Evol., 1*:101-123, 1968.

Scalia, F., M. Halpern, H. Knapp, and W. Riss:

The efferent connexions of the olfactory bulb in the frog: a study of degenerating unmyelinated fibres. *J. Anat., 103*:245-262, 1968.

Schmidt, R.F.: The Functional Organization of Presynaptic Inhibition of Mechanoreceptor Afferents. In von Euler, C., S. Skoglund, and U. Söderberg (Eds.): *Structure and Function of Inhibitory Neuronal Mechanisms.* Oxford, Pergamon, 1968, pp. 227-233.

Schmidt, R.F., J. Senges, and M. Zimmermann: Presynaptic depolarization of cutaneous mechanoreceptor afferents after mechanical skin stimulation. *Exp. Brain Res., 3*:234-247, 1967.

Schneider, D., and R.A. Steinbrecht: Checklist of Insect Olfactory Sensilla. In Carthy, J.D., and G.E. Newell (Eds.): *Invertebrate Receptors.* Symp. Zool. Soc. Lond., No. 23, New York, Academic, 1968, pp. 279-297.

Sefton, A.J., and W. Burke: Mechanism of recurrent inhibition in the lateral geniculate nucleus of the rat. *Nature, 211*:1276-1278, 1966.

Seifert, K., and G. Ule: Die Ultrastruktur der Riechschleimhaut der neugeborenen und jugendlichen weissen Maus. *Z. Zellforsch., 76*: 147-169, 1967.

Shevelev, I.A.: Population characteristics of the neurons of the lateral geniculate body of the cat. *Biofizika, 13*:1080-1084, 1968.

Shevelev, I.A., and L.H. Hicks: Characteristics of temporal summation in different levels of the visual system in anesthetized cats by the thresholds of primary evoked potentials. *Zh. Vyssh. Nerv. Deyat. Pavlov., 18*:650-659, 1968.

Shimazu, H., and W. Precht: Inhibition of central vestibular neurons from the contralateral labyrinth and its mediating pathway. *J. Neurophysiol., 29*:467-492, 1966.

Silakov, V.L.: Changes in the evoked potentials of subcortical formations of the visual system after switching off the cerebral cortex. *Zh. Vyssh. Nerv. Deyat. Pavlov., 18*:160-162, 1968.

Sjöstrand, F.S.: The Synaptology of the Retina. In de Reuck, A.V.S., and J. Knight (Eds.): *Color Vision, Physiology And Experimental Psychology,* Ciba Found. Symp., Boston, Little, Brown, 1965, pp. 110-151.

Skrebitskii, V.G.: Intracellular records of the single unit activity of the visual cortex in nonanaesthetized rabbits. *Zh. Vyssh. Nerv.*

Deyat. Pavlov., *16*:864-873, 1966.

Skrebitskii, V.G.: Auditory suppression of the postsynaptic inhibition in photically evoked responses. *Zh. Vyssh. Nerv. Deyat. Pavlov.*, *17*:158, 1967.

Slifer, E.H., J.J. Prestage, and H.W. Beams: The chemoreceptors and other sense organs on the antennal flagellum of the grasshopper (*Orthoptera; Acrididae*). *J. Morphol.*, *105*:145-191, 1959.

Smith, C.A.: Morphological Features of Axo-Dendritic Relationships Between Efferent and Cochlear Nerves in the Cochlea of Mammal and Pigeon. In Euler, C. von, S. Skoglund, and U. Söderberg (Eds.): *Structure and Function of Inhibitory Neuronal Mechanisms.* Oxford, Pergamon, 1968, pp. 141-146.

Smith, C.A., and G.L. Rasmussen: Recent observations on the olivo-cochlear bundle. *Ann. Otol.*, *72*:489-506, 1963.

Smith, C.A., and F.S. Sjöstrand: Structure of the nerve endings on the external hair cells of the guinea pig as studied by serial sections. *J. Ultrastruct. Res.*, *5*:523-556, 1961.

Snigula, F., and O.-J. Grüsser: Vergleichende verhaltensphysiologische und neurophysiologische Untersuchungen am visuellen System von Katzen. I. Die simultane Helligkeitsschwelle. *Psychol. Forsch.*, *32*:14-42, 1968.

Snyakin, P.G.: The Interaction of Analysors During Process of Perception of Stimuli. In *Current Problems of Physiology and Pathology of the Nervous System.* Moscow, Meditsina, 1965. Also *Ref. Zh. Biol.*, *7*:320, 1966.

Sohmer, H.: The effect of contralateral olivo-cochlear bundle stimulation on the cochlear potentials evoked by acoustic stimuli of various frequencies and intensities. *Acta Oto-laryng.*, *60*:59-70, 1965.

Sokolov, E.N., and V.P. Dulenko: Neuronal responses of *Helix pomatia* to tactile stimulation. *Zh. Vyssh. Nerv. Deyat. Pavlov.*, *18*:113-119, 1968.

Sokolov, E.N., V.B. Polyanskii, and A. Bagdonas: Stabilization of reactions in individual neurons of the visual cortex in nonanesthetized rabbits during repeated light stimulation. *Zh. Vyssh. Nerv. Deyat. Pavlov.*, *18*:701-707, 1968.

Spinelli, D.N.: Receptive field organization of ganglion cells in the cat's retina. *Exp. Neurol.*, *19*:291-315, 1967.

Spinelli, D.N., A. Starr, and T.W. Barrett: Auditory specificity in unit recordings from cat's visual cortex. *Exp. Neurol.*, *22*:75-84, 1968.

Spinelli, D.N., and M. Weingarten: Afferent and efferent activity in single units of the cat's optic nerve. *Exp. Neurol.*, *15*:347-362, 1966.

Spoendlin, H.: The Organization of the Cochlear Receptor. In *Advances in Oto-Rhino-Laryngology.* Basel, S. Karger, 1966, vol. 13.

Sprague, J.M.: Interaction of cortex and superior colliculus in mediation of visually guided behavior in the cat. *Science*, *153*:1544-1547, 1966.

Starr, A., and J. S. Wernick: Olivocochlear bundle stimulation: Effects on spontaneous and tone-evoked activities of single units in cat cochlear nucleus. *J. Neurophysiol.*, *31*:549-564, 1968.

Steinberg, R.H.: Oscillatory activity in the optic tract of cat and light adaptation. *J. Neurophysiol.*, *29*:139-156, 1966.

Steinberg, R.H.: Ganglion cell response characteristics from the area centralis in the intact eye of the cat. NAMI-1031 and USAARU 68-5, Naval Aerospace Medical Institute, Pensacola, Fla., 1968a.

Steinberg, R.H.: Central inhibition of retinal function? *Vision Res.*, *8*:317-318, 1968b.

Steriade, M., and M. Demetrescu: Simulation of peripheral sensory input by electrical pulse trains applied to specific afferent pathways. *Exp. Neurol.*, *19*:265-277, 1967.

Stevens, C.F.: Structure of cat frontal olfactory cortex. *J. Neurophysiol.*, *32*:184-192, 1969.

Stone, H., E.J.A. Carregal, and B. Williams: The olfactory-trigeminal response to odorants. *Life Sci.*, *5*:2195-2201, 1966.

Stone, H., B. Williams, and E.J.A. Carregal: The role of the trigeminal nerve in olfaction. *Exp. Neurol.*, *21*:11-19, 1968.

Stopp, P.E., and I.C. Whitfield: Unit responses from brain-stem nuclei in the pigeon. *J. Physiol. (London)*, *158*:165-177, 1961.

Sudakov, K.V., and S.K. Rogacheva: The afferent and efferent activity of the gastric fibers of the vagus nerve during fasting and after taking food. *Fed. Proc.*, *22*:T306-10, 1963.

Suga, N.: Single unit activity in cochlear nucleus and inferior colliculus of echo-locating bats. *J. Physiol. (London)*, *172*:449-474, 1964.

Suga, N.: Analysis of frequency-modulated sounds by auditory neurones of echo-locating bats. *J. Physiol. (London)*, *179*:26-53, 1965.

Sukhov, A.G.: Cortical inhibitory neurons. *Fiziol. Zh. SSSR Sechenov.,* 54:270-275, 1968.

Supin, A. Ya.: Mechanism of reticulo-cortical activation. *Fiziol. Zh. SSSR Sechenov.,* 54:893-898, 1968.

Suzuki, H., and M. Ichijo: Tonic inhibition in cat lateral geniculate nucleus maintained by retinal spontaneous discharge. *Jap. J. Physiol.,* 17:599-612, 1967.

Suzuki, H., and E. Kato: Cortically induced presynaptic inhibition in cat's lateral geniculate body. *Tohoku J. Exp. Med.,* 86:277-289, 1965.

Suzuki, H., and E. Kato: Binocular interaction at cat's lateral geniculate body. *J. Neurophysiol.,* 24:909-920, 1966.

Tamar, H.: The movements and responses of *Halteria grandinella. Acta Protozool.,* 4:365-381, 1967.

Teramoto, S., and R.S. Snider: Modification of auditory responses by cerebellar stimulation. *Exp. Neurol.,* 16:191-200, 1966.

Toyama, K., and K. Matsunami: Synaptic action of specific visual impulses upon cat's parastriate cortex. *Brain Res.,* 10:473-476, 1968.

Toyoda, J.-I., and R.M. Shapley: The intracellularly recorded response in the scallop eye. *Biol. Bull.,* 133:490, 1967.

Trujillo-Cenoz, O.: Some aspects of the structural organization of the arthropod eye. In *Sensory Receptors. Cold Spring Harbor Symposia on Quantitative Biology,* 30:371-382, 1965.

Tsuchitani, C., and J.C. Boudreau: Single unit analysis of cat superior olive S segment with tonal stimuli. *J. Neurophysiol.,* 29:684-697, 1966.

Tucker, D.: Olfactory cilia are not required for receptor function. *Fed. Proc.,* 26:544, 1967.

Tucker, D., and J.C. Smith: The chemical senses. *Ann. Rev. Psychol.,* 20:129-158, 1969.

Ungiadze, A.A.: Electrical activity of the hippocampus during peripheral stimulation. *Fiziol. Zh. SSSR Sechenov.,* 52:1420-1427, 1966.

Van der Horst, G.J.C., and M.A. Bouman: On searching for "Mach band type" phenomena in colour vision. *Vision Res.,* 7:1027-1029, 1967.

Vasil'ev, A.G., and D.P. Matyushkin: Response of auditory system of bats to ultrasonic stimuli. *Fiziol. Zh. SSSR Sechenov.,* 53:1407-1413, 1967.

Vastola, E.F.: Steady-state effects of visual cortex on geniculate cells. *Vision Res.,* 7:599-609, 1967.

Vatter, O.: Efferente Potentiale in der Retina des Kaninchens. *Naturwissenschaften (Berlin),* 54:618-619, 1967.

Verzeano, M.: Evoked response and neuronal discharge. Second Annual Winter Conference on Brain Research.

Veselý, C., and L. Faltýnek: Reakce sluchového analyzátoru ma zatizeni hlukem za podminek funkčni dekortikace sirici se korovou depresi. *Sborn. Ved. Prac. Lek. Fak. Králov. Univ.,* 7:635-640, 1964.

Voronkov, G.S., and K.G. Gusel'nikova: Presynaptic inhibition in the frog olfactory bulb. *Zh. Vyssh. Nerv. Deyat. Pavlov.,* 18:909-911, 1968.

Wall, P.D.: The laminar organization of dorsal horn and effects of descending impulses. *J. Physiol. (London),* 188:403-423, 1967.

Warr, W.B.: Fiber degeneration following lesions in the posteroventral cochlear nucleus of the cat. *Exp. Neurol.,* 23:140-155, 1969.

Watanabe, T., T.T. Liao, and Y. Katsuki: Neuronal response patterns in the superior olivary complex of the cat to sound stimulation. *Jap. J. Physiol.,* 18:267-287, 1968.

Watanabe, T., and K. Ohgushi: FM sensitive auditory neuron. *Proc. Japan Acad.,* 44:968-973, 1968.

Watanabe, T., K. Yanagisawa, J. Kanzaki, and Y. Katsuki: Cortical efferent flow influencing unit responses of medial geniculate body to sound stimulation. *Exp. Brain Res.,* 2:302-317, 1966.

Webster, W.R.: Auditory habituation and barbiturate-induced neural activity. *Science,* 164:970-971, 1969.

Webster, W.R., C.W. Dunlop, L.A. Simons, and L.M. Aitkin: Auditory habituation: A test of a centrifugal and a peripheral theory. *Science,* 148:654-656, 1965.

Weingarten, M., and D.N. Spinelli: Retinal receptive field changes produced by auditory and somatic stimulation. *Exp. Neurol.,* 15:363-376, 1966.

Wersäll, J.: Efferent Innervation of the Inner Ear. In Euler, C. von, S. Skoglund, and U. Söderberg (Eds.): *Structure and Function of Inhibitory Neuronal Mechanisms.* Oxford, Pergamon, 1968, pp. 123-139.

Westerman, R.A., and J.A.F. Wilson: The fine structure of the olfactory tract in the teleost *Carassius carassius* L. *Z. Zellforsch.,* 91:186-199, 1968.

Westheimer, G.: Spatial interaction in human

cone vision. *J. Physiol. (London)*, 190:139-154, 1967.

Westheimer, G.: Bleached rhodopsin and retinal interaction. *J. Physiol. (London)*, 195:97-105, 1968.

Whitfield, I.C.: Behaviour of auditory cortical neurones in response to complex sound stimuli. Final Tech. Rept. DA-91-591-EUC-3636. U.S. Army, 1966.

Whitfield, I.C.: *The Auditory Pathway*. London, Edward Arnold, 1967a.

Whitfield, I.C.: The Pharmacological Behaviour of the Cochlear Nucleus. In Herxheimer, A. (Ed.): *Drugs and Sensory Functions*. London, Churchill, 1967b.

Whitfield, I.C., and S.D. Comis: A Reciprocal Gating Mechanism in the Auditory Pathway. In Oestreicher, H.L., and D.R. Moore (Eds.): *Cybernetic Problems in Bionics*. New York, Gordon and Breach, 1967.

Wickelgren, B., and P. Sterling: Receptive fields in cat superior colliculus. *Physiologist*, 10:344, 1967.

Widén, L., and C. Ajmone-Marsan: Effects of corticipetal and corticifugal impulses upon single elements of the dorsolateral geniculate nucleus. *Exp. Neurol.*, 2:468-502, 1960.

Wiederhold, M.L., and W.T. Peake: Efferent inhibition of auditory-nerve responses: Dependence on acoustic-stimulus parameters. *J. Acoust. Soc. Amer.*, 40:1427-1430, 1966.

Wiederhold, M.L., and S.H. Swift: Electrical stimulation of the crossed olivo-cochlear bundle—its effect on responses of auditory-nerve fibers to tone bursts. *J. Acoust. Soc. Amer.*, 41:1585-1586, 1967.

Wiesel, T.N., and D.H. Hubel: Spatial and chromatic interactions in the lateral geniculate body of the rhesus monkey. *J. Neurophysiol.*, 29:1115-1156, 1966.

Wilska, A., and H.K. Hartline: The origin of "off-responses" in the optic pathway. *Amer. J. Physiol.*, 133:491-492, 1941.

Wilson, V.J., R.M. Wylie, and L.A. Marco: Organization of the medial vestibular nucleus: Synaptic inputs to cells in the medial vestibular nucleus. *J. Neurophysiol.*, 31:166-185, 1968.

Wolbarsht, M.L., H.G. Wagner, and E.F. Mac Nichol, Jr.: The Origin of "On-" and "Off-" Responses of Retinal Ganglion Cells; Receptive Fields of Retinal Ganglion Cells. In Jung, R. and H. Kornhuber (Eds.): *The Visual System: Neurophysiology and Psychophysics*. Berlin, Springer-Verlag, 1961, pp. 163-175.

Wolbarsht, M.L., and S.S. Yeandle: Visual processes in the *Limulus* eye. *Ann. Rev. Physiol.*, 29:513-542, 1967.

Wolf, G.: Projections of thalamic and cortical gustatory areas in the rat. *J. Comp. Neurol.*, 132:519-530, 1968.

Wolf, G., and J. Sutin: Fiber degeneration after lateral hypothalamic lesions in the rat. *J. Comp. Neurol.*, 127:137-156, 1966.

Wolter, J.R.: The centrifugal nerves in the human optic tract, chiasm, optic nerve, and retina. *Trans. Amer. Ophthal. Soc.*, 63:678-707, 1965.

Wuttke, W., and O.-J. Grüsser: Die funktionelle Organisation der rezeptiven Felder von on-Zentrum-Neuronen der Katzenretina. *Pflügers Arch. Ges. Physiol.*, 289:R83, 1966.

Yamamoto, C.: Olfactory bulb potentials to electrical stimulation of the olfactory mucosa. *Jap. J. Physiol.*, 11:545-554, 1961.

Yamamoto, C., T. Yamamoto, and K. Iwama: The inhibitory system in the olfactory bulb studied by intracellular recording. *J. Neurophysiol.*, 26:403-415, 1963.

Yasuda, M., and K. Hiwatashi: A model of retinal neural networks and its spatio-temporal characteristics. NHK Labs. Note, no. 116, Broadcast. Sci. Res. Labs., Tokyo, 1968.

Yokota, T., A.G. Reeves, and P.D. Mac Lean: Intracellular olfactory response of hippocampal neurons in awake, sitting squirrel monkeys. *Science*, 157:1072-1074, 1967.

Zaiko, N.S., and E.S. Lokshina: Reflex reaction of the taste receptors of the tongue to direct stimulation of the gastric receptors. *Byul. Eksp. Biol. Med. (USSR)*, 53:9-11, 1963.

Zimmermann, M.: Dorsal root potentials after C-fiber stimulation. *Science*, 160:896-898, 1968.

Zotterman, Y. (Ed.): *Sensory Mechanisms, Progress in Brain Research*. Amsterdam, Elsevier, 1967, vol. 23.

SUGGESTED READING

Cogan, D.G.: *Neurology of the Visual System*. Springfield, Charles C Thomas, 1969.

Creutzfeldt, O.D.: Some Principles of Synaptic Organization in the Visual System. In Schmitt,

Principles of Sensory Physiology

F.O., G.C. Quarton, T. Melnechuk, and G. Adelman (Eds.): *The Neurosciences—Second Study Program.* New York, Rockefeller U. Pr., 1970, pp. 630-647.

Goldberg, J.M., and R.A. Lavine: Nervous system: Afferent mechanisms. *Ann. Rev. Physiol., 30*:319-358, 1968.

Granit, R.: The development of retinal neurophysiology. *Science, 160*:1192-1196, 1968.

Halpern, B.P.: Some Relationships Between Electrophysiology and Behavior in Taste. In Kare, M.R., and O. Maller (Eds.): *The Chemical Senses and Nutrition.* Baltimore, Johns Hopkins, 1967, pp. 213-241.

Hartline, H.K., F. Ratliff, and W.H. Miller: Inhibitory Interaction in the Retina and Its Significance in Vision. In Florey, E. (Ed.): *Nervous Inhibition,* Proceedings of Second Friday Harbor Symposium, Oxford, Pergamon, 1961, pp. 241-284.

Kennedy, D.: Inhibition in visual systems. *Sci. Amer., 209*:122-130, 1963.

Lohman, A.H.M., and H.J. Lammers: On the Structure and Fibre Connections of the Olfactory Centres in Mammals. In Zotterman, Y. (Ed.): *Sensory Mechanisms, Progress in Brain Research.* Amsterdam, Elsevier, 1967, vol. 23, pp. 65-82.

Mac Gregor, R.J.: Neural organization in the primate retina. Memorandum RM-4912-ARPA, Rand Corp., Santa Monica, Calif., 1967.

Nieuwenhuys, R.: Comparative Anatomy of Olfactory Centres and Tracts. In Zotterman, Y. (Ed.): *Sensory Mechanisms, Progress in Brain Research.* Amsterdam, Elsevier, 1967, vol. 23, pp. 1-64.

Oakley, B., and R.M. Benjamin: Neural mechanisms of taste. *Physiol. Rev., 46*:173-211, 1966.

Ottoson, D., and G.M. Shepherd: Experiments and Concepts in Olfactory Physiology. In Zotterman, Y. (Ed.): *Sensory Mechanisms, Progress in Brain Research.* Amsterdam, Elsevier, 1967, vol. 23, pp. 83-138.

Rall, W.: Dendritic Neuron Theory and Dendrodentritic Synapses in a Simple Cortical System. In Schmitt, F.O., G.C. Quarton, T. Melnechuk, and G. Adelman (Eds.): *The Neurosciences—Second Study Program.* New York, Rockefeller U. Pr., 1970, pp. 552-565.

Ratliff, F.: Inhibitory Interaction and the Detection and Enhancement of Contours. In Rosenblith, W.A. (Ed.): *Sensory Communication.* New York, M.I.T. Pr. and John Wiley, 1961, pp. 183-203.

Spoendlin, H.: *The Organization Of the Cochlear Receptor. Advances in Oto-Rhino-Laryngology.* Basel, Karger, 1966, vol. 13.

Straatsma, B.R., M.O. Hall, R.A. Allen, and F. Crescitelli (Eds.): *The Retina: Morphology, Function and Clinical Characteristics.* Berkeley, U. of California Pr., 1968.

Whitfield, I.C.: *The Auditory Pathway.* London, Edward Arnold, 1967.

Wolbarsht, M.L., and S.S. Yeandle: Visual processes in the *Limulus* eye. *Ann. Rev. Physiol., 29*:513-542, 1967.

Chapter V

Initial Events

The first effect which a stimulus exerts must be different in its details for each type of receptor, for herein lies the basis of the differentiation of receptors in receptor evolution. We know little of this initial step, of the first molecular events, except in the case of the visual receptors.

VISUAL RECEPTION

Visual Pigments

In visual receptors, both rods and cones, there is present one or another visual pigment. All these pigments contain some type of opsin, a protein. The apoprotein opsin is attached, presumably at several sites, to a carotenoid prosthetic group, either retinal-1 or the slightly different retinal-2 (Hubbard and Kropf, 1967).

By combining rapidly with either retinal-1 or retinal-2, opsin determines the rate of retinal formation and thus of visual pigment formation.

Retinal-2, first discovered in freshwater fish (Wald, 1937), has a second double bond in its 6-carbon ring (Fig. 5-1). While retinal-1 complexed with rod opsins forms retinene-1 pigments (rhodopsins), the combinations of retinal-2 and rod opsins are known as retinene-2 pigments (porphyropsins).

Both retinals may be present in one species, as in the brook char (*Salvelinus fontinalis*) (McFarland and Munz, 1965) and Lake Windermere char (*Salvelinus willughbii*) (Bridges, 1967). Schwanzara (1967a), in a study of thirty-four purely freshwater tropical fish, found 60 per cent of the species to contain both retinals. Retinene-1 pigments alone and retinene-2 pigments alone were each present in 20 per cent of the species. The presence of these pigments is correlated with the photic environment (Schwanzara, 1967b).

The salmon, eel and other euryhaline fish produce both retinals but use primarily porphyropsins (retinene-2 rod pigments) if they spawn in fresh water; the euryhaline alewife and white perch contain a very preponderant quantity of retinal-2 (Wald, 1941-42). Young sea lampreys (*Petromyzon marinus*) chiefly produce rhodopsin, but shift to porphyropsin when they mature and before they swim up a river to spawn (Wald, 1956-57). Bullfrogs change their rod pigment at metamorphosis; while the tadpole uses porphyropsin, the adult frog possesses rhodopsin (Wald, 1945-46).

Marine fish living at great depths contain a modified rhodopsin which has its maximum sensitivity at a shorter wavelength (Denton and Warren, 1956; Munz, 1957; Wald, Brown and Brown, 1957). European eels shift to this deep-sea rhodopsin shortly before swimming to the Sargasso Sea for spawning (Carlisle and Denton, 1957).

Only retinal-1 has been identified in invertebrate eyes (Wald, 1960).

The opsins (apoproteins) of vertebrate eyes form two major groups, one found in rods and the other in cones. While the aforementioned rod pigments, rhodopsins and porphyropsins, result respectively from the combination of retinal-1 and of retinal-2 with rod opsins, two other vertebrate visual pigments are based on cone opsins. The junction of retinal-1 with cone opsins gives rise to iodopsins, and the union of retinal-2 with cone opsins produces cyanopsins (Wald, 1968).

The vertebrate visual pigments show their typical maximum sensitivity at the following wavelengths: rhodopsin—500 mμ, deep-sea rhodopsin—approximately 480 mμ, porphyropsin—522 mμ, iodopsin—562 mμ, and cyanopsin—620 mμ.

In the prawn (*Palaemonetes vulgaris*) two eye visual pigments have been identified (Goldsmith, Dizon and Fernandez, 1968). The crayfish *Procambarus* and *Orconectes* also have two eye visual pigments (Wald, 1967), as does the fly *Calliphora* (Langer and Thorell, 1966). *Procambarus* in addition has a pair of light sensitive neurons in the sixth abdominal ganglion which contain a visual pigment (Bruno and Kennedy, 1962). The light reception of a dinoflagellate protozoan species appears to depend on phytochrome or phytochrome functioning in conjunction with a blue-absorbing pigment (Forward and Davenport, 1968).

Opsins, being proteins, differ among species. Also, several opsins may be present in one species; this is the case in man.

The retinals ($C_{20}H_{28}O$) are produced when vitamin A (an alcohol) loses two hydrogen atoms and are aldehydes. De Witt, Goodman and Huang (1965), using rat intestinal mucosa homogenates, obtained retinal by means of a reaction of β-carotene with molecular oxygen.

The process requires the breaking of β-carotene's central double bond to yield two retinal molecules.

Retinals can exist in either the cis or trans configuration. The cis isomer is bent in such a manner at C_{11} that the end of a line of carbons, C_{11}-C_{15}, is twisted out of the plane of the main portion of the molecule (Fig. 5-1). On the other hand, the trans isomer's molecule is essentially all in one plane. Visual pigments, such as the rhodopsin of the rods, consist of 11-cis retinal (retinal-1 or retinal-2), the chromophore, attached to an opsin.

When a quantum of light is absorbed by cattle or frog rhodopsin, it changes the 11-cis retinal to the straight trans retinal in approximately 60 per cent of the cases. Light effects the cis-trans isomerization in all investigated visual pigments. Thus light converts iodopsin (with 11-cis retinal) to the all-trans prelumi-iodopsin (Yoshizawa and Wald, 1967).

A means of reconverting some of the trans-retinal to the cis-form is also present in all

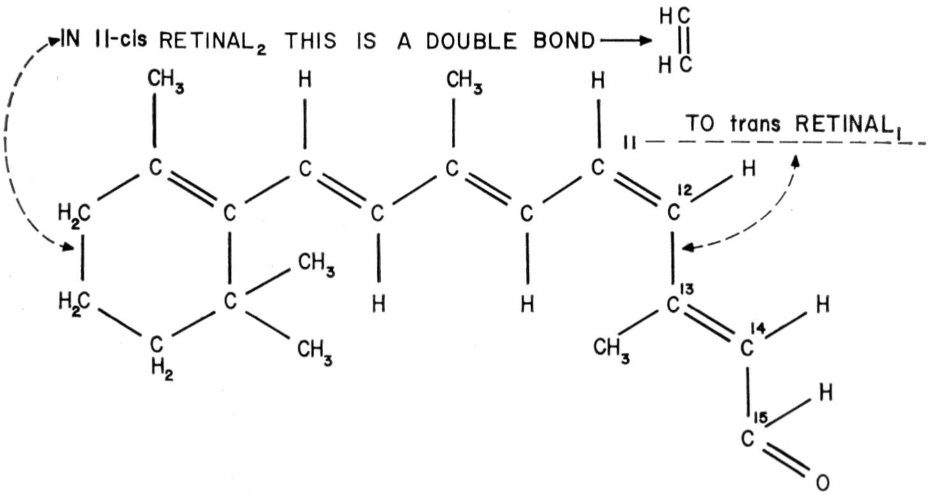

11-cis RETINAL₁ ($C_{19}H_{27}CHO$)

FIGURE 5-1. The "cis" isomer of retinal-1. A quantum of light, by causing the end of the line of carbons, C_{11}-C_{15}, to go into the plane of the rest of the molecule, can transform the "cis" into the "trans" isomer (broken arrows at right). Retinal-2 differs from retinal-1 in having a second double bond in its 6-carbon ring (broken arrows at left).

visual systems. Thus in the case of the rhodopsin system, the enzyme isomerase catalyzes conversions between the trans- and cis-forms of retinal.

By using radioactively labeled amino acids, Hall, Bok and Bacharach (1968) have shown rhodopsin to be constantly formed in the frog.

The outer segment of the albino rat's rod receptor contains about 3 or 4×10^7 rhodopsin molecules to insure a high rate of quantum absorption and a proportional amount of cis-trans isomerization. The retinal prosthetic group or chromophore of rhodopsin has been reported to lie in a plane parallel to the transverse axis of the rod (Denton, 1954), and light absorption measurements indicate that 80 per cent of the rhodopsin extinction takes place in this plane (Wald, Brown and Gibbons, 1963).

Rhodopsin is estimated to have a molecular weight of about 40,000, and a molecular diameter of perhaps 35 to 45 Å. However, Millar *et al.* (1967), by determining the amino acids composing the opsin, have found the molecular weight of rhodopsin to be considerably beneath the generally quoted value. Wald (1968) describes the chromophore group, retinal, as forming an unexpectedly large portion of rhodopsin. The chromophore is said to have a molecular weight of 282 and a length of 20 Å. Azuma and Kito (1967) report rhodopsin to contain more acidic amino acid residues than basic ones, and to be rich in the hydrophobic amino acid phenylalanine.

Human experiments show that the visual threshold of the dark-adapted eye is reached when 25 to 75 quanta of light at 507 mμ enter the retina. Of these, only 5 to 15 quanta are actually absorbed by rhodopsin (Pirenne, 1967).

The cis-trans retinal conversion is the first step in the bleaching of the purplish red rhodopsin, and produces the highly colored prelumirhodopsin. Further transformations then lead to lumirhodopsin and the deep orange metarhodopsin I (Fig. 5-2). The latter is converted to the light yellow metarhodopsin II in a reversible reaction probably involving

the loss of a hydrogen ion (proton) from the primary retinal-opsin bond (Hubbard, Bownds and Yoshizawa, 1965). Abrahamson and Ostroy (1967) describe the metarhodopsin I–metarhodopsin II conversion as very rapid at body temperatures and as requiring important changes in protein configuration, which result in a sizable protein unfolding.

Donner and Reuter (1967) have suggested that the first phase of dark adaptation in rods depends on the accumulation of metarhodopsin II, but Frank and Dowling (1968) discount the possibility of intermediate products of rhodopsin bleaching affecting the rods' sensitivity.

After isomerization the trans-retinal maintains its attachment to the opsin at least throughout the stages of the rhodopsin bleaching process which culminate in the formation of metarhodopsin II. During this portion of the bleaching process it is therefore possible

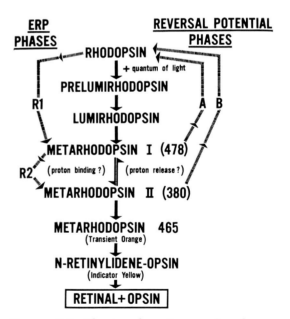

FIGURE 5-2. The transformations and early receptor potentials of vertebrate rhodopsin bleaching. Possible regenerative potentials are illustrated on the right. The thermal decay sequence beyond prelumirhodopsin ends with the separation of retinal from opsin. The last two substances may recombine to form rhodopsin, or retinal may be reduced to vitamin A.

for an absorbed photon, by producing the trans-cis retinal isomerization, to bring about the instantaneous reformation of rhodopsin.

In vertebrates metarhodopsin II is then hydrolyzed to trans-retinal and opsin, according to the scheme of Matthews *et al.* (1963-64), and these products separate. However, Ostroy, Erhardt and Abrahamson (1966) report that metarhodopsin II gives rise to metarhodopsin 465, identical with transient orange and regarded as a side product by Matthews *et al.* (1963-64), and that metarhodopsin 465 in turn is transformed to N-retinylidene-opsin (NRO), also known as indicator yellow (Fig. 5-2). In vertebrates the NRO is then hydrolyzed to retinal and opsin, and Abrahamson and Ostroy (1967) state that the rapidity of this hydrolysis at neutral pH's explains why NRO was not observed by some investigators.

The hydrolysis of metarhodopsin II, or probably more correctly NRO, has been found in cattle rhodopsin to involve the breaking of the bond between the aldehyde group of the 11-trans retinal and the E-amino group of a lysine molecule in the opsin (Bownds, 1966). This is the primary attachment of retinal to opsin and is a Schiff base

$$\overset{\text{H}}{\underset{|}{}}$$

linkage (retinyl $\cdot$ C $=$ N $\cdot$ opsin). Bownds (1967) has further determined the amino acids adjacent to the lysine molecule in opsin; together with the retinal-bound lysine they form a decapeptide segment.

Secondary side chain retinal-opsin interactions must also exist to produce the color of the original and intermediate visual pigments. A secondary retinal-opsin link is believed to be stereospecific, to have a stabilizing effect, and to be involved in a bathochromic shift in the absorption spectrum of rhodopsin. The retinal is asymmetrically attached to opsin (Kito *et al.*, 1968a).

In most investigated lower animals—the squid (*Loligo pealii*), the cuttlefish (*Sepia officinalis*), the octopus (*Octopus vulgaris*), and the lobster (*Homarus americanus*)—the trans-retinal remains attached to the opsin in

a metastable state. This metastable attachment is maintained in the aforementioned invertebrates up to a temperature of 20°C and below 20°C must be broken with denaturing organic solvents. The metastable attachment observed between trans-retinal and opsins from invertebrates is probably dependent on the particular protein conformation, especially near the points of retinal-opsin linkage, of invertebrate rhodopsins (Kito *et al.*, 1968b).

The given conversions beyond the formation of prelumirhodopsin involve changes in the retinal-opsin relationship, do not require light and are referred to as a thermal decay sequence. The intermediate pigments have been investigated only at low temperatures, since at normal temperatures they are unstable and have only a fleeting existence. However, it is generally assumed that the above series of changes also takes place in the functional retina.

Abrahamson and Ostroy (1967), on the basis of kinetic and chemical data, suggest that *in vivo* a distinction between lumirhodopsin and metarhodopsin I does not apply or that instead a pathway bypassing lumirhodopsin may exist.

Following the isomerization of the retinal, the opsin also undergoes changes in configuration during rhodopsin bleaching. These changes take place in consecutive steps, each producing a loss of protein organization. The rearrangements of opsin appear to be involved in the formation of metarhodopsin II and 465. The alterations in opsin configuration, which expose new ionizing or ion-binding groups, may play a role in the separation of the retinal from the opsin.

Crescitelli, Mommaerts and Shaw (1966) have shown optically that the attachment of the opsin to the retinal gives the first a helical conformation and the latter a specific dissymmetry. Both of these properties are lost in bleaching. According to Kito *et al.* (1968b), the isomerization of retinal leads to the disorganization of the α-helical structure of the opsin in cattle rhodopsin but not in squid rhodopsin. Close to 30 per cent of rhodopsin has a helical structure (Azuma and Kito, 1967).

Abrahamson and Ostroy (1967) have written a detailed review of our knowledge of photopigments and their transformations. Other, similar reviews are those of Gribakin and Govardovskii (1966), Bonting (1967), Mote (1967), and Wald (1968).

It is still not certain how the photochemical process described above leads to the development of a receptor or generator potential. In fact, it is still possible that the approximately 50 per cent of the light quanta which are absorbed by rhodopsin but do not isomerize retinal play a role.

Thus it has been hypothesized that light excitation of the chromophores causes the formation of electric charge carriers which then move along an electric gradient or through an electric field to produce a current. In this hypothesis the isomerization of retinal and the following steps in the bleaching of rhodopsin are regarded as portions of an adaptive mechanism which competes with the given excitatory process (Rosenberg, 1966).

In order to gain some idea of the energy and quantum efficiency which would be needed to produce a moving charge carrier from rhodopsin, Rosenberg and Harder (1967) have determined the semiconduction and photoconduction activation energies of a series of crystalline (?) and melted retinals. They found that the combination of retinal with opsin by means of a Schiff's base could be significant in appreciably lowering the semiconduction and photoconduction activation energies beneath those required with the separated chromophore. The necessity of a triplet state as kinetic intermediate in the formation of a moving charge carrier has been suggested, but apparently retinal would show insufficient energy in this condition. Therefore, Rosenberg and Harder have turned to studies of the activation energy needed for retinal when it is found in a host solid solution.

On the other hand, Kropf (1967) has shown

that excitation energy is sometimes transferred from the apoprotein (opsin) of rhodopsin to the chromophore to produce cis-trans isomerization. Ultraviolet light is primarily absorbed by the opsin, but one of every four ultraviolet photons so absorbed causes the bleaching of the recipient rhodopsin molecule (a little over half of the photons absorbed by the retinal produce bleaching).

It is very possible, however, that rhodopsin bleaching is the key to receptor excitation, and that the energy originally involved in isomerizing retinal is highly amplified before a change in cellular potential occurs. Ebrey and Platt (1967) found that the energy of a threshold retinal quantum absorption may be amplified by 10^5 to 10^7 to produce the nerve impulse, and that the process involved takes tens of milliseconds. Hubbard, Bownds and Yoshizawa (1965) have postulated that the exposure of ionizing or ion-binding groups (sulfhydryl groups, or a proton-binding group) may be the immediate source of cell excitation. Even more attractive as a source of excitation to these investigators is a possible redistribution of charges on the opsin due to the isomerization of the retinal, followed by opsin conformational changes. It now appears that the charge redistribution by itself might trigger electrical events, an alternative which was also stated by Hubbard, Bownds and Yoshizawa (1965).

The Early Receptor Potential

It seems that the a-wave of the electroretinogram develops during the existence of the metarhodopsin II. An early receptor potential (ERP) has been identified in monkey, cat, rat, frog and goldfish retinas which first appears before the formation of metarhodopsin I.

This ERP consists of two parts, an earlier phase R1, and a later, slower phase R2. Pak (1965) describes the first, R1 phase as positive and R2 as negative, but Brown and Murakami (1964) report R1 as negative and R2 as positive, and the polarity seems to depend on the method of recording. Cone

(1967) refers to the R1 as cornea-positive and the R2 as cornea-negative.

Evidence has been presented that the R1 phase itself consists of two components (Arden et al., 1966).

Yonemura and Kawasaki (1967) have obtained indications of the existence of a third portion of the ERP with the same sign as R1.

Brown, Watanabe and Murakami (1965) found the R1 to have a latency of not more than 25μsec, and Cone (1967), employing a flash duration of 0.7μsec, noted no latent period preceding the rising phase of R1. Cone (1967) states that such a latent period would have to be shorter than 0.5μsec at 25°C. The R1 reaches its peak in about 100μ sec.

In the retina of the rat, made up almost entirely of rods, the action spectra of both phases of the ERP agree well with the absorption spectrum of rhodopsin (Pak and Cone, 1964). Such matching of the ERP action spectrum with the photopigment absorption spectrum has also been demonstrated for the pure-cone retina of the ground squirrel (Pak and Ebrey, 1966), and the eyes of the squid (Hagins and McGaughy, 1967) and the horseshoe crab (Brown, Murray and Smith, 1967).

The ERP can normally be obtained only by employing very strong lights (Smith and Brown, 1966) and saturates at the higher flash energies.

The ERP is resistant to low temperatures, is not eliminated by anoxia (Brown and Murakami, 1964) and is only enhanced, especially its later phase, by immersion of the frog retina in isotonic potassium chloride (Pak, 1965). Brindley and Gardner-Medwin (1966) have confirmed that the ERP is not reduced by changes in medium ion concentration.

The findings given above indicate that the ERP is produced by an early, fast change in the molecule of the visual pigment and does not involve an ion flow or a membrane depolarization. Since isotonic potassium chloride should block the synapse between the visual receptor cell and the next cell of the visual pathway, the bipolar cell, the observation of

the ERP after one hour's immersion in KCl is also further evidence of its origin in the receptor. The increased height of the R2 phase in isotonic potassium chloride is probably only due to a greater external current flow resulting from reduced membrane resistance (Lettvin, General Discussion, 1965).

The R1 of the ERP is less sensitive to temperature reduction than the R2. Below 5°C the R2 peak is eliminated, while the R1 peak has been observed at −35°C (Pak and Ebrey, 1965). The temperature resistance of the R1 by itself shows that the R1 is called forth either by the transformation of prelumirhodopsin to lumirhodopsin or the lumirhodopsin-metarhodopsin I conversion.

The R2 may also be separately abolished in the toad by repetitive light stimulation (Brown, 1965). It is depressed by low pH, while the R1 is enhanced and prolonged by low pH (Pak, Rozzi and Ebrey, 1967). These results also indicate that the R1 and R2 potentials result from different processes.

The peak of the R2 appears after approximately 1 msec, and the full duration of the ERP is 7 msec (Brown, Watanabe and Murakami, 1965).

In the vertebrate retina only the R1 and R2 peaks of the ERP are linear potentials. Stimulus intensity and the extent of visual adaptation do not determine their form. The size of R1 and R2 reflects the total of excited pigment molecules, and, for a certain stimulus intensity, the percentage of pigment in the receptor cells. Therefore, each responding pigment molecule must increase these potentials by the same amount. Approximately 10^5 pigment molecules need to be excited in each albino rat retinal rod to produce noticeable potentials (Cone, 1965). The amplitude of the ERP, which may reach 1 mV in the rat, no longer increases linearly with flash intensity after each pigment molecule has absorbed one photon. Pak (1968) presents evidence that the generating unit of the ERP is indeed the single pigment molecule. Fuortes and Yeandle (1964) suggest that brief increases in the membrane conductance of xiphosuran (*Limu-*

lus) visual cells result from the absorption of individual photons, and it appears that the absorption of single quanta may produce small potentials in locust retinulae (Scholes, 1965).

Under similar conditions larger ERP's are produced by predominantly rod eyes than by purely cone eyes. The former's threshold of response is approximately one log unit lower, and excessive light reduces the mainly rod eye potentials more easily than those of cone eyes (Pak and Ebrey, 1966). These observations can be attributed to the differences in light sensitivity between rods and cones. Also, the R2 phase seems to be shorter and reaches its peak sooner in all-cone eyes, and cooling has a much smaller effect on the R2 of cone eyes.

The outer segments of rods and cones are filled with double-membrane discs layered one above the other. A number of studies indicate that the visual pigment molecules themselves make up a portion of the disc membrane.

Thus Azuma and Kito (1967) believe the α-helical portion of rhodopsin (near 30%), and the amino acid residues which compose primarily nonpolar side chains of this pigment, to be located in the interior of membranes. Retinal, considered a lipid, is probably also situated in membrane interiors.

The double-membrane discs, which are rich in phospholipids, arise from the cell plasma membrane and remain connected with it in all of the outer segment of lower vertebrates. In adult mammals the discs remain in contact with the cell plasma membrane in the basal portion of the outer segment. However, in most of the outer segment of the adult mammal, the hollow discs seem to separate from the plasma membrane and apparently have no connection with it or other discs (Dowling, 1967).

Lettvin (General Discussion, 1965) is inclined to doubt the last arrangement on an electrical basis, for in the rods, for instance, it would cause the individual rhodopsin molecules' contributions to the ERP to cancel each other. Instead, Lettvin suggests that the discs may be connected in some consistent manner to a continuous membrane and that the inter-

nal space of each disc is still in contact with the protoplasmic fluid external to it.

Clark and Branton (1967) found that the internal surfaces of the discs are opposed, but Dowling (1967) considers a similar phenomenon to be an artifact of hypertonic fixation. Dowling (1967) does, however, believe, on the basis of osmotic responses, that the internal space of the discs is to be considered intra-, and not extra-cellular.

McConnell (1967) reports that outer segments of cattle visual receptors containing undamaged discs pick up protons on exposure to light. This process requires unbleached rhodopsin. The regenerative transformation of the subsequently bleached pigment to rhodopsin, by dark incubation of the outer segments with 11-cis retinal, produces a release of the previously captured protons.

McConnell's (1967) findings integrate well with a statement by Falk and Fatt (1966) that a flash of light causes rhodopsin to quickly bind a proton. Falk and Fatt (1966) suggest that this binding takes place during the conversion of metarhodopsin I to metarhodopsin II. Cone's work (1967) shows the metarhodopsin I-metarhodopsin II transformation to give rise to the R2 of the ERP (Fig. 5-2). He has also identified a B response, of opposite polarity to R2 and produced by the photoregeneration of metarhodopsin II to rhodopsin, which is presumably linked to the release of a proton (Fig. 5-2).

Ebrey and Platt (1967) report that metarhodopsin I but not metarhodopsin II breaks down fast enough at the rat's body temperatures to perhaps be part of the excitation process.

Abrahamson and Ostroy (1967) also add their voices to those who consider the metarhodopsin I–metarhodopsin II conversion to be most closely correlated with the development of a visual potential.

Cone (1967) believes the ERP to develop from charge displacements as the rhodopsin molecule (or a nearby molecule) goes through configurational changes. He interprets the two phases of the ERP as indicative of two sepa-

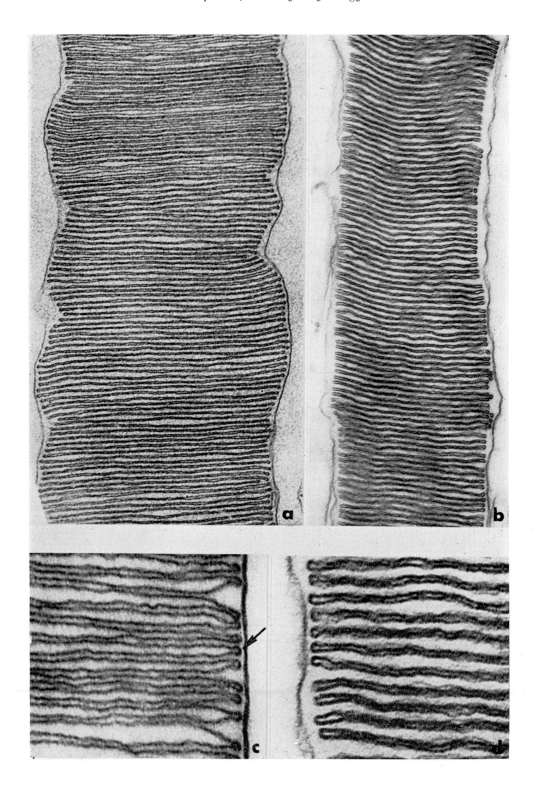

rate or successive charge displacements, a view which is shared by Brindley and Gardner-Medwin (1966). Cone (1967), using the albino rat, has identified the R1 of the ERP with the formation of metarhodopsin I, and a potential of the opposite polarity, denoted as A, with the photoregeneration of rhodopsin from metarhodopsin I (Fig. 5-2).

In rats metarhodopsin I appears virtually immediately following a saturating light flash and then *in vivo* breaks down during several milliseconds. Under physiological conditions metarhodopsin II appears with a half-time of a millisecond and only breaks down over several minutes.

Arden and Ikeda (1965) have seemingly also reported the A potential as a fast regenerative potential. Pak and Boes (1967) have corroborated Cone's findings that the A regenerative potential, of opposite polarity to R1, probably results from metarhodopsin I's photoregeneration to rhodopsin, while the B regenerative potential, of opposite polarity to R2, very likely originates in metarhodopsin II's photoregeneration to rhodopsin (some of the B potential could develop from the metarhodopsin II–metarhodopsin 465 conversion). Pak and Boes (1967)combine the A and B potentials under the term *reversal potential* and found that at 0°C only the A phase develops (as is also true of its "bleaching mate," R1).

Ebrey and Platt (1967) have confirmed Cone's (1967) and Pak and Boes' (1967) reports that the intermediate pigments formed in rhodopsin bleaching in turn produce photovoltages on exposing the preparation to its second flash of light. Ebrey and Platt's photovoltages probably were indicative of the photoregeneration of rhodopsin.

Hagins and McGaughy (1967), using squid retinas, found that light flashes caused rhodopsin to produce a photovoltage which they also suggest originates in a shift of molecular charges. They offer evidence that the rhodopsin photovoltage signals the conversion of rhodopsin to acid metarhodopsin (with the aid of thermal reactions) and that an acid metarhodopsin photovoltage indicates reversion to rhodopsin by a return to its charge distribution.

The photovoltage of rhodopsin was smaller by a factor of 10^9 than the receptor current of the live retina, and the photovoltage's magnitude was proportional to the number of excited rhodopsin molecules. The rhodopsin photovoltage is eliminated by freezing and thawing which does not break down rhodopsin. Hagins and McGaughy make no attempt to relate this last fact to a membrane disorganization, nor do they in this paper relate the rhodopsin photovoltage to the ERP in mammals.

Light flashes also called forth photovoltages from basic metarhodopsin and isorhodopsin.

Rosenberg (1966) described photovoltaic effects emanating from sheep visual rods and from carotenoid pigments and suggested that rhodopsin and other visual pigments bound to the disc membranes of the visual receptor outer segments may be in a system restricting water entrance.

Falk and Fatt (1966) found that the light-induced resistance changes in the outer segments of frog rods and in rhodopsin solutions were greatly dependent on pH. However, Crawford, Gage and Brown (1967) report that the ERP in frog retinas remained extant at

◄ FIGURE 5-3. Longitudinal sections of a rod and a cone. In neither the rat rod (a, c) or the monkey foveal cone (b, d) can the discs be seen to be connected with the plasma membrane or each other. In rods the internal surfaces of the double-membrane discs are separated by a wider space than in cones. The thinner appearance of the rod discs' membranes may be an artifact. The typical button ending of rod discs is indicated by an arrow (c). a, b, ×50,000; c, d, ×150,000. (Fig. 5, page 196, from chapter by John E. Dowling in Allen, John M. [Ed.]: *Molecular Organization and Biological Function*. New York, Harper and Row, 1967.)

pH's of 1 and 13. These pH's should disorganize the disc membranes; therefore, these results appear to be at variance with Hagins and McGaughy's (1967) freezing-thawing findings on the squid retina.

McConnell (1967) found that the disorganization of the outer segment membranes of cattle rods by means of a detergent abolishes the light-produced proton uptake only at pH's above 6. This also seems to show that an organized membrane may not be essential for the ERP. At higher pH's protons are released, indicating that nevertheless protein groups normally buried in the outer segment membranes are involved in the proton uptake.

However, Cone and Brown (1967) state that the rhodopsin molecules are highly oriented in the lamellar membranes of receptor outer segments.

Two papers indicate that the ERP arises from the receptor cell plasma membrane itself.

Smith and Brown (1966) have recorded a potential similar to the ERP from retinular cells, the visual receptors of the horseshoe crab, *Xiphosura polyphemus*. With these invertebrate photoreceptors an early depolarizing potential of 0.5 to 1.5 mV and a latency of under 0.5 msec was obtained. In numerous experiments this potential was followed, after the light flash, by hyperpolarization.

Smith and Brown found their early invertebrate potential to reverse in sign when they shifted from extracellular to intracellular recording. They also changed the retinular cell's membrane potential by passing current through an intracellular microelectrode and found that the early potential's polarity and amplitude varied with the membrane potential. These findings implied that the source of the early potential was the cell membrane. Smith and Brown even ventured the suggestion that the possibly involved rhodopsin molecules might be constituents of the cell membrane.

If the source of their early potential is indeed rhodopsin, Smith and Brown state, the action of light on the pigment molecules could cause the last to act on other membrane structures which control membrane permeability to ions.

Since the polarity of the early potential is determined by the membrane potential, a component of the early potential is probably associated with or produced by a conductance change in the membrane, according to Smith and Brown. The fact that the early potential's polarity cannot, however, be reversed is a sign of an initial phase unaffected by the membrane potential.

Smith and Brown were also able to obtain their early potential from the eccentric cell of the *Xiphosura* (*Limulus*) ommatidium. This cell is a neuron, the apical dendrite of which is surrounded by the retinular cells. They also recorded their early potential from what were presumably pigment cells surrounding the ommatidium and obtained it from pigmented and possibly pigmented cells in ganglia of *Aplysia* the sea hare, an opisthobranch mollusk.

Hagins and McGaughy (1968) supply evidence that the fast photovoltage of the ERP of the squid photoreceptor arises from a charge displacement in the electrical capacitance of the plasma membrane surrounding the outer segment of the receptor. Their results indicate that a light flash produces a localized charge displacement in the illuminated portion of the plasma membrane itself, and that the dipoles thus created must be normal to the cell surface (Fig. 5-4). The fact that the photovoltage arises only in one surface zone of the receptor, in its outer segment (i.e. that the receptor is electrically asymmetric), causes this membrane polarization to be reduced only by a current flow parallel to the longitudinal axis of the receptor into the interior of the retina. This results in a net transretinal voltage.

The concept that the source of the ERP resides in the plasma membrane itself is supported by the facts that the rhodopsin photovoltage in vertebrates is eliminated by disorienting the rod rhodopsin through heating

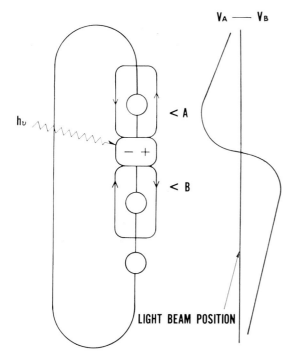

V_A —— V_B

< A

− +

< B

LIGHT BEAM POSITION

$h\upsilon$

FIGURE 5-4. A model for the production of fast photovoltages in a cell layer by intramolecular charge displacements in the cell membranes. (A, B) Sites of electrodes; (V_A-V_B) voltage at A minus voltage at B. On the left a diagrammatic sample cell plasma membrane contains unpolarized (circles), and photochemically polarized (oval) rhodopsin molecules. The produced molecular dipoles are normal to the cell membrane. On the right is illustrated the longitudinal voltage gradient which should result within a cell layer from currents produced by the membrane charge displacements. The interelectrode voltage would be largest with a light beam at A, minimal with the beam at B, and it would reverse with the beam at an intermediate location. Such results were obtained experimentally. (Adapted from Hagins, W.A., and R.E. McGaughy: Membrane origin of the fast photovoltage of squid retina. *Science*, 159:3811, 213-215, 1968 [Copyright 1968 by the American Association for the Advancement of Science].)

to 58°C (Cone and Brown, 1967), that this photovoltage in the squid can be abolished by freezing and thawing without disrupting the rhodopsin molecule (Hagins and McGaughy, 1967), and that the photovoltages of the squid

and of vertebrates are basically alike, although their receptor plasma membranes differ in folding and orientation.

Hagins and McGaughy's (1968) findings show that the charge displacement in the plasma membrane must cause its exterior to become positive to its inner surface when rhodopsin is transformed to acid metarhodopsin. The reconstitution of rhodopsin is accompanied by a reversal in sign of the membrane potential.

Vinnikov (1965) invokes electron movement related to ATP reconstitution as a stage in the origin of the ERP in the rod outer segment membranes. These membranes carry not only pigment molecules but also succinic oxidase and cytochrome oxidase. Vinnikov also reports a release of potassium ions and some sodium ions from a rod outer segment fraction on illumination. He suggests a change in ion balance may be involved in ERP generation.

Shukolyukov (1967) did not find succinic dehydrogenase activity and cytochrome oxidase activity in outer segments to be high. Pearse and McConnell (1966) have located a redox compound in retinal outer segment discs which could play a role in electron transport.

Research by Buckser and Diamond (1966), Bonting (1966), and Bonting and Bangham (1967) indicates that sodium ions are taken up by photoreceptors upon illumination. Kikuchi and Takeda (1966) found indications that sodium ions play a role in the development of retinal slow potentials elicited by illumination.

Smith, Stell and Brown (1968), using xiphosuran retinular cells, present evidence that the receptor potential is not the result of an increase in cell membrane ion permeability. Instead, partly because light and electric current have similar effects on the membrane potential, they take the view that the investigated visual cells have a source of current, a constant current generator, in their cell membranes. Stimulation with light would affect this membrane generator. Smith, Stell and Brown regard the increase in cell membrane permeability to sodium and other ions following light stimulation as secondary; this increased permeability could result from the nonlinear current-voltage relation of the retinular cell membrane.

Smith, Stell, Brown, Freeman and Murray's (1968) findings indicate that the mentioned constant current generator in the photoreceptor membrane is an electrogenic sodium pump.

A membrane pump is described as electrogenic when the quantity of sodium ions actively pushed out through the membrane differs from the amount of potassium ions actively taken into the cell. Such a pump, which moves a greater number of charges in one direction, can give rise to a current.

The electrogenic sodium pump helps to maintain the normal membrane potential and, of course, its energy is provided by the ATP-ATPase system. Light is said to effect changes in the pump, which result in the appearance of the receptor potential. These changes may consist of a modification of the pump's electrogenicity or its rate. A reversal of pumping direction is less likely.

Verification of the hypothesis that the retinular cell receptor potential stems from the modification of function of a membrane electrogenic pump would cast the role of rhodopsin (and probably other visual pigments) in a new light. It would next have to be determined how the light-induced alterations in rhodopsin in turn affect the sodium pump.

Recently some investigators, such as Bonting (1967), Abrahamson and Ostroy (1967), and Pak (1968) have downgraded the significance of the ERP in visual stimulation. Thus Pak (1968) points out that the apparent small amplitude of the ERP (2-3 mV at most by extracellular recording) indicates it probably could not directly initiate receptor cell excitation. Moreover, the potentials evoked from the thermal decay intermediates of rhodopsin bleaching resemble the ERP phases but do not produce excitation. Nevertheless, Pak (1968) agrees that the ERP reflects the effect of light on the visual pigment and is aware that the ERP may initiate unknown processes (amplifications?) which may lead to receptor response.

Arden (1968) has written a good review of work on the early receptor potential and similar responses.

Results With Pigment Epithelium

An early potential similar to the ERP, but of relatively smaller amplitude, has also been observed to arise from the retinal pigment epithelium of anurans (Brown, 1965; Brown and Crawford, 1967a; Brown and Gage, 1966; Crawford, Gage and Brown, 1967) and mammals (Arden, Ikeda and Siegel, 1966).

The pigment epithelium lies immediately behind the photoreceptor layer of the retina, as viewed from the direction of entering light and the vitreous humor, and by villous processes extends between the receptors' outer segments. It contains many melanin granules, a few receptor outer segment sections undergoing digestion, and in lower vertebrates some possibly light-sensitive myeloid bodies (Dowling, 1967).

The early potential of the pigment cells, like the ERP, consists of two phases of opposed polarity. However, both pigment cell potential phases show only slight light adaptation, and the threshold for eliciting them is over one log unit above that of the ERP (Pak and Ebrey, 1966).

The first phase is unaffected by dehydration of the pigment cells (Brown and Gage, 1966), by lowered temperature, or by pH (Crawford, Gage and Brown, 1967), and may be dependent on solid state phenomena (Crawford, Gage and Brown, 1967). The first phase has itself been reported to consist of two components (Brown and Crawford, 1967b).

The second phase falls faster than the first phase on injury to the cell membrane and seems to be generated across it (Brown and Crawford, 1967a).

The early potential of the pigment cells gives rise to a third response, comparable to the late RP, which is dependent on ion movement and shows poor light adaptation (Brown and Gage, 1966).

A c-wave which emanates from the pigment cell layer seems to actually have its origin in the rhodopsin of retinal photoreceptors (Brown and Crawford, 1966).

The very broad action spectra of all three phases of the pigment cell response show it to originate in a single photopigment, melanin (Brown and Crawford, 1967b). This conclusion is corroborated by the fact that the pigment cell response appears in pigmented rat eyes but not in albino rat eyes (Arden, Ikeda and Siegel, 1966; Brown and Crawford, 1967b). There are indications the response results from a change in the charge across oriented dipoles.

Photovoltaic potentials have been obtained from synthetic melanin under various conditions (Crawford, Gage and Brown, 1967). The results with melanin support the view that at least the first phase potential, which can be elicited from pigment cells at extreme pH's, is a solid state phenomenon.

Ebrey and Platt (1967) found that a flash of light causes all organismic, oriented pigments to emit potentials of millisecond duration.

In the earlier papers Rosenberg and his co-workers (Rosenberg, 1962; Rosenberg, Heck and Aziz, 1964, 1965) reported that isolated carotenoid pigments showed changes in photopotential with wavelength which paralleled the order of chromatic potentials obtained by Svaetichin from the fish retina. Also, β-carotene cells were found to produce a true color response (mixture of short and long wavelengths had the effect of selected single mid-spectral wavelengths). β-carotene is a dimer of retinal which has lost its aldehyde group.

The findings on the retinal pigment cell responses, and on synthetic melanin and other biological pigments, parallel to a considerable extent the results obtained with the ERP. They show that the origin of the ERP of visual receptors can be understood in terms of the properties of light-sensitive pigments.

Their results prompt Crawford, Gage and Brown (1967) to suggest that the ERP may be based on solid state phenomena. They therefore consider that the ERP develops from photovoltaic events, and state that it could be produced by dipoles oriented in some relationship to the receptor cell. They also indicate that it is possible that the chromophores supply energy to the membrane protein.

The fact that Arden, Bridges, Ikeda and Siegel (1966a) could record photovoltaic responses from rat and guinea pig retinas which had been treated with glutaraldehyde is additional evidence for solid state events in the retina.

Potentials similar to the ERP have also been recorded on illuminating whole green leaves (Arden, Bridges, Ikeda and Siegel, 1966b; Ebrey, 1967). Leaf sections which lack chlorophyll or other leaf pigments do not yield such responses. The electrode at a green leaf's apex becomes negative to the electrode at the leaf's base, indicating that the source of the voltage is oriented longitudinally in the leaf. Arden *et al.* (1966b) state that the leaf potentials originate from oriented dipoles.

Becker and Cone (1966), by using an intense light flash, succeeded in obtaining an early potential from the skins of all organisms tested. This potential was increased by a contribution from any present skin melanin. A later response from frog skin, elicited by short wavelengths, may depend on another skin pigment.

All ERP-type responses generate as dipoles normal to their tissue source and emanate from oriented structures. Thus the rat rhodopsin ERP arises from radially arranged current dipoles. In leaves, where the chloroplasts are not oriented, the responses originate from the cell surface; the surface offers an arrangement —it is all in the same plane. Why the charges flow from the interior light-sensitive pigments to the cell surface remains undetermined (Arden, 1968).

Although almost 90 per cent of the frog's visual pigment is rhodopsin, the frog's ERP is generated primarily by the cone pigment iodopsin and also apparently receives contributions from other cone pigments. This unexpected origin of the frog's ERP may be related to the fact that frog rhodopsin, unlike iodopsin, is found in lamellae that make no contact with the extracellular space (Goldstein, 1968).

The Late Receptor Potential

Brown, Watanabe and Murakami (1965), using the cynomolgus monkey (*Macaca irus*), investigated an early part of the electroretinogram (ERG). This preliminary ERG potential, the first portion of which gives origin to the ERG's a-wave (or may be considered the rising phase of the a-wave), is now known as the late receptor potential, or late RP. The late RP was found to have a minimal latent period of approximately 1.5 msec and could be eliminated with anoxia, leaving the ERP. The whole receptor is traversed by the extracellular current of the late RP, and the late RP potential may reach 5.0 mV. The greatest amplitude of the R2 phase of the ERP is found at the same depth of the retina as the greatest amplitude of the late RP. The ERP precedes, and may give rise to the late RP, and the last in turn is followed by the a- and b-waves of the ERG. The b-wave seems to arise in radially oriented neurons of the retina's inner nuclear layer; it may be affected by convergent pathways coming from widely separated receptors (Arden and Brown, 1965).

Tomita (1965) believes the late RP's he recorded from the carp retina, which were always negative, to have originated in the cone inner segment. He divides them into three groups according to the most stimulating wavelength (and thus according to the three cone types). Tomita *et al.* (1967) and Kaneko and Hashimoto (1967) later confirmed that these negative potentials, 5 mV or less in amplitude, arise in the inner segments of cones.

The view that the late RP does not develop in the vicinity of visual pigment molecules suggests that the ERP may be conducted to the late RP site. If the ERP is only the external sign of an electric conduction, then the mechanism of this conduction could not be similar to that of nerve impulse conduction, since the ERP is not accompanied by either a membrane depolarization or ion movement. Perhaps a first conduction is intracellular, by way of the ciliary filaments or neurofibrils (Brown and Murakami, 1964). Cohen (1961) describes the fibrils in the postnuclear stalks of visual receptors as suggestive of neurofibrils and also observed striated filaments (ciliary rootlets) in the rod inner segment.

While the ERP is linear and not amplified, the late RP is a highly amplified potential which at average stimulus intensities may exceed the ERP by a factor of two million.

Wald (1965) has suggested, although without supporting evidence, a series of amplification stages in the visual rod. Each of these stages would involve the activation of a proenzyme to an enzyme, and the system could start with the exposure of a catalyst in rhodopsin by the light isomerization of the 11-cis retinal to the 11-trans form. Such a photomultiplier effect could occur even in the partially solid state of the plasma membrane by surface adsorptions, and the plasma membrane also has liquid interfaces.

Seegers (1966), on the other hand, regards Wald's view of the blood clotting process, the source of Wald's amplification suggestion, as incorrect.

The ERP is only "adapted" by the bleaching of the visual pigment. On the other hand, the late RP and the b-wave show true or neural adaptation, since they decrease significantly after a period of light stimulation which does not cause appreciable bleaching of the visual pigment. Therefore, neural processes must intercede between the ERP and the late RP (Cone, 1965).

During the late RP the extracellular current has been described as traveling from the zone of the inner segments of the monkey's (*Macaca irus*) visual receptors toward the axon endings. This current could develop as a result of active hyperpolarization in the region of the inner segments, but according to Brown,

Watanabe and Murakami (1965), it is more likely that it results from an active depolarization of the axon endings. Tomita *et al.* (1967) found the late RP's they recorded from cone inner segments of the carp to be hyperpolarizing potentials. They hypothesize that while vertebrate photoreceptors show hyperpolarizing responses, invertebrate photoreceptors are depolarized. Insect photoreceptors appear to be depolarized (Naka and Eguchi, 1962). Bortoff and Norton (1967) suggest that the proximal flow of the photoreceptor current is due to active hyperpolarization of the outer segments on illumination, a concept which is reminiscent of Hagins and McGaughy's (1968) observations on the squid ERP.

In any case, the current flows in the opposite direction from that taken by generator potentials. Thus it appears that the late RP of mammals cannot operate like a generator potential. However, since it enters the axon endings, it could supplant a visual receptor generator potential in mammals and initiate nerve impulses.

The late RP of cones has a greater amplitude than that of rods.

While the late RP of cones falls rapidly after strong stimuli, as observed in the fovea of the cynomolgus monkey (*Macaca irus*), the late RP of rods declines quite slowly following such stimuli, as seen in the night monkey (*Aotus trivirgatus*). This difference appears to be another illustration of the duplicity theory. The rapid decrease of the cone late RP indicates that the cones are the source of the retinal ganglion cells' "off" responses (see Chap. IV) to intense stimuli. However, at low stimulus intensities the rod late RP drops fairly rapidly, possibly making the rods now capable of initiating "off" responses (Brown, Watanabe and Murakami, 1965).

As the intensity of a light flash is raised, the cone late RP first reaches a maximum amplitude, and then, by increasing delay of its decay, its duration lengthens (Brown and Murakami, 1967). The delay of the late RP's decay does not affect the rate of the cone's

rapid decay phase itself. Brown and Murakami (1967) conclude from this that the part of the cone membrane which produces the late RP develops a stable activated state, the length of which depends on the stimulus intensity.

No matter what the extent of delay of the cone late RP's decay, the d.c. component of the ERG, produced by neurons of the inner nuclear layer, decays only immediately after the late RP's decay (Brown and Murakami, 1967). As this ERG d.c. component emanates from a higher level of the visual pathway, the above finding tends to establish the importance of the late RP in the train of receptor events which lead to visual perception.

The a- and b-waves of the ERG quickly disappear in isotonic potassium chloride and more slowly in a Ringer's solution lacking sodium ion (Pak, 1965). It thus appears that these later potentials are, like most neural processes, dependent on ion movements.

It has been shown that the b-wave plays no role in at least primary visual transmission but may be significant in later processes (Wolin and Massopust, 1966).

The above description of the series of potentials arising in visual receptors following light stimulation holds, however, only for mammals. Thus squid photoreceptors differ both structurally and functionally from their mammalian counterparts. Squid photoreceptors possess long, branched axons from which action potentials have been recorded (Mac Nichol, Jr. and Love, 1960). Their local currents do not flow in the direction of the current which develops in the mammalian visual receptor during its late RP but rather flow in the same direction as that of a normal generator potential (Hagins, Zonana, and Adams, 1962).

Illumination causes the squid photoreceptors' outer segments to become negative to the basal portions of the receptors. The potential which is produced fluctuates with light intensity. The current flow increases by approximately 40,000 electronic charges per photon of light, and it has been established that light energy and other available energy together produce the receptor current (Hagins, 1965).

Summary

It thus seems that the first steps in visual reception may at least be partly known. The absorption of quanta of light by visual pigment molecules located in the membranes of the outer segments of visual receptors leads to an isomerization. This photoisomerization and consequent thermal decay transformations result in charge displacements which give rise to the R1 and R2 phases of the early receptor potential (ERP).

At least the first of these ERP phases appears to be based on a solid state phenomenon and can be correlated with the photovoltaic events culminating in the formation of metarhodopsin I. The important second phase of the ERP is associated with the conversion of metarhodopsin I to metarhodopsin II, and this transformation is considered by some investigators to be most intimately related to receptor excitation. However, precisely how the ERP phases arise from the photochemical and thermochemical processes which precede them or how transduction occurs is not yet understood. Perhaps the changes produced by light in a visual pigment in turn lead to a modification of the membrane molecules controlling the electrogenic sodium pump.

The significance of our knowledge of the ERP lies in the fact that this potential may be the first immediate product of a receptor transduction of chemical to electrical energy which has been discovered and successfully studied. It might be profitable to look for early potentials resembling the ERP in other types of receptors.

By a method which has not yet been fully determined, the ERP gives rise to the late receptor potential (late RP). The development of the late RP, unlike that of the ERP, involves a membrane ion conductance and a membrane depolarization, and it is a highly amplified potential which shows true adaptation. The late RP's extracellular current, which in mammals, and so on, flows in the opposite direction to that of a normal generator potential, then apparently initiates nerve impulses in neuron axon endings (the bipolar cells). The late RP also gives rise to the a-wave of the electroretinogram.

As yet little is known of how the energy of the ERP is amplified to the energy level of the late RP, if indeed the ERP itself is part of the process leading to the late RP. Wald (1965) has suggested a search in visual rods for a multistage amplification system based on enzymes.

An alternative hypothesis of visual excitation states that light excitation of the chromophore results in the formation of an electric charge carrier which is capable of movement through an electric field or along a gradient of charges and thus becomes a current. The proponents of this hypothesis regard cis-trans isomerism and the consequent bleaching transformations as portions of an adaptive mechanism which competes with the above excitatory process (Rosenberg, 1966).

It is not yet certain what produces the extracellular current which travels to the bipolar cells' axons during the late RP.

Further, there may also exist dissipative processes which permit rhodopsin to fall from the excited state to its original energy level. Guzzo and Pool (1968) suggest fluorescence (that of rhodopsin lies at 575 mμ), phosphorescence, radiationless transfer, exciton formation and simple heat dissipation as possible candidates for this role.

Parallel studies on the potentials which can be elicited by light flashes from retinal pigment cells and biological pigments have given us greater insight into the early events which take place in visual receptors.

Wald (1968) notes the advantages the retina offers for sensory research. Because the retinal visual receptors form a single layer and their types can easily be differentiated by sensitivities and absorption spectra, each receptor cell and receptor type can be separately investigated. Furthermore, the visual pigment molecules are arrayed in a well-ordered, two-dimensional grid. The isomerization of a single pigment molecule can excite its receptor cell, and the ERP linearly reflects the responses of the pigment molecule population.

RECEPTION BY THE PACINIAN CORPUSCLE

Another receptor type which has yielded much information on the nature of the receptor response is the large pacinian corpuscle. In the case of this end organ, however, the first steps in excitation are less understood than the subsequent development of potentials and impulses.

Method

Loewenstein (1960a) and others used the easily accessible pacinian corpuscles in the mesenteric membrane of the cat to study the development of the receptor (generator) potential, which in normal mammalian mechanoreceptors appears at a millisecond after stimulation. The corpuscle, plus a length of the afferent myelinated axon innervating it, was dissected free from the mesentery. Such a preparation of a corpuscle and a portion of its attached axon remains viable in Ringer's solution and in Kreb's solution for several hours.

Loewenstein and his co-workers stimulated intact and decapsulated corpuscles mechanically with a glass stylus affixed to a piezoelectric crystal. The mechanical deflection of the crystal could be delicately controlled by varying the voltage applied to it, and the amplitude of this deflection was monitored photoelectrically. Pulses of varying waveform were applied across the crystal—square pulses of 1 msec to 1 second length produced mechanical deflections with rise time constants of 0.5 to 0.7 msec. The amplitudes of the mechanical deflections in the crystal increased linearly with the employed electric pulses over a broad range of voltages, making it easier to apply carefully graded and measured stimuli. The amplitude of the mechanical deflection varied from 0.7μ to 80μ, and in one group of experiments use was made of styli with tips ranging from 5μ to 600μ in diameter. Similar techniques were later employed by Ozeki and Sato (1964) and by Il'Inskii and Volkova (1966).

The generator (receptor) potential and the impulses produced by the corpuscle as a response to mechanical stimulation passed up the innervating axon and were picked up by an electrode at the point where the axon leaves the corpuscle. Therefore, the generator (receptor) potentials, since they developed in the nerve ending, had to decay exponentially along the myelinated axon in its course through the corpuscle for an average distance of 450μ before reaching the electrode. Nevertheless, these potentials still had a size of 15μV to 100μV, and could easily be recorded. More direct records were also obtained by placing recording electrodes on the exposed sensory nerve terminal (Fig. 5-5).

It was possible to pick up generator potentials from beyond the corpuscle without the complicating action potentials (nerve impulses) by blocking the last with tetrodotoxin or procaine or by stretching or compressing the myelinated axon within the corpuscle. The use of tetrodotoxin was most effective.

A more complete picture of the described experimental techniques can be obtained from Loewenstein (1961a), Loewenstein and Mendelson (1965), Ishiko and Loewenstein (1961), and Loewenstein and Ishiko (1960).

Results

Loewenstein and Rathkamp (1958) demonstrated that the pacinian corpuscle's ability to respond to mechanical stimuli resides either in the innermost lamellae surrounding the nerve ending or the afferent nerve ending itself, and probably the latter. Hebel and Schweiger (1967) examined pacinian-type corpuscles in the skin of the nasal-mouth zone of cattle with the electron microscope. They found the distal portion of the sensory nerve ending to give rise to fingerlike projections.

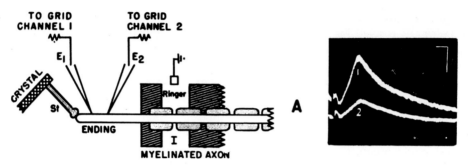

FIGURE 5-5. Loewenstein's technique for recording localized potentials from the Pacinian corpuscle's nonmyelinated nerve ending. (*St*) Stylus, (E_1, E_2) microelectrodes transmitting to different amplifier channels. E_1 is about 20μ from *St* and 350μ from E_2. The first node of Ranvier (*I*) has been grounded and insulated from the nerve ending. Trace *1* is the negative potential recorded from E_1, and trace *2* the potential from E_2, upon one mechanical stimulus by the stylus. The potential recorded by the closer electrode E_1 has a larger amplitude and a faster rate of rise. Scale: 50μV; 1 msec. (From Loewenstein, W.R.: The generation of electric activity in a nerve ending. *Ann. N.Y. Acad. Sci.*, 81:367-387, 1959.)

Mitochondria and vesicles are massed at the bases of these projections. These surface structures and organelles of the distal portion of the nerve ending suggest that it is the site of the transformations involved in excitation.

It has been implied by some investigators that acetylcholine may play a role in the development of the pacinian corpuscle's generator (receptor) potential. Loewenstein and Molins (1958) found a high concentration of acetylcholinesterase in the sensory nerve ending of the pacinian corpuscle but almost none in its lamellae. Shanthaveerappa and Bourne (1966) also report the corpuscle's nerve fiber to contain considerable quantities of cholinesterases, and found the inner core and the lamellar cells to be lacking in cholinesterase activity.

On the other hand, Hebel and Schweiger (1967) determined acetylcholinesterase to be concentrated specifically at the surface of the nerve ending and at the surface membranes of all the lamellae of their cattle corpuscle. These workers even hypothesize that in their pacinian-type corpuscle the vesicles at the bases of the nerve-ending projections might contain acetylcholine.

However, the demonstration of acetylcholine or other transmitters in the sensitive endings

of receptors, although the subject of many studies, has been only partially successful. It can be said that acetylcholine has been found to at least temporarily increase the excitability of cutaneous thermal and mechanoreceptors (Bing and Skouby, 1950; Dodt *et al.*, 1953; Jarrett, 1956).

In any case, it appears fairly certain that the pacinian corpuscle's high sensitivity to mechanical stimuli is due to the fact that deformation of the nerve-ending membrane leads in some manner to a drop in electrical resistance and to increased ion permeability and thus to depolarization or the generator potential.

Il'Inskii and Volkova (1966) report that there is an increase in the membrane surface area of the pacinian corpuscle's nerve terminal during depolarization. Hyperpolarization in turn is said to be associated with a reduction in the surface area of the nerve-ending membrane. The results of these investigators, and the findings of Il'Inskii, Volkova and Cherepnov (1968), suggest that the membrane is stretched by an effective stimulus. Such stretching could in turn result in greater ion permeability.

The pacinian corpuscle is not sensitive to increased uniform hydrostatic pressure, even of great magnitude, but only to a differential effect or strain (Loewenstein, 1965). However, a mechanical pulse which reduces the nerve ending's 2μ to 3μ diameter by 0.4μ to 0.8μ elicits a clear-cut generator (receptor) potential (Loewenstein, 1961a).

Similar results have been obtained with the ampulla of Lorenzini.

The degree of deformation of the sensory nerve ending of a pacinian corpuscle produced by a known stimulus is partially determined by the fluid layers and lamellae which surround the ending and also by the connections between the lamellae. The lamellae and their interconnections represent elastic elements, while the fluid layers form viscous elements (Loewenstein, 1965). The stimulus energy is transmitted relatively accurately by the viscous fluid, but much of it is lost during passage through the elastic components of the corpuscle. Therefore, the stimulus energy acting on the nerve ending differs in magnitude and time course from the mechanical energy which was originally exerted on the surface of the corpuscle. According to Loewenstein's computations, under 3 per cent of an outside pressure is transmitted through the corpuscle to the core enclosing the sensory nerve ending.

Loewenstein and Skalak (1966) stress a particularly great elasticity on the part of the interconnections between the lamellae.

The mechanics of pressure transmission are also the basis of the pacinian corpuscle's being phasic and an "on-off" receptor. If the corpuscle is subjected to a compression of 20μ reaching its peak in 2 msec, the core pressure is a large fraction of the surface pressure until the peak pressure is reached. Then, with the beginning of the static period of stimulation, the core pressure quickly falls to zero because of a parallel drop in the pressure transmitted by the viscous elements as the elasticity of the lamellae and their interconnections comes into play. It might be said that the pacinian corpuscle has an elastic filter. Also important is the cessation of fluid velocities in the system. The viscous forces which transmit the stimulus energy to the sensory nerve ending depend on

the stimulus velocity and follow it fairly closely. Transmission in the pacinian corpuscle can be said to be very dependent on velocity, and stimuli of insufficient velocity have no effect.

The capsule of the pacinian corpuscle can also be viewed as a filter for low frequencies (Loewenstein and Skalak, 1966). The corpuscle's frequency threshold for acoustic stimuli has been found to lie at 112 to 117 cps (Mirkin, 1966).

When the stimulus becomes static, both fluid velocity and core pressure fall to zero, their rate of fall determining the rate of adaptation. As the core pressure drops to zero, the generator potential decays exponentially, and impulses cease to emanate from the corpuscle. Loewenstein (1965) considers the conversion of mechanical to electric energy, or the transducer process, to occur from the appearance of the response to the time when its decay is entirely exponential.

The fact that the adaptation rate and the phasic nature of the corpuscle are dependent on the filtering action of the outer corpuscle can be proven by stripping off the lamellae down to the 20μ to 30μ diameter inner core. After this is done, the corpuscle core responds like a slowly adapting receptor, and the time span of the generator potential can be increased to over 70 msec (Loewenstein and Mendelson, 1965). During much of its course such a long potential follows the time course of the applied stimulus to a high degree. The inner core can then once more be surrounded by an artificial capsule of layers of mesothelium to return it to a fast adaptation rate. To provide the effect of a natural capsule such an artificial capsule must be composed of many thin and elastic layers separated by fluid (Loewenstein and Mendelson, 1965).

In both complete pacinian corpuscles and their bare nerve endings the generator potential's rate of increase accelerates almost linearly with an acceleration in the rise of the applied compression. The magnitude of the receptor potential also grows with an acceleration of the rate of compression, and its latent period falls (Nishi and Sato, 1968).

If the compression rises more rapidly than a critical slope, an action potential develops. This slope has a value of 1.1-1.2 rheobase/msec (Nishi and Sato, 1968).

A decapsulated corpuscle core develops a generator potential on application of a stimulus but does not respond to stimulus cessation with a generator potential.

How is the "off" generator response of the pacinian corpuscle to be explained? As the stimulus is removed, the corpuscle returns to its original circular cross-section because of the elastic rebound of the lamellae and their interconnections. This rebound produces new viscous forces, and once more the inner core is subjected to pressure. This pressure can approach that produced by the application of the stimulus if the fluid velocity is high enough. Although "off" compression occurs at right angles to that created during stimulus application, according to Loewenstein (1965) and Loewenstein and Skalak (1966) this has no effect on the transducer action. If the corpuscle is now decapsulated, no "off" response is obtained, showing that the energy stored in the elastic lamellae and their interconnections during stimulus application is necessary for this response.

Loewenstein has shown that the generator potential appears only in the stimulated portion of the nerve ending's surface. When a 20μ area was mechanically distorted, the potential fell exponentially with distance from the point of stimulation (Fig. 5-5). The potential dropped with distance at the same rate as a passive potential produced by imposing an electric charge on the same area. Similarly, reduced ability to form a generator potential is restricted to a site subjected to high frequencies.

The generator potential decays exponentially with time, the time constant being about 3 to 5 msec.

If two nearby points of the nerve ending are stimulated at the same time, the resulting generator potentials sum (Loewenstein, 1959; Ozeki and Sato, 1964). Therefore, increasing

mechanical distortion produces generator potentials which cover a proportionately larger area. A generator potential called forth by mechanical distortion of the intact pacinian corpuscle represents the sum of the individual generator potentials developing at many separate, scattered receptor sites. In the intact corpuscle the capsule should act to spread the stimulus over the whole nerve ending, and the responding receptor sites should therefore be distributed over the entire surface of the nerve membrane. The increase in amplitude of generator potential seen to follow greater strength of mechanical stimulation is at least mainly the consequence of an increase in the area of excited membrane (Fig. 5-6).

The relationship between the area of nerve ending membrane stimulated and the peak values of the generator potential, assuming a drop in resistance of the excited portion of the membrane to one tenth of its resting value at infinite time, is expressed by the equation

$$\text{generator potential } V = k \, \frac{E \cdot bx}{1 + bx}$$

in which k is a constant determined by the distance between stimulating and recording sites, E is the resting potential, $1 + b$ is the ratio between resting potential and the minimum value to which this potential can be brought by a mechanical stimulus, and x is the proportion of the membrane which has been excited. This equation describes a nonlinear function in which with equal increases in the excited membrane area, the successive additions to the generator potential become progressively smaller (Loewenstein, 1961b).

As would be expected, there is also summation between successively produced generator potentials, if the time interval is sufficiently short.

The latent period of the pacinian corpuscle's generator potential is about 0.2 msec.

An increase in the intensity of the stimulus applied to a decapsulated terminal raises both the magnitude and the duration of the receptor potential. As the stimulus intensity is elevated further, the potential's magnitude reaches a final, saturation level, but the potential's decay

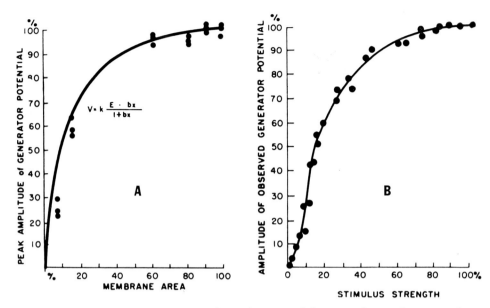

FIGURE 5-6. A. The generator potential as a function of the area of excited nerve ending. The abscissa values represent the increasing areas of ending membrane excited by progressively larger stylus diameters. The excited area which gives rise to the maximum potential is assigned a value of 100 per cent. The generator potentials, after spreading electrotonically, were recorded from the nerve fiber. The experimental values (solid circles) agree with the curve (solid line) obtained from the given equation.
B. The generator potential as related to stimulus amplitude. An intact corpuscle is subjected to increasingly large mechanical pulses and the elicited generator potentials are recorded from the nerve fiber. The resulting curve resembles that of A, suggesting that increasing stimuli act to excite larger membrane areas. (From Loewenstein, W.R.: Excitation and inactivation in a receptor membrane. *Ann. N.Y. Acad. Sci.*, 94:510-534, 1961.)

continues to be prolonged (Ozeki and Sato, 1965).

The generator current, as differentiated from the generator potential which it immediately creates, rises to its peak within 1 msec and decays completely in one more millisecond (Ozeki and Sato, 1964). The generator current is the immediate consequence of the action of a mechanical stimulus on the nerve ending. It is a localized inward current which is graded in size and rate of increase like the generator potential. The last, in fact, is really only the generator current after it has spread with exponential decay and while it is maintained by the capacitance and resistance of the nerve membrane.

The generator current is not only dependent on the resting potential of the stimulated membrane, but also is determined by temperature. The generator potential rises more rapidly and reaches a higher amplitude with greater membrane polarization (Fig. 5-7), and the generator current also shows both a faster rate of rise ($Q_{10} = 2.5$) and a larger amplitude ($Q_{10} = 2.0$) with increasing temperature (Fig. 5-8). Higher temperature may increase the ion permeability of the nerve terminal membrane. According to Ishiko and Loewenstein (1961), the rise of, and the amplitude of the pacinian corpuscle's generator potential at various temperatures indicate that the transducer process requires activation energies in the range of 16,000 cal/mole.

The generator potential is also surprisingly resistant to the action of tetrodotoxin and other drugs.

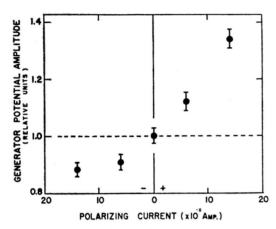

FIGURE 5-7. The effects of polarizing current on the generator potential. While identical mechanical stimuli are used to produce generator potentials, the nerve ending is subjected to hyperpolarizing (inward, +) and depolarizing (outward, −) constant currents of different intensities. The generator potential values are multiples of the generator potential's value at the resting membrane potential. Each value represents the average relative amplitude of 50 generator potentials, and the limits of the standard error of every value are indicated. The amplitude of the generator potential varies directly with hyperpolarizing currents, and almost linearly over a considerable range of current strengths. (From Loewenstein, W.R., and N. Ishiko: Effects of polarization of the receptor membrane and of the first Ranvier node in a sense organ. *J. Gen. Physiol.*, 43:981-998, 1960.)

These observations and also the failure of the generator potential to be actively transmitted along the receptor membrane indicate that the formation of the generator current differs basically from the production of a nerve action potential or nerve impulse.

The generator potential shows fluctuations with time which are much greater than those met in nerve and muscle fiber action potentials. Loewenstein (1961b) believes these fluctuations to be due to a continuous statistical variation in the number of active receptor sites on the nerve terminal membrane. The fluctuations increase with stimulus strength and thus with the area of membrane excited, up to a maximum point. The fluctuation in

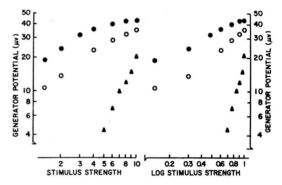

FIGURE 5-8. The effects of temperature on the generator potential. Solid circles, 35°C; open circles, 25°C; solid triangles, 15°C. The ordinates and abscissae are plotted logarithmically. The abscissa of the right-hand graph is on a log log scale. (From Ishiko, N., and W.R. Loewenstein: Effects of temperature on the generator and action potentials of a sense organ. *J. Gen. Physiol.*, 45: 105-124, 1961.)

excited sites could be expected to be proportional to the total area of excited membrane. Then, with a further rise in stimulus strength, the fluctuations fall again. This reduction probably occurs because, as the generator potential shows progressively smaller increases per additional equal area of excited membrane, it finally reaches a point where it is less affected by proportionately equivalent changes in the number of excited membrane sites (see Fig. 5-6A). The extent of fluctuation may be sufficient to give a generator potential a standard deviation of 8 per cent of its average amplitude.

The amplitude of the generator potential is a linear function of the logarithm of the sodium concentration in the fluid around the corpuscle's nerve ending. On this basis Diamond, Gray and Inman (1958) believe a cross-membrane transfer of charges, primarily by sodium ions, to give rise to the generator potential. Ozeki and Sato (1964) also consider the generator potential to be associated with membrane depolarization and to result from an increased membrane permeability to sodium and other ions.

Nishi (1968a) perfused the pacinian corpuscle with saline solutions modified by the absence of sodium, by the substitution of lithium for sodium, or by changing the concentration of potassium chloride or calcium chloride. Nishi observed that the sodium-free solution first raised the threshold for mechanical stimulation and prevented impulse formation in less than 8 minutes after the start of corpuscle perfusion. Lithium solution also elevated the threshold, but impulse generation terminated only 22 minutes after the initial employment of the solution. Calcium and potassium ions did not appear to have a direct effect on the generator potential.

It was thus shown that sodium and lithium ions have a very significant role in the development of the generator potential. However, the absence of sodium probably brings about the abolition of impulses by directly affecting the impulse-generating mechanism rather than by producing a large decrement in the generator potential.

When Sato, Ozeki and Nishi (1968) replaced the normal saline solution around an almost decapsulated pacinian core with choline solution, the amplitude of the generator potentials fell 50 to 75 per cent in 60 to 90 minutes. If lithium solution was used, the generator potentials decreased only 30 per cent in amplitude during the same time span. These findings seem to confirm that lithium ions can replace sodium ions in the initiation of the generator potential. Lithium ions are thought to reduce the generator potential by accumulating inside the sensory ending.

The inner core of the pacinian corpuscle, which surrounds the nerve ending, is composed of the processes of lamellar cells. These processes contain a large number of vacuoles, ranging from 250 to 600 Å in diameter. In functional corpuscles the vacuoles contribute their contents to the capsular fluid surrounding the nerve ending. This may affect the ionic composition of this fluid and change the ending's level of excitability (Cherepnov, 1968a, b).

Since the generator potential follows a drop in the electrical resistance of the membrane and an increase in its ion permeability, as is the case for nerve action potentials, the active receptor sites may perhaps best be thought of as openings in the membrane. Thus any mechanical deformation of the nerve-ending membrane resulting in distension could cause pores to open in the membrane. A greater distension or increase in the surface area of the membrane would then produce a greater number of open pores and result in a larger amount of ion movement and a greater generator potential. In this way the amplitude of the generator potential could reflect the strength of the stimulus.

Unlike the case in nerve axon membranes and sarcolemma, in the nerve terminal membrane of the pacinian corpuscle the scattered receptor sites are functionally independent. These sites of the transduction of mechanical to electrical energy also cannot be activated by passing a current through them.

Loewenstein and Cohen (1959a, b) found that continued high-frequency stimulation of the pacinian corpuscle can produce its inactivation. Thus after 180 identical stimuli at a frequency of 500/sec, the generator potential may be only 20 per cent of its original amplitude, and it may cease to appear after 10,000 such stimuli. This depression of the generator potential, i.e. of charge transfer, can be called forth with subthreshold stimuli, is independent of the resting membrane potential and is completely reversible. Depression of the potential becomes greater with increased stimulus strength, frequency and duration. The depressive effect was shown to be due to inactivation, apparently of localized sites, in the nerve terminal membrane.

Il'Inskii (1965) observed that while depolarization is called forth by a stimulus in one corpuscle position, hyperpolarization is evoked after a rotation of 90 degrees.

Il'Inskii, Volkova and Cherepnov (1968) noted that primary hyperpolarization could be produced only by mechanical stimulation of the corpuscle along the greater transverse axis of the nerve ending. Nishi and Sato (1968), while mechanically stimulating the decapsulated nerve ending, found direction to have a similar significance. When compression was applied along the short axis of the bare nerve ending, depolarization was obtained. Compression along the long axis produced hyperpolarization.

Il'Inskii (1965) has offered, and extensively confirmed (Il'Inskii, 1966a), an explanation for the significance of stimulus orientation. He indicates that when compression is applied along the short axis of the elliptically cylindrical nerve ending, an increase in the surface area of the neural membrane is produced. This results in the opening of pores and in depolarization. However, compression exerted along the long axis of the sensory ending, by lowering the ratio of the long axis to the short axis, reduces the membrane's surface area. The consequence is hyperpolarization.

Presumably a reduction in the membrane surface would lead to a somewhat lower sodium permeability. The magnitude of the depolarization far exceeded the extent of the obtained hyperpolarizations.

The bilaterally symmetrical structure of the pacinian corpuscle's inner core is more suitable for compression along the short axis, this evoking the depolarizing potential (Nishi and Sato, 1968).

According to Nishi and Sato (1968), when a mechanical stimulus which has elicited a depolarizing potential in the complete pacinian corpuscle is terminated, hyperpolarization ensues, and vice versa. Il'Inskii (1966b) postulates that a rebound of the ending membrane is responsible for these phenomena. Thus, when the ratio of the long axis to the short axis of the membrane has been elevated by the stimulus, causing an increase in surface, the poststimulatory rebound of the elastic lamellae would temporarily reduce the said ratio and the ending's membrane surface to below the normal level.

However, Loewenstein (1965) and Nishi and Sato (1968), unlike Il'Inskii (1966b), have observed hyperpolarization following the removal of a depolarizing mechanical stimulus from a decapsulated ending. The first two groups of investigators may not have removed

all the lamellae of the inner core.

The hyperpolarization which appears even on the gradual termination of compression may in turn be succeeded by depolarization. The last may result in an action potential, the "off" response (Nishi and Sato, 1968). In the view of Nishi and Sato the "off" response of the pacinian corpuscle is a "posthyperpolarization" response.

After the cessation of a depolarizing mechanical stimulus, a period of reduced responsiveness, or of hyperpolarization, is evident as well in tonic mechanoreceptors.

A period of depression (hyperpolarization) which appears shortly after the start of a single, maintained depolarizing stimulus in intact pacinian corpuscles may also be analogous to the release phenomenon of tonic mechanoreceptors (Loewenstein, 1965). Such a period of lower reactivity in the intact corpuscle marks the termination of the dynamic phase of stimulation, the end of the last being due to the effects of the elastic components of the capsule.

A normal refractory period does not follow a generator potential in the corpuscle's receptor membrane (Discussion, Loewenstein, 1965).

Il'Inskii and Volkova (1966) found the orientation of the corpuscle relative to the stimulus to affect the observed latent period. They reported that if a pacinian corpuscle is oriented in respect to the mechanical stimulus so as to result in the shortest latent period, a longitudinal rotation of 90 degrees produces the longest latent period. Further rotation through 180 degrees is followed by a return to the original duration of the latent period. Il'Inskii, Volkova and Cherepnov (1968) observed stimulation along the small transverse axis of the elliptical sensory nerve ending to result in the shortest latent periods.

The variation in latent period with orientation of the pacinian corpuscle is probably consequent to the development of unlike responses, depolarizing or hyperpolarizing, at different corpuscle-to-stimulus orientations.

Further, noticeably higher thresholds are

obtained if the pacinian corpuscle is stimulated along its longitudinal axis (Il'Inskii, Volkova and Cherepnov (1968).

Summary and Discussion

It thus appears that a mechanical stimulus impinging on the pacinian corpuscle is transformed by the elements of the capsule and that this modified mechanical force then acts to deform the membrane of the nerve terminal. This membrane is the transducer site; it translates a mechanical deformation into the electrical energy of the receptor (generator) potential.

Goldman (1965) generalizes the above scheme to all mechanoreceptors and suggests that the transducer is active, or supplies energy to produce its output. Receptor potentials are known to be greatly dependent on oxygen supply and to be affected by metabolic inhibitors.

Goldman also points out that differences in the sensitivities of the various kinds of mechanoreceptors can be due to the nature of their external, surrounding transformer elements. For example, the external, nonnervous elements of a receptor may diffuse, concentrate, or change the direction of a mechanical stimulus. They may transform mechanical pressure into a shearing force.

In the case of the crustacean stretch receptor (see Chap. II, The Crustacean Stretch Receptor—An Examination), as in the pacinian corpuscle, elastic transformer elements bring about a loss of stimulus energy. In the tonic stretch receptor these elements consist of elastic, reversible stretch components of the muscle. Irreversible, plastic stretching further produces a reduction in the sensitivity of the stretch receptor (Wendler, 1963).

Differences in sensitivity may further rest on the relation of the transducer membrane to the transformer structures. Thus in crustacean statocysts and stretch receptors, the sensory neuron may be so attached in the sense organ that an impinging mechanical force will cause the transducer membrane to be stretched.

Julian and Goldman (1962) applied sub-

threshold mechanical (compressive) stimuli to lobster (*Homarus*) giant axons and concluded that these act by stretching the axon membrane. Recent findings also indicate that effective mechanical stimuli act on pacinian corpuscles by causing their transducer membranes to stretch (Il'Inskii and Volkova, 1966; Il'Inskii, Volkova and Cherepnov, 1968).

Such stretching would result in increased ion permeability and thus lead to a receptor potential.

Wolbarsht (1960) infers that mechanical distortion of the insect mechanoreceptor hair leads to increased nerve membrane permeability. Thurm (1965) suggests that a mechanical stimulus distorts the nerve ending of the bee's hair plate sensillum by compression through the cuticular cap. Stimuli probably also act by compression on the chordotonal and campaniform receptors of arthropods. Görner (1965) believes that in the case of the trichobothria of *Tegenaria* spiders, the stimulus acts by inclining the nerve ending over the edge of the hair helmet. Ottoson and Shepherd (1965) indicate that the membrane of the sensory terminals of the muscle spindle also shows increased ion permeability and charge transfer (primarily by sodium ions) on stimulation, this resulting in a depolarization.

That the receptor sites of the pacinian corpuscle's transducer membrane cannot be stimulated with an electric current can be shown by sending an antidromic electrical impulse into the nerve terminal and by direct electrical stimulation of the nerve ending. This nonreactivity of the pacinian corpuscle's transducer membrane to electrical stimulation mirrors the similar resistance of a large group of transducer membranes. Thus Terzuolo and Washizu (1962) showed that an antidromic impulse does not reach or excite the sensory terminals of the stretch receptor of the crayfish (*Cambarus*). In fact, one can state that generally the receptor region of sensory neurons cannot be excited electrically (Grundfest, 1965). The resistance of such transducer membranes to electrical stimulation may keep their own receptor potentials from affecting their responses.

However, a portion of the receptor sites of some transducer membranes are responsive to electrical stimuli, and these may be reactive not only to depolarization but to hyperpolarizing stimuli as well. The result may be increased permeability in the case of an activating process or reduced permeability consequent to an inactivating process (Grundfest, 1965).

The resistance of the pacinian corpuscle's generator potential to pharmaceuticals also reflects the nature of receptor generator potentials as a group.

The Origin of the Nerve Impulse in the Pacinian Corpuscle

A number of researchers, including Loewenstein (1960a), have indicated that the nerve impulse emanating from the pacinian corpuscle originates at the first node of Ranvier, on a portion of myelinated nerve fiber within the corpuscle. Thus Diamond, Gray and Sato (1956) report only a graded generator potential at the unmyelinated nerve ending, followed by all-or-nothing action potentials at the first and second nodes of Ranvier.

However, Hunt and Tackeuchi (1962) and Ozeki and Sato (1964) report that the unmyelinated nerve ending in the pacinian corpuscle is the site of formation of the all-or-nothing nerve impulse. Ozeki and Sato found this action potential to be transmitted over the nerve ending at an average speed of 1.6 meters/sec. The amplitude of the action potential was inversely related to the stimulus strength.

The above relationship is based on the shunting action of the ending's membrane, its

permeability to sodium ions increasing with the magnitude of the stimulus.

The absolute refractory period of the bare nerve ending has been determined to be close to 2 msec, and its relative refractory period to be approximately 10 msec.

According to Ozeki and Sato (1964), impulse formation at the bare terminal follows the flow of a graded generator current across the nerve membrane.

Ozeki and Sato suggest that the cause of the failure of previous investigators to observe the formation of the action potential at the bare nerve ending lies in the electrical peculiarities of the receptor.

On perfusing pacinian corpuscles with 0.03 per cent procaine, Nishi (1968b) noted that impulses from the corpuscle were quickly blocked, while the threshold for mechanical stimuli was not significantly elevated for several minutes. Nishi concluded that the formation of generator potentials is probably less affected by local anesthesia than the initiation of impulses at the corpuscle's terminal, and that the receptor potential—and impulse—generating mechanisms differ.

Similar results have been reported from frog muscle spindles (Ottoson, 1965) and from crayfish stretch receptors (Eyzaguirre and Kuffler, 1955).

The action of calcium ions on impulse initiation appears to compete with that of procaine. The effect of procaine on impulse formation was enhanced by lowering the calcium ion concentration and reduced by raising the calcium ion concentration (Nishi, 1968b). Such competitive action between calcium and procaine has also been observed in the nervous system.

GUSTATORY RECEPTION

General

Taste receptors may be sensory neurons (insect chemoreceptors) or secondary sense cells (vertebrate taste cells). In the case of the former the dendrites of the gustatory neurons extend to the tip of a chemosensory hair,

where they are exposed to gustatory stimuli through the distal orifice of the hair. The taste cells of vertebrates possess distal processes or microvilli (2.0μ x 0.1μ in mammals) which extend into the taste pore superficial to the taste cells of a taste bud. In higher vertebrates these microvilli are exposed to the saliva.

It is therefore at the distal ends of the dendrites of insect sensory neurons and at the microvilli of the taste cells of vertebrates that gustatory stimulation must mainly take place. According to Farbman (1965), the microvilli are specialized in having an unusually thin surface plasma membrane; it measures only 90 Å in comparison with the 120 to 130 Å thickness of the plasma cell membrane lining the rest of the taste cell. However, Murray and Murray (1967) did not observe such differential membrane widths.

In vertebrates bare nerve endings located between taste cells and close to the taste pore may also subserve gustation. Thus Kimura and Beidler (1961) have found discrepancies between the responses to salts of single taste cells and those recorded from their subjacent taste nerve fibers. If 1.0M barium chloride is flown over the rat's tongue, a steady level of response is soon obtained, but then the nerve activity begins to rise. If the barium chloride is now rinsed off, the discharge falls only very slowly. These observations suggest that after an interval barium chloride may reach subsurface nerve endings. Alcohol also may act directly on bare fibers, those of the trigeminal portion of the lingual nerve (Hellekant, 1967). Such bare nerve endings may be able to display some specificity in their responses, as is true of olfactory trigeminal nerve endings.

Beidler (1965), in order to study the responses of the rat tongue's bare nerve endings, removed the tongue's epithelium with collagenase. Most normal taste stimuli did not now evoke a response in the chorda tympani nerve; only very concentrated inorganic salts and sometimes sugars and acids did. The responses to these effective stimuli appeared after a long latent period and continued to rise until the stimuli were rinsed off. Continued stimulation produced a temporary loss of sensitivity.

The lingual nerve carries the fibers which form bare nerve endings in the tongue. Recordings from the lingual nerve of the normal rat's tongue also showed that only very con-

centrated stimuli elicit responses in these fibers. Such responses again had a lengthy latent period, and they rose until the stimulus was washed off.

Certain organisms may obtain considerable chemosensory information from free nerve endings. In fish like the sea robin free nerve endings serving the fins seem to have a gustatory function.

However, for the purposes of the present discussion the responses of bare nerve endings are not relevant.

Kare (1968) and other investigators have found evidence that taste substances are directly absorbed from the oral cavity and then quickly go to the brain. The esophagus of experimental rats was tied off and their trachea was cannulated prior to introducing radioactively labeled glucose and sodium into their oral cavity. After waiting for one, two or three minutes, the rats were sacrificed and autopsied, and radioactivity was found in their brain. If the animals were sacrificed one or two minutes after the labeled taste stimuli were placed in their mouth, all radioactivity was localized in the brain. When the same labeled taste solutions were introduced into the gut of control rats, radioactivity was primarily noted in the liver and the blood, and there was very little of it in the brain.

Kare *et al.* (1969) determined that in rats ^{14}C-glucose travels from the oropharynx to the intracranial cavity by way of all the tissues of the head. No preferential pathway to the brain could be identified, and typically the parts of the brain nearest the oropharynx contained the greatest concentration of labeled glucose.

Perfusion of the head region after 4 minutes with normal saline introduced into the ascending aorta failed to affect the distribution of the radioactivity. Also, little radioactivity was present in a 4-minute cardiac blood sample. These observations contraindicate a circulatory route for craniad movement of the glucose.

Apparently taste particles travel directly from the oropharynx to the brain by nonspecific diffusion. Kare (1968) reported that oral stimulants seem to move to the brain within fifteen seconds.

Nevertheless, taste stimuli act primarily at a surface of the taste receptor. This surface, like the other surfaces of the receptor cell, is formed by the cell plasma membrane. It is therefore the composition and structure of the cell membrane, and in particular of that portion of it at the surface exposed to taste stimuli, which determines the nature of the first step in the taste response.

The Cell Membrane

Cell membranes, according to the Danielli model, appear to be basically composed of two inner layers of radially oriented phospholipid molecules and two surface layers of tangentially oriented protein molecules. The hydrophobic, hydrocarbon ends of the phospholipid molecules point inward, are adjacent to each other and are held together by London and Van der Walls forces. The hydrophilic, polar groups of the phospholipids, consisting of their organic phosphate portions, face outward. They are attached at the inner and the outer surface of the cell membrane to the tangentially oriented surface protein molecules by means of dipole or ionic attractions or by hydrogen bonds.

The interior double layer of primarily phospholipid, and also some cholesterol, molecules is estimated to be about 51 Å thick. The erythrocyte membrane's lipid, by dry weight, is 65 per cent phospholipid and 24 per cent cholesterol. The negatively charged phosphate groups of the phospholipids of taste receptor membranes can apparently bind ions and molecules. A similar action has also been proposed for the positively charged nitrogen bases in the organic phosphates of the phospholipids.

The inner bimolecular lipid layer of cell membranes permits the ready passage of many fat-soluble substances and gives cell membranes an electrical capacitance of approximately $1\mu F/cm^2$. However, there may also be water-filled spaces between the lipid molecules which permit water-soluble molecules and ions to cross the cell membrane; or perhaps, instead, water-soluble molecules simply slip between the phospholipid molecules. Pinocytosis too may sometimes play a role. Electron microscope studies show a honeycomb type of ultrastructure in some cell membranes (also beneath the outer envelope in the nuclear membrane of *Amoeba proteus*), and no interlipid spaces have been observed (above a 7 Å limit of resolution).

At a 1967 meeting Wallach offered a hypothetical submolecular cell membrane structure in which protein helixes at the inner and outer surfaces of the membrane present their hydrophobic groups to the membrane's interior phospholipids; there would be considerable interaction between these hydrophobic protein portions and the phospholipids. The hydrophilic parts of the protein chains penetrate through the interior of the membrane and form pores. The last would permit the passage of water and water-soluble substances.

Optical rotatory dispersion and circular dichroism spectra of the membranes of *Bacillus subtilis* and human erythrocytes indicate that approximately one third to one quarter of their protein is in a helical shape, while the rest may form random coils. There is evidence that these features are common to the proteins of different membrane systems (Lenard and Singer, 1966).

Electron microscope studies have demonstrated protein structures in the interior of biological membranes. Also, a "red shift" has been noted in the spectra of proteins *in situ* within the membrane. This means that the minima, maxima and inversion points of these spectra are displaced several millimicrons in the direction of longer wavelengths when compared to the spectra of α-helical proteins in solution. The spectra of the membrane proteins further have a lesser peak-to-peak amplitude. Korn believes that the two hypotheses offered for the "red shift" both demand that α-helixes of membrane protein lie within a comparatively hydrophobic zone (Bernhard, 1969).

A modification of Wallach's proposed membrane structure has been advanced by Sjöstrand. He suggested that the membrane phospholipids extend into spaces within the hydrophobic sections of the helix proteins. This would hold the two major components of the membrane together (Chance, 1968).

The last hypothesis is supported by what has been learned of the structure of cytochrome c, which is found in membranes. X-ray diffraction has shown that a hydrophobic space is located on the inner surface of this enzyme (Chance, 1968).

Green has proposed a membrane model which would allow the cell membrane to assume three distinct conformations (Bernhard, 1969).

At the surfaces of the cell membrane the parallel protein chains are attracted to each other by dipole or ionic forces or are bound together by hydrogen bonds. Between these protein chains are groups of water molecules. In myelin the protein chains appear to be 9.8 Å apart, and a distance of 3.33 Å has been calculated to separate their side chains (Vandenheuvel, 1965). The protein molecules contain numerous amino acid groups that are charged and could interact with stimulating ions and molecules. There are more anionic than cationic amino acid groups.

It has been pointed out that changes at the level of interactions between protein molecules or some other membrane subunit reorganization might be involved in the transmission of negative membrane potentials (Chance, 1968).

Cell membranes may further contain polysaccharide molecules, which are probably chiefly associated with the hydrophilic ends of the phospholipid layer pointing toward the outer surface.

Although cell membranes are primarily lipoprotein membranes and generally have the basic composition described above, they may differ between cell types and species in the kinds and proportions of their proteins, lipids and polysaccharides. It has even been shown that different portions of a single cell membrane may be unlike. The cell membrane has been described as a mosaic of heterogeneous functional units which often shows regional variations in thickness, stratification and enzyme activities.

That the inner and outer surfaces of cell membranes are not identical has been demonstrated with divalent ions and tetrodotoxin. Divalent ions kill the nerve cell membrane only if they approach it from the inside, while tetrodotoxin has its effect only when it reaches the membrane from the outside.

The Origin of the Gustatory Receptor Potential

It is generally believed that in taste receptors the receptor potential arises, like in mechanoreceptors, as a result of increased ion permeability on the part of the active cell membrane. How this greater ion permeability comes about is still not known, but it has been hypothesized that the ions or molecules of chemical stimuli loosely combine or react with receptor sites in the exposed taste receptor cell membrane. Such combination could produce a small, localized change in the structure of the macromolecule forming the receptor site and thus result in the opening of a pore, initiating charge transfer.

Potentials across presumably the cell plasma membranes of mammalian taste cells have been measured both before and during the application of a chemical stimulus to the tongue, by inserting ultra-microelectrodes into taste buds (Kimura and Beidler, 1961; Tateda and Beidler, 1964). It was found that the interiors of what were considered hamster and rat taste cells are normally negative to the outside, and that there exists a 10 to 50 mV potential across the presumed unstimulated taste cell membrane. A chemical stimulus (cocaine, iron chloride) produced a depolarization of this membrane. However, this depolarization reached its peak amplitude slowly, was long lasting, and cannot clearly be described as a receptor potential. Since the microelectrode could not be placed with precision, it can only be said that stimulation resulted in a depolarization, i.e. a considerable increase in the permeability, of the presumed taste cell membrane at some distance from the microvilli. The process resulting in the recorded depolarization must then have travelled at least 15μ to 30μ from the microvilli within some milliseconds. A response was produced by all applied chemicals, but the degree of membrane depolarization, which never exceeded 40 mV, varied with the chemical stimulus employed. It would thus appear that the ionic concentration gradient across the membrane of the gustatory receptor is the source of the original energy required for a taste response, as holds true for instance for mechanoreceptors.

But how could the opening of cell membrane pores, i.e. increased membrane permeability, lead to the original depolarization of the microvilli or the distal tip of the dendrite of a sensory neuron? Here a difficulty is encountered, for while nerve axons or mechanoreceptors are bathed in tissue fluid, the solution outside the microvilli or the sensory dendrite tip may only be water or contain only large nonelectrolyte molecules. Yet in the case of the flesh fly (*Boettcherisca peregrina*) water applied to the tip of the chemosensory hair elicits a response from both the water receptor and the salt receptor (Morita, 1967).

Morita (1967) deals with this problem by hypothesizing that when for instance water or a sucrose solution is applied to the chemosensory hair tip, ions diffuse from the extracellular fluid within the hair to outside the receptor surface of the sensory dendrite's distal end. The cations which are now found outside the receptor membrane can move through it when pores open in the membrane as a consequence of stimulus action, and this entrance of cations results in depolarization and represents the receptor membrane current. Morita's findings indicate the dendrite tip's membrane is permeable to all cations. As evidence for his hypothesis Morita cites that dissolving sucrose in concentrations of less than one molal sodium chloride enhanced the response in proportion to the chemical potential of the sodium chloride present.

Beidler (1961b, 1963) has postulated that

when pores open in the receptor membrane surface, potassium ions diffuse out of the receptor.

Beidler (1967), dealing with the mammalian taste cell, however, instead suggests that the cell plasma membrane of the microvilli may differ from the membrane of other regions of the cell and is impermeable to electrolytes. He bases himself on the consideration that otherwise, when the potassium chloride concentration outside the cell is equal to that inside, the membrane potential should drop to zero. Further, potassium chloride levels above or below this concentration should respectively increase or reduce taste responses. In reality, however, as the concentration of a stimulating potassium chloride solution is raised, the response continues to increase until at higher concentrations saturation of the receptors is attained and the response-concentration curve levels off.

Duncan (1964) has proposed that taste stimulation deforms the cell membrane of the vertebrate taste receptor's microvilli, but thus only initiates a series of steps resulting in an increase in the permeability of the lateral membrane, outside of which is tissue fluid.

Beidler (1953), by electrophysiologically recording the results of stimulating the rat's tongue with sodium chloride, found that the primary taste reaction must take place at the surface of the taste cell, since, after application of 0.2M sodium chloride, a latent period of only 50 msec elapsed before the response. Protein and nucleic acid molecules are good candidates for the receptor molecules on the cell surface. The role of such molecules in taste responses is made all the more likely by the marked species differences in taste. Proteins are known to be highly species specific.

The time for response to taste solutions on the tongue has even been shortened to 20 to 25 msec by later observations (Beidler, 1965). The chemosensory neurons of the blowfly may show a latent period of only 3 msec (Browne and Hodgson, 1962), but this very low value partially reflects the absence of an intervening secondary sense cell. Additional evidence for a primary taste response on the cell's sur-

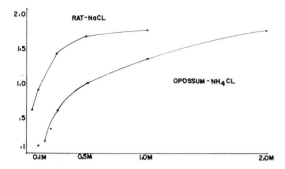

FIGURE 5-9. Response-concentration curves of the rat and the opossum for their respective most stimulating salts. Ordinate, values of ratios of integrated chorda tympani response to response called forth by standard of 0.1M sodium chloride (rat) or 0.5M ammonium chloride (opossum). See Figures 5-11 and 5-12. Abscissa, molar concentration. The rat's response to 1.0M sodium chloride was made equal to the opossum's response to 2.0M ammonium chloride to facilitate comparison of the curves. The rat is more sensitive to dilute solutions of its most stimulating salt, and its receptors are saturated at a lower concentration. The two low-concentration values not included in the opossum's curve suggest that this curve may be S-shaped.

face membrane is the fact that 0.1M sodium cyanide, a rapidly acting poison, can elicit a taste response (Beidler, 1961a, b). Further, 0.1M sodium cyanide, 10 mM strychnine and acids with a pH of 2.5 can all produce a taste response without destroying the receptor cell if they are quickly washed off.

A loose combination of the stimulus molecule with the receptor structure is indicated by the complete and rapid reversibility of gustatory responses (Beidler, 1954). Beidler (1953) also found taste responses to be time independent, determined primarily by the cation of a compound, and to approach a maximum level, or saturation, with increasing stimulus concentration (Fig. 5-9). The concentration producing saturation varies between salts as well as between sugars and between bitter substances.

Taste Equations

Beidler (1954) developed a hyperbolic equation which permits one to determine the entire curve of response versus concentration (Fig. 5-9) for many simply acting taste stimuli and also the equilibrium constant (usually about 8-15 liter/mole, but sometimes as high as 1500 liter/mole), provided one knows two points on the said response-stimulus curve. This equation is based on the mass action law and the assumption that the employed stimulating molecules or ions are each subject to adsorption by one of only a definite number of similar, unfilled receptor sites. A monomolecular reaction is considered to take place. The use of Beidler's equation also rests on the apparently correct supposition that taste responses reach a condition of equilibrium rather than a steady state. The equation can be expressed as:

$$KC = \frac{S}{T-S} \qquad (1)$$

in which K is the equilibrium constant, and has a value directly related to the affinities of the receptor sites for the stimulus, C is the concentration of the taste stimulus, S represents the number of receptor sites which have adsorbed the taste molecules or ions, and T is the total number of receptor sites present and subject to the stimulus.

Beidler then assumes that the extent of the neural response is proportional to the number of receptor sites S at which adsorption has taken place, or

$$Response\ R = x\ S$$

in which x is a constant.

Similarly, the greatest possible neural response, at saturation of all the available receptor sites, should be proportional to the total number of sites T subject to stimulation, or

$$Greatest\ Response\ Rg = x\ T$$

Substituting R for S and Rg for T in equation (1) (the proportionality constants cancel), we get

$$KC = \frac{R}{Rg-R} \qquad (2)$$

which can easily be converted into the final form of Beidler's fundamental equation,

$$\frac{C}{R} = \frac{C}{Rg} + \frac{1}{KRg} \qquad (3)$$

This equation expresses the relationship between the concentration of a taste stimulus and the size of the neural response. If the ratio concentration divided by response (C/R) is graphed against concentration (C), a straight line should be obtained if the equation is correct. Its slope should be 1/Rg, and it should intercept the ordinate at 1/KRg. Beidler found the curves obtained by use of his fundamental equation to closely coincide with those he drew from experimental data, with the exception of the curves for potassium chloride stimulation. The steady-level integrated activity of the many fibers of the mammalian taste nerve is the source of Beidler's experimental data.

Evans and Mellon, Jr. (1962b), who used chemoreceptor hairs of the blowfly (*Phormia regina*), also found Beidler's fundamental equation to provide response-stimulus curves which correlate well with experimental results. These authors, as well as Dethier (1962), share Beidler's view that the first step in the gustatory response involves the adsorption of stimulating molecules by receptor sites on the surface of the taste cell membrane.

On the other hand, Beidler himself reported the poor application of his equation to responses elicited by potassium chloride. He attempted to explain the divergence between the computations obtained by use of his equation and the experimental results of potassium chloride stimulation by hypothesizing two separate, different sites for potassium chloride adsorption. Yamashita, Akaike and Sato (1963) also found the results from Beidler's equation to be in poor agreement with experimental data from potassium chloride and from calcium chloride stimulation of the rat's tongue.

Tateda (1967) reported that stimulus-response curves obtained by electrophysiological recording from the rat's chorda tympani nerve of that animal's responses to stimulation with D-fructose and D-glucose did not coincide with those obtained from Beidler's equation. However, the sucrose stimulus-response curve for lower concentrations did seem to verify the Beidler equation. Diamant, Funakoshi, Ström and Zotterman (1963) recorded responses to sucrose from man's chorda tympani, and these results also coincided with those predicted by the Beidler equation. The results obtained by recording the rat's responses to α-amino acids do not fit well with Beidler's taste equation (Halpern, Bernard and Kare, 1962). Some of the possible causes for the above discrepancies will be explored in the second part of this section, on membrane surface events.

Stone (1967) has rearranged Beidler's equation into the form

$$\frac{R}{Rg} = \frac{CK}{CK + 1}$$

in order that graphing it will produce a straight line with a slope of one. Stone's results from psychophysical taste testing of amino acids on man appear to verify the correctness of the Beidler equation.

Tateda (1967) has modified Beidler's fundamental taste equation to develop an equation for the case where all the stimulated receptor sites are not combined with just one molecule, but different percentages of the receptor sites are each complexed, respectively, with one, two, or more stimulus molecules. Thus stimulation of receptor sites on the rat's tongue with glycine may result in unstable receptor site-glycine combinations which are amenable to complexing with additional glycine molecules. Tateda states his equation as

$$\log \frac{R}{R_h - R} = n \log C + \log K$$

in which R_h is the greatest response produced by a high concentration of the stimulus and n represents a whole number.

An equation describing the behavior of a taste stimulus in the presence of another which competes with it for the same receptor sites has also been given (Beidler, 1961a). If there is competitive inhibition of the response to substance X by substance Z, the response to X can be described by:

$$\text{Response to } X(R_x) = \frac{Rg_x K_x C_x}{1 + K_x C_x + K_z C_z}$$

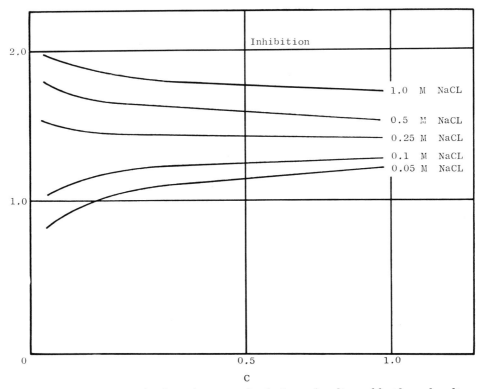

FIGURE 5-10. Responses (ordinate) to mixed solutions of sodium chloride and sodium butyrate at different concentrations (*C*) of sodium butyrate. As the concentration of sodium butyrate is raised, the response to the more concentrated sodium chloride solutions falls because of competition between the chloride and butyrate anions. (From Beidler, L.M.: Taste receptor stimulation. *Progr. Biophys. Biophys. Chem.,* 12:107-151, 1961 [Pergamon Press].)

A like equation would indicate the response to substance Z, and the full response to the mixed stimuli would be obtained by adding the values calculated from each equation.

Competitive inhibition becomes noticeable only when the total of stimulating molecules and/or ions exceeds the number of similar receptor sites with which both substances can interact (Fig. 5-10). Therefore high concentrations of stimuli are used for the investigation of possible competitive inhibition.

The higher the equilibrium constant K (or the affinity for the receptor sites) of a substance, and the lower its maximum response, the greater will be its observed inhibition of the response to the competing stimulus.

The reverse situation, in which a substance reacts with two different types of taste cells,

and the total response to the substance is therefore a sum of the responses from the two groups of receptors, has been given an interesting treatment by Yamashita *et al.* (1967b).

Since in the hamster saccharin combines with both sodium chloride-sensitive receptors and the clearly different sucrose receptors, the total response to saccharin (T) was viewed as the combination of the separate responses to sucrose (U) and to sodium chloride (S), or

Total saccharin response $T = mU + nS + p$ The partial correlation coefficients were determined between, respectively, the level of the responses to 0.02M saccharin and to 0.1M sodium chloride, and the magnitude of the responses to 0.02M saccharin and to 0.5M sucrose. There was a close correlation between the responses to saccharin and to sodium chloride, and a good correlation between the responses to saccharin and to sucrose. Yamashita *et al.* conclude that the nerve impulses produced by a concentration of saccharin are equivalent to the sum of a number of impulses elicited by sodium chloride and a number of sucrose-produced impulses. Thus saccharin must call forth a salty-sweet taste in the hamster, although the ratio of salty to sweet in the total taste effect can change with the saccharin concentration. Yamashita *et al.* suggest that their approach may be generally valid for the case of substances which stimulate more than one type of receptor cell.

Beidler (1961a) has formulated the minimum concentration C_m of a stimulus needed to produce a steady threshold response as being related to the reciprocal of the equilibrium constant K multiplied by the greatest response Rg produced by the stimulus at saturation concentration. Thus

$$C_m \sim \frac{1}{KRg}$$

The steady level threshold response is conceived of as an electrophysiological phenomenon. It should be just discernable with electronic instrumentation or would be barely above the innate noise level of the equipment.

The threshold concentration of a taste stimulus is thus determined by the degree of binding of the stimulus to its receptor sites (as indicated by the equilibrium constant) and by the number of available receptor sites.

Deutsch and Hansch (1966) used an equation which had previously been successfully employed to describe other biological systems (Hansch and Fujita, 1964) to elucidate the factors involved in producing the sweet taste. In this formulation the observed relative sweet taste (ST) is a function of the constant for hydrophobic bonding (B), the free energy-related Hammett constant (H), and rate or equilibrium constants $(a, a^1, a^{11}, a^{111})$ for the stimulus-receptor site interaction. Thus

$$\log ST = -aB^2 + a^1B + a^{11}H + a^{111}$$
$$(4)$$

As is true of the Hammett constant (H), B is related to free energy. It reflects the relative change in free energy which results from transferring a derivative into a different phase. B is equal to the log of the ratio of the partition coefficient between octanol and water (C_d) of a derivative of the substance in question to the partition coefficient between octanol and water (C_q) of the substance itself, or

$$B = \log \frac{Cd}{Cq} \qquad (5)$$

Deutsch and Hansch used equation (4) to determine the role of hydrophobic bonding and basic groups in producing the sweet taste.

The change in free energy, ΔE, involved in taste responses can be determined from the equation

$$\Delta E = -Rt \ln K$$

in which t represents time (Beidler, 1963). The change in free energy is indicative of the strength by which the stimulus is bound to the receptor, and this free energy usually has values of several kilocalories per mole. These free-energy values support the conception that the first step of the taste response consists of a combination of the stimulus with a surface receptor site. They also indicate that the stimulus-receptor site interaction is a weak one.

The change in entropy is positive. This could mean a loss of water of hydration or a configurational change in the receptor molecules, or both, during a taste response.

Selected Aspects of Taste Responses

Nejad (1961) has suggested that several steps are involved in taste responses and that a number of the later steps are of an enzymatic nature. He found that the application of not only mercuric chloride ($HgCl_2$), but also of iodoacetic acid to the tongue prevented taste responses. Iodoacetic acid reacts with sulfhydryl (SH) groups, and if the tongue was immersed in cysteine, which can provide sulfhydryl groups, before the application of iodoacetic acid, the last did not block taste responses. Nejad (1961) therefore indicated that a secondary process in the gustatory response involves sulfhydryl groups. The role of sulfhydryl groups in the gustatory response was further established by Yur'eva (1961). This investigator showed that guanidine, a substance which acts to expose masked sulfhydryl groups, greatly increases the size and length of taste responses when applied to the frog's tongue. The enhancing action of guanidine could be counteracted by use of cadmium chloride ($CdCl_2$), which reacts with sulfhydryl groups. The effect of cadmium chloride could in turn be eliminated by the addition of compounds supplying sulfhydryl groups. Duncan (1964) has hypothesized that in the taste cell sulfhydryl groups cause ATPase to initiate the breakdown of ATP, releasing energy for the receptor potential.

It has also been suggested, on the basis of experimental evidence (Nejad, 1961; Pfaffmann, 1959), that a later, secondary step among those making up the gustatory response is significantly affected by temperature.

In the cat, taste sensitivity seems to be greatest at or a little above 30°C (Sato, 1963; Yamashita *et al.*, 1964), while human behavioral studies show man to have the highest taste sensitivity at generally 30° to 40°C. The lowest human thresholds for quinine and for 6-n-propylthiouracil have been said to appear at about 22°C (Fischer, Griffin and Rockey, 1966). There appears to be no optimum temperature for taste sensitivity in the poikilothermic frog.

Iwayama and Nada (1967a) investigated ATPase activity in the circumvallate, foliate and fungiform papillae of rats. They found ATPase to be most concentrated at the surface membranes of all the cells of each taste bud. The region of the microvilli showed especially great activity. However, ATPase activity was also very high in the cores of the papillae, where it was presumably centered in capillary walls and nervous tissue. These results could be confirmed for the rat

and rabbit (Iwayama and Nada, 1967b). In the rat and rabbit ganglion cells, nerve fibers (Schwann cells?) and blood vessel walls of the lamina propria showed considerable ATPase activity.

When PCMB, a specific SH group inhibitor, was previously applied to the sections, ATPase was totally inactivated (Iwayama and Nada, 1967b).

The significance of ATP for taste responses is discussed in The General Mechanism Of The Receptor Response, Chapter III.

Cholinesterases have been observed to be localized at the bases of taste buds in both the vallate papillae of rats and the foliate papillae of rabbits (Tsuchiya, Suzuki and Okui, 1969a). Two different cholinesterases could be identified. As the mentioned taste papillae contain large quantities of cholinesterases and hold many other esterases, it seems quite possible that esterases have a part in the gustatory process (Tsuchiya, Suzuki and Okui, 1969b).

Since cholinesterase activity in the vicinity of rat taste buds is inhibited by a number of bitter taste substances, Tsuchiya and Aoki (1967) suggest that such inhibition of the action of cholinesterase may be involved in the bitter taste. The degree of bitterness of such bitter substances to man somewhat parallels their ability to inhibit cholinesterase. The acetylcholinesterase activity of rabbit serum and the cholinesterase activity of human plasma are also inhibited by bitter substances, although each to different degrees. Sweet taste stimulants do not inhibit cholinesterases (Tsuchiya and Okui, 1966), nor does phenylthiocarbamide, known as PTC (Tsuchiya and Aoki, 1967).

The possible role of acetylcholine in the initiation of taste nerve impulses is treated in The General Mechanism Of The Receptor Response, Chapter III.

Some evidence has been obtained that at least certain taste substances may enter the taste cell. If radioactively-labeled (^{14}C) glycine is put on the surface of the rat's tongue for several minutes, the interiors of taste cells show increased radioactivity at the end of three minutes (Halpern, in Discussion, Hodgson, 1967). This time span is also the one required for glycine to elicit a full response.

The mammalian taste bud response potential recorded by Kimura and Beidler (1961) and Tateda and Beidler (1964) was also investigated by Nejad (1961). By stimulating the rat's tongue with 0.1M sodium chloride, Nejad found this taste bud response potential to reach its greatest amplitude only in 10 to 15 seconds. No early phase of the response potential, which it might be possible to link to the initiation of nerve impulses, was observed. Action potentials appear in the afferent innervating axons within 30 msec after taste cell stimulation.

That there may be no direct relationship between the recorded taste bud potentials and taste nerve impulses is also indicated by the fact that chemicals resulting in varying rates of impulse adaptation call forth taste bud potentials with identical time courses. Further, increasing sodium chloride concentrations sometimes reverse the polarity of the taste bud potentials.

It is possible that microelectrodes inserted into taste buds might pick up potentials produced by the application of stimulating solutions to the tongue surface.

Cocaine, which blocks taste nerve impulses, reversed the polarity of the taste bud response potential and decreased the taste buds' resting potential. Acetylcholine and gamma-amino butyric acid produce no change in taste bud potentials.

Pfaffmann (1959) studied the frequency of the nerve impulses elicited in single chorda tympani fibers of the rat and hamster in response to 0.1M and 1.0M sodium chloride solutions. He found that the impulse frequency varied greatly with time and sometimes fell below a tenth of its previous level in less than half a second. However, the integrated responses of a rat's whole chorda tympani nerve to 0.1M sodium chloride may show only a 5 to 10 per cent variation in their relative amplitudes during a period of 18 hours (Beidler, 1961a).

Stürckow (1967), while stimulating the labellar chemoreceptive hairs of the blowfly *Calliphora*, noticed a viscous, sticky material at the hair tips which had previously been seen in the butterflies *Vanessa* and *Leptinotarsa*. She found that this material could fill the pore at the tip of the hair and that its outward movement, by carrying away the stimulus, could prevent excitation. Stürckow also hypothesized that the sticky fluid might contribute to taste reception by moistening the surface of the sensory neurons. Observed irregularities in response and unusually long latent periods were probably the result of the extrusion of the sticky substance.

Hodgson (1967) and his collaborators have employed tritiated water to study the fate of taste stimuli located on the sensory neuron membranes of the blowfly. When the tritiated water was placed on the ends of the labellar chemoreceptive hairs, it did not appear to remain there. Upon injection into the proboscis of the blowfly, behind the labellum, such labeled water slowly travelled into the chemoreceptive hairs. Cutting off the ends of the sensilla accelerated this movement. These findings indicated to the researchers that in the blowfly stimuli are washed from the sensory neuron membranes by a slowly, continuously moving fluid. This fluid, presumably Stürckow's viscous substance, could affect stimulation, adaptation, and other parameters of receptor activity.

In many species the sustentacular cells surrounding the olfactory receptors are thought to be secretory. There is also reason to believe that mammalian gustatory cells may secrete a fluid.

Von Békésy (1964a) found that the tastes evoked by stimulation of the human tongue with electric pulses were "purer" than chemical tastes. Thus the sweetness produced was very mild and resembled that called forth by glycine (an amino acid without isomers). The sweet taste did not vary with the stimulating frequency or with location on the tongue.

The salty and sour tastes were best produced by 0.5 msec dc pulses at 30-40 cps, while bitter was maximal at 100 cps, and sweet at 70 cps.

With the use of 0.5 msec pulses, the sour and salty sensations were found to become continuous at 3 to 4 cps, while for sweet and bitter the fusion frequency was 7-10 cps.

The taste sensations evoked by electrical pulses develop differently from normal gustatory responses. Thus 0.5 msec pulses emitted at 100 cps from 3 mm electrodes caused the electrical taste response to reach its maximum magnitude in approximately 0.15 seconds. With point electrodes the bitter and sweet sensations rose faster to their maxima than sour and salty. Also, the increase in the sweet sensation produced by doubling the voltage on a point electrode was on occasion equivalent to the increase resulting from an eightfold elevation of the concentration of a sugar solution.

Apparently electrical taste is evoked by direct depolarization of the taste cells or the associated nerve fibers.

An anodal current calls forth responses from both insect chemoreceptive hairs and mammalian taste cells (Wolbarsht, 1958; Pfaffmann, 1955), although it hyperpolarizes nerve. Anodal current was found to particularly stimulate receptors when it was applied with a pipette filled with hydrochloric acid. This finding indicates that when anodal current is employed the actual stimulus may be the electrophoretic movement of cations into the receptors.

Fischer and Griffin (1964) have found a relation between the taste threshold to a drug and its general body activity; a lower threshold is paralleled by more biological activity. It is suggested that the taste threshold of a drug is correlated with its systemic activity because both are dependent on the degree of affinity or adsorption of the drug to biological (receptor) surfaces. If the toxicity of two drugs differs by a factor of two, the level of their taste thresholds will vary by a factor of three.

As an example of threshold-activity relationships Fischer and Griffin cite the lower thresholds shown to the physiologically more active l-quinine than to d-quinine, the free base of quinine, or its sulphate and chloride. Similarly, the thresholds to the systemically more potent D-amphetamine are lower than the thresholds to L-amphetamine. The sulphoxide of chlorpromazine is more toxic and produces lower taste thresholds than chlorpromazine itself, while the less potent drug imipramine has higher thresholds.

Membrane Surface Events

There is general agreement that at least the first step in the taste response consists of a combination of the stimulus ion or molecule with a receptor site in the membrane surface. Therefore, the nature of the membrane surface and the interactions between the stimulus ions or molecules and structures on the membrane surface are of paramount interest to the student of gustation.

The Membrane Charge

One of the significant aspects of the membrane surface in terms of stimulus adsorption is its charge. The surface membranes of cells generally contain an excess of anionic over cationic groups, and these membranes therefore carry a negative charge. The excess anionic groups are sufficiently concentrated to produce a surface potential, and this should in turn give rise to a layer of counterions on the outside of the cell surface. The rate at which the cell surface potential drops in the outside medium with distance from the surface depends on the concentration of ions in the medium.

The negative charge of cell membranes is due to the excess anionic groups, and if one knows the density of these groups, the charge per unit surface can be arrived at. There are indications that the membrane anionic groups may be amino acid side chains and the phosphate groups of phospholipids. Vandenheuvel (1965) has found that there is one amino acid residue per area of 32.6 Å^2 in myelin. It has been estimated that 8.2 per cent of the amino acid residues are excess anionic groups. Therefore, if cell surface membranes generally resemble myelin and the above estimates are correct, there should be at least one excess anionic site per 400 Å² of membrane surface, and it should have a charge density of at least the order of magnitude of 2.5×10^{13} charges/cm² (Beidler, 1967). Hodgkin and Chandler (1965) estimate a density of 1.4×10^{13} electronic charges per centimeter squared for the surface membrane of squid nerve axon, produced by phosphate or carboxyl groups.

If an electrolyte solution comes in contact with a cell surface membrane, the excess anionic groups bind cations; therefore, the surface charge falls.

The surface charges in a cell membrane affect the voltage gradient across it and may thus influence its internal structure. The molecular configurations of receptor sites may be affected by the surface charges.

Cation- and Anion-Receptor Site Interactions

It is believed that the cations of a taste solution primarily combine with anionic membrane sites composed of the phosphate groups of phospholipids. Alkali cations and hydrogen ions may also combine with some amino acid groups, but these last combinations are thought to play only an insignificant role in producing a normal taste response. Hydrogen ions combine with membrane receptor sites only at high hydrogen ion concentrations (low pH's), and pK measurements show that most of the amino acid groups are not these hydrogen ion receptor sites.

If amino acid groups were the chief receptor sites for taste stimuli, changes in pH, which greatly affect the nature of amino acid groups, should have a profound effect on taste reception. Actually, in both vertebrate and insect preparations changes in pH between 3 and 11 have had little effect on taste responses.

Lifson (1957) has indicated that ion-binding on the taste cell membrane may involve combination with a single or with multiple reactive groups or even interactions with membrane electrostatic fields. A single receptor group may be a polyelectrolyte or a polyphosphate.

The approximate usual range of the values of the equilibrium constants (8-15 liters/mole) and of the relative free energy (about 2-3 kcal/mole) encountered in taste responses agree well with those for the binding of salts by polyelectrolytes.

The investigations of Eisenman (1962) on glass electrodes strongly suggest that electrostatic fields emanating from negatively charged anionic groups in the taste cell membrane chiefly determine the relative abilities of cations to interact with membrane receptor sites.

The ability of receptor sites to discriminate between sodium and potassium ions has been said to be based only on the difference in extent of hydration of the ions when they reach the receptor site. Sodium ions lose some of their water of hydration if they approach an anionic receptor site with a strong electrostatic field. The sodium ions can then approach the receptor site more closely than can potassium ions (Ling, 1962). However, since the cations with the larger halos of water of hydration lose their water of hydration earlier, only a reduced number of levels of cation stimulating-propensity exist.

Sodium and lithium have similar stimulating abilities because their hydrated ions resemble one another. Potassium, rubidium and cesium ions also form a single group of stimuli for a similar reason. All of the above ions appear to react with the same receptor sites. Potassium, rubidium and cesium ions, however, may also combine with other receptor sites.

The extent to which the above ions are bound to anionic receptor sites seems to depend on the strength of the electrostatic field of these receptor sites. Such differences in receptor site electrostatic fields may explain why rodents have many more single taste fibers in their chorda tympani nerve which show a stronger response to sodium chloride than to potassium chloride solutions, and thus have a much higher chorda tympani response to sodium chloride, while the opposite is true of carnivores. In the species of these two orders which have been studied there are some chorda tympani fibers which give the opposite sodium-potassium response ratio to that of the majority of the chorda tympani fibers of the organism. In the different taste cells of an organism, there may be different proportions of receptor sites reacting either more strongly with sodium or more fully with potassium.

If a change in the environment of an amino acid carboxyl group affects its electrostatic field strength, it may thereby also produce an alternation in the relative reactivities of this carboxyl group to cations (Beidler, 1967). Whether the structure and receptor site properties of taste cell membranes change with age has not yet been fully determined.

Generally, most chemical groups show higher reactivity to potassium than to sodium. However, polyelectrolytes with many phosphate groups interact more strongly with sodium ions (Strauss and Ross, 1959).

The chorda tympani response to sodium chloride has been observed to fall during experiments on the bat (*Myotis*), although there was no decrease in the responses to salts of other cations (Tamar, 1957). Such a decline in sodium chloride and in sugar responses has also been reported by Beidler (1963).

Stürckow (1963) found that in a fly the salt-sensitive neuron's response to a dilute salt solution became increasingly lower in consecutive tests. Salt has also been noticed to have a partially irreversible action in the fly (Evans and Mellon, 1962b).

The interaction of receptor sites with the monovalent ammonium ion shows basic similarities to the binding by these sites of the monovalent ions mentioned previously. However, in all the species investigated ammonium chloride is a strong taste stimulus.

The combination of divalent ions, such as calcium and magnesium, with membrane receptor sites appears to be a separate process from monovalent ion binding. Sato and Kusano (1960) found evidence for this by taste stimulation of the frog's tongue while recording from single fibers of its glossopharyngeal nerve. A divalent ion is able to attach to two anionic membrane receptor sites at the same time (Beidler, 1967). The adaptation of taste cells to calcium chloride has but little effect on the response to subsequent stimulation with sodium chloride.

In the blowfly calcium ions inhibit the salt receptor and also at very low concentrations the response of the sugar receptor to 0.2 molal sucrose. On the other hand, in the frog calcium chloride, as well as barium chloride, may produce more spontaneous activity and enhance the effects of both taste substances and mechanical stimuli (Koketsu and Kimura, 1953; Rapuzzi *et al.*, 1961). Koketsu and Kimura (1953), Kusano (1959) and others have also found sodium chloride to inhibit responses to calcium chloride, although the action of these two salts is different.

When an organism's taste cells are stimulated with salt solutions, these receptors are exposed not only to cations but also to a large number of anions.

Beidler (1952) learned, by recording from the rat's chorda tympani nerve (Fig. 5-11), that in the rat the cation of a salt primarily determines the taste response-concentration curve. The anion also has an effect on the elicited taste response, but in the rat this effect is clearly secondary to that of the cation. As a result, Beidler obtained "families" of response-concentration curves, each "family" consisting of the curves for the salts formed by the union of different anions with a certain cation. The cation of the salts determined the general level of their response-concentration curves.

Morrison (1967) has behaviorally confirmed Beidler's conclusion that cations are chiefly responsible for the taste of salts to the rat. His results suggest that the substitution of one cation for another can produce not only intensity but also qualitative differences in taste.

Morita (1967) determined that in the flesh fly (*Boettcherisca peregrina*) the magnitude of the taste response depends only on the cation and not on the anion of a salt.

Anions were found to inhibit the production of a taste response by cations in rodents (Beidler, 1967). Therefore, in such mammals the greater the affinity of a salt's anion for its cationic receptor sites in the membrane, the larger will be the reduction of the magnitude of the taste response to the salt.

If in an organism cation binding has an excitatory effect and anion binding is inhibitory, the magnitude of a taste response could be determined both by the proportion of cationic to anionic receptor sites reached by an ionized stimulus and the ability of these sites to interact with the stimulating ions. The nature of the receptor sites and the ratio of anionic to cationic sites can vary between receptor cells and species.

Beidler (1967) indicates that in the rat the extent of the taste response thus depends on the total of positively charged receptor sites (anionic sites combined with the positively charged cations and positively charged cationic sites not combined with anions). The same applies to spontaneous activity. The normal, low amount of spontaneous activity in the rat's chorda tympani nerve can be reduced by flowing low concentrations of potassium benzoate over its tongue. This is true because in the rat the potassium cation only weakly excites the majority of the anionic receptor sites found on the anterior tongue, which is innervated by chorda tympani fibers,

while the benzoate anion is strongly inhibiting. Only the benzoate ions combine well and occupy many cationic sites. Thus the relative number of positively charged sites is reduced. Higher concentrations of potassium benzoate affect a proportionately greater number of anionic sites, since most of the cationic sites are already filled at low concentrations, and elicit taste responses.

Klotz (1953) discovered that the capacity of organic anions to combine with the protein albumin increases with both the chain length and the size of the anion. This finding appears to be in agreement with the results obtained by stimulating mammalian tongues with a series of organic sodium salts of increasing anionic chain length, while recording the integrated responses of the whole chorda tympani nerve. Thus Beidler (1954) stimulated the rat using the salts of sodium with the anions formate, acetate, propionate and butyrate. Each anion in this series contains one carbon atom more than its predecessor. Beidler found that each increase in chain length of the anion was accompanied by a decrease in the amplitude of the integrated taste response. Similar results, given in Table I, were obtained with the opossum (*Didelphys virginiana*) by Tamar (1957). The last investigator further found that in the cat (*Felis domesticus*) 0.5M ammonium formate elicits over three times the taste response called forth by 0.5M ammonium acetate (formate = 0.79, acetate = 0.22). The taste response of the frog also decreases with increasing chain length of the organic anions of sodium salts, and with longer chain length of organic acids and amino acids (Nejad, 1959). Apparently

FIGURE 5-11. Method of recording taste impulses from the chorda tympani nerve. Views of a rat preparation from above (top) and from the side (bottom). An operative opening has been made on the ventral side of the rat's jaw. The chorda tympani nerve was then partly dissected free, cut proximally, and lifted onto one of two electrodes (*E*). The other electrode rests on exposed tissue, and the preparation is grounded. The tongue has been inserted into a flow chamber (*FC*) and is being stimulated by taste solutions alternated with water rinses. The amplified action potentials are sent from an oscilloscope into an integrator and then a recorder. (Courtesy of Dr. Irving Y. Fishman, Grinnell College, Grinnell, Iowa. Top view in Beidler, L.M.: *Ann. Otol.*, 69:398-409, 1960.)

the greater binding ability of the anions with the longer chain length is accompanied by a smaller amplitude of taste response, since the effect of these anions is inhibitory.

However, other results show that in some species certain anions may have a great excitatory effect, and that anions may have at least as much of an effect on the level of

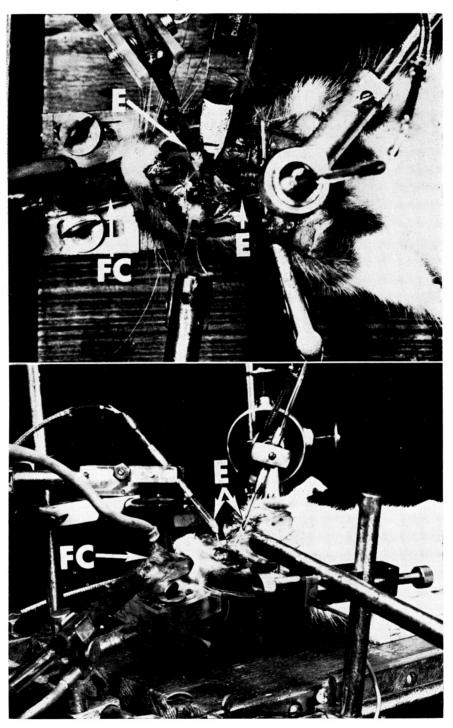

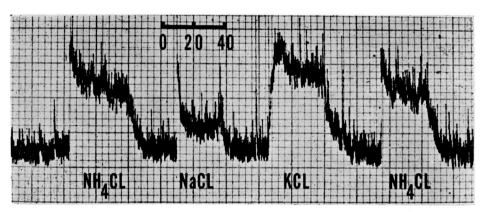

FIGURE 5-12. Record of chorda tympani taste responses from a bat (*Myotis austrori-parius*). This record was obtained through the technique illustrated in Figure 5-11. One-molar salt solutions were alternated with water rinses. Each response consists of the integrated action potentials from the whole nerve. The scale indicates time in seconds. (From Tamar, H.: Taste reception in the opossum and the bat. *Physiol. Zoöl.*, 34:86-91, 1961 [U. Chicago Pr., Copyright 1961 by the University of Chicago].)

response as cations. Konishi (1967) determined that in the carp (*Cyprinus carpio*) the magnitude of response to dilute salts rises with the valence of the anion. The integrated response of the whole palatine nerve to the optimum concentration of $Na_4Fe(CN)_6$ is several times as high as the response to the optimum concentration of sodium chloride. The optimum concentration of Na_2SO_4 also produces a noticeably higher response than that called forth by the optimum concentration of sodium chloride. Konishi's results make it clearly evident that it is not the number of cation atoms in each molecule of the mentioned highly stimulating salts which is responsible for their powerful action on the carp. The given dilute salts act on a separate receptor system highly sensitive to dilute electrolytes with monovalent cations, and concentrations of the mentioned salts greater than their optimum concentrations result in a reduced response. A relationship exists between the normality of the salt solutions and their optimum concentrations.

Konishi further indicated that the size of response may depend primarily on the nature of the anion, particularly its valence.

Tamar (1961) reported that in the opossum (*Didelphys virginiana*) 0.5M Na_2CO_3 and 0.5M Na_2SO_4 elicit higher integrated chorda tympani responses than both 0.5M and 1.0M sodium chloride. However, 0.5M $NaNO_3$ produces a chorda tympani taste response of only one-sixth the amplitude of that called forth by 0.5M sodium chloride. The cat (*Felis domesticus*) shows an unusually high chorda tympani response to 0.5M Na_2CO_3, five times as high as that to 0.5 M sodium chloride. The solution of 0.5M Na_2CO_3 had a pH of 11, but water given a pH of 11 with sodium hydroxide elicited no response, and 0.5M $NaHCO_3$, with a pH of 8, called forth only a very small response. The cat, like the opossum, gives only a small response to 0.5M $NaNO_3$.

Cohen *et al.* (1955) also found anions to play a major role in taste responses of the cat, and similar observations have been made on the frog (Kusano and Sato, 1957, 1958). Gillary (1966) reported anions to significantly stimulate the blowfly, and Steinhardt (1966) discovered the not-always-present fifth sensory neuron of the labellar chemoreceptive hairs of *Phormia regina* to be an anion receptor.

Konishi (1967) deals with the problem of how anions could interact with the surface membrane to produce stimulation. He suggests that if receptor sites carry a positive charge,

TABLE I
EFFECT OF 0.5M SALTS OF INCREASING CHAIN LENGTH ON THE OPOSSUM'S TASTE RESPONSE

Name	Sodium Chloride	Sodium Formate	Sodium Acetate	Sodium Propionate	Sodium Butyrate
Formula	NaCl	NaCHO₂	NaC₂H₃O₂	NaC₃H₅O₂	NaC₄H₇O₂
Salt response / 0.5M NH₄Cl response	0.30	0.29	0.20	0.13	0.11
Water response	None	None	None	Small	Larger

the stimulating anions could be adsorbed to the inner portion of the double counterion layer in the solution outside the receptor surface. Such anions could then significantly affect the Stern potential at the membrane surface. If the response to stimulating anions is really the consequence of such a change in potential, the valence of the anions should significantly influence the size of the response.

Large organic ions, including choline, may also combine with membrane receptor sites to produce a taste response. In the cat 0.5M choline chloride elicits about as large a chorda tympani taste response as 0.5M sodium chloride (Tamar, 1957).

The salty sensation stems from inorganic salts, especially distinctly from many having chlorine, bromine, sulfate and nitrate anions. As the atoms making up a salt become larger and heavier, it becomes increasingly bitter. For example, potassium iodide has a more clearly bitter taste than potassium bromide (Moncrieff, 1967).

"Nonelectrolyte"-Receptor Site Interactions

A considerable number of nonelectrolytes have been observed to produce taste responses. The work of Klotz (1953) suggests that such stimulating molecules may bind to proteins or lipids in the receptor membrane surface. Beidler (1967) stated that the molecules might be bound to protein side chains by means of hydrogen bonds. Such hydrogen bonding would lend additional significance to the steric configuration of the nonelectrolyte molecules. The formation of the hydrogen bonds would cause configurational or other changes in the membrane surface and lead

to the opening of pores and a taste response.

The response to sucrose may rise slowly for some time before the maximum neural activity is reached.

Shallenberger and Acree (1967) and Shallenberger (1968) develop the thesis that sweet taste is dependent on the formation of two hydrogen bonds between the sweet molecule and the receptor site. One proton would be supplied by the sweet compound, the other, by the receptor site on a protein molecule. However, London dispersion, the most significant factor in hydrogen bonding, rather than proton transfers, would contribute to the interaction. Shallenberger and Acree indicate that sweet compounds must therefore possess a somewhat acidic proton which lies only a certain distance (about 3 Å) from an electronegative orbital that would bond with a proton from the receptor site. The receptor site must have a similar structural arrangement.

The above conceptualization correlates well with the view that the sweetness of sugars is reduced by hydrogen bonds within the glycol portion of their molecules. A larger number of intramolecular hydrogen bonds would leave fewer hydrogen atoms available for intermolecular bonding. It is considered that vicinal OH groups of the glycol structure must lie in a staggered conformation to permit a sweet taste to develop, and that inactive OH groups are likely to be attached through intramolecular hydrogen bonds.

Shallenberger (1968) shows how sour and salty substances could also interact with the receptor site for sweet.

Konishi and Niwa (1964), using the carp, found a direct correlation between the stimulating efficacy of nonelectrolytes and the number of their polar groups.

Dastoli and Price (1966) extracted a protein from the fungiform papillae at the tip of the cow's tongue which combined weakly with sugars and saccharin. This protein fraction, which was homogeneous, and soluble in 20 per cent ammonium sulfate but insoluble in 40 per cent, interacted with low concentrations of sugars. The strengths of combination fell into the same order as the sweetness of the sugars for man and the dog, and the reactions were not time dependent. The combination of fructose with the protein was nearly unaffected by pH's between 5.5 and 9.6, but was inhibited by lower pH's, as is true of taste responses to sugars. The complexing of the sugars by the protein fitted Beidler's fundamental equation, and plots of C/R versus C yielded straight lines (indicating unimolecular reactions). It is quite possible that the reactive protein fraction, whose behavior was studied by refractometry and ultraviolet-difference spectroscopy, was composed of the bovine receptor molecules for sugars.

Dastoli, Lopiekes and Price (1968) have assigned the above protein a molecular weight of about 150,000, and an isoionic point of 9.1.

The findings of Dastoli and Price (1966) have essentially been corroborated by Hiji, Kobayashi and Sato (1968), who identified a similar sugar-complexing protein in extracts from the rat tongue. The extract fraction containing this rat protein showed a 1.4-fold increase in spectral absorbancy at 280 mμ, the wavelength of its maximum absorbancy, when 0.5M sucrose was added. Positive results were not obtained with control extracts from the tongue of the cat (which shows low sensitivity to sugars) nor with rat muscle or intestinal epithelium extracts. Only small amounts of sugar-complexing protein were indicated in extracts from the tongues of colchicine-injected rats (colchicine inhibits the multiplication of taste cells).

A study of a bitter-sensitive protein has also been performed. Dastoli, Lopiekes and

Doig (1968) extracted the epithelial tissue from the posterior portion of over fifteen pig (*Sus*) tongues. One extract fraction was found to form complexes with bitter substances. The strengths of these complexes appeared to parallel the relative bitterness of the employed compounds to man. The obtained ΔF values indicate that the observed complexing was based on weak physical interactions. The ΔF values are also in accordance with the formation of hydrogen bonds. Exposure of extract fractions from the tip of the tongue to bitter compounds produced no results, nor did any posterior tongue fraction interact with sugars.

Hydra littoralis possesses primitive, but highly specific, receptors for the tripeptide reduced glutathione. The glutathione-receptor interaction appears to take place through the agency of ionizable receptor groups. If a protein is the receptor, two β-carboxyl groups of peptide aspartic acid or α-carboxyl groups of peptide glutamic acid, an imidazole group and an end α-amino group may be involved. There is reason to believe that charged structures at the receptor site bind complementary charged groupings on the glutathione molecule. These charged receptor structures could comprise one of the carboxyl groups and the terminal α-amino group (Lenhoff, 1968).

It has been determined that the main tripeptide chain of glutathione must be present for a reaction, and that the free, positively charged α-amino group of the glutamyl portion of glutathione is directly involved in linkage to the receptor (Lenhoff, 1968).

Water Responses

When certain taste stimuli are removed from the tongues of some species by flowing water over the tongue, an increased level of nerve activity is noted. Such nerve taste responses to the replacement of a solution by water are known as water responses. The last have been observed in monkeys (Fishman, 1959; Gordon *et al.*, 1959), the cat, dog, pig, rabbit, rat, opossum, chicken and pigeon (Kitchell, Ström and Zotterman, 1959), frog (Nejad, 1959;

Nomura and Sakada, 1965), fish (Konishi and Zotterman, 1963; Konishi, 1967), butterfly and flesh fly. Morita (1967) has recorded impulses from the separate water receptor of the flesh fly (*Boettcherisca peregrina*). Water produces over 50 impulses/sec in the half-second following its application to the water-sensitive neurons of the blowfly's (*Phormia's*) labellar chemoreceptive hairs.

Water responses vary in different species. They are quite large in the chorda tympani of the rabbit, but those recorded from the chorda tympani of the cat are smaller (Nejad, 1959). Only flowing water elicits a water response in the cat (Cohen *et al.*, 1955). The water response of the dog is weak, and there is none in man (Diamant, Funakoshi, Ström and Zotterman, 1963). Water calls forth only a minimal discharge in the glossopharyngeal nerve of the frog (Nomura and Sakada, 1965). In general, water responses are frequently noted after stimulation with many acids and the salts of citrate, benzoate, acetate and butyrate.

The water receptor of the blowfly (*Phormia regina*) is inhibited by dilute salt and sugar solutions and perhaps is inhibited under normal conditions by the extracellular fluid of the chemosensory hair (Wolbarsht, 1965).

Nomura and Sakada (1965) state that distilled water does not call forth the water response in the frog. They indicate that the frog's water response is really a response to low concentrations of calcium ions and that the involved receptors respond to a threshold concentration of less than 0.05 mM of calcium ions. The given results do not have a bearing on the significance of its water response to the frog, since there is a considerable quantity of calcium ions in normal natural waters.

Hodgson (1967) considers the low osmotic pressure of water to be a likely real stimulus of the water receptor discharge. He points out that this explanation of the water response is in agreement with the inhibitory effect of solutes.

Beidler (1967) has advanced a hypothesis proposing that water responses consist of spontaneous activity resulting from an excess of positively charged, cationic receptor sites in the membrane. If there are a greater number of cationic than anionic receptor sites in the membrane, application of a salt will result in a greater binding of the salt's anions than cations, and the amount of spontaneous activity (water response) will drop. Then, when most of the cationic sites have bound anions, the cation of the salt will interact with the membrane's anionic receptor sites, and a taste response will develop.

According to this hypothesis, the effectiveness of a salt in reducing spontaneous activity should be related to the extent to which its anion interacts more readily and more strongly with membrane receptor sites than its cation. In the rabbit potassium benzoate, with its highly reactive benzoate ion, indeed reduces spontaneous activity more than potassium chloride does.

On the other hand, the application of water to the tongue has been reported to reduce the spontaneous activity of salt fibers in the rat (Pfaffmann, 1965).

If the opossum is stimulated with sodium chloride, sodium formate, and sodium acetate, the water wash following these salts does not result in the appearance of a noticeable water response. However, the water washes following sodium propionate and sodium butyrate respectively call forth a smaller and a larger water response (Table I). Here the anions with the greatest chain length and highest binding ability are most successfully used to subsequently call forth a water response. These results suggest that the degree of inhibition of spontaneous activity produced by an anion is related to the ability of a subsequent water rinse to elicit a water response. The propionate anion, and even more the butyrate anion, by highly inhibiting spontaneous activity in the opossum's taste receptors, may eliminate any adaptive influences to which the spontaneous activity has been subjected. Therefore, following the removal of these highly inhibitory anions, the spontaneous activity temporarily rises to new heights.

The above suggestion is supported by the chorda tympani responses obtained by Beidler (1961a) when he alternately applied potassium benzoate and water rinses to the tongue of the rat. In the frog the amplitude of the water response obtained on rinsing after the application of acetic acid rises with the concentration of the acetic acid (Yamashita, 1964). This also suggests that the water response is a type of postinhibitory discharge.

In vertebrates the water response often lasts for a full minute.

In the cat, dog and rat ethyl alcohol produced an initial depression of chorda tympani activity, followed by a slowly rising response. The subsequent water rinse then resulted in a water response (Hellekant, 1967).

Konishi (1967) observed that of two taste receptor systems in the carp the system which is very sensitive to dilute electrolytes with monovalent cations can also show high activity upon a water rinse. To initiate this high activity, distilled water must be flown over the receptors after they are subjected to a salt solution (having a monovalent cation) which is sufficiently concentrated to depress chemoreception. Konishi named this response to a distilled water rinse the "distilled water effect," or DWE.

An increase in the concentration of the previously applied salt solution, which is accompanied by a further reduction in the magnitude of the resultant taste response, leads also to a larger DWE, until the last attains a maximum size. Beyond this point a further increase in salt concentration results in a reduced response to the subsequent distilled water rinse. There is a relationship between both the DWE and the optimum salt concentration for producing a maximum response on the one hand and the normality of the salt solution on the other. Water rinses following salts with polyvalent cations never call forth a DWE in the carp.

Konishi hypothesizes that the washing away of cations from the receptor site surfaces produces DWE's. If the cationic strength say, in the double counterion layer over the receptor

sites, is sufficient to depress the taste response, perhaps by a screening effect (holding off the interacting anions), then washing away of the cations should lead to a potential. The above hypothesis is strengthened by the observation that when the concentration of salts with monovalent cations is raised beyond the level resulting in a maximum DWE, the time necessary for the DWE to reach its peak is lengthened. Since there is a continuous flow of distilled water during this development of the DWE, this observation suggests that greater amounts of distilled water are now needed to wash away a significant portion of the larger quantity of effective cations supplied by the excessively concentrated salt solution.

The positive hydrogen ion appears to depress the DWE better than the negative hydroxyl ion, and polyvalent cations are more depressant than monovalent cations by a factor of twenty or thirty. As would be expected, nonelectrolytes such as sucrose do not depress the DWE but act like distilled water.

However, in the carp previous stimulation with nonelectrolytes results in a water response on rinsing (Konishi and Zotterman, 1963).

Effects of Acids and Hydrocarbons

If a solution of low pH is applied to taste receptors, many of its hydrogen ions will bind to the proteins in the receptor membrane. This will increase the membrane's positive surface charge and reduce the binding of further hydrogen ions. Anions combine separately with other receptor sites, and Beidler (1967) suggests that the extent of the response to acids should be determined by their anions.

A solution of mixed 0.1M acetic acid and 0.01M sodium acetate elicits almost as high a taste response as that called forth by 0.1M acetic acid alone. Although in the first, mixed buffer solution the hydrogen ion concentration is only one seventh or less of that in pure 0.1M acetic acid, the buffer solution contains about eight times as many acetate anions. Beidler explains the surprisingly high response to the buffer solution on the basis of an increased anion binding reducing the positive membrane charge and permitting more hydrogen binding. Beidler believes that an acid solution's sourness depends on the reactivity of the acid's anions with cationic receptor sites.

Carbon dioxide gas has been reported to produce considerable activity in acid, salt and cold nerve fibers of cats, dogs and rats (Kawamura and Adachi, 1967). However, in view of the unusually strong effect of Na_2CO_3 in the cat (Tamar, 1961), the possibility of a unique action by H_2CO_3 should not be overlooked.

Hodgson and Steinhardt (1967) studied the effect of straight-chain hydrocarbons on the labellar chemoreceptors of the blowfly (*Phormia regina*). They found that at noninjurious concentrations lower alcohols and long chain amines produce a reversible inhibition of the salt, water and sugar receptors. Octylamine had a similar action on amino acid receptors in the spiny lobster (*Panulirus argus*).

In the blowfly the salt receptor is most sensitive to the octylamine and higher alcohol molecules, followed by the sugar receptor and then the water receptor. While in the case of the salt and water receptors there is a linear relationship between octylamine concentration and the produced inhibition, this does not hold true for the sugar receptor.

The action of hydrocarbons on the salt and water receptors appears to resemble a narcosis, as of nerve, although a denaturation of protein receptor sites is also possible. In the case of the sugar receptors denaturation seems more plausible, partly because of the nonlinear inhibition-concentration relation. Inhibition of the sugar receptor by octylamine is prevented by glycerol, which is known to stabilize proteins.

At higher concentrations long-chain hydrocarbons injure the receptors.

The effect of natural chelators on some responses causes the suspicion that certain receptor sites are normally occupied or covered, and must be "cleared" to enable them to fully interact with taste stimuli. Thus, if citric acid is flown over the tongue of the rat, later responses to 0.1M sodium chloride have a greater magnitude (Beidler, 1966).

Hellekant (1969) has studied the effect produced by the addition of menthol to stimulating solutions containing different concentrations of acetic acid. He concludes that menthol, a saturated alcohol of the cyclic terpene type, like alcohol, causes a slow, partial depolarization of gustatory receptors. If the receptor is at this time exposed to a weak stimulus, the depolarization produced by it will sum with that due to menthol, and an enhanced response will be obtained. If, on the other hand, a strong stimulus is used, the partial depolarization elicited by menthol will be significant in having reduced the degree of depolarization which can still occur in the cell membrane. Therefore, menthol depresses the neural responses to strong stimuli.

Menthol exerts its apparent cooling effect on the tongue by partially exciting, or depolarizing, thermoreceptors.

It is possible that menthol enters the cell.

Receptor Differences

It has been mentioned earlier in this book that a spectrum of different receptor sites is found on one taste cell, and that the types and proportions of receptor sites vary from one taste cell to another. Furthermore, receptor sites may differ greatly from one species to another, and similar kinds of receptor sites may show a totally different distribution in separate species.

Receptor site differences may be subtle. Thus taste receptor sites have been shown to have varying stereoselectivities, indicating fine variations in molecular configurations. Also, delicate differences in electrochemical properties exist between receptor sites.

Such variation in receptor sites shows itself in species differences in gustation (Fig. 5-9), such as the near reversal of sodium-potassium chorda tympani response ratios between rodents and carnivores (Beidler, Fishman and Hardiman, 1955). Among the rodents the hamster and guinea pig have a much greater chorda tympani response to 0.5M sucrose than the rat.

Von Frisch (1934) tested honeybees (*Apis mellifica*) with thirty-four substances sweet to man and found that they responded to only nine. Saccharin was not accepted by bees at low concentrations and repelled them at higher concentrations. However, acetyl-saccharose, which is bitter to man, was accepted by the bees.

Not only are the taste thresholds of fish lower than those of man, but the minnow (*Phoxinus phoxinus* L.) is more sensitive to the trisaccharide raffinose than to many other sugars (Glaser, 1966). Man does not find raffinose very sweet.

Differences in taste response have also been discovered between Swedish and Japanese carp (*Cyprinus carpio*) by Konishi and Zotterman (1963). They found that Swedish carp showed high integrated palatine nerve responses to sucrose and weak ones to quinine, while the opposite was true of Japanese carp. Japanese carp were also much more sensitive to saliva, milk and silkworm pupa extract.

A highly specific carp receptor was also found, which responds only to saliva and probably also related substances in milk and pupa fluid. Fractionation studies indicate that the substances which stimulate the saliva receptor are lipid in nature.

The inactivation of the carp's taste receptors by the lytic agents digitonin and sodium cholate, which act on lipids, indicates that lipids form important components of the receptor membrane. The sweet and saliva receptors are the first to become inexcitable under the action of sodium cholate, while the salt and the acid receptors are the most resistant. The receptors show a similar order of susceptibility to gymnemic acid.

Not only are there major differences in gustatory reception between populations of a species, but significant taste differences of genetic origin exist between individuals of a single population. Thus taste thresholds in a Caucasian population for the bitter phenylthiourea group of antithyroid substances show a bimodal distribution, and this distribution has been used to divide the tested individuals into tasters and "nontasters." Taste thresholds for the phenylthiourea group of compounds are under considerable genetic control.

The taste thresholds in the population for most compounds, however, follow a gaussian distribution. An individual's taste thresholds for these more numerous compounds tend to resemble each other in that all show either a lower or higher relative degree of sensitivity. Only the threshold for hydrochloric acid does not follow this last generalization. There is less genetic control of taste thresholds for "gaussian-distribution" compounds (Fischer, 1967).

Fischer and Griffin (1964) have suggested that sensitive tasters of phenylthiourea compounds and the substances whose thresholds follow a gaussian distribution (quinine, etc.) possess a greater number of receptor sites per unit receptor cell surface (and volume?) than do poor tasters.

The distribution of PTC tasters and "nontasters" among great apes and monkeys is similar to that in man.

Individual differences in the reception and perception of sweet substances are large in man (Cameron, 1947; Borg *et al.*, 1967).

Among the suckling pigs of the same litter, some accepted saccharin at every concentration they could perceive, while others were indifferent to it and a number rejected saccharin (Kare, 1968).

It has been possible to select out two strains of quail (*Colinus virginianus*) in respect to the response to ferric chloride. One strain rejects this compound, while the other consumes high concentrations.

Considerable variations in taste may also be found between discrete regions in one individual. Thus the differential distribution of the bitter quality at the back of the human tongue, sweet at its tip, sour at its sides, and salty at the tip and sides is well known. In the blowfly (*Phormia*) the tiny gustatory pegs of the interpseudo-tracheal papillae contain salt receptors and sugar receptors which differ in their sensitivities from their counterparts in the chemosensory hairs of the fly's labellum. The salt-sensitive neurons of the gustatory pegs, unlike those of the hairs, respond to calcium chloride and d- and l-arabinose. Also, while of the polyhydric alcohols only inositol acts on the hair sugar receptor, another polyhydric alcohol without a ring structure, sorbitol, evokes responses from the sugar neuron of the gustatory peg (Dethier and Hanson, 1965).

The extent of the excitation evoked by stimuli in a group of receptors may change with time. The size of the responses by the cat's taste receptors may show a positive relation with variations in the taste nerves' spontaneous activity (Ishiko and Amatsu, 1964). Seasonal changes in taste responses have been observed in the frog (Kusano, 1960) and the carp (Konishi and Niwa, 1964). Thus in spring preparations of the carp (*Cyprinus carpio*) the maximum salt responses appeared at higher concentrations. Glaser (1966) reports that fish have higher absolute taste thresholds in the fall and early winter and that their taste sensitivities become keener once more in the spring. He presents evidence that temperature is not responsible for these sensitivity changes. Age, nutritional condition, and the sugars in the food of the larva can apparently affect the blowfly's responses (Wolbarsht, 1957; Evans, 1961).

Molecular Structure, Properties and Taste—Sweet and Bitter

Investigations on sweet receptors and work with sweet-tasting substances have especially illuminated the significance of molecular structures and configurations in producing gustatory excitation. Studies on the sweet taste have also brought out species differences.

It has been learned that the methyl group (CH_3) often acts to stimulate the bitter taste. Thus the conversion of p-anisonitrile to p-ethoxybenzonitrile by the addition of a methyl group (which also increases the molecular weight) changes the taste from sweet to bitter (Beidler, 1961a).

The alkylation of saccharin by the addition of a methyl group causes it to convert from sweet to tasteless.

Moving the methyl group to different positions on the aromatic ring of tolylurea affects the taste of this molecule. In the sweet p-tolylurea the methyl group is on one end of the aromatic ring and a $NHCONH_2$ group on the other. In the bitter m-tolylurea only one carbon atom of the aromatic ring is between the two groups, and in the tasteless o-tolylurea the methyl group is adjacent to the $NHCONH_2$ group. Similarly, transforming the symmetry of dimethylurea from the α- to the s-form by a shift in the position of one of the two methyl groups changes its taste from very sweet to bitter. While α-dimethylurea has two methyl groups on one side of the molecule and an exposed amine (NH_2) group on the other, s-dimethylurea has an exposed methyl group on each end of the molecule.

The presence of an amine group may produce a sweet taste. While acetic acid (CH_3-$COOH$) is quite sour, glycine (NH_2CH_2-$COOH$) is sweet.

Ferguson and Childers (1960) describe the —$COOH$ and —SO_2NH_2 groups as evoking sweetness. The addition of basic groups is also considered to increase the sweet taste.

The effectiveness of a taste stimulus can often be raised by the addition of side chains. Thus 4-nitro-2-amino-phenyl alkyl ethers become sweeter as their side chain is lengthened to the propyl derivative, after which, with further additions, the stimulating propensities of the ethers are reduced. Gallic acid esters become more bitter as their carbon chain is increased from the methyl to the butyl form.

Many compounds possessing an aromatic ring or other ring structures call forth strong taste sensations. This is true of some amino acids, alkyl ethers, saccharin and alkaloids.

The nature and intensity of the evoked taste is highly dependent on the place of attachment to the cyclic structure and on the position in space of substituent polar groups. While 1.2-dinitrobenzene is sweet, 1.3- and 1.4-dinitrobenzene are bitter. These compounds produce no mixed tastes at any concentrations; their taste is strictly determined by the specific configuration.

The groups attached to a compound's ring structure may imbue it with greater stimulus effectiveness, may affect the distribution of charges on the molecule and modify the action of other substituents or may reduce taste effectiveness by providing steric hindrance.

Deutsch and Hansch (1966) indicate that the level of sweetness is dependent on the extent of hydrophobic bonding. Another significant factor is the water solubility of a substance. Thus substitutions on the isothiazole nucleus which result in a reduction of water solubility also produce a decrease in sweetness. The negative charges on a molecule, or how easily it forms hydrogen bonds with water, play a role in water solubility.

When a substance is dissolved in water, its sweetness is then determined by the partition coefficient for its adsorption to the receptor sites. Such combination with the receptor sites is influenced not only by hydrophobic bonding but also by the polarity of the molecule, the extent of charge separation, the electron density of the substance at its reactive surfaces and steric configuration.

The benzene ring may play a role in hydrophobic bonding with receptor molecules; amino acids with an aromatic ring are strong taste stimuli for man (Solms *et al.*, 1965). The position of substituted groups and their effect on electron distribution in the benzene ring largely determine the sweetness of members of the 2-amino-4-nitrobenzene group. Electron-supplying groups taking a para position to the nitro group or groups which take electrons occupying a para position to the amino group will affect the charge distribution of a molecule. Such groups are —COOH and —SO$_2$NH$_2$, described as sweet. The sweet substances sucaryl, 5-benzyl-2-furfuraldoxime and dulcin all must undergo a separation of charges to gain sufficient water solubility and an adequate degree of hydrophobic bonding ability.

Deutsch and Hansch envision the receptor site as composed of a location for hydrophobic bonding and also of a place for electronic bonding.

Marcström (1965) reported, on the basis of psychophysical studies on man, that the stimulating propensities of sweet, bitter-sweet and bitter substances can be correlated with their water solubility and their steric configurations.

Marcström (1967) investigated the relationship between the absolute taste thresholds (considered equivalent to stimulating efficacies) of sweet, bitter-sweet and bitter compounds in man and their solubilities in water. Solubility was measured by the number of moles dissolved in a unit volume of a saturated aqueous solution. The pH and temperature were considered in making a number of solubility determinations.

Marcström found that while no threshold-solubility relationship could be obtained by examining the results for all his compounds together, the stimulus thresholds of bitter compounds alone were nearly directly proportional to their water solubilities. He therefore divided all his compounds into five groups on the basis of a number of factors—taste quality, the region of the tongue stimulated, the effect of pH and temperature on taste thresholds, and the relation between stimulus intensity and magnitude of sensation. After the threshold values for each of the five groups were corrected according to the factors listed above, Marcström noted the logarithms of the average thresholds of the compounds to be apparently linearly related to the logarithms of their solubilities. Marcström sought to explain the significance of his five groups of compounds by hypothesizing that the members of different groups may have to actually enter differing solutions and therefore be involved in different phase equilibria before they can interact with their receptor molecules.

Considerable variations were found in the taste thresholds reported in the literature. Individual differences (number of receptors, condition of the subject, etc.), training and formation of taste "memories," and methodology may be responsible for some of these disparities.

In this connection it might also be mentioned that close to the normal threshold there is enough adaptation to continuously change the threshold (von Békésy, 1966).

McBurney and Pfaffmann (1963) determined, by avoiding water rinses with human subjects, that the threshold for sodium chloride always just exceeds the sodium concentration in the saliva. If the receptors were adapted to a higher concentration of sodium chloride, the threshold was raised to a level slightly over this concentration; if the tongue was rinsed with a concentration of sodium chloride below that in the saliva, the threshold dropped accordingly to a point just over this lower concentration. Washing the tongue with water resulted in a threshold of about .001 molar sodium chloride, only a hundred's of the normal threshold.

That the sodium chloride threshold is dependent upon the nature of the fluid covering the tongue has also been shown by electrophysiological recording from the chorda tympani nerve of man, the dog and the rat. A sodium chloride concentration below that of an adapting solution causes a drop in the existing impulse discharge.

Odor stimulation may lower a high threshold for sour taste, raise a low threshold, or have little effect on a medium threshold (Schutz and Pilgrim, 1953).

Tongue movements may result in greater gustatory sensitivity and, according to Ishiko and Amatsu (1965), increase the magnitude of the taste responses recorded from the cat's chorda tympani nerve. Beidler (1953) has suggested that tongue movements may produce their beneficial effect by continuously changing the stimulus concentrations acting on the taste cells, thus preventing rapid adaptation of these receptors. However, in the case of the circumvallate papillae, movement may primarily enable the stimulus to reach the receptors. This is true because the taste buds of the circumvallate papillae are located around a poorly accessible trench at the base of each papilla. In goats, sheep and calves movement of the circumvallate papillae produces greater taste responses in the glossopharyngeal nerve (Bell and Kitchell, 1966).

Direct stimulation of the sympathetic nerves, or anything which affects the autonomic nervous system, may at least to some degree modify sense responses. Thus the magnitude of the taste responses in the frog's glossopharyngeal nerve may be increased by stimulating the sympathetic innervation of the tongue. Stimulation of the tortoise's cervical sympathetic nerve, by changing the thickness of the nasal mucosa and the size of the lumen in the nasal cavity, may markedly influence its olfaction.

If a sense affects the autonomic nervous system, it could thereby modify other senses (Moulton, 1967). It has been found that gustatory and olfactory stimuli can increase secretion by the parotid gland and alter heart function and respiration, all of which are regulated by the autonomic nervous system. Parotid secretion appears to be particularly stimulated through the nose's trigeminal innervation.

Increased parotid secretion is paralleled by greater salivary sodium content, which in itself could somewhat affect gustation.

Taste thresholds may be affected by many aspects of physiology. The taste threshold of 6-n-propylthiouracil (PROP) may be altered by hormone therapy, menstruation (Kaplan et al., 1963), stress and pregnancy (Fischer and Griffin, 1961). The PROP threshold may also change on taking aspirin.

Olfactory acuity has also been reported to vary with the menstrual cycle. Some evidence indicates that hormones and drugs may indirectly affect olfactory sensitivity by producing changes in the nasal mucosa, or acting on the sympathetic nervous system (Moulton, Discussion in Hoshishima, 1967).

Shaber et al. (1967) determined the taste threshold of the rat for saccharin by means of a conditioned suppression behavioral technique in which hypothalamic stimulation through implanted electrodes served as a reward. Their reported threshold was four times lower than that established earlier with a different methodology, a two-choice preference experiment.

It should also be remembered, as Marcström himself points out, that thresholds may not be indicative of relative stimulating abilities over the whole range of concentrations if different stimulus-receptor site interactions are involved.

Evans (1963) has written an outstanding paper on the nature of the carbohydrates which elicit a behavioral taste response in the blowfly (*Phormia regina*). He points out that while chemicals of widely divergent structure can produce the sweet sensation, among a group of compounds having a similar structure only those with certain specific configurations elicit a sweet taste. Thus glucose, sucrose, glycogen, polyhydric alcohols, D-amino acids, saccharin, sucaryl sodium, sucaryl calcium, and even heavy metal salts of lead and beryllium, all can call forth the sweet taste, but in insects saccharin, dulcin, most carbohydrates, the amino acids, and inorganic salts do not produce a sweet response. A few carbohydrates are the only sweet stimuli for insects.

Another peculiarity of the sweet sensation is its close relationship to the bitter taste. The chemical structures of some sweet substances resemble the structures of certain bitter compounds. Thus, when the oxygen attached by a double bond to a carbon in dulcin, sweet to man, is replaced by sulfur, the bitter substance p-ethoxy-phenylthiocarbamide is obtained. Also, sweet substances like saccharin call forth a bitter aftertaste in man. In the rhesus monkey glycerol, ethylene glycol and saccharin call forth responses in both "sweet" and "bitter" taste nerve fibers, although sucrose acts on the "sweet" receptors alone (Gordon *et al.*, 1959). In the dog, on the other hand, saccharin combines only with sites on the "bitter" receptors (Andersson *et al.*, 1950). In the carp also the "sweet" fiber is stimulated by all the effective sweet substances except saccharin (Konishi and Zotterman, 1963).

In the hamster saccharin interacts both with the receptors for sucrose (Fig. 5-15) and the receptors which are reactive to sodium chloride (Yamashita *et al.*, 1967b). These two receptor types are clearly separable in the hamster, and the response to sucrose is generally inversely related to the response to sodium chloride (Fig. 5-14). The sucrose-sensitive receptors show a considerable rise in response level as the concentration of saccharin is raised from 0.0003M to 0.01M-0.03M and, after a maximum response at the latter concentration, the response falls again with further concentration increases. However, the salt receptors instead exhibit a low rate of rise in response with increasing saccharin concentrations and show their highest response at greater concentrations than the 0.03M level.

In the rat saccharin has similar stimulating effects on the corresponding but less clearly distinguished receptor types (Fig. 5-13). The receptors primarily responsive to sodium chloride show a typical salt response-concentration curve for saccharin. The receptors in which sucrose elicits the highest responses have, like their counterparts in the hamster, a fast rate of rise in response with increasing saccharin concentration, to a maximum response at 0.03M (Yamashita *et al.*, 1967b).

In the hamster there are very good correlations between, respectively, the responses to 0.02M saccharin and to 0.1M sodium chloride, and the responses to 0.02M saccharin and to 0.5M sucrose. Apparently in the hamster saccharin elicits both a sweet and a salty taste, although the ratio of these two evoked taste qualities may change with the concentration of saccharin.

In man potassium chloride and ammonium chloride also have been reported to evoke two tastes, salty and bitter, at the same time (Renquist, 1919).

The high equilibrium constant of about 1,700 liters/mole for the combination of saccharin with human taste receptor sites shows that this substance must be strongly held to its receptor sites in man. It is very possible that in man saccharin interacts with a different group of receptor sites from those which are reactive to sucrose.

The bitter sensation, like the sweet, is brought about by a considerable variety of substances—alkaloids, heavy salts such as bile salts, salts of magnesium and of ammonium, picric acid, and some glucosides.

Sweet taste stimuli were found to interact with different kinds of receptor sites in the blowfly (*Phormia regina*), indicating how substances of widely differing structures could all elicit the sweet taste. It was learned that fructose and mannose act on one type of receptor site, mannose interacting much less strongly, and that glucose combines with another kind of receptor site (Evans, 1963). If blowfly larvae were supplied with either fructose or glucose during development, the adults showed a relatively lower response to the sugar on which they had been reared, indicat-

ing an organic ability to differentiate these sugars. In glucose-reared flies, fructose was thirty-seven times as stimulating as glucose, while in fructose-reared specimens this ratio was reduced to less than one. Changes in the response to sucrose paralleled the changes in the fructose response, showing that both these sugars act on the same receptor site (Evans, 1961).

Tateda (1967) has suggested that fructose, sucrose and glycine may act on the same receptor sites in the rat.

Experimental evidence also indicates that there is more than one type of sweet receptor site and more than one type of bitter receptor site in man.

Thus one of two observers had a noticeably lower threshold to the sweet compounds sucrose, hydroquinone, m-nitrophenol and p-nitrophenol, while the other observer exhibited

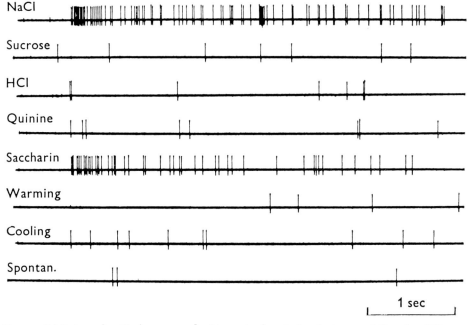

FIGURE 5-13. Impulse discharges evoked in a single rat chorda tympani fiber by different stimuli. The tongue was stimulated, at 25°C, with 0.1M sodium chloride, 0.5M sucrose, 0.01N hydrochloric acid, 0.02M quinine hydrochloride, and 0.02M sodium saccharin. Water at 40°C was used for warming, and water at 20°C for cooling. The spontaneous discharge is shown in the bottom trace. Both sodium chloride and saccharin excited sizeable responses. (From Ogawa, H., M. Sato, and S. Yamashita: Multiple sensitivity of chorda tympani fibres of the rat and hamster to gustatory and thermal stimuli. *J. Physiol.* [London], 199:223-240, 1968.)

a greater sensitivity to the sweet o-nitro-phenol. Both observers were equally sensitive to other sweet substances. This suggests that unlike groups or kinds of receptor sites, represented to different degrees in two observers, were involved in the taste responses (Marc-ström, 1967).

If equivalent increases in the strengths of equally intense stimuli do not result in similar increases in the observed intensity of sensation for every subject, different receptor mechanisms may be at work. Therefore, the relationship between the logarithm of the stimulus intensity and the logarithm of the magnitude of the evoked sensation was plotted for a group of sweet compounds. The slopes of the resulting curves were similar for nitrobenzene, 1,2-dinitrobenzene and resorcinol, but the slopes for these compounds clearly differed from the slopes for phoroglucinol, phenol, p-nitrophenol, and so on. These results indicate that different stimulus-receptor site interactions are taking place (Marcström, 1967).

Similar observations were made with bitter compounds. The curve of the log of the stimulus versus the log of the resulting sensation has a considerably steeper slope for the lesser concentrations of phenylthiourea than do the equivalent portions of the curves for additional bitter compounds (1.3-dinitrobenzene, etc.).

Also, the bitter pyrogallol primarily stimulates receptors on the posterior margins, rather than at the base, of the human tongue. It is quite probable that these receptors for pyrogallol, since they occupy a different location from the other bitter receptors, are also of another nature.

It was discovered that the disaccharide maltose, consisting of two glucose units, is thirty-three times more stimulating than the single glucose molecule to the blowfly. Chemical evidence indicates that the greater combining ability of maltose is probably not due to a spatial juxtaposition of groups of two glucose receptor sites. Instead, it appears likely that the glucose receptor site is larger than a single hexose molecule.

Evans (1963) deduces from the available experimental evidence that apparently the hydroxyl groups on carbon atoms 3 and 4 of glucose are entirely responsible for stimulation in the blowfly. These two hydroxyl groups have the trans configuration, but in the effective Cl conformation of the glucose molecule, the C_3 hydroxyl group lies at an angle of 19 degrees above the plane of the molecule, and the C_4 group has a 19 degree downward inclination. The glucose molecule thus attaches to its receptor site at two separate points. Further specificity could be supplied by β steric hindrance due to β substituents of effective size which are found in various glucose derivatives.

Generally α-pyranose, or six-membered ring compounds (with the C_3 and C_4 hydroxyl groups), were about as stimulating as glucose. This included a compound having the stable ether linkage.

Dethier (1955) was able to generalize that to elicit a taste response in the blowfly a carbohydrate molecule must fall within a certain size range; only pentoses, hexoses, and di- and tri-saccharides are stimulating.

It can also be said that linear polyols can at the most call forth only relatively weak responses.

Dethier (1963) has further suggested that effective sugar molecules may weakly combine with their receptor sites by such means as Van der Waal forces.

Andersen *et al.* (1963) studied the mechanisms of sugar taste stimulation by electrophysiologically recording from the whole chorda tympani nerve and single chorda tympani fibers of the dog. They discovered that while some chorda tympani fibers showed activity upon application to the dog's tongue of all the mono- and di-saccharides tested, other fibers responded only to fructose. The nerve fibers which responded to all the sugars showed the highest responses to D-fructose and the next highest to sucrose. The stimulating propensities of the disaccharides sucrose, maltose and lactose reflected their monosaccharide composition. In the whole chorda tympani the most stimulating sugar was D-fructose, followed by sucrose, 1-sorbose, d-mannose, d-glucose, maltose, d-galactose and lactose in that order. The order of stimulating ability for the dog was similar to that found for man in psychophysical studies.

The relative water solubility of each of the tested sugars parallels the order of their stimulating efficacy in the dog and man. Andersen *et al.* suggest that both of these properties of a sugar may depend on the same molecular structures. The disaccharides are apparently not split prior to interaction with their receptor sites.

Actually sugars have a relatively low position on the scale of sweetness.

Single taste nerve fibers in the rat have been observed to show regularly repeated, short bursts of impulse activity in response to sucrose (Beidler, 1953; Pfaffmann, 1955; Fishman, 1957). The rate of the impulses was comparatively slow.

Investigations on sweet substances have also brought to light that receptor sites can show a high level of stereospecificity. The stereoselectivity of certain receptor sites is evidenced by the fact that the α-anomers of a number of sugar molecules and their derivatives are perceived as sweeter by man than the β-anomers, some of which elicit a bitter taste. The opposed tastes of these α- and β-stereoisomers indicates that certain "sweet" and "bitter" receptors have complementary structures (Beidler, 1963).

It has been known for over a decade that 6-α-D-glucopyranosyl-D-glucose tastes sweet, while the 6-β isomer of this substance is bitter. Pangborn and Gee (1961) investigated the taste of the hexose sugars D-glucose and D-galactose and reported that their α-anomers are sweeter than their β-anomers. Dethier (1955) found that generally the alpha glucosidic derivatives of substances are considerably better taste stimulants for the blowfly than the beta derivatives. On the other hand, for man β-fructose and β-L-rhamnose are sweeter than the corresponding α-anomers (Tsuzuki and Yamazaki, 1953). Pangborn and

Chrisp (1966), after working with six human subjects, reported that the α-anomer of D-xylose was more sweet than the equilibrium solution at lower concentrations, but that both had equal sweetness at 0.666 molar concentration. They corroborated their earlier finding that the β-anomer of D-fructose tastes more sweet than a D-fructose equilibrium mixture, and found the α-anomer of L-rhamnose less sweet than its equilibrium mixture. Although the α-form of D-mannose had a sweeter flavor than a D-mannose equilibrium mixture, α-D-mannose by itself produced both a sweet and a bitter taste.

Steinhardt *et al.* (1962) carried out a study of the human taste response to the monosaccharide D-mannose. They suggested that the ambiguous, mixed taste of D-mannose is due to the difference in taste of the two anomers which compose this sugar. The α-anomer seems to be sweet, and has a higher threshold than the β-anomer, and the β-anomer apparently is bitter. Probably as a consequence of the dual composition of D-mannose and individual differences, some human subjects taste D-mannose as sweet, others as bitter, and a large number of subjects perceive it as first sweet and then bitter or vice versa.

The two anomers of D-mannose are stereoisomers, and differ only in the reversed positions of a hydrogen and a hydroxyl group at one end of the six-carbon ring.

It has also been learned from taste experiments involving homologous series of substances that increasing molecular weight in a chemical series is sometimes associated with a shift in taste from sweet to bitter. This phenomenon was observed with amino acids by Stone (1967). It is possible that the reduced ability to evoke the sweet taste which is associated with greater molecular weight may be related to lower water solubility. Increased molecular weight seems to generally result in lower water solubility.

Marcström (1967) reports that the washing from the human tongue of a number of substances elicits the sweet sensation, although the presence of these substances does not produce a sweet taste. Thus rinsing the bitter pyrogallol from the tongue evokes the sweet quality (at the tip of the tongue), as does washing benzyl alcohol from the tongue. The rinsing from the tongue of buffers such as mixed solutions of primary and secondary phosphate also has this effect. If medium concentrations of certain electrolytes are washed from the tongue, a sweet taste results (Renquist, 1919).

However, low concentrations of the above electrolytes may themselves call forth a sweet sensation. Furthermore, most of the halides of alkali metals may produce the sweet quality at their lower effective concentrations, up to 0.02M to 0.04M (Renquist, 1919). Sodium nitrite has a metallic taste at higher concentrations but like potassium nitrite also is sweet at lower concentrations (Marcström, 1967). Very low concentrations of sodium chloride have also been reported to sometimes have a sweet taste (Indow, 1966). This raises the possibility that the mentioned substances taste sweet only at low concentrations, and that washing higher concentrations of these compounds from the tongue at first only reduces their concentrations to the sweet-tasting range.

Another possible explanation for the sweet taste of sodium chloride at low concentrations may lie in the reported mediation in many mammals of sugar responses and salt responses by the same taste nerve fibers. At sufficient sodium chloride concentrations the cross-correlation pattern of impulses in all the salt-responsive fibers, the proper ratios of impulses in all the parallel units, would evoke the salty sensation. But Pfaffmann (1965) suggests that at insufficient salt concentrations the less sensitive salt-responsive fibers would not react or react well and thus would not contribute properly to the formation of the salt-pattern input. Thus an inadequate afferent input would be called forth by low concentrations of sodium chloride, an input which could be centrally interpreted as a sweet input, just as could impulses from a single sugar-salt fiber.

Konishi (1958) noted not only that heavy metal solutions block the sweet sensation on the human tongue but also that rinsing off these heavy metals produces a sweet taste.

Von Békésy (1966) did not find a change in taste sensation with concentration during his experimental stimulations of single human taste papillae. He suggests that changes in the taste of a substance involve the interaction of neural activity from different types of taste papillae. If a substance acted on several papillae, the adaptation of the taste cells of one papilla to the substance's primary taste quality could permit an observer, as the concentration was increased, to notice chemical side effects capable of exciting other papillae.

At higher concentrations the side effects of compounds may be sufficiently strong to evoke new taste sensations.

Adaptation to sodium chloride was found to cause concentrations of this salt below the adapting concentration to excite sour and bitter "antitastes" (Bartoshuk *et al.*, 1964). These tastes, which appeared in the absence of the salty sensation, increased with dilution of the sodium chloride further below the adapting concentration and were clear-cut and lasting. After salt adaptation water evoked the strongest "antitastes."

Water produces a sweet sensation after adaptation to acids (Pfaffmann, 1965).

Marcström (1967) has written an exhaustive paper on taste stimulation by sweet and bitter compounds. After a complete review of gustatory discrimination and of previous concepts and findings on those features of sweet and bitter compounds which are involved in gustation, Marcström deals with the psychophysical technique of taste threshold determination. He describes his studies on some possible weaknesses in the experimental method developed by him. Thus pH, the type of water used to make up the solutions (pH differences?) and the temperatures of the solutions all had some effect on taste thresholds. The rapid oxidation of some compounds had no effect on the observed thresholds. Marcström's findings concerning the interaction of various sweet compounds (and similarly of a number of bitter compounds) with different types of receptor sites and his correlation of thresholds with water solubilities are dealt with earlier in this portion of the chapter.

Of considerable interest in relation to sweet reception is the action of "gymnemic acid" in reversibly blocking sweet taste. This sweet inhibitor is obtained from an Indian plant, *Gymnema sylvestre*. The actual chemical structure of the active principal is not yet known, but Yackzan (1966) believes it to be a water-soluble, heat-stable large molecule containing hydroxyl, carboxyl and glycosyl groups. Borg *et al.* (1967), by recording from the human chorda tympani and by psychophysical tests, found "gymnemic acid" to reversibly block only sweet reception in man, confirming results obtained in a similar manner by Diamant, Oakley *et al.* (1965), but the substance has in the past also been reported to affect the bitter taste. The spectacular action of this blocking agent can easily be demonstrated to students by asking them to chew *Gymnema* leaves and then eat sugar.

Electrophysiological recordings from dogs and hamsters support the view that "gymnemic acid" exerts its action on the taste cells; it may inhibit the excitation of sweet receptor sites.

In rats the drinking of "gymnemic acid" does not affect later selection of sucrose but does prevent the selection of saccharin (Lovell *et al.*, 1961).

A red berry, the "miraculous fruit" (*Synsepalum dulcificum*) of West Africa, contains a substance which causes man to taste otherwise sour food products as sweet. The berry, obtained from a shrub, is used by the local population to overcome the flavor of sour palm wine, beer and maize bread. Even dilute organic and mineral acids taste sweet after the berry's mucilaginous content has been chewed. A sour taste inhibitor is probably responsible for the effect of "miraculous fruit" (Beidler, 1966).

Kurihara and Beidler (1968) extracted the active principle of "miraculous fruit." They found it to be a basic glycoprotein and estimated its molecular weight at 44,000. When the purified protein, which itself has no taste, was mixed with a sour substance, the taste of the mixture in the mouth gradually changed from sour to sweet in approximately one minute. A sweetening of acids was discernible at a protein concentration of 5×10^{-8}M, and the maximum sweetening was produced by 4×10^{-7}M.

Molecular Structure, Properties and Taste—Amino Acids

The research done on amino acids has also brought out the high level of specificity attained by some receptor sites. As in the case of sugars, stereoselectivity is involved in the differing taste effects of the two forms, the D- and L-isomers, in which the common amino acids, with the exception of glycine, are found.

All amino acids except glycine possess an asymmetric α-carbon atom and therefore have stereoisomers. The letters D and L are prefixed to the names of amino acids to denote their steric configuration. When they are part of a protein molecule in nature, the amino acids seem to all be of the L-form.

As has been true in the research on sugar taste, investigations of the taste responses to amino acids have been hampered by problems of chemical purity and purity of the D- or L-enantiomorphs of the employed amino acids. Furthermore, the concentrations of amino acids, like those of sugars, may affect the taste responses to them.

Lawrence and Ferguson (1959) observed the D-forms of the amino acids asparagine and tryptophan to have a sweet taste, while the L-forms did not.

Solms *et al.* (1965) found the D-isomers of histidine, leucine, phenylalanine, tryptophan and tyrosine to primarily have a weak to strong sweet taste, while their respective L-isomers mainly had a weak to strong bitter taste. These results corroborate the work of Berg (1953). L-alanine and the amino acid glycine were sweet. The named amino acid isomers also possessed their own distinctive flavors. The D- and L-enantiomorphs of a number of other amino acids were almost tasteless, while the isomers of an additional group of amino acids produced complex taste sensations. A number of amino acids, among them those containing an aromatic ring structure, proved to be strong taste stimuli for man.

The crab *Carcinides maenas*, when some of its chemoreceptors were stimulated with the D- and L-forms of glutamic acid and leucine, showed different nerve responses to the different stereoisomers (Case and Gwilliam, 1961).

Halpern, Bernard and Kare (1962), by recording from the rat's chorda tympani nerve, found that in this organism the D-, L- and mixed DL-stereoisomers of the amino acid alanine called forth their maximum amplitude of response after different time periods. In behavioral experiments also rats differentiated between these stereoisomers. L-alanine was selected over D-alanine, and in further research there seemed also to be some preference for D-tryptophan over L-tryptophan. The rats preferred low concentrations of DL-alanine and glycine, accepted low concentrations of DL-methionine, and rejected all concentrations of DL-valine.

When the stimulus concentrations of glycine and DL-alanine were raised, the rat's chorda tympani showed a considerably increased response, and a noticeably longer time period elapsed before the maximum response was reached.

The responses to alanine and glycine showed attributes of the responses to sugars. These were the slow development of the response, its low amplitude, and the significance of steric configuration. However, there is rapid adaptation to sugar responses, while to high concentrations of glycine and alanine there was only a very slow adaptation.

Although the neural effects of glycine and alanine differed from that produced by sodium chloride, all three of these substances may interact with the same receptor sites. This is indicated by the fact that after stimulation with high concentrations of the mentioned amino acids, the response to 0.1M sodium chloride dropped by 63 per cent, and was still depressed 20 hours later. The responses to the amino acids remained unaffected.

Stone (1967) performed psychophysical tests with L-amino acids and glycine on human subjects. The responses to all amino acids increased with concentration. The taste of most of the amino acids was complex, and secondary taste elements were detected as the concentrations were raised. The sweet taste of glycine tended to corroborate previous views that the basic $C(NH_2)COOH$ structure alone produces the sweet modality. L-valine was primarily bitter, as was expected from its possession of two CH_3 groups, since these are considered bitter stimuli. However, L-threonine, in which one of valine's CH_3 groups is replaced by an OH group, also evoked various degrees of bitterness in different subjects. Three persons described threonine as primarily sweet but with an underlying bitterness.

Both aspartic and glutamic acid possess two COOH groups, but glutamic acid also has a CH-OH (or CH_2) grouping between its two COOH groups. Glutamic acid was a weaker stimulus than aspartic acid and was less sour and more sweet and salty. Stone believes the taste differences between aspartic and glutamic acid to originate from the CH-OH moiety.

An increase in amino acid chain length, although linked with a shift from sweetness to bitterness, did not result in a more intense bitter taste.

Yoshida *et al.* (1966) determined the tastes and taste thresholds of a series of L- and DL-amino acids, and of one D-amino acid. The taste thresholds of amino acids for man varied from 0.1×10^{-3}M to 30×10^{-3}M. There was no consistent relationship between the thresholds for the amino acids and their steric configurations or molecular weights. However, acidic and basic amino acids usually had a low stimulus threshold, while neutral amino acids usually had a high one. The amides of acidic amino acids had a higher threshold than the acidic amino acids themselves.

The L-isomers of aspartic acid, glutamic acid and histidine-HCl had a sour taste. Stone (1967) also reported the first two L-amino acids to be sour.

Beidler (1961a) states that while most α-amino acids may be sweet, those with the amine (NH_2) group on the β- or the γ-carbon atom are normally not sweet.

Bardach, Fujiya and Holl (1967), by electrophysiologically recording from nerve bundles, determined that some fish also have highly specific receptor sites for amino acids. Thus cysteine was very stimulating for two species of catfish (*Ictalurus*), the sea robin (*Prionotus carolinus*) and the tomcod (*Microgadus tomcod*), but homocysteine, which has only one more carbon atom in its carbon chain, called forth no impulses in nerve bundles of sea robins. The response of the catfish species and the tomcod to homocysteine was doubtful, but after a rinse these fish gave strong responses to stimulation with cysteine.

The stimulating propensity of a substance for fish taste receptors is not always dependent on its water solubility. Charged lipids, such as cholesterol and inositides, which have low water solubility, were effective on catfish barbels.

Enhancing and Inhibiting Effects

The fact that quite unlike substances may act on the same receptor sites is illustrated by the phenomenon of competitive taste inhibition. Some additive effects in turn indicate that the substances involved act on different receptor sites of the taste cell.

Evidence has also been obtained that different substances may combine at one time with the same receptor sites to produce synergistic effects. Enhancement of the response due to such multimolecular combination has been observed by simultaneous stimulation with a sugar and an amino acid, and with 5'-ribonucleotides and monosodium glutamate. Furthermore, in the case of some substances, a second molecule of the substance may ap-

parently interact with a receptor site with which one molecule of the same material has already combined.

Tateda (1967) recorded from the rat's chorda tympani nerve while applying sugars, amino acids, and combinations of the two to its tongue. He determined that the responses to D-fructose, D-glucose and sucrose could once more be increased by use of very high concentrations of these sugars after a saturation level of stimulation had already been reached with normal concentrations. This indicates that a second molecule of the mentioned sugars can interact with an already occupied receptor site. Tateda describes such a double combination with sucrose molecules as a (sucrose)$_2$-receptor site complex. Presumably the affinity of a single sucrose molecule-receptor site complex for an additional sucrose molecule is less than the affinity of an empty receptor site for a first sucrose molecule.

Tateda's response-concentration curve for glycine also shows a second increase in response and a second saturation level. It is possible that a number of different complexes can form between glycine molecules and a receptor site.

In another experiment quantities of sucrose were dissolved in solutions of glycine, and these mixed solutions were then applied to the rat's tongue. For some concentrations of such mixtures the resulting responses were three to five times as high as the sum of the responses to separate, individually applied glycine and sucrose solutions of the same concentrations. The response to a sucrose-glycine mixture was therefore not a sum of the separate effects of the contained sucrose and glycine but instead demonstrated considerable enhancement. This synergism can be explained as due to the combination of both sucrose and glycine with the same receptor sites. Perhaps a glycine-receptor site complex interacts better with a sucrose molecule than does a single sucrose molecule-receptor site complex. The sucrose-glycine-receptor site complex may produce a higher response than a receptor site–single molecule combination, as is true of the (sucrose)$_2$-receptor site complex.

Tateda also found evidence that glycine and fructose act on the same receptor sites.

Sato, Yamashita and Ogawa (1967), continuing the work of Sato and Akaike (1965), studied the enhancement produced in the rat's neural response to monosodium glutamate by the addition of 5'-ribonucleotides. They recorded from single fibers of the rat's chorda tympani and also from the whole nerve while applying experimental taste solutions to the rat's tongue.

The results showed that when sodium 5'-guanylate (5'-GMP) or sodium 5'-inosinate (5'-IMP) are added in optimal amounts to monosodium glutamate (MSG), they produce a fivefold enhancement in the total chorda tympani response. Even the addition of the above two ribonucleotides in a quantity 1/100 as great as the amount of MSG resulted in noticeable enhancement.

Single fibers showing good responses to sucrose exhibited much greater response enhancement when 5'-ribonucleotides were added to MSG than did sodium chloride-sensitive fibers. In fact, the response to a solution of MSG and 5'-GMP apparently is linearly related to a fiber's sucrose response. Also, the ratio of the potentiation produced by adding 5'-GMP or sodium 5'-uridylate (5'-UMP) to MSG is closely correlated with a fiber's sucrose–sodium chloride response ratio.

Sodium chloride reduced the enhancement resulting from the addition of 5'-ribonucleotides to MSG. Thus mixing one of the 5'-ribonucleotides and MSG in 0.1 per cent sodium chloride rather than in water caused the observed synergism to fall by approximately one half. This indicates some type of competitive action by sodium chloride.

The nerve fibers exhibiting a considerably enhanced response to a 5'-ribonucleotide-MSG mixture also responded to these substances when they were applied to the tongue separately. Thus neither the 5'-ribonucleotide or

MSG required the presence of the other to react with sites on the involved taste cells.

In the cat salt fibers have been observed to react to IMP-MSG and GMP-MSG mixtures with enhanced responses (it is known that there are few sucrose fibers in the cat). When one of the ribonucleotides or monosodium glutamate was added to 0.5M sodium chloride, the response of the salt fiber increased accordingly. However, adding these substances to 0.005M quinine noticeably reduced the quinine fiber's response (Adachi *et al.*, 1967a). The effect on the quinine fiber's response suggests some sort of competition on the part of IMP, GMP and MSG with quinine.

Mixtures of sodium 5'-inosinate (5'-IMP) and amino acids were applied to the tongue of the rat by Adachi *et al.* (1967b), and the integrated responses of the chorda tympani were electrophysiologically recorded. The mixtures of 5'-IMP and mono-aminodicarboxylic acids always produced enhancement. However, mixtures of 5'-IMP with L-valine or with L-histidine only produced responses equivalent to the sum of the effects of the components of the solutions. The 5'-IMP-sodium succinate mixtures also only showed additive effects. On the basis of these findings the authors suggest that both the amine and dicarboxyl groups of amino acids may play a role in producing synergism when amino acid-5'-IMP mixtures are used as taste stimuli.

Integrated responses from the cat's chorda tympani show that in this organism a 2.5M ethyl alcohol solvent causes the response to 0.02M quinine hydrochloride (from the anterior portion of the tongue) to fall by a factor of 2.5. This suggests competition between ethyl alcohol and quinine. The responses to salt and to acetic acid fell slightly. However, the response to 1M sucrose increased if this sugar was dissolved in 2.5M ethyl alcohol (Hellekant, 1967). It is not clear whether bona fide synergism was involved in this increase.

Mixtures of quinine and 6-n-propylthiouracil have been reported to produce synergism, and other mixtures inhibition (Fischer and Griffin, 1964).

Combination With Two Receptor Sites

A chemical stimulus may in turn also combine with two different kinds of receptor sites. Such dual affinities often produce mixed tastes, and lead to results which can be treated mathematically only by use of two equilibrium constants. The full responses are calculated for a dual-site stimulus by applying Beidler's taste equation separately to responses from each set of receptor sites and then adding the obtained values.

Beidler (1961a, b) cites ammonium chloride as a substance which interacts with two types of receptor sites in the rat. The combination of ammonium chloride with one of these sets of receptor sites, making up about 10 per cent of the total, has an equilibrium constant of 86. The interaction with the other 90 per cent of the receptor sites has an equilibrium constant of 0.8. The 10 per cent of the sites for which K equals 86 are reactive at lower stimulus concentrations and have a lower level of response saturation than the other receptor site group. Ammonium chloride may taste salty to man at low concentrations but is bitter at great concentrations. At medium concentrations it produces both tastes.

Potassium chloride also combines with two kinds of receptor sites in the rat. In man it is sweet at 0.009M concentration, bitter at a molarity of 0.03, and bitter, salty and sour at 0.02 moles (von Skramlik, 1926).

If a substance combines with more than one type of receptor site, the set of receptor sites for which combination has the highest equilibrium constant is the set of greatest significance at threshold concentrations. This is true because a high equilibrium constant indicates a strong interaction between the stimulus and the receptor sites. More powerful interaction will in turn result in a greater amount of filling of the receptor sites at low concentrations.

For substances combining with two or more types of receptors the threshold for response

is not indicative of the responses to higher concentrations.

Second Receptor Systems

Some organisms possess more than one taste receptor system, and each group of receptors has its unique properties.

This is brought out by the work of Konishi (1967), who recorded from both single palatine fibers and the whole palatine nerve of the carp (*Cyprinus carpio*).

In this freshwater fish one receptor system is highly sensitive to very dilute inorganic electrolytes with monovalent cations. Polyvalent anions increase the magnitude of response elicited from this receptor system, which is nonreactive to pure water. The responses of the system are marked by a slow rise to the maximum activity evoked by the stimulus. As an optimum concentration of the electrolyte stimulus, related to its normality, is passed, the elicited response magnitude falls once again.

A second receptor system is stimulated by high concentrations of electrolytes, reacts primarily to their cations and responds well to polyvalent cations, which call forth little activity in the first system described above. The second receptor system therefore gives its greatest responses to concentrations of electrolytes which also severely depress activity in the first, dilute-electrolyte receptor system.

As a result of the presence of these two systems, the carp's response-concentration curve for an electrolyte with a monovalent cation has an inverse S-shape. It rises as the electrolyte approaches its optimum concentration for the dilute-electrolyte receptor system, and then falls again, as this concentration is passed. Then the curve rises a second time as the concentration of the electrolyte becomes sufficiently high to adequately stimulate the second receptor system.

A depression of responses was also produced by middle concentrations of most nonelectrolytes, including sucrose and quinine (Konishi and Niwa, 1964).

That there are indeed two taste receptor

systems in the carp is shown by the results of subjecting the palatal organ to polarizing currents.

An anodal current noticeably lowers the threshold for the rapid type of response to higher concentrations which is characteristic of the second, high-concentration receptor system, and augments the magnitude of the responses coming from this system. At the same time an anodal current reduces the slowly developing responses to dilute electrolytes which originate in the dilute-electrolyte receptor system. As would be expected, an anodal current also greatly enhances the response to polyvalent-cation compounds such as calcium chloride.

On the other hand, a cathodal current reduces the rapid responses of the high-concentration receptor system and produces little change or sometimes an increase in the responses emanating from the dilute-electrolyte receptor system.

Thus polarizing currents by their effects clearly differentiate between two kinds of response mechanisms.

Konishi believes that stimulation of the dilute-electrolyte receptor system may require an electrokinetic process and related phenomena. Previous treatment with alkali, which should result in negative ionization of the receptor sites, reduces the responses from this system, and an application of acid subsequent to alkali treatment prevents such response depression. This indicates that the dilute-electrolyte receptors are stimulated when the negatively charged anions of an electrolyte interact with positively charged radicals at the receptor membrane.

The increase in response occasionally observed after several applications of a dye cation may result from the combination of the dye cations with anion groups on the receptor sites. Such neutralization of negatively charged anion groups should increase the affinity of the stimulus anions for the receptor sites. Calcium chloride sometimes had the same action as a dye cation.

A higher concentration of an electrolyte, or a mixture of two dilute electrolytes which separately are effective stimulants, depresses the response of the dilute-electrolyte receptor system. Depression rather than saturation takes place because the now greater concentration of ions in the applied taste solution may reduce the Stern potential at the receptor surface. The Stern potential is produced by ions adsorbed to the receptor surface or the double counterion layer just above it and determines the extent to which ions will be attracted to the receptor site.

The cations of polyvalent cation compounds added in sufficient concentration to dilute electrolytes may depress responses by gathering at the inner surface of the double counterion layer. This could have a screening effect against the oppositely charged anions and prevent them from coming to the receptor surface. It could also decrease the Stern potential through reducing the thickness of the double counterion layer.

A similar arrangement of two electrolyte receptor systems, with one of them sensitive to water, has been suggested for the cat (Cohen, Hagiwara and Zotterman, 1955).

In the chorda tympani taste response of the rat, there is an early, transient component which is not used in the determination of the magnitude of the response. It consists of an irregular discharge which falls in frequency within 2 seconds. Tateda (1967) suggests that this early, fast response, which precedes the more stationary and normally investigated response, may be produced by the stimulation of different receptor sites from those which contribute to the "stationary" response. This is indicated by the fact that, at higher levels of stimulus concentration, the fast response did not rise as rapidly with increasing concentration of taste solutions as did the "stationary" response. Beidler (1961a) stated that the early, fast response is thought to originate from the nerve fibers themselves.

Taste Modalities

As might be expected from the considerable spectrum of taste receptor sites which has been found to exist in an individual organism, the classification of taste into four taste qualities is now considered archaic by many investigators. It is no longer generally believed that any, even the most unusual tastes, can be duplicated by mixing some or all of the four basic taste qualities in the proper proportions.

However, some scientists continue to speak of the four basic taste modalities. Moncrieff (1967) points out that if this concept is accepted, the metallic and alkaline tastes would have to be attributed to the common chemical sense, which is chiefly mediated by the trigeminal nerves. The metallic taste in particular is well known, and a good idea has been obtained of the concentrations of metal ions needed to reach the threshold for the metallic taste.

Von Békésy (1964a) used 0.3 mm gold point electrodes to produce taste sensations by electrical stimulation of the human tongue. He was able to elicit only each of the four basic taste qualities (sour, salty, sweet, bitter) and obtained no gustatory sensation at all from some spots. Von Békésy indicated that this result appears to represent a confirmation of the original four taste modalities concept. Using cooperative subjects, he also only found purely salty, sour, sweet, and bitter taste papillae and even describes differences in the anatomical structure of these papilla types! The tastes sensed from the papillae did not vary with the frequency of the applied d.c. pulses.

Using chemical stimulation of individual human taste papillae, von Békésy (1966) was able to confirm the results he obtained with electrical stimulation. Each papilla responded with the same single taste quality to both chemical and electrical stimulation. A few larger papillae were apparently formed by the fusion of two or three individual papillae, and these responded with different taste qualities on their several aspects. Such larger papillae were most frequent at the tongue's edge and on the palate.

On the other hand, how is the observation that each normal human papilla responds with only one of the four taste qualities to be correlated with the discovery of single chorda tympani fibers conveying several taste qualities in the rat (Fishman, 1957; Erickson, 1963; Yamashita *et al.*, 1967a), the hamster (Fishman, 1957; Yamashita *et al.*, 1967b) and the cat (Pfaffmann, 1941; Pfaffmann, 1955; Cohen *et al.*, 1955; Nagaki *et al.*, 1964)? Further, how can von Békésy's results be related to the findings that individual rat and hamster taste cells are sensitive to multiple taste qualities (Kimura and Beidler, 1961; Tateda and Beidler, 1964)? Von Békésy points to the possibility of a major species difference in this regard between man and the other mentioned mammals. He also notes (1966) that electrophysiological techniques have their limitations. Von Békésy states that it is not certain that most of the preparations described in the many purported single fiber studies really consisted of only one active nerve fiber. He instead prefers to lay greater weight on the microelectrode studies of rat taste buds. Also, the possibility of various efferent and other inhibitory connections and feedbacks could complicate the analysis of taste fiber responses.

It appears unlikely, however, that many single fiber preparations in reality contained two or more active fibers. The impulse discharge of a single fiber is identified by equal spike height and duration and by the presence of regular intervals between the impulses. Also, the electrophysiological findings of Erickson (1963) on the impulse frequency elicited in single taste fibers by stimulation with several salts, to be described shortly, have been verified by behavioral experiments.

Erickson (1965), referring to von Békésy's (1964b) statement of a duplexity theory of taste, suggests that further efforts would have to be made to find taste units responsive to multiple stimuli. One possibility might be to make use of new taste substances, or perhaps smaller responses to additional taste qualities might still be discovered.

Erickson (1967, Discussion) reports that he and his co-workers have also chemically stimulated single human taste papillae, using a specially constructed flow chamber and more concentrated compounds than those employed by von Békésy. They found that while certain papillae appeared to be specific, others responded to several or all of the four taste modalities used.

Erickson (1967, Discussion) also states that he does not have an understanding of what is happening when a major portion of a sensory system is directly excited with an electric current, as is the case in von Békésy's research. Little knowledge can be gained in this manner if the biological systems under study have a heterogeneous innervation. Erickson feels that a whole taste papilla is not the type of separate unit which is subject to profitable analysis.

Pfaffmann (Discussion, in Erickson, 1967), in commenting on the discrepancy between von Békésy's results and those of electrophysiologists, points out that von Békésy has not reported the impulse discharge in the neural elements innervating a human taste papilla but has made psychophysical findings on the final sensations produced. It is well known that electrophysiological and psychophysical (or behavioral) results are difficult to correlate. Perhaps there is a funneling (see introduction to Chap. IV) or integration of the evoked neural activity in the brain. But first more electrophysiological results on man should tell us whether we have as broad fiber sensitivities as have primates and other animals. Erickson (1967, Discussion), however, discounts the possibility of funneling in man to the point of giving us cortical neurons which are each receptive to only one of the four taste qualities, since this would only supply us with the taste information available to insects.

Beidler (Discussion in Erickson, 1967) has echoed the possibility that one hundred odd broadly sensitive taste fibers innervating the taste buds of a single papilla could together, by integration, produce a single taste quality. He also points to the fact that von Békésy used unusually dilute stimuli.

Von Békésy (1964b) developed a duplexity theory of taste based on his findings that the interactions between certain taste qualities and temperature senses formed these modalities into two separate groups. If any two of the stimuli were applied simultaneously, one to each side of the human tongue, bitter, sweet and warm interacted only with each other, just as salty, sour and cold formed an interacting group.

In the cat, dog and rat, carbon dioxide gas has been observed to produce responses in separate fibers respectively mediating each of the three sensations in the latter group given above (Kawamura and Adachi, 1967).

Cross-fiber Neural Patterns

Yamashita *et al.* (1967a, b) found that in single chorda tympani fibers of the rat and the hamster, there was a direct relation between the responses to sour (HCl), bitter (quinine) and cooling. Fibers which responded well to one of these three modalities also gave good responses to the other two (Fig. 5-14). Yamashita *et al.* (1967a) suggest that this correlation may mean that HCl, quinine and cooling induce similar nerve activity, already indicated for the rat by Erickson, Doetsch and Marshall (1965), and also that the responses to the three types of stimuli may interact in the nervous system. That responses to HCl, quinine and cooling are transmitted by the same nerve fibers and the likelihood that they go to the same general destination in the nervous system could be a parallel phenomenon to the interacting stimulus groups found by von Békésy (1964b) in man. The difference in the makeup of the interacting stimulus groups for man and for the rat could well be due to a species difference.

Morrison (1967) found the rat's behavioral responses to sucrose to more closely resemble those to sodium chloride than those to hydrochloric acid or quinine. The responses to quinine resembled those to sodium chloride rather than those to sucrose, and this was also true of the responses to hydrochloric acid. The reactions to hydrochloric acid were relatively

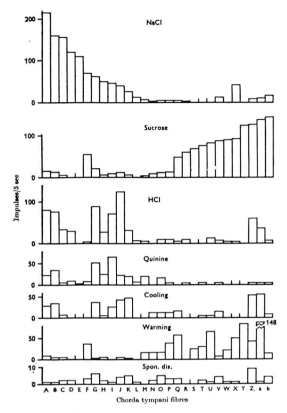

FIGURE 5-14. Response profiles of twenty-eight hamster chorda tympani fibers. Half are arranged according to their response to 0.1M sodium chloride, the other half by the degree of responsiveness to 0.5M sucrose. Stimuli: 0.1M sodium chloride, 0.5M sucrose, 0.01N hydrochloric acid, 0.02M quinine hydrochloride, water at 20°C (cooling to tongue at 40°C) and water at 40°C (warming to tongue at 20°C). The level of spontaneous discharge is shown at the bottom. Many units gave similar responses to hydrochloric acid, quinine and cooling. A number of units responded well to both sucrose and warming. In general the fibers reactive to sodium chloride differed from those discharging to sucrose, and some units gave a significant response only to sucrose. (From Ogawa, H., M. Sato, and S. Yamashita: Multiple sensitivity of chorda tympani fibres of the rat and hamster to gustatory and thermal stimuli. *J. Physiol. [London], 199:* 223-240, 1968.)

more similar to the quinine responses than to the responses shown to sodium chloride or sucrose. This last behavioral observation appears to be in good agreement with the neural results given in the previous paragraph.

In the hamster (Yamashita *et al.*, 1967b) the chorda tympani fibers which carry a high frequency of responses to sucrose also mediate the main impulse activity in response to warming (Figs. 5-14, 5-15).

A single rat chorda tympani unit, which did not respond to either cooling or warming alone, was adapted to a 0.1M sodium chloride solution at a temperature of 30°C. When the same solution, but at a temperature of 10°C, was flown over the tongue without the intervening application of a water rinse, it produced a significant increase in the response. The reverse experiment, in which the adapting 0.1M sodium chloride solution was warmed from 10°C to 30°C, only produced a decrease in the impulse frequency.

These effects of temperature were clearly not the result of an influence on the interaction between the stimulating sodium chloride and its receptor sites, since a rise in temperature facilitates the stimulus-receptor site combination. Instead, Yamashita *et al.* (1967a) suggest that in this case a stimulating action of cooling summed with the effect of the taste stimulus to produce a greater receptor cell membrane depolarization. This would indicate that the reactivity of single taste nerve fibers to several different qualities of stimuli need not be a consequence of their branching to several receptor cells but instead could result from the multiple sensitivity of a single taste cell.

According to Ogawa, Sato and Yamashita (1968) the temperature-sensitive chorda tympani fibers of the rat and hamster resemble those of the cat in showing low thermal sensitivity and rapid adaptation to temperature stimuli. Temperature variations elicited an average change in impulse rate of —0.42 impulses/sec °C in nineteen rat taste fibers sensitive to cooling. The response of such units dropped to the resting level in just a few seconds. The impulse rate of the rat chorda tympani fibers was minimal at a temperature of 35°C.

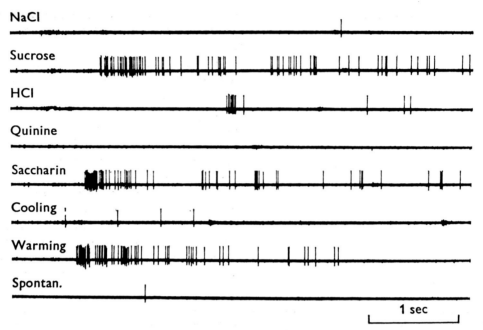

NaCl

Sucrose

HCl

Quinine

Saccharin

Cooling

Warming

Spontan.

1 sec

FIGURE 5-15. Responses of a single hamster chorda tympani fiber. Stimuli: 0.1M sodium chloride, 0.5M sucrose, 0.01N hydrochloric acid, 0.02M quinine hydrochloride and 0.02M sodium saccharin, all at 25°C. Also water at 20°C and at 40°C. Spontaneous activity at the bottom. Sizeable discharges were elicited by sucrose, saccharin and warming. (From Ogawa, H., M. Sato, and S. Yamashita: Multiple sensitivity of chorda tympani fibres of the rat and hamster to gustatory and thermal stimuli. *J. Physiol. [London]*, 199:223-240, 1968.)

In rats and hamsters the responses to hydrochloric acid and to quinine are generally carried in the same nerve fibers, and in hamsters the responses to sodium chloride and to quinine are also linked (Fig. 5-14). Thus particular groups of taste fibers are composed of units which each either serve individual receptors sensitive to special combinations of gustatory stimuli or branch to receptors which are individually sensitive to one or another of the linked stimuli or both. Conversely, the rat and hamster taste fibers which convey the impulses evoked by sucrose do not carry many of the impulses elicited by sodium chloride, and vice versa (Fig. 5-14).

Erickson (1963) found that the rat chorda tympani fibers which fire frequent impulses in response to potassium chloride are also often highly excited by ammonium chloride, while sodium chloride most strongly affects a different group of taste fibers. Therefore, potassium chloride and ammonium chloride (and also calcium chloride) call forth similar neural patterns, whereas sodium chloride (and lithium chloride) produce a different neural pattern.

The cross-fiber correlation of the responses to potassium chloride and to ammonium chloride, and the observation that the chief effect of sodium chloride is exerted on other fibers, were corroborated by behavioral experiments. Rats which learned to avoid potassium chloride solution because of an electric shock also did not drink much ammonium chloride, and vice versa. However, such avoidance was poorly generalized to sodium chloride, nor was the avoidance of sodium chloride linked with any considerable depression of the consumption of the other two salt solutions or any discrimination between them.

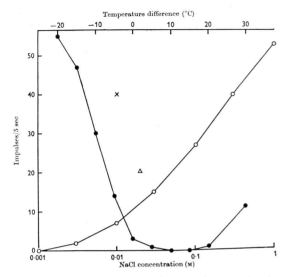

FIGURE 5-16. Responses of a single rat chorda tympani fiber to sodium chloride (open circles) and to temperature (solid circles). Ordinate, number of impulses fired within 5 seconds after stimulation. Upper abscissa, difference in temperature between applied water and tongue. Cross, response to 0.01N hydrochloric acid; triangle, response to 0.02M quinine hydrochloride. A decrease of 20°C in the temperature of the tongue's surface evoked a discharge of about the same magnitude as that following stimulation with 1M sodium chloride. (From Ogawa, H., M. Sato, and S. Yamashita: Multiple sensitivity of chorda tympani fibres of the rat and hamster to gustatory and thermal stimuli. *J. Physiol.* [*London*], 199:223-240, 1968.)

The close cross-correlation between the impulse discharges to sodium chloride and to lithium chloride has also been verified by behavioral studies. Nachman (1963) observed that naive rats which were briefly exposed to sodium chloride and to lithium chloride drank both with equal eagerness. After suffering from the toxic effects of lithium chloride, these rats then generalized their newly developed aversion to lithium chloride primarily to sodium chloride, less to ammonium chloride, and least to potassium chloride.

However, Nachman, unlike Erickson (1963), presented the mentioned salts to his rats in equal molar concentrations. Therefore, his methodology does not make it possible to distinguish between the qualitatively different effects and the intensity effects of the tested salts.

Morrison (1967) as well found that sodium salts and lithium chloride give rise to like behavioral responses in the rat. Further, the behavioral responses to magnesium salts, potassium salts, ammonium chloride and distilled water resembled each other. These results correlate well with those obtained by Erickson, Doetsch and Marshall (1965) from the rat's chorda tympani on stimulation with magnesium chloride, potassium chloride and ammonium chloride. Reasons are given for believing that not only the intensity aspects of the evoked taste sensations but also qualitative aspects play a role in the taste groupings of salts.

Morrison (1967) observed some differences between the behavioral responses to calcium chloride, ammonium chloride and potassium chloride. These observations do not jibe with the across-fiber patterns Erickson (1963) recorded from the chorda tympani. However, in relating electrophysiological data from the chorda tympani nerve with behavioral results, it should be remembered that the glossopharyngeal nerve serving the posterior tongue of mammals often has a different order of integrated responses from the chorda tympani.

Papers by Pfaffmann, Fisher and Frank (1967) and by Yamada (1967) deal with the integrated responses of the glossopharyngeal nerve in the mammal and contrast these responses to those recorded from the chorda tympani.

In rats sodium chloride receptor sites predominate in the tongue region served by the chorda tympani, while in hamsters sucrose sites and hydrochloric acid sites are most numerous. A few chorda tympani fibers in the hamster responded only to sucrose (Fig. 5-14). About one fourth of the chorda tympani taste fibers investigated in either the rat or the hamster were responsive to all four taste modalities (Ogawa, Sato and Yamashita, 1968).

The cross-fiber pattern of neural coding first described by Erickson (1963) for the rat has been verified for the opossum (*Didelphys virginiana*) by Marshall (1968). Marshall, however, found he could only obtain the inverse relationship between the similarity of the cross-fiber response to substances and the ability to behaviorally discriminate between these substances by recording the second second of chorda tympani activity. Erickson (1963) used the first second of neural activity in his work on the rat. Marshall employed differential positive reinforcement in the form of a reward of drinking water to cause his opossums to discriminate between test stimuli.

Tapper and Halpern (1968) have used ionizing radiation to produce a high and maintained aversion in rats to gustatory stimuli. They found that rats so conditioned against either D1-alanine or sodium saccharin also avoided the other of these substances, as well as glycine. However, they did not discriminate against D-glucose or potassium chloride.

Tapper and Halpern (1968) employed a wide range of concentrations of each test substance to demonstrate a high degree of intrachemical generalization.

Unconditioned rats select the conditioning solutions of sodium saccharin, Dl-alanine and glycine over distilled water.

The greater sensitivity to potassium chloride than to sodium chloride of such carnivores as the dog apparently means that in these animals a predominant number of taste nerve fibers at least chiefly innervate either receptor cells which possess an excess of surface membrane receptor sites for potassium chloride, have only such receptor sites, or both. There is therefore no basis for expecting the greater potassium chloride versus sodium chloride response of the dog or other carnivores to be reflected in the sensitivities of other tissues of the species to these two salts.

Molecular Imprinting

Fischer and Griffin (1964) observed that tasting practice could lower taste thresholds for quinine and PROP considerably. Furthermore, a drop in threshold for 1-quinine was accompanied by lower thresholds for PROP, sucrose and hydrochloric acid.

These findings, suggestive of taste "memory," are explained in terms of the imprinting of molecular configurations on the taste receptor. Analogous imprinting has been produced in silica gel by preparing it in a quinine mixture and then extracting the quinine. Low, threshold or subthreshold concentrations of the imprinting molecules are optimal, perhaps because a bimolecular stimulus-receptor site complex does not give rise to an effective imprint. The taste thresholds of poor 1-quinine tasters showed a greater drop, but fell more slowly, than the thresholds of good tasters.

Since carbons 3, 4, 8 and 9 of 1-quinine are asymmetric, PROP, without any asymmetric carbons, might fit into the imprint of 1-quinine with the least difficulty, followed by sucrose with one asymmetric carbon and d-quinine with two. This is the actual order of the extent of the threshold decrease after taste practice with 1-quinine.

A return to the original thresholds after an interval without taste practice is related by the authors to the replacement of the imprinted taste cells by new ones. The faster than normal drop in thresholds following a second practice after a forgetting interval is tied to the possible existence of a neural or central taste memory.

In connection with taste imprinting, it is interesting that the minnow (*Phoxinus phoxinus* L.) learns a behavioral response fastest with saccharose, followed by acetic acid, sodium chloride and quinine-hydrochloride in that order (Glaser, 1966).

The Role of the Saliva

The influence of the saliva on gustation has also been investigated by Fischer and Griffin (1964). They determined that one's own saliva is essential for tasting the tested compounds [PTC, 6-n-propylthiouracil (PROP), quinine] and that boiling the saliva eliminates its gustatory function. The saliva of persons with low sensitivity to quinine and PROP had twice the oxidation rate of the saliva of good tasters, primarily because of the presence of hydrogen peroxide. On the other hand, the saliva of good

PROP tasters showed more catalase activity. Fischer and Griffin do not believe that such salivary differences are mainly responsible for the different taste thresholds of "tasters" and "nontasters."

The above material should give some indication of the complexity of various aspects of taste reception. It is striking how fine molecular structural details at different receptor sites act to determine the gustatory sense of an organism.

The book *Taste and Olfaction III*, edited by Carl Pfaffmann and published by the Rockefeller University Press in 1970, and the two preceding volumes of the series, are good sources of material pertaining to taste reception. The review "The Chemical Senses," by Benjamin *et al.* is also recommended.

REFERENCES

Abrahamson, E.W., and S.E. Ostroy: The photochemical and macromolecular aspects of vision. *Progr. Biophys.*, 17:179-215, 1967.

Adachi, A., M. Funakoshi, and Y. Kawamura: Neurophysiological Studies on Taste Effectiveness of Chemical Taste Enhancers. In Hayashi, T. (Ed.): *Olfaction and Taste, Proceedings of the Second International Symposium*. Oxford, Pergamon, 1967a, pp. 411-413.

Adachi, A., J. Okamoto, T. Hamada, and Y. Kawamura: Taste effectiveness of mixtures of sodium 5'-inosinate and various amino acids. *J. Physiol. Soc. Jap.*, 29:65-71, 1967b.

Andersen, H.T., M. Funakoshi, and Y. Zotterman: Electrophysiological Responses to Sugars and Their Depression by Salt. In Zotterman, Y. (Ed.): *Olfaction and Taste, Proceedings of the First International Symposium*. Oxford, Pergamon, 1963, pp. 177-192.

Andersson, B.B., S. Landgren, L. Olsson, and Y. Zotterman: The sweet taste fibres of the dog. *Acta Physiol. Scand.*, 21:105-119, 1950.

Arden, G.B.: Recent Work on the Early Receptor Potential and Related Rapid Responses. In *The Clinical Value of Electroretinography*. ISCERG Symp. Ghent. Basel-New York, Karger, 1968, pp. 51-59.

Arden, G.B., and K.T. Brown: Some properties of components of the cat electroretinogram revealed by local recording under oil. *J. Physiol. (London)*, 176:429-461, 1965.

Arden, G.B., and H. Ikeda: A new property of the early receptor potential of rat retina. *Nature*, 208:1100-1101, 1965.

Arden, G.B., H. Ikeda, and I.M. Siegel: New components of the mammalian receptor potential and their relation to visual photochemistry. *Vision Res.*, 6:373-384, 1966.

Arden, G.B., C.D.B. Bridges, H. Ikeda, and I.M. Siegel: Isolation of a new fast component of the early receptor potential. *J. Physiol. (London)*, 186:123P-124P, 1966a.

Arden, G.B., C.D.B. Bridges, H. Ikeda, and I.M. Siegel: Rapid light-induced potentials common to plant and animal tissues. *Nature, 212*: 1235-1236, 1966b.

Azuma, M., and Y. Kito: Studies on optical rotation, circular dichroism and amino acid composition of rhodopsin. *Ann. Rep. Biol. Works, Fac. of Sci., Osaka University*, 15:59-69, 1967.

Bardach, J., M. Fujiya, and A. Holl: Investigations of External Chemoreceptors of Fishes. In Hayashi, T. (Ed.): *Olfaction and Taste, Proceedings of the Second International Symposium*. Oxford, Pergamon, 1967, pp. 647-665.

Bartoshuk, L.M., D.H. Mc Burney, and C. Pfaffmann: Taste of sodium chloride solutions after adaptation to sodium chloride: Implications for the "water taste." *Science, 143*:967-968, 1964.

Becker, H.E., and R.A. Cone: Light-stimulated electrical responses from skin. *Science, 154*: 1051-1053, 1966.

Beidler, L.M.: Our taste receptors. *Sci. Monthly*, 75:343-349, 1952.

Beidler, L.M.: Properties of chemoreceptors of tongue of rat. *J. Neurophysiol.*, 16:595-607, 1953.

Beidler, L.M.: A theory of taste stimulation. *J. Gen. Physiol.*, 38:133-139, 1954.

Beidler, L.M.: Taste receptor stimulation. *Prog. Biophys. Biophys. Chem.*, 12:107-151, 1961a.

Beidler, L.M.: Biophysical approaches to taste. *Amer. Sci.*, 49:421-431, 1961b.

Beidler, L.M.: Dynamics of Taste Cells. In Zotterman, Y. (Ed.): *Olfaction and Taste, Proceedings of the First International Symposium*. Oxford, Pergamon, 1963, pp. 133-148.

Beidler, L.M.: Comparison of gustatory receptors, olfactory receptors and free nerve endings.

In *Sensory Receptors. Cold Spring Harbor Symposia on Quantitative Biology*, 30:191-200, 1965.

Beidler, L.M.: A physiological basis of taste sensation. *J. Food Sci.*, 31:275-281, 1966.

Beidler, L.M.: Anion Influences on Taste Receptor Response. In Hayashi, T. (Ed.): *Olfaction and Taste, Proceedings of the Second International Symposium.* Oxford, Pergamon, 1967, pp. 509-534.

Beidler, L.M., I.Y. Fishman, and C.W. Hardiman: Species differences in taste responses. *Amer. J. Physiol.*, 181:235-239, 1955.

Békésy, G. von: Sweetness produced electrically on the tongue and its relation to taste theories. *J. Appl. Physiol.*, 19:1105-1113, 1964a.

Békésy, G. von: Duplexity theory of taste. *Science*, 145:834-835, 1964b.

Békésy, G. von: Taste theories and the chemical stimulation of single papillae. *J. Appl. Physiol.*, 21:1-9, 1966.

Bell, F.R., and R.L. Kitchell: Taste reception in the goat, sheep and calf. *J. Physiol. (London)*, 183:145-151, 1966.

Benjamin, R.M., B.P. Halpern, D.G. Moulton, and M.M. Mozell: The chemical senses. *Ann. Rev. Psychol.*, 16:381-416, 1965.

Berg, C.: Physiology of the D-amino acids. *Physiol. Rev.*, 33:145-189, 1953.

Bernhard, R.: Conference on cell membranes: seeds of rebellion. *Sci. Res.*, 4, no. 5:25-26, 1969.

Bing, H.I., and A.P. Skouby: Sensitization of cold receptors by substances with acetyl-choline effect. *Acta Physiol. Scand.*, 21:286-302, 1950.

Bonting, S.L.: Development and mode of action of the rhodopsin system in the photoreceptor cell. *Ophthalmologica*, 152:527-529, 1966.

Bonting, S.L.: Physiological chemistry of the eye. *Arch. Ophthal.*, 78:803-819, 1967.

Bonting, S.L., and A.D. Bangham: On the biochemical mechanism of the visual process. *Exp. Eye Res.*, 6:400-413, 1967.

Borg, G., H. Diamant, B. Oakley, L. Ström, and Y. Zotterman: A Comparative Study of Neural and Psychophysical Responses to Gustatory Stimuli. In Hayashi, T. (Ed.): *Olfaction and Taste, Proceedings of the Second International Symposium.* Oxford, Pergamon, 1967, pp. 253-264.

Bortoff, A., and A.L. Norton: An electrical model of the vertebrate photoreceptor cell. *Vision Res.*, 7:253-263, 1967.

Bownds, D.: The site of attachment of the rhodopsin chromophore. *Fed. Proc.*, 25, Pt. 1:787, 1966.

Bownds, D.: Site of attachment of retinal in rhodopsin. *Nature*, 216:1178-1181, 1967.

Bridges, C.D.B.: Photopigments in the char of Lake Windemere (*Salvelinus willughbii* Gunther, forma *autumnalis* and forma *vernalis*). *Nature*, 214:205-206, 1967.

Brindley, G.S., and A.R. Gardner-Medwin: The origin of the early receptor potential of the retina. *J. Physiol. (London)*, 182:185-194, 1966.

Brown, J.E., J.R. Murray, and T.G. Smith: Photoelectric potential from photoreceptor cells in ventral eye of *Limulus*. *Science*, 158:665-666, 1967.

Brown, K.T.: An early potential evoked by light from the pigment epithelium-choroid complex of the eye of the toad. *Nature*, 207:1249-1253, 1965.

Brown, K.T., and J.M. Crawford: Intracellular recording of rapid light-evoked responses from pigment epithelium cells of the frog eye. *Physiologist*, 9:146, 1966.

Brown, K.T., and J.M. Crawford: Intracellular recording of rapid light-evoked responses from pigment epithelium cells of the frog eye. *Vision Res.*, 7:149-163, 1967a.

Brown, K.T., and J.M. Crawford: Melanin and the rapid light-evoked responses from pigment epithelium cells of the frog eye. *Vision Res.*, 7:165-178, 1967b.

Brown, K.T., and P.W. Gage: An earlier phase of the light-evoked electrical response from the pigment epithelium-choroid complex of the eye of the toad. *Nature*, 211:155-158, 1966.

Brown, K.T., and M. Murakami: A new receptor potential of the monkey retina with no detectable latency. *Nature*, 201:626-628, 1964.

Brown, K.T., and M. Murakami: Delayed decay of the late receptor potential of monkey cones as a function of stimulus intensity. *Vision Res.*, 7:179-189, 1967.

Brown, K.T., K. Watanabe, and M. Murakami: The early and late receptor potentials of monkey cones and rods. *Cold Spring Harbor Symposium on Quantitative Biology*, 30:457-482, 1965.

Browne, L.B., and E.S. Hodgson: Electrophysiological studies of arthropod chemoreception. IV. Latency, independence, and specificity of labellar chemoreceptors of the blowfly, *Lu-*

cilia. *J. Cell. Comp. Physiol.*, 59:187-202, 1962.

Bruno, M.S., and D. Kennedy: Spectral sensitivity of photoreceptor neurons in the sixth ganglion of the crayfish. *Comp. Biochem. Physiol.*, 6: 41-46, 1962.

Buckser, S., and H. Diamond: Increase in Na concentration of the isolated frog retina after light stimulation. *Biochem. Biophys. Res. Commun.*, 23:240-242, 1966.

Cameron, A.T.: The taste sense and the relative sweetness of sugars and other sweet substances. Scientific Rep., Ser. No. 9. Sugar Research Foundation, New York, 1947.

Carlisle, D.B., and E.J. Denton: A change in visual pigments in the life of the fresh-water eel. *J. Physiol. (London)*, 139:8P, 1957.

Case, J., and G.F. Gwilliam: Amino acid sensitivity of the dactyl chemoreceptors of *Carcinides maenas*. *Biol. Bull.*, 121:449-455, 1961.

Chance, B.: Biological membranes: Regulatory functions (Meetings). *Science*, 160:1261-1266, 1968.

Cherepnov, V.L.: Ultrastructure of the inner core of the Pacinian corpuscles (cat). *Zh. Evol. Biokhim. Fiziol.*, 4:91-96, 1968a.

Cherepnov, V.L.: Effect of mechanical stimulation on ultrastructure of the internal bulb of Pacinian bodies. *Dokl. Akad. Nauk. SSSR, 178:* 947-948, 1968b.

Clark, A.W., and D. Branton: Fracture faces of frozen outer segments from the guinea pig retina. *J. Cell Biol.*, 35:2, *part 2,*23A, 1967.

Cohen, A.I.: The fine structure of the extrafoveal receptors of the rhesus monkey. *Exp. Eye Res.*, 1:128-136, 1961.

Cohen, M.J., S. Hagiwara, and Y. Zotterman: The response spectrum of taste fibres in the cat: A single fibre analysis. *Acta Physiol. Scand.*, 33: 316-332, 1955.

Cone, R.A.: The early receptor potential of the vertebrate eye. *Cold Spring Harbor Symposia on Quantitative Biology*, 30:483-491, 1965.

Cone, R.A.: Early receptor potential: photoreversible charge displacement in rhodopsin. *Science*, 155:1128-1131, 1967.

Cone, R.A., and P.K. Brown: Dependence of the early receptor potential on the orientation of rhodopsin. *Science*, 156:536, 1967.

Crawford, J.M., P.W. Gage, and K.T. Brown: Rapid light-evoked potentials at extremes of pH from the frog's retina and pigment epithe-lium, and from a synthetic melanin, *Vision Res.*, 7:539-551, 1967.

Crescitelli, F., W.F. Mommaerts, and T.I. Shaw: Circular dichroism of visual pigments in the visible and ultraviolet spectral regions. *Proc. Nat. Acad. Sci. U.S.A.*, 56:1729-1734, 1966.

Dastoli, F.R., D.V. Lopiekes, and A.R. Doig: Bitter-sensitive protein from porcine taste buds. *Nature, 218:*884-885, 1968.

Dastoli, F.R., D.V. Lopiekes, and S. Price: A sweet-sensitive protein from bovine taste buds. Purification and partial characterization. *Biochemistry*, 7:1160-1164, 1968.

Dastoli, F.R., and S. Price: Sweet-sensitive protein from bovine taste buds: Isolation and assay. *Science*, 154:905-907, 1966.

Denton, E.J.: On the orientation of molecules in the visual rods of *Salamandra maculosa. J. Physiol. (London), 124:*17-18P, 1954.

Denton, E.J., and F.J. Warren: Visual pigments of deep-sea fish. *Nature*, 178:1059, 1956.

Dethier, V.G.: The physiology and histology of the contact chemoreceptors of the blowfly. *Quart. Rev. Biol.*, 30:348-371, 1955.

Dethier, V.G.: Chemoreceptor mechanisms in insects. *Soc. Exp. Biol. Symp.*, 16:180-196, 1962.

Dethier, V.G.: *The Physiology of Insect Senses.* New York, John Wiley, 1963.

Dethier, V.G., and F.E. Hanson: Taste papillae of the blowfly. *J. Cell. Comp. Physiol.*, 65:93-100, 1965.

Deutsch, E.W., and C. Hansch: Dependence of relative sweetness on hydrophobic bonding. *Nature, 211:*75, 1966.

De Witt, S., M. Goodman, and S. Huang: Biosynthesis of vitamin A with rat intestinal enzymes. *Science*, 149:879-880, 1965.

Diamant, H., M. Funakoshi, L. Ström, and Y. Zotterman: Electrophysiological Studies on Human Taste Nerves. In Zotterman, Y. (Ed.): *Olfaction and Taste, Proceedings of the First International Symposium.* Oxford, Pergamon, 1963, pp. 193-203.

Diamant, H., B. Oakley, L. Ström, C. Wells, and Y. Zotterman: A comparison of neural and psychophysical responses to taste stimuli in man. *Acta Physiol. Scand.*, 64:67-74, 1965.

Diamond, J., J.A.B. Gray, and D.R. Inman: The relation between receptor potentials and the concentration of sodium ions. *J. Physiol. (London)*, 142:382-394, 1958.

Diamond, J., J.A.B. Gray, and M. Sato: The site

of initiation of impulses in Pacinian corpuscles. *J. Physiol. (London)*, *133*:54-67, 1956.

Dodt, E., A.P. Skouby, and Y. Zotterman: The effect of cholinergic substances on the discharges from thermal receptors. *Acta Physiol. Scand.*, *28*:101-114, 1953.

Donner, K.O., and T. Reuter: Dark-adaptation processes in the rhodopsin-rods of the frog's retina. *Vision Res.*, *7*:17-41, 1967.

Dowling, J.E.: The Organization of Vertebrate Visual Receptors. In Allen, J.M. (Ed.): *Molecular Organization and Biological Function*. New York, Harper and Row, 1967, pp. 186-210.

Duncan, C.J.: The transducer mechanism of sense organs. *Naturwissenschaften*, *51*:172-173, 1964.

Ebrey, T.G.: Fast light-evoked potential from leaves. *Science, 155*:1556-1557, 1967.

Ebrey, T.G., and J.R. Platt: First-stage electrical effects in vision. Nat. Acad. Sci. Abstr., *Science, 158*:527, 1967.

Eisenman, G.: Cation selective glass electrodes and their mode of operation. *J. Biophys.*, *2*: 259-332, 1962.

Erickson, R.P.: Sensory Neural Patterns and Gustation. In Zotterman, Y. (Ed.): *Olfaction and Taste, Proceedings of the First International Symposium*. Oxford, Pergamon, 1963, pp. 205-213.

Erickson, R.P.: Duplexity theory of taste (letter). *Science, 147*:890, 1965.

Erickson, R.P.: Neural Coding of Taste Quality. In Kare, M.R., and O. Maller (Eds.): *The Chemical Senses and Nutrition*. Baltimore, Johns Hopkins, 1967, pp. 313-327.

Erickson, R.P., G.S. Doetsch, and D.A. Marshall: The gustatory neural response function. *J. Gen. Physiol.*, *49*:247-263, 1965.

Evans, D.R.: Depression of taste sensitivity to specific sugars by their presence during development. *Science, 133*:327-328, 1961.

Evans, D.R.: Chemical Structure and Stimulation by Carbohydrates. In Zotterman, Y. (Ed.): *Olfaction and Taste, Proceedings of the First International Symposium*. Oxford, Pergamon, 1963, pp. 165-176.

Evans, D.R., and D. Mellon, Jr.: Electrophysiological studies of a water receptor associated with the taste sensilla of the blowfly. *J. Gen. Physiol.*, *45*:487-500, 1962a.

Evans, D.R., and D. Mellon, Jr.: Stimulation of a

primary taste receptor by salts. *J. Gen. Physiol.*, *45*:651-661, 1962b.

Eyzaguirre, C., and S.W. Kuffler: Processes of excitation in the dendrites and in the soma of single isolated sensory nerve cells of the lobster and crayfish. *J. Gen. Physiol.*, *39*:87-119, 1955.

Falk, G., and P. Fatt: Rapid hydrogen ion uptake of rod outer segments and rhodopsin solutions on illumination. *J. Physiol.*, *183*:211-224, 1966.

Farbman, A.I.: Fine structure of the taste bud. *J. Ultrastruct. Res.*, *12*:328-350, 1965.

Ferguson, L.N., and L.G. Childers: Ultraviolet spectroscopic studies of some sweet and non-sweet m-nitroanilines. *J. Org. Chem.*, *25*:1971-1975, 1960.

Fischer, R.: Genetics and Gustatory Chemoreception in Man and Other Primates. In Kare, M.R., and O. Maller (Eds.): *The Chemical Senses and Nutrition*. Baltimore, Johns Hopkins, 1967, pp. 61-81.

Fischer, R., and F. Griffin: "Taste-blindness" and variations in taste-threshold in relation to thyroid metabolism. *J. Neuropsych.*, *3*:98-104, 1961.

Fischer, R., and F. Griffin: Pharmacogenetic aspects of gustation. *Arzneimittelforschung* (Drug Res.), *14*:673-686, 1964.

Fischer, R., F. Griffin, and M.A. Rockey: Gustatory chemoreception in man: multidisciplinary aspects and perspectives. *Perspect. Biol. Med.*, *9*:549-577, 1966.

Fishman, I.Y.: Single fiber gustatory impulses in rat and hamster. *J. Cell. Comp. Physiol.*, *49*: 319-334, 1957.

Fishman, I.Y.: Gustatory impulses of the white-faced, ringtail monkey. *Fed. Proc.*, *18*:45, 1959.

Forward, R., and D. Davenport: Red and far-red light effects on a short-term behavioral response of a dinoflagellate. *Science, 161*:1028-1029, 1968.

Frank, R.N., and J.E. Dowling: Rhodopsin photoproducts: effects on electroretinogram sensitivity in isolated perfused rat retina. *Science, 161*:487-489, 1968.

Frisch, von, K.: On the taste sense in bees. *Z. Vergl. Physiol.*, *21*:1-156, 1934.

Fuortes, M.G.F., and S. Yeandle: Probability of occurrence of discrete potential waves in the eye of *Limulus. J. Gen. Physiol.,* 47:443-463, 1964.

Gillary, H.L.: Quantitative electrophysiological studies on the mechanism of stimulation of the salt receptor of the blowfly. Thesis. The Johns Hopkins University, 1966.

Glaser, D.: Untersuchungen über die absoluten Geschmacksschwellen von Fischen. *Z. Vergl. Physiol.,* 52:1-25, 1966.

Goldman, D.E.: The transducer action of mechanoreceptor membranes. *Cold Spring Harbor Symposia on Quantitative Biology,* 30: 59-68, 1965.

Goldsmith, T.H., A.E. Dizon, and H.R. Fernandez: Microspectrophotometry of photoreceptor organelles from eyes of the prawn *Palaemonetes. Science, 161:* 468-469, 1968.

Goldstein, E.B.: Visual pigments and the early receptor potential of the isolated frog retina. *Vision Res.,* 8:953-963, 1968.

Gordon, G., R. Kitchell, L. Ström, and Y. Zotterman: The response pattern of taste fibres in the chorda tympani of the monkey. *Acta Physiol. Scand.,* 46:119-132, 1959.

Görner, P.: A proposed transducing mechanism for a multiply-innervated mechanoreceptor (trichobothrium) in spiders. *Cold Spring Harbor Symposia on Quantitative Biology,* 30:69-73, 1965.

Gribakin, F.G., and V.I. Govardovskii: Structure, visual pigments and optical properties of photoreceptors. *Usp. Sovr. Biol.,* 62:120-138, 1966.

Grundfest, H.: Electrophysiology and pharmacology of different components of bioelectric transducers. *Cold Spring Harbor Symposia on Quantitative Biology,* 30:1-14, 1965.

Guzzo, A.V., and G.L. Pool: Visual pigment fluorescence. *Science, 159:*312-314, 1968.

Hagins, W.A., H.V. Zonana, and R.G. Adams: Local membrane current in the outer segments of squid photoreceptors. *Nature,* 194:844-847, 1962.

Hagins, W.A.: Electrical signs of information flow in photoreceptors. *Cold Spring Harbor Symposia on Quantitative Biology,* 30:403-418, 1965.

Hagins, W.A., and R.E. Mc Gaughy: Molecular and thermal origins of fast photoelectric effects in the squid retina. *Science,* 157:813-816, 1967.

Hagins, W.A., and R.E. Mc Gaughy: Membrane origin of the fast photovoltage of squid retina. *Science, 159:*213-215, 1968.

Hall, O.M., D. Bok, and A.D.E. Bacharach: Visual pigment renewal in the mature frog retina. *Science, 161:*787-789, 1968.

Halpern, B.P., R.A. Bernard, and M.R. Kare: Amino acids as gustatory stimuli in the rat. *J. Gen. Physiol.,* 45:681-701, 1962.

Halpern, B.P., in Discussion, Hodgson, E.S.: Chemical Senses in the Invertebrates. In Kare, M.R., and O. Maller (Eds.): *The Chemical Senses and Nutrition.* Baltimore, Johns Hopkins, 1967, pp. 7-18.

Hansch, C., and T. Fujita: p-σ-π analysis. A method for the correlation of biological activity and chemical structure. *J. Chem. Soc.,* 86: 1616-1626, 1964.

Hebel, R., and A. Schweiger: Zur Feinstruktur und Funktion sensibler Rezeptoren. *Zbl. Vetinaermed.* [A], 14:15-25, 1967.

Hellekant, G.: Action and Interaction of Ethyl Alcohol and Some Other Substances on the Receptors of the Tongue. In Hayashi, T. (Ed.): *Olfaction and Taste, Proceedings of the Second International Symposium.* Oxford, Pergamon, 1967, pp. 465-479.

Hellekant, G.: The effect of menthol on taste receptors. *Acta Physiol. Scand.,* 76:361-368, 1969.

Hiji, Y., N. Kobayashi, and M. Sato: A "sweet-sensitive protein" from the tongue of the rat. *Kumamoto Med. J.,* 20:137-139, 1968.

Hodgkin, A.L., and W.K. Chandler: Effects of changes in ionic strength on inactivation and threshold in perfused nerve fibers of *Loligo. J. Gen. Physiol.,* 48:27-30, 1965.

Hodgson, E.S.: Chemical Senses in the Invertebrates. In Kare, M.R., and O. Maller (Eds.): *The Chemical Senses and Nutrition.* Baltimore, Johns Hopkins, 1967, pp. 7-18.

Hodgson, E.S., and R.A. Steinhardt: Hydrocarbon Inhibition of Primary Chemoreceptor Cells. In Hayashi, T. (Ed.): *Olfaction and Taste, Proceedings of the Second International Symposium.* Oxford, Pergamon, 1967, pp. 737-748.

Hubbard, R., D. Bownds, and T. Yoshizawa: The chemistry of visual photoreception. In *Sensory Receptors. Cold Spring Harbor Symposia on Quantitative Biology,* 30:301-315, 1965.

Hubbard, R., and A. Kropf: Molecular isomers in vision. *Sci. Amer.,* 216:64-76, 1967.

Hunt, C.C., and A. Takeuchi: Response of the nerve terminal of the Pacinian corpuscle. *J. Physiol. (London), 160*:1-21, 1962.

Il'Inskii, O.B.: Process of excitation and inhibition in single mechanoreceptors (Pacinian corpuscles). *Nature, 208*:351-353, 1965.

Il'Inskii, O.B.: Some morphophysiological properties of single mechanoreceptors (Pacinian corpuscles). *Proc. Acad. Sci. USSR, 171*:494-497, 1966a.

Il'Inskii, O.B.: "On" and "off" responses in mechanoreceptors. *Fiziol. Zh. SSSR Sechenov, 52*:948-952, 1966b.

Il'Inskii, O.B., and N.K. Volvoka: Certain morphological and physiological characteristics of single mechanoreceptors (Pacinian corpuscles). *Dokl. Akad. Nauk SSSR, 171*:494-497, 1966.

Il'Inskii, O.B., N.K. Volkova, and V.L. Cherepnov: Structure and function of Pacini's corpuscles (cat). *Fiziol. Zh. SSSR Sechenov., 54*:295-302, 1968.

Indow, T.: A general equi-distance scale of the four qualities of taste. *Jap. Psych. Res., 8*:136-150, 1966.

Iriuchijima, J., and Y. Zotterman: Conduction rates of afferent fibres to the anterior tongue of the dog. *Acta Physiol. Scand., 51*:283-289, 1961.

Ishiko, N., and W.R. Loewenstein: Effects of temperature on the generator and action potentials of a sense organ. *J. Gen. Physiol., 45*:105-124, 1961.

Ishiko, N., and M. Amatsu: Effects of stretch of the tongue on taste responses in glossopharyngeal and chorda tympani nerves of cat. *Kumamoto Med. J., 17*:5-17, 1964.

Ishiko, N., and M. Amatsu: Changes in the chorda tympani nerve responses to taste stimuli associated with movement of the tongue in cat. *Jap. J. Physiol., 15*:623-637, 1965.

Iwayama, T., and O. Nada: Histochemically demonstrable ATPase activity in the taste buds of the rat. *Exp. Cell Res., 46*:607-608, 1967a.

Iwayama, T., and O. Nada: Histochemical observation on the phosphatases of the tongue, with special reference to taste buds. *Arch. Histol. Jap., 28*:151-163, 1967b.

Jarrett, A.S.: The effect of acetylcholine on touch receptors in frog's skin. *J. Physiol. (London), 133*:243-254, 1956.

Julian, F.J., and D.E. Goldman: The effects of mechanical stimulation on some electrical properties of axons. *J. Gen. Physiol., 46*:297-313, 1962.

Kaneko, A., and H. Hashimoto: Recording site of the single cone response determined by an electrode marking technique. *Vision Res., 7*:847-851, 1967.

Kaplan, A.R., W. Powell, R. Fischer, and R. Marsters: Re-examination of genetic aspects of taste thresholds for thioureas. *Proceedings, the XI Intl. Congress of Genetics,* The Hague, 1963.

Kare, M.R.: Tele-lecture to the sensory physiology class at Indiana State University, Terre Haute, Indiana, 1968.

Kare, M.R., P.J. Schechter, S.P. Grossman, and L.J. Roth: Direct pathway to the brain. *Science, 163*:952-953, 1969.

Kawamura, Y., and A. Adachi: Electrophysiological Analysis of Taste Effectiveness of Soda Water and CO_2 Gas. In Hayashi, T. (Ed.): *Olfaction and Taste, Proceedings of the Second International Symposium.* Oxford, Pergamon, 1967, pp. 431-437.

Kikuchi, R., and Y. Takeda: Effect on retinal potentials of intracellularly applied tetra-ethyl-ammonium ions. *Naturwissenschaften, 53*:227-228, 1966.

Kimura, K., and L.M. Beidler: Microelectrode study of taste receptors of rat and hamster. *J. Cell. Comp. Physiol., 58*:131-140, 1961.

Kitchell, R.L., L. Ström, and Y. Zotterman: Electrophysiological studies of thermal and taste reception in chickens and pigeons. *Acta Physiol. Scand., 46*:133-151, 1959.

Kito, Y., T. Suzuki, M. Azuma, and Y. Sekoguti: Absorption spectrum of rhodopsin denatured with acid. *Nature, 218*:955-956, 1968a.

Kito, Y., M. Azuma, and Y. Maeda: Circular dichroism of squid rhodopsin. *Biochim. Biophys. Acta, 154*:352-359, 1968b.

Klotz, I.M.: Protein Interactions. In Neurath, H., and K. Bailey (Eds.): *The Proteins.* New York, Academic, 1953, vol. 1, part A, pp. 727-806.

Koketsu, K., and K. Kimura: Effect of some salt ions upon chemoreceptors in the mucous membrane of a frog's palate. *Kyushu Mem. Med. Sci., 3*:233-241, 1953.

Konishi, J.: On the sweet taste sensation. *Rep. Fac. Fish., Pref. Univ. Mie, 3*:101-103, 1958.

Konishi, J.: Studies on the Stimulation of Chemoreceptors of Freshwater Fish by Dilute Solutions of Electrolytes. In Hayashi, T. (Ed.): *Olfaction and Taste, Proceedings of the Second International Symposium.* Oxford, Pergamon, 1967, pp. 667-692.

Konishi, J., and H. Niwa: Some properties of taste receptors in freshwater fish: Responses to weak solutions. *Jap. J. Physiol., 14*:328-343, 1964.

Konishi, J., and Y. Zotterman: Taste Functions in Fish. In Zotterman, Y. (Ed.): *Olfaction and Taste, Proceedings of the First International Symposium.* Oxford, Pergamon, 1963, pp. 215-233.

Kropf, A.: Intramolecular energy transfer in rhodopsin. *Vision Res., 7*:811-818, 1967.

Kurihara, K., and L.M. Beidler: Taste-modifying protein from miracle fruit. *Science, 161*:1241-1243, 1968.

Kusano, K.: The influence of cations on the activity of gustatory receptors. III. Effects of Ca Cl_2, $MgCl_2$, $SrCl_2$ and $BaCl_2$. *Kumamoto Med. J., 12*:28-38, 1959.

Kusano, K.: Analysis of the single unit activity of gustatory receptors in the frog tongue. *Jap. J. Physiol., 10*:620-633, 1960.

Kusano, K., and M. Sato: Properties of fungiform papillae in frog's tongue. *Jap. J. Physiol., 7*: 324-338, 1957.

Kusano, K., and M. Sato: The influence of anions on the activity of gustatory receptors. *Jap. J. Physiol., 8*:254-274, 1958.

Langer, H., and B. Thorell: Microspectrophotometry of single rhabdomeres in the insect eye. *Exp. Cell Res., 41*:673-677, 1966.

Lawrence, A.R., and L.N. Ferguson: Exploratory physicochemical studies on the sense of taste. *Nature, 183*:1469-1471, 1959.

Lenard, J., and S.J. Singer: Protein conformation in cell membrane preparations as studied by optical rotatory dispersion and circular dichroism. *Proc. Nat. Acad. Sci. USA, 56*:1828-1835, 1966.

Lenhoff, H.M.: Behavior, hormones and hydra. *Science, 161*:434-442, 1968.

Lettvin, J.Y.: General discussion: Early receptor potential. In *Cold Spring Harbor Symposia on Quantitative Biology, 30*:501-504, 1965.

Lifson, S.: Potentiometric titration, association phenomena, and interaction of neighboring groups in polyelectrolytes. *J. Chem. Phys., 26*: 727-734, 1957.

Ling, G.N.: *A Physical Theory of the Living State.* New York, Blaisdell, 1962.

Loewenstein, W.R.: Properties of a receptor membrane: Spatial summation of electrical activity in a non-myelinated nerve ending. *Nature, 183*:1724-1725, 1959.

Loewenstein, W.R.: Biological transducers. *Sci. Amer., 203*:98-108, 1960a.

Loewenstein, W.R.: Mechanisms of nerve impulse initiation in a pressure receptor (Lorenzinian Ampulla). *Nature, 188*:1034-1035, 1960b.

Loewenstein, W.R.: On the specificity of a sensory receptor. *J. Neurophysiol., 24*:150-158, 1961a.

Loewenstein, W.R.: Excitation and inactivation in a receptor membrane. *Ann. N.Y. Acad. Sci., 94*:510-534, 1961b.

Loewenstein, W.R.: Facets of a transducer process. In *Cold Spring Harbor Symposia on Quantitative Biology, 30*:29-43, 1965.

Loewenstein, W.R., and S. Cohen: After-effects of repetitive activity in a nerve ending. *J. Gen. Physiol., 43*:335-345, 1959a.

Loewenstein, W.R., and S. Cohen: Post-tetanic potentiation and depression of generator potential in a single non-myelinated nerve ending. *J. Gen. Physiol., 43*:347-376, 1959b.

Loewenstein, W.R., and N. Ishiko: Effects of polarization of the receptor membrane and of the first Ranvier node in a sense organ. *J. Gen. Physiol., 43*:981-998, 1960.

Loewenstein, W.R., and M. Mendelson: Components of receptor adaptation in a Pacinian corpuscle. *J. Physiol. (London), 177*:377-397, 1965.

Loewenstein, W.R., and D. Molins: Cholinesterase in a receptor. *Science, 128*:1284, 1958.

Loewenstein, W.R., and R. Rathkamp: The sites for mechano-electric conversion in a Pacinian corpuscle. *J. Gen. Physiol., 41*:1245-1265, 1958.

Loewenstein, W.R., and R. Skalak: Mechanical transmission in a Pacinian corpuscle. An analysis and a theory. *J. Physiol. (London), 182*: 346-378, 1966.

Lovell, M.R.C., C.G. Gross, and L.A. Weizkrantz: A note on the effects of gymnemic acid on taste perception. *Anim. Behav., 9*:31-33, 1961.

Mac Nichol, Jr., E.F., and W.E. Love: Electrical responses of the retinal nerve and optic ganglion of the squid. *Science, 132*:737-738, 1960.

Marcström, A.: Psychophysical taste response experiments with sodium chloride and sucrose. *Ark. Zool., 17*:537, 1965.

Marcström, A.: Studies on the connection between physicochemical properties and stimulating abilities of some sweet and bitter compounds. *Ark. Zool.*, 19:421-535, 1967.

Marshall, D.A.: A comparative study of neural coding in gustation. *Physiol. Behav.*, 3:1-15, 1968.

Matthews, R.G., R. Hubbard, P.K. Brown, and G. Wald: Tautomeric forms of metarhodopsin. *J. Gen. Physiol.*, 47:215-240, 1963-64.

McBurney, D.H., and C. Pfaffmann: Gustatory adaptation to saliva and sodium chloride. *J. Exp. Psychol.*, 65:523-529, 1963.

Mc Connell, D.G.: The light-induced proton uptake in bovine retinal outer segment fragments. *J. Cell Biol.*, 35:part 2, 89A, 1967.

Mc Farland, W.N., and F.W. Munz: Codominance of visual pigments in hybrid fishes. *Science, 150*:1055-1056, 1965.

Millar, P.G., J. E. Shields, E.C. Dinovo, R.A. Henriksen, and R.L. Kimbel: The homogeneity and molecular weight of bovine rhodopsin. *Fed. Proc.*, 26:822, 1967.

Mirkin, A.S.: The reaction of isolated mechanoreceptors of the Paccini body to acoustic pressure. *Dokl. Akad. Nauk SSSR, 170*:227, 1966.

Moncrieff, R.W.: *The Chemical Senses.* 3rd ed., London, L. Hill, 1967.

Morita, H.: Effects of Salts on the Sugar Receptor of the Fleshfly. In Hayashi, T. (Ed.): *Olfaction and Taste, Proceedings of the Second International Symposium.* Oxford, Pergamon, 1967, pp. 787-798.

Morrison, G.R.: Behavioural response patterns to salt stimuli in the rat. *Canad. J. Psychol./Rev. Canad. Psychol., 21*:141-151, 1967.

Mote, F.A.: Visual sensitivity. *Ann. Rev. Psychol., 18*:41-64, 1967.

Moulton, D.G.: The Interrelations of the Chemical Senses. In Kare, M.R., and O. Maller (Eds.): *The Chemical Senses and Nutrition.* Baltimore, Johns Hopkins, 1967, pp. 249-261.

Moulton, D.G., in Discussion, Hoshishima, K.: Endocrines and Taste. In Kare, M.R. and O. Maller (Eds.): *The Chemical Senses and Nutrition.* Baltimore, Johns Hopkins, 1967, pp. 139-153.

Munz, F.W.: Photosensitive pigments from retinas of deep-sea fishes. *Science, 125*:1142-1143, 1957.

Murray, R.G., and A. Murray: Fine structure of taste buds of rabbit foliate papillae. *J. Ultrastruct. Res., 19*:327-353, 1967.

Nachman, M.: Learned aversion to the taste of lithium chloride and generalization to other salts. *J. Comp. Physiol. Psychol., 56*:343-349, 1963.

Nagaki, J., S. Yamashita, and M. Sato: Neural response of cat to taste stimuli of varying temperatures. *Jap. J. Physiol., 14*:67-89, 1964.

Naka, K., and E. Eguchi: Spike potentials recorded from the insect photoreceptor. *J. Gen. Physiol., 45*:663-680, 1962.

Nejad, M.S.: An electrophysiological investigation of the taste receptors of the frog. *Fed. Proc., 18*:112, 1959.

Nejad, M.S.: Factors involved in the mechanism of stimulation of gustatory receptors and bare nerve endings on the tongue of the rat. Doctoral thesis, Florida State Univ., Tallahassee, Fla., 1961.

Nishi, K.: Modification of the mechanical threshold of the Pacinian corpuscle after its perfusion with solutions of varying cation content. *Jap. J. Physiol., 18*:216-231, 1968a.

Nishi, K.: Abolition of impulse initiation at the Pacinian corpuscle by local anesthetics. *Jap. J. Physiol., 18*:536-550, 1968b.

Nishi, K., and M. Sato: Depolarizing and hyperpolarizing receptor potentials in the nonmyelinated nerve terminal in Pacinian corpuscles. *J. Physiol. (London), 199*:383-396, 1968.

Nomura, H., and S. Sakada: On the "water response" of the frog's tongue. *Jap. J. Physiol., 15*:433-443, 1965.

Ogawa, H., M. Sato, and S. Yamashita: Multiple sensitivity of chorda tympani fibres of the rat and hamster to gustatory and thermal stimuli. *J. Physiol. (London), 199*:223-240, 1968.

Ostroy, S.E., F. Erhardt, and E.W. Abrahamson: Protein configuration changes in the photolysis of rhodopsin. II. The sequence of intermediates in the thermal decay of cattle metarhodopsin in vitro. *Biochim. Biophys. Acta., 112*:265-277, 1966.

Ottoson, D.: The action of calcium on the frog's isolated muscle spindle. *J. Physiol. (London), 178*:68-79, 1965.

Ottoson, D., and G.M. Shepherd: Receptor potentials and impulse generation in the isolated spindle during controlled extension. In *Cold Spring Harbor Symposia on Quantitative Biology, 30*:105-114, 1965.

Ozeki, M., and M. Sato: Initiation of impulses at the non-myelinated nerve terminal in Pacinian corpuscles. *J. Physiol. (London), 170*:167-185, 1964.

Ozeki, M., and M. Sato: Changes in the membrane potential and the membrane conductance associated with a sustained compression of the non-myelinated nerve terminal in Pacinian corpuscles. *J. Physiol. (London), 180*: 186-208, 1965.

Pak, W.L.: Some properties of the early electrical response in the vertebrate retina. In *Cold Spring Harbor Symposia on Quantitative Biology, 30*:493-499, 1965.

Pak, W.L.: Rapid photoresponses in the retina and their relevance to vision research. *Photochem. Photobiol., 8*:495-503, 1968.

Pak, W.L., and R.J. Boes: Rhodopsin: responses from transient intermediates formed during its bleaching. *Science, 155*:1131-1133, 1967.

Pak, W.L., and R.A. Cone: Isolation and identification of the initial peak of the early receptor potential. *Nature, 204*:836-838, 1964.

Pak, W.L., and T.G. Ebrey: Visual receptor potential observed at sub-zero temperatures. *Nature, 205*:484-486, 1965.

Pak, W.L., and T.G. Ebrey: The early receptor potentials of rods and cones in rodents. *J .Gen. Physiol., 49*:1199-1208, 1966.

Pak, W.L., V.P. Rozzi, and T.G. Ebrey: Effect of changes in the chemical environment of the retina on the two components of the early receptor potential. *Nature, 214*:109-110, 1967.

Pangborn, R.M., and R.B. Chrisp: Gustatory responses to anomeric sugars. *Experientia, 22*: 612-622, 1966.

Pangborn, R.M., and S.C. Gee: Relative sweetness of alpha and β-forms of selected sugars. *Nature, 191*:810-811, 1961.

Pearse, A.G.E., and D.G. Mc Connell: Cytochemical localization of redox compounds in isolated bovine retinal outer segment disks. *Nature, 212*:1367-1368, 1966.

Pfaffmann, C.: Gustatory afferent impulses. *J. Cell. Comp. Physiol., 17*:243-258, 1941.

Pfaffmann, C.: Gustatory nerve impulses in rat, cat and rabbit. *J. Neurophysiol., 18*:429-440, 1955.

Pfaffmann, C.: The Sense of Taste. In Field, J. (Ed.): *Handbook of Physiology.* Washington, D.C., American Physiological Society, 1959, Vol. I, Sect. I, pp. 507-533.

Pfaffmann, C.: De Gustibus. *Amer. Psychol., 20*: 21-33, 1965.

Pfaffmann, C. (Ed.): *Taste and Olfaction III, Proceedings of the Third International Symposium.* New York, Rockefeller U. Pr., 1970.

Pfaffmann, C., G.L. Fisher, and M.K. Frank: The Sensory and Behavioral Factors in Taste Preferences. In Hayashi, T. (Ed.): *Olfaction and Taste II, Proceedings of the Second International Symposium.* Oxford, Pergamon, 1967, pp. 361-381.

Pirenne, M.H.: *Vision and the Eye.* London, Chapman and Hall, 1967.

Rapuzzi, G., B. Taccardi, and C. Casella: L'action du $BaCl_2$ sur les récepteurs de la langue de Grenouille. *J. Physiol. (Paris), 53*:669-678, 1961.

Renquist, Y.: Über den Geschmack. *Skand. Arch. Physiol., 38*:97-201, 1919.

Rosenberg, B.: Electronic charge transport in carotenoid pigments and a primitive theory of the electroretinogram. *Photochem. Photobiol., 1*:117-129, 1962.

Rosenberg, B.: A Physical Approach to the Visual Receptor Process. In Augenstein, L.G., R. Mason, and M.R. Zelle (Eds.): *Advances in Radiation Biology.* New York, Academic, 1966, Vol. II, pp. 193-241.

Rosenberg, B., and H. C. Harder: Semiconduction and photoconduction activation energies of the retinals. *Photochem. Photobiol., 6*:629-641, 1967.

Rosenberg, B., R.J. Heck, and K. Aziz: Color responses in an organic photoconductive cell. *J. Opt. Soc. Amer., 54*:1018-1026, 1964.

Rosenberg, B., R. J. Heck, and K. Aziz: A physical basis for the chromatic S-potentials in color vision. *Photochem. Photobiol., 4*:351-357, 1965.

Sato, M.: The Effect of Temperature Change on the Response of Taste Receptors. In Zotterman, Y. (Ed.): *Olfaction and Taste, Proceedings of the First International Symposium.* Oxford, Pergamon, 1963, pp. 151-164.

Sato, M., and N. Akaike: 5'-ribonucleotides as gustatory stimuli in rats. Electrophysiological studies. *Jap. J. Physiol., 15*:53-70, 1965.

Sato, M., and K. Kusano: Electrophysiology of Gustatory Receptors. In *Electrical Activity of Single Cells.* Hongo, Tokyo, Igakushoin, 1960, pp. 77-95.

Sato, M., M. Ozeki, and K. Nishi: Changes produced by sodium-free condition in the receptor potential of the nonmyelinated terminal in Pacinian corpuscles. *Jap. J. Physiol.,* 18:232-237, 1968.

Sato, M., S. Yamashita, and H. Ogawa: Patterns of Impulses Produced by MSG and 5'-Ribonucleotides in Taste Units of the Rat. In Hayashi, T. (Ed.): *Olfaction and Taste, Proceedings of the Second International Symposium.* Oxford, Pergamon, 1967, pp. 399-410.

Scholes, J.: Discontinuity of the excitation process in locust visual cells. In *Cold Spring Harbor Symposia on Quantitative Biology, 30*:517-527, 1965.

Schutz, H.G., and F.J. Pilgrim: Psychophysiology in food acceptance research. *J. Amer. Diet. Ass.,* 29:1127-1128, 1953.

Schwanzara, S.A.: Visual pigments of tropical freshwater fishes. *Life Sci., 6*:157-162, 1967a.

Schwanzara, S.A.: The visual pigments of freshwater fishes. *Vision Res.,* 7:121-148, 1967b.

Seegers, W.H.: Visual excitation and blood clotting. *Science,* 151:841, 1966.

Shaber, G.S., J.A. Rumsey III, B.C. Dorn, and R.L. Brent: Saccharin behavioral taste threshold in the rat. *Fed. Proc.,* 26:543, 1967.

Shallenberger, R.S.: Die chemischen Grundlagen des Geschmacks. *Umschau Wiss. Tech., 14*: 445, 1968.

Shallenberger, R.S., and T.E. Acree: Molecular theory of sweet taste. *Nature, 216*:480-482, 1967.

Shanthaveerappa, T.R., and G.H. Bourne: Histochemical studies on the Pacinian corpuscle. *Amer. J. Anat.,* 118:461-470, 1966.

Shukolyukov, S.A.: Oxidative systems in the outer segments of retina (bull). *Zh. Evol. Biokhim. Fiziol.,* 3:200-205, 1967.

Skramlik, E. von.: I. Physiologie des Geruchs und Geschmackssinnes. In Handbuch Der Physiologie Der Niederen Sinne. Leipzig, Georg Thieme, 1926, pp. 346-520.

Smith, T.G., and J.E. Brown: A photoelectric potential in invertebrate cells. *Nature, 212*:1217-1219, 1966.

Smith, T.G., W. K. Stell, and J.E. Brown: Conductive changes associated with receptor potentials in *Limulus* photoreceptors. *Science,* 162:454-456, 1968.

Smith, T.G., W.K. Stell, J.E. Brown, J.A. Freeman, and G.C. Murray: A role for the sodium pump in photoreception in *Limulus. Science,* 162:456-458, 1968.

Solms, J., L. Vuataz, and R.H. Egli: The taste of L- and D-amino acids. *Experientia,* 21:692-697, 1965.

Steinhardt, R.A.: Physiology of labellar electrolyte receptors of the blowfly, *Phormia regina.* New York, Columbia University, unpublished thesis, 1966.

Steinhardt, Jr., R.G., A.D. Calvin, and E.A. Dodd: Taste structure correlation with α-D-mannose and β-D-mannose. *Science, 135*:367-368, 1962.

Stone, H.: Gustatory Response to L-Amino Acids in Man. In Hayashi, T. (Ed.): *Olfaction and Taste, Proceedings of the Second International Symposium.* Oxford, Pergamon, 1967, pp. 289-306.

Strauss, V.P., and P.D. Ross: Counterion binding by polyelectrolytes. II, IV. *Amer. Chem. Soc. J., 81*:5292-5295, 5299-5302, 1959.

Stürckow, B.: Electrophysiological studies of a single taste hair of the fly during stimulation by a flowing system. *Proc. XVI Int. Congr. Zool.,* 3:102-104, 1963.

Stürckow, B.: Occurrence of a Viscous Substance at the Tip of the Labellar Taste Hair of the Blowfly. In Hayashi, T. (Ed.): *Olfaction and Taste II, Proceedings of the Second International Symposium.* Oxford, Pergamon, 1967, pp. 707-720.

Tamar, H.: The taste sense of the opossum and the bat. Doctoral thesis, Florida State Univ., Tallahassee, Fla., 1957.

Tamar, H.: Taste reception in the opossum and the bat. *Physiol. Zool.,* 34:86-91, 1961.

Tapper, D.N., and B.P. Halpern: Taste stimuli: a behavioral categorization. *Science, 161*:708-710, 1968.

Tateda, H.: Sugar Receptor and Alpha-Amino Acid in the Rat. In Hayashi, T. (Ed.): *Olfaction and Taste, Proceedings of the Second International Symposium.* Oxford, Pergamon, 1967, pp. 383-397.

Tateda, H., and L.M. Beidler: The receptor potential of the taste cell of the rat. *J. Gen. Physiol.,* 47:479-486, 1964.

Terzuolo, C.A., and Y. Washizu: Relation between stimulus strength, generator potential, and impulse frequency in stretch receptor of Crustacea. *J. Neurophysiol.,* 25:56-66, 1962.

Thurm, U.: An insect mechanoreceptor: Part I: Fine structure and adequate stimulus. In *Cold*

Spring Harbor Symposia on Quantitative Biology, 30:75-82, 1965.

Tomita, T.: Electrophysiological study of the mechanisms subserving color coding in the fish retina. in *Cold Spring Harbor Symposia on Quantitative Biology.* 30:559-566, 1965.

Tomita, T., A. Kaneko, M. Murakami, and E.L. Pautler: Spectral response curves of single cones in the carp. *Vision Res.,* 7:519-531, 1967.

Tsuchiya, S., and T. Aoki: Cholinesterase activities in the gustatory region of the rat tongue and their inhibition by bitter-tasting substances. *Tohoku J. Exp. Med.,* 91:41-52, 1967.

Tsuchiya, S., and S. Okui: Studies on bitter-tasting drugs. I. Effect of bitter tasting drugs on cholinesterase activities. *Pharmacy (Japan),* 26:279-284, 1966.

Tsuchiya, S., Y. Suzuki, and S. Okui: Esterases in the taste papilla of tongue. II. Electrophoretic separation of cholinesterases. *Yakugaku Zasshi,* 89:496-500, 1969a.

Tsuchiya, S., Y. Suzuki, and S. Okui: Esterases in the taste papilla of tongue. III. Multiple forms of esterases. *Yakugaku Zasshi,* 89:501-505, 1969b.

Tsuzuki, Y., and J. Yamazaki: Sweetness of fructose and of some other sugars, especially its variation with temperature. *Biochem. Z.,* 323: 525-531, 1953.

Vandenheuvel, F.A.: Structural studies of biological membranes: the structure of myelin. *Ann. N.Y. Acad. Sci.,* 122:57-76, 1965.

Vinnikov, J.A.: Fine structure of the taste bud. *J. Ultrastruct. Res.,* 12:328-350, 1965.

Wald, G.: Visual purple system in freshwater fishes. *Nature,* 139:1017-1018, 1937.

Wald, G.: The visual systems of euryhaline fishes. *J. Gen. Physiol.,* 25:235-245, 1941-42.

Wald, G.: Chemical evolution of vision. *Harvey Lect., Ser., 41*:117-160, 1945-46.

Wald, G.: The metamorphosis of visual systems in the sea lamprey. *J. Gen. Physiol.,* 40:901-914, 1956-57.

Wald, G.: The Distribution and Evolution of Visual Systems. In Florkin, M., and H.S. Mason (Eds.): *Comparative Biochemistry,* New York, Academic, 1960, Vol. I, p. 311.

Wald, G.: Visual excitation and blood clotting. *Science, 150*:1028-1030, 1965.

Wald, G.: Visual pigments of crayfish. *Nature, 215*:1131-1133, 1967.

Wald, G.: Molecular basis of visual excitation. *Science, 162*:230-239, 1968.

Wald, G., P.K. Brown, and P.S. Brown: Visual pigments and depths of habitat of marine fishes. *Nature, 180*:969-971, 1957.

Wald, G., P.K. Brown, and I.R. Gibbons: The problem of visual excitation. *J. Opt. Soc. Amer., 53*:20-35, 1963.

Wendler, L.: Über die Wirkungskette zwischen Reiz und Erregung. Versuche an den abdominalen Streckreceptoren des Flusskrebses. *Z. Vergl. Physiol., 47*:279-315, 1963.

Wolbarsht, M.L.: Water taste in *Phormia. Science, 125*:1248, 1957.

Wolbarsht, M.L.: Electrical activity in the chemoreceptors of the blowfly. II. Responses to electrical stimulation. *J. Gen. Physiol., 42*:413-428, 1958.

Wolbarsht, M.L.: Electrical characteristics of insect mechanoreceptors. *J. Gen. Physiol., 44*: 105-122, 1960.

Wolbarsht, M.L.: Receptor sites in insect chemoreceptors. In *Sensory Receptors. Cold Spring Harbor Symposia on Quantitative Biology,* 30:281-288, 1965.

Wolin, L.R., and L.C. Massopust: Selective cooling of the eye. *Arch. Ophthal., 76*:723-728, 1966.

Yackzan, K.S.: Biological effects of *Gymnema sylvestre* fractions. *Alabama J. Med. Sci., 3*: 1-9, 1966.

Yamada, K.: The Glossopharyngeal Nerve Response to Taste and Thermal Stimuli in the Rat, Rabbit and Cat. In Hayashi, T. (Ed.): *Olfaction and Taste II, Proceedings of the Second International Symposium.* Oxford, Pergamon, 1967, pp. 459-464.

Yamashita, S.: Chemoreceptor response in frog, as modified by temperature change. *Jap. J. Physiol., 14*:488-504, 1964.

Yamashita, S., N. Akaike, and M. Sato: Stimulation of taste receptors of rat by certain salts. *Kumamoto Med. J., 16*:184-193, 1963.

Yamashita, S., H. Ogawa, and M. Sato: Multimodal sensitivity of taste units in the rat. *Kumamoto Med. J., 20*:67-70, 1967a.

Yamashita, S., H. Ogawa, and M. Sato: Analysis of responses of hamster taste units to gustatory and thermal stimuli. *Kumamoto Med. J., 20*: 159-162, 1967b.

Yamashita, S., K. Yamada, and M. Sato: The effect of temperature on neural taste response of cats. *Jap. J. Physiol., 14*:505-514, 1964.

Yonemura, D., and K. Kawasaki: The early receptor potential in the human electroretinogram. *Jap. J. Phys., 17*:235-244, 1967.

Yoshida, M., T. Ninomiya, S. Ikeda, S. Yamaguchi, T. Yoshikawa, and M. Ohara: Studies on the taste of amino acids. Part I. Determination of threshold values of various amino acids. *Nippon Nogei Kagaku Kaishi J. Agr. Chem. Soc. Jap., 40*:295-299, 1966.

Yoshizawa, T., and G. Wald: Photochemistry of iodopsin. *Nature, 214*:566-571, 1967.

Yur'eva, G. Yu.: New data on the role of protein sulfhydryl groups in taste sensitivity. *Biophysics (USSR) (English Transl.), 6*:29-32, 1961.

Zotterman, Y.: Thermal Sensations. In Field, J. (Ed.): *Handbook of Physiology*. Washington, D. C., American Physiological Society, Vol. I, Sect. I, 1959a, pp. 431-458.

Zotterman, Y.: The nervous mechanism of taste. *Ann. N.Y. Acad. Sci., 81*:358-366, 1959b.

SUGGESTED READING

Abrahamson, E.W., and S.E. Ostroy: The photochemical and macromolecular aspects of vision. *Progr. Biophys., 17*:179-215, 1967.

Beidler, L.M.: Anion Influences on Taste Receptor Response. In Hayashi, T. (Ed.): *Olfaction and Taste II, Proceedings of the Second International Symposium*. Oxford, Pergamon, 1967, pp. 509-534.

Beidler, L.M., and W.E. Reichardt: Sensory transduction. *Neurosci. Res. Progr. Bull., 8*: 459-560, 1970.

Békésy, G. von: Taste theories and the chemical stimulation of single papillae. *J. Appl. Physiol., 21*:1-9, 1966.

Benjamin, R.M., B.P. Halpern, D.G. Moulton, and M.M. Mozelle: The chemical senses. *Ann. Rev. Psychol., 16*:381-416, 1965.

Brown, K.T., K. Watanabe, and M. Murakami: The early and late receptor potentials of monkey cones and rods. In *Sensory Receptors. Cold Spring Harbor Symposia on Quantitative Biology, 30*:457-482, 1965.

De Reuck, A.V.S., and J. Knight (Eds.): *Touch, Heat and Pain*. Ciba Foundation Symp., Boston, Little, Brown, 1966.

Hubbard, R., D. Bownds, and T. Yoshizawa: The chemistry of visual photoreception. In *Sensory Receptors. Cold Spring Harbor Symposia on Quantitative Biology, 30*:301-315, 1965.

Hubbard, R., and A. Kropf: Molecular isomers in vision. *Sci. Amer., 216*:64-76, 1967.

Loewenstein, W.: Biological transducers (Pacinian corpuscle). *Sci. Amer., 203*:98-108, 1960.

Loewenstein, W.R. (Ed.): *Handbook of Sensory Physiology*. Vol. 1, *Principles of Receptor Physiology*. New York, Springer-Verlag, 1971.

Ogawa, H., M. Sato, and S. Yamashita: Multiple sensitivity of chorda tympani fibres of the rat and hamster to gustatory and thermal stimuli. *J. Physiol. (London), 199*:223-240, 1968.

Pfaffmann, C. (Ed.): *Olfaction and Taste III*. Proc. Third Int. Symp., New York, Rockefeller U. Pr., 1970.

Tosteson, D.C. (Ed.): *The Molecular Basis of Membrane Function*. Englewood Cliffs, Prentice-Hall, 1969.

Tucker, D., and J.C. Smith: The chemical senses. *Ann. Rev. Psychol., 20*:129-158, 1969.

Wald, G., P. K. Brown, and I.R. Gibbons: The problem of visual excitation. *J. Opt. Soc. Amer., 53*:20-35, 1963.

Wolken, J.J.: *Vision. Biophysics and Biochemistry of the Retinal Photoreceptors*. Springfield, Charles C Thomas, 1966.

Wolken, J.J.: *Invertebrate Photoreceptors. A Comparative Analysis*. New York, Academic Press, 1971.

Chapter VI

Nervous Transmission

The responses excited by stimuli in various receptor cells are mediated to the brain by neurons. The bulk of our knowledge of receptor cell responses has, with the possible exception of vision, been obtained by recording from the nerves innervating the receptors. It is therefore important for the student of sensory physiology to understand the structure and function of nerve cells. The present chapter is intended to provide a brief review of the salient features of these subjects.

STRUCTURE AND BASIC RELATIONSHIPS

The Neuron

The basic unit of the nervous system is the nerve cell or neuron.

A neuron may consist of a cell body or perikaryon containing a nucleus and nucleolus, of dendrites or branches of the cell body which carry nerve messages to it and of a long fiber or axon which conveys nerve impulses away from the cell body. Axons have diameters of about 0.0008 to 0.8 mm, and the giant axons of squid even reach diameters of 1 mm. Axons, as well as sensory neuron dendrites, may attain a length of over 3 feet.

The cytoplasm of a neuron contains neurofibrils or neurofilaments (80-100 Å) of unknown function. These could have a role in nerve impulse transmission.

A system of neurotubules (200-400 Å) appears to transport proteins, and so on, from the cell body to all parts of the neuron. This view is reinforced by the fact that colchicine, which is known to destroy neurotubules, significantly reduces the rapid movement of protein within the axons of retinal ganglion cells (Karlsson and Sjöstrand, 1969). Colchicine also appears to interfere with the transport of amine granules in adrenergic nerves (Dahlström, 1968).

Mitochondria are most numerous in the cell body and at both the receptor and transmitter endings of the neuron, where there are particularly great needs for energy.

With the exception, in some neurons, of a portion of the cell body adjoining the axon known as the axon hillock, the cell soma is dotted with ribonucleoprotein (ribosome) aggregates, the Nissl substance. Dendrites also contain ribosomes. These ribonucleoprotein particles, which carry on protein synthesis, presumably play a role in nerve regeneration. They decrease in number if a neuron endowed with a neurilemma membrane is injured and regenerates. Separated axons, which are devoid of ribosome aggregates, degenerate.

Sensory neurons, motor neurons and internuncial neurons each form a significant group of nerve cells. Sensory neurons are nerve cells which convey impulses from sites of origin in either their own free terminal dendritic branches, in neuronal receptor structures or at synapses with receptors to higher nervous centers (Fig. 6-1). In many sensory neurons a single dendrite extends from a receptor on the periphery to the cell body in the dorsal root ganglion, and this sensory dendrite may equal an axon in length. However, some authorities emphasizing the point of impulse origin over the location of the perikaryon consider the perikaryon of such sensory neurons to lie along the length of an axon beginning behind the peripheral branchings (Fig. 6-1).

The dendritic endings of sensory neurons have a less extensive and simpler arrangement than those of the most sizeable neurons of the brain.

Investing Membranes

The Myelin Sheath

The axons of numerous neurons, including many sensory neurons, are surrounded by a

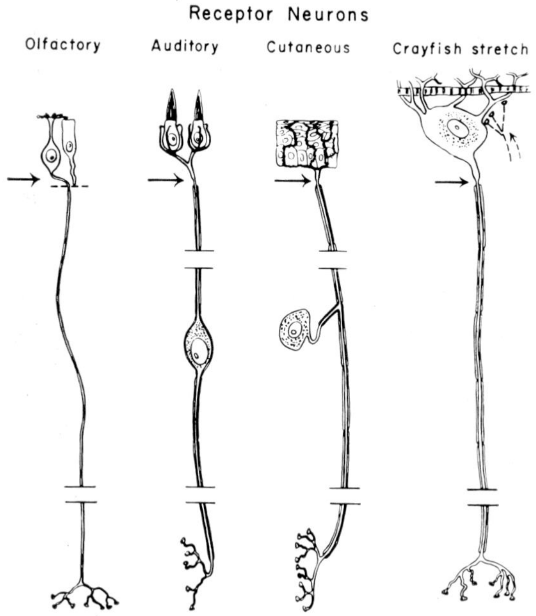

FIGURE 6-1. Schematic drawing of four kinds of sensory neurons. Olfactory neurons possess specialized peripheral receptor structures, while the cutaneous neurons transmitting pain terminate in free nerve endings. Auditory neurons synapse with hair sense cells, and crayfish stretch receptor neurons innervate muscle bundles. The large arrows mark the point of impulse origin, the nerve fiber central to this point being here considered the axon, irrespective of the location of the perikaryon. (Adapted from Bodian, D.: Neurons, Circuits, and Neuroglia. In Quarton, G.C., T. Melnechuk, and F.O. Schmitt [Eds.]: *The Neurosciences—A Study Program.* New York, Rockefeller U. Pr., 1967, pp. 6-24.)

myelin sheath composed primarily of phospholipids. The long dendrites (also considered distal portions of the axons) of these sensory neurons are also invested by myelin. The myelin sheath, where present, does not extend over a proximal portion of the axon or over the terminal branches of the axon or the long sensory dendrite.

The proximal or initial segment of myelinated axons is frequently constricted and is then known as the axon neck.

Myelinated nerve fibers are characterized by higher speeds of nerve impulse transmission than other fibers. The myelin sheath increases the impulse speed by about a factor of ten. Myelin also has insulating properties and reduces the energy required for the transmission of nerve impulses by approximately a factor of ten.

The rate of impulse propagation further varies directly with the diameter of the nerve fiber.

The myelin sheath of nerve fibers is segmented by recurrent gaps, the nodes of Ranvier. These occur at fairly regular intervals of one to several millimeters. It is at the nodes of Ranvier that the nerve impulses in myelinated fibers are regenerated. They thus maintain their original amplitude by jumping from node to node.

Although the lamellae of myelin have been believed to each consist of two unit membranes, Di Carlo (1967a, b) has shown that myelin, axolemma and other animal membranes are composed of osmiophilic granules surrounded by osmiophobic globules. His results indicate an organization of polyhedric blocks, each made up of six osmiophobic globules around an osmiophilic granule.

In the peripheral nervous system the formation of the myelin sheath is a function of a satellite cell of the nervous system, the Schwann cell. Each segment of the myelin sheath is produced by one Schwann cell. At the start of myelin formation, as observed by Geren (1954), the Schwann cell grows around the nerve fiber. After the two processes of the cell meet, one process continues to wind around the fiber, beyond the other, in several spirals. As it does so, it comes to contain the bulk of the cell's cytoplasm. When the multiple envelopment of the nerve fiber is completed, the Schwann cell's nucleus and cytoplasm are lost, and the windings of the cell membrane combine to form the strong myelin sheath.

The Schwann cell nucleus has also been observed to travel around the nerve fiber during myelination.

Peripheral nerve fibers which do not possess a myelin sheath are nevertheless generally surrounded by Schwann cells. The function of these encompassing Schwann cells, when they are not constituents of the neurilemma membrane, is not yet known; they do not undergo potential changes during the passage of a nerve impulse.

The Neurilemma

An outer membrane layer of Schwann cells and other satellite cells of the neuroglia type, which may be present around both myelinated and unmyelinated fibers, is known as the neurilemma. The neurilemma membrane is essential for nerve regeneration; its absence in the case of the nerve fibers of the spinal cord means that a break in the spinal cord results in permanent paralysis of the muscles functionally dependent on motor neuron fibers which leave the spinal cord below the point of injury.

Neuroglia

In addition to Schwann cells, various neuroglial cells are found around and between neurons.

Neuroglia containing numerous fibrils, known as skeletal neuroglia, act as the supporting tissue of the nervous system. In addition to providing structural support, skeletal neuroglia may insulate nerve cell processes and synapses and allow various substances (oxygen, water, ions, etc.) to pass through them to the neurons. Also, it has been suggested that skeletal neuroglia may in certain

repects be metabolically coupled with adjacent neurons.

Another group of neuroglial cells, the oligodendrocytes, give rise to the myelin sheaths of central nerve fibers. Like Schwann cells, these cells contain large numbers of ribosomes.

Oligodendrocytes and Schwann cells are found in intimate contact with neurons, especially with the cell bodies of neurons in sensory ganglia. This intimate physical relationship with adjacent sensory neurons may be indicative of some close functional interrelations (Bodian, 1967).

In tissue culture both oligodendrocytes and Schwann cells show slow pulsatile activity.

Other neuroglia, the microglia, have been believed to phagocytize degenerating neurons. No basic role in healthy nerve tissue has yet been assigned to microglia.

After observing electrical coupling between nonfiring neurons and neuroglia *in vitro,* Walker and Hild (1969) have suggested that low-resistance junctions between neurons and neuroglia might be responsible for temporarily "silent" neurons and other phenomena. Adey (1969) reports that Hertz has postulated a temporary uptake of excess extracellular potassium ions by neuroglia. The spreading depression of brain cells has been ascribed to the successive release of potassium ions by contiguous neurons.

Maintenance of Nerve Fibers

Nerve fiber regeneration always proceeds by growth from the part of the fiber proximal to a place of section (closest to the perikaryon).

If a nerve fiber is transected, the portion distal to the cut finally degenerates in a number of days. However, this distal portion can be employed for experimental work for two days or more before it deteriorates and will transmit tens of thousands of action potentials. Portions of frog sciatic nerves in frog Ringer's solution may be temporarily maintained by cooling in a refrigerator.

NERVE FUNCTION

The transmission of impulses by nerve cells must be explained in terms of an underlying potential difference across the cell membrane based both on a differential distribution of ions and on the resulting feasible ion movement. Also, impulse transmission is the consequence of interrelated changes in the potential difference across the cell membrane and this membrane's ion permeability.

The Resting Potential

When the neuron is in a resting state, its interior is about 60 to 70 mV negative in respect to the external solution. This resting potential is the immediate result of an outward movement of positively charged potassium ions across the cell membrane, a movement which in turn can only be understood against a background of ion distributions on both sides of the cell membrane.

Although the cell membrane separates two aqueous solutions of similar conductivity, which contain about equal numbers of ions, the chemical makeup of these solutions is strikingly different.

The outside solution (interstitial fluid) in its inorganic constituents resembles seawater or blood. In the extracellular solution more than 90 per cent of the ions consist of the positively charged sodium ions and the negatively charged chloride ions.

The intracellular solution's ionic makeup has been less fully determined. However, it appears that sodium ions and chloride ions together do not even form 10 per cent of the dissolved contents of the intracellular fluid. Instead, positively charged potassium ions and a mixture of negatively charged organic ions compose most of the ionic complement of the internal solution.

While sodium ions are about 10 times as concentrated outside the cell than inside, and there appear to be 14 times as many chloride ions outside, there are approximately 30 times as many potassium ions inside the cell.

Hodgkin (1965) estimates that in the giant axon of the squid (*Loligo pealii*) there are 400 millimoles of potassium ion, 50 of sodium ion and 40 to 150 of chloride ion, while for the surrounding fluid the respective figures are 20, 440 and 560 millimoles.

The ions on both sides of the semipermeable cell plasma membrane would, if able to do so, diffuse along their concentration gradients, each at a rate proportional to the difference in its concentration between the two sides of the membrane. However, the large negatively charged organic ions inside the neuron cannot diffuse out because the cell membrane is not permeable to them. The membrane has some, but only low permeability, to the positively charged sodium ions and the negatively charged chloride ions. Only the positively charged potassium ions can diffuse relatively easily along their steep concentration gradient from the inside to the outside of the neuron.

It is the outward movement of some positively charged potassium ions which causes the interior of the neuron to have a negative electric potential in respect to the outside.

Most of the remaining potassium ions inside the neuron are held there by the 60 to 70 mV negative potential, but the 30 times higher internal potassium ion concentration would, in the absence of an expenditure of cellular energy, be possible only if the interior was 90 mV negative to the outside (the potassium ion equilibrium potential). Apparently the cell plasma membrane performs work to bring potassium ions into the cell and maintain the high internal potassium ion concentration. But there is still a small net loss of potassium ions.

Cellular energy must also be expended to force out sodium ions against their concentration gradient and a potential gradient. Although the permeability of the membrane to sodium is low, an unbalanced inward diffusion (osmosis) of sodium ions would eventually result in a much greater internal than outside concentration of sodium ions. This is true because the original 60 to 70 mV interior-exterior negative potential would act to hold sodium ions in the neuron.

Thus the cell expends metabolic energy (supplied by ATP) to pull in potassium ions and force out sodium ions against their concentration gradients. In the case of sodium ions the cell must also oppose a potential gradient, since the excess negative charge of the protoplasm attracts the positively charged sodium ions. This phenomenon, the "pumping" of sodium ions and potassium ions by the cell, in which the sodium ion is exchanged for the potassium ion, is referred to as the sodium pump.

Since the quantities of potassium ions and sodium ions which diffuse through the cell membrane at any one time make up only a minute fraction of the amounts of these ions inside the neuron, a nerve cell can function for a long period without an active sodium pump.

Birks and Cohen (1968) ascribe the effects of applying a cardiac glycoside to skeletal muscle to the poisoning of the sodium pump in the terminal portions and endings of the motor nerve axons. They describe these slowly developing effects.

Cellular energy does not need to be employed to maintain the concentration gradient of the negatively charged chloride ions, since the relative negative resting potential of the cell interior tends to repel chloride ions which might start to enter the cell and acts to push out some of the chloride ions which are present inside. The 60 to 70 mV potential drop across the cell membrane appears to be adequate to prevent a change in the chloride ion concentration ratio across the cell membrane or keeps the rates of osmosis in either direction equal. The resting potential thus represents the chloride ion equilibrium potential.

Experimental variation of the media into which dissected-out nerve axons have been immersed has shown that normal resting potentials require the maintenance of the normal potassium concentration gradient across the cell membrane. Increased potassium ion concentrations in the outside medium resulted in reduced resting potentials. Similarly, Hodgkin and Baker (Baker, 1966) found that when they replaced most of an axon's internal protoplasm with an experimental solution, the last had to contain a high concentration of potassium ions and a low amount of sodium ions in order for a normal resting potential to be attained. The other ions present *in vivo* were found to be of less significance. If, however, the internal potassium ion concentration was brought down to the level of the external concentration, the resting potential was totally eliminated.

In fact, when the external potassium ion concentration was raised considerably over the internal concentration, the resting potential was reversed, or the inside of the axon was positive to the exterior. This finding shows that the cell membrane is highly permeable to potassium ions in both directions, and that the magnitude and direction of the potassium concentration gradient are what determine the resting potential.

The perfusion experiments of Hodgkin and Baker also showed that the proper concentrations of potassium and sodium ions inside and outside the axon membrane are all that is required to produce a resting potential; no other source of energy is necessary.

A resting potential based entirely on ionic concentration differences and ion movements across a semipermeable membrane can be described by the Goldman equation. A simplified form of this equation is applicable to typical cells, in which the product of the internal potassium ion concentration and the cell membrane's permeability to potassium ions greatly exceeds the product of internal sodium ion concentration and membrane permeability to sodium ions, and in which chloride ion movement is a negligible factor (Moreton, 1968). This simplified form of the Goldman equation may be stated as follows:

$$P = \frac{RT}{F} \ln \frac{K_s + (M_{Na}/M_K)\ Na_s}{K_c}$$

in which P represents the resting potential, R the gas constant, T the absolute temperature, and F the Faraday constant. K_s and Na_s, respectively, are the potassium ion and the sodium ion concentrations in the surrounding fluid, and K_c is the potassium ion concentration within the cell. M_{Na} and M_K, respectively, represent the membrane's permeability to sodium ions and to potassium ions.

Electrogenic Sodium Pumps

In addition to ionic gradients and permeabilities, the resting potential of a cell membrane may also be determined by the operation of an electrogenic sodium pump and other factors.

A number of different neurons, as well as muscle fibers, have been reported to possess an electrogenic sodium pump.

An electrogenic pump is a cellular "pump" in which the active movement of potassium ions into the cell is not linked with the active expulsion of an equal number of sodium ions through the cell membrane. If the ratio of actively entering potassium ions to actively removed sodium ions is more than one, the cell's plasma membrane will be depolarized. Conversely, if an excess of sodium ions is actively pushed out through the cell membrane, the last will be hyperpolarized. A pump which expulses a net excess of sodium ions is known as an electrogenic sodium pump.

The extent to which an electrogenic sodium pump hyperpolarizes the cell membrane by producing a potential difference above that due to ionic concentration gradients alone depends on the membrane's resistance. At a constant rate of sodium ion transport, the membrane hyperpolarization varies directly with the membrane resistance.

Electrogenic sodium pumps are believed to produce hyperpolarization in *Aplysia* neurons (Carpenter and Alving, 1968) and in the lobster giant axon (Senft, 1967), and posttetanic hyperpolarization in nonmyelinated mammalian nerve fibers (Rang and Ritchie, 1968) and in the stretch receptor neuron of the crayfish (Nakajima and Takahashi, 1966). The electrogenic sodium pump also appears to be required for a slow inhibitory postsynaptic potential in the bull frog's sympa-

thetic ganglion cells (Nishi and Koketsu, 1967) and for a lasting inhibitory postsynaptic potential in abdominal ganglion cells of the opisthobranch gastropod *Aplysia* (Pinsker and Kandel, 1969). Nakajima and Takahashi (1966) and Kerkut and Thomas (1965) obtained hyperpolarization by injection of sodium ions into, respectively, the stretch receptor neuron of the crayfish and ganglion cells of the snail.

Multiple observations indicate that electrogenic sodium pumps are indeed responsible for the investigated hyperpolarization effects.

Thus Carpenter and Alving (1968) determined that their resting membrane potential rose with higher temperatures, sometimes as much as 2 mV/°C, and that it could increase by as much as 50 per cent between 5°C and room temperature. At normal temperatures the resting membrane potential could be noticeably higher than the cell membrane's equilibrium potential for potassium ions. Senft (1967), who observed a great warmth-induced increase in hyperpolarization, found his lobster axon membrane to reach the potassium equilibrium potential. Nishi and Koketsu (1967) noted their inhibitory postsynaptic potential to be highly reduced at lower temperatures.

Carpenter and Alving found their temperature results to be in agreement with the expected increase in active sodium ion transport with higher temperatures. In one cell, as the resting potential showed a temperature-induced increase, the equilibrium potential for potassium ions and the electrical resistance of the membrane both underwent comparatively little change. There was similarly no change in the potassium equilibrium potential at the time of the posttetanic hyperpolarizations studied by Nakajima and Takahashi (1966). The last researchers believe that this finding, and a lack of change in membrane resistance, are the best evidences that potassium ion permeability and movement are not involved in their hyperpolarizations. Nishi and Koketsu (1967) echo the opinion that a hyperpolarization potential not associated with the membrane's potassium equilibrium potential cannot be based on potassium ion concentration changes. Furthermore, the membrane ionic gradient cannot change sufficiently fast to produce the noted rapid rises in membrane potential (Carpenter and Alving, 1968; Senft, 1967). All the mentioned researchers agree that the fast hyperpolarizations of the membrane with increasing temperature are most likely produced by an electrogenic ion pump.

Ouabain, a cardiac glycoside, is known to specifically inhibit both active sodium ion transport (Carpenter and Alving, 1968; Rang and Ritchie, 1968) and the action of the sodium ion– and potassium ion–dependent adenosine triphosphatase, which is essential for releasing energy from ATP for sodium pumps (Baker, 1965). All the investigators who subjected their preparations to ouabain (Carpenter and Alving, Rang and Ritchie, Senft, and Nishi and Koketsu) found that it eliminated membrane hyperpolarization. Nishi and Koketsu (1967) noted that ouabain's action on their inhibitory (hyperpolarizing) postsynaptic potential was highly specific; there was no effect on other potentials or on excitatory synaptic transmission. Senft (1967) determined that ouabain eliminated that portion of the membrane potential which varies with temperature; the remaining potential corresponded to the value expected for a potassium ion potential and showed the normal ion diffusion potential changes with increases in absolute temperature.

The metabolic inhibitors 2, 4 dinitrophenol, sodium cyanide and sodium azide had less drastic and less specific effects on membrane hyperpolarization, and considerably lowered ATP levels.

Changes in the ionic composition of the medium reduced membrane hyperpolarization if they also acted adversely on sodium ion transport. Replacing sodium ions by lithium ions, which are probably only slowly expelled from the cell, eliminated membrane hyperpolarization (Carpenter and Alving, Rang and Ritchie, Nakajima and Takahashi). Both Carpenter and Alving, and Rang and Ritchie, report that a small amount of potassium ions had to be present in the outside medium for their membrane hyperpolarizations to take place. Carpenter and Alving suggest that the potassium is essential because it may be required on the outer membrane surface for the Na^+-K^+ ATPase system.

Rang and Ritchie (1968) and Nakajima and Takahashi (1966) have suggested that the electrogenic sodium pump may operate only in conjunction with a coupled (Na^+-K^+) pump, perhaps at some specific ratio of activity. Carpenter and Alving (1968) also mention some active potassium ion transport.

It has been possible to divide the resting potential of a molluscan neuron into ionic gradient and electrogenic sodium pump components. Marmor and Gorman (1970) found the resting potential of the giant neuron in the gastroesophageal ganglion of *Anisodoris nobilis* to fundamentally vary with external potassium ion concentration in accordance with the ionic hypothesis (Goldman equation). However, the hyperpolarization produced by 10 mM of external potassium ion increased with temperature to a value far beyond that which could be attributed to the temperature dependence of the Goldman equation. Higher temperatures did not call forth these unexpectedly great hyperpolarizations if the intracellular sodium ions were depleted or if ouabain was applied. The last observations indicate that the described effect of temperature is mediated through an electrogenic sodium pump.

Marmor and Gorman point out that active, electrogenic sodium ion transport may also contribute to the resting potential of other excitable cells.

Nakajima and Takahashi (1966) state that the "off" effect observed in stretch receptor neurons and in muscle spindles is at least partially produced by electrogenic sodium pumps. The "off" effect consists of a drop in the impulse rate below the maintained normal level following a high response.

Electrogenic sodium pumps appear to have a wide distribution in nature, and may be significant in nervous integration.

Other Possible Contributing Factors

There may be an increase with rising temperature in the ratio of the membrane permeability for sodium ions to the membrane permeability for potassium ions. Evidence for such a temperature-dependent change in the ratio of ionic permeabilities has been obtained with neurons of the mollusca *Anisodoris nobilis* and *Aplysia*. Membrane resting potentials may also be regulated by this factor (Marmor and Gorman, 1970).

It appears that a number of mechanisms may interact to give rise to the resting membrane potentials of complexly structured cell membranes.

Membrane Potentials in Other Cells

The differences in ionic composition between the internal and the external solution which were described earlier for the nerve cell also hold true for cells in general. Other cells, such as muscle cells, also have resting potentials. Preceding their function they exhibit action potentials which are comparable to the impulses carried by nerve cells. However, only in the case of the neuron does the specialized function of the cell, the transmission of nerve impulses, depend directly on the ionic concentration gradients between the interior and the exterior.

The Action Potential

The nature of the nerve impulse or action potential has been elucidated by electrically stimulating nerve fibers, which are sensory dendrites or more usually the axons of neurons, and recording the resulting changes in potential. Such studies can be performed by placing a nerve (the sciatic nerve of the frog, etc.) into a lucite chamber, stimulating it with a stimulator through a pair of stimulating electrodes, and recording from another portion of the nerve with a pair of recording electrodes connected to amplifiers and an oscilloscope. A monophasic action potential can be obtained by killing the nerve over the more distant recording electrode with potassium chloride.

If transmembrane potential changes or currents must be measured, a glass microelectrode connected to a cathode-follower amplifier is inserted into the neuron. Such a microelectrode is commonly filled with 3M potassium chloride, has a tip diameter between 0.5μ and 1μ, and has a resistance of from 10 to 20 megohms.

The application of voltage clamps has been of outstanding value in studying the processes involved in the propagation of an action potential. In this procedure the axon's resting potential is quickly changed by means of a microelectrode, and the new, impressed potential is maintained through a feedback system. Now the current passing through a unit area of cell membrane at the new, selected membrane potential can be determined.

When a nerve fiber is stimulated with an electric pulse which is below the threshold necessary to call forth a true, propagated action potential, the produced potential (really a reduction in the resting potential or a partial depolarization) falls rapidly and disappears after traversing only several millimeters of the nerve fiber. Similarly, *in vivo* the passage of a single or too few nerve impulses to a summating neuron, or of an insufficient quantity of a chemical mediator to a neuron, calls forth a local potential of subimpulse amplitude which dies away after covering only a short distance (see page 331).

If, however, a section of the nerve fiber is stimulated with an electric pulse whose amplitude exceeds the critical threshold for the initiation of an action potential, there begin mutually reinforcing changes in membrane potential and the involved membrane's permeability to sodium. The now sufficiently large reduction in the resting potential for some unknown reason quickly increases the membrane's permeability to sodium ions. The entrance of the positively charged sodium ions into the nerve fiber section's interior reduces the resting potential further, which in turn results in the entrance of still larger quantities of sodium ions, until the interior of the nerve fiber section is not only no longer negative to the exterior but has a relative positive potential of 30 to 50 mV. Thus a 90 to 120 mV change in potential takes place. This reversal of the involved cell membrane's resting potential is the action potential or nerve impulse, and is maintained for approximately 1 msec at any one nerve fiber locus (Fig. 6-2). Since the resting potential breaks down at the site of the nerve impulse, the last can also be described as a propagated depolarization of the nerve cell membrane.

A reduction in the positive charge on the exterior of the membrane will tend to excite the nerve, while an increase in the external positive charge will have an inhibitory effect.

The threshold drop in membrane resting potential which must be produced to initiate an action potential seems to range around 10 to 18 mV. Since the nerve cell membrane's capacity approximates $1\mu F/cm^2$, about 1.2×10^{-7} coulombs of charge should be required to effect a potential change of 120 mV. During an impulse a minimum of 1.2×10^{-12} moles of monovalent ions must cross each square centimeter of membrane (Eyring, 1967).

It has been suggested that the membrane pores through which sodium ions can enter the cell are negatively charged and thus do not permit the smaller chloride ions to move through them.

How is the action potential transmitted along the length of the nerve fiber? The interior of the fiber at the site of the action potential is now positively charged in respect to the adjoining fiber interior next in the path of the impulse. A current, the action current, therefore flows from this positive region to the adjacent negative one (the electrons actually move in the opposite direction) and then completes its circuit by traveling in a circular pathway through the cell membrane and the exterior solution to its region of origin (Fig. 6-2). In passing through the cell membrane this current reduces the resting potential, an effect which once again increases sodium permeability and culminates in the development of an action potential. The last continues to advance in this manner.

At the location of the action potential the exterior of the nerve fiber is negative to the outside surface of the adjacent membrane regions with an extant resting potential. Therefore, a nerve impulse may be described as a wave of electrical negativity or a propagated negative potential.

The amplitude of this continuously self-regenerating potential, the nerve impulse, usually does not vary as it moves along the nerve fiber. If a portion of the fiber is cooled with ice, the action potential exhibits a reduced amplitude as it passes along this fiber portion, but regains its original amplitude as soon as it once again enters a normal part of the fiber. Generally the action potentials in any particular fiber show a characteristic amplitude which remains the same provided the same conditions (of pH, osmotic pressure, temperature, etc.) prevail.

The velocity of nerve impulse transmission varies directly with nerve fiber diameter, is much higher in myelinated nerves and differs greatly among fiber types. Some nerve impulses progress at under a meter per second. The impulses of thin, nonmyelinated vertebrate fibers (1μ-2μ) travel only a few meters per second, while those of the thickest myelinated vertebrate fibers (near 20μ in diameter) move at close to 100 meters/sec. The sensory fibers from the organs of equilibration are among the nerve fibers with the highest speeds of impulse transmission.

As is true of the resting potential, the nerve action potential's development is dependent upon the internal solution having a high content of potassium ions and a low concentration of sodium ions. As in the case of the resting potential, the potassium ion and sodium ion concentration gradients are a sufficient source of energy for the formation of the action potential.

The extent to which the internal solution becomes positively charged during the action potential is directly correlated with the value of the sodium ion concentration gradient; injection of sodium ions into the nerve fiber decreases the amplitude of the following action potentials.

When in Hodgkin and Baker's perfusion experiments (Baker, 1966) an internal solution's potassium sulfate was exchanged for a sugar concentration of the same osmotic pressure, the internal positive voltage reached by the action potential was raised. Apparently the internal potassium ions reduce the inward movement of sodium ions, or act somewhat like internal sodium ions.

If a nerve axon membrane is depolarized and an ensuing cross-membrane potential of zero is maintained with the voltage clamp, an inward current is first noted but is quickly followed by a lasting outward current. The inward current appears to be due to a fast movement of external sodium ions through the membrane, which has temporarily become permeable to them. The later outward current is probably due to the outward movement of potassium ions when the membrane becomes and remains permeable to these ions.

When, in the above experiment, an external solution lacking sodium ions is employed so that the internal sodium ion concentration is higher, the first, brief current is outward. Sodium ions should now be leaving the axon.

Extracellular potassium ions exert a depolarizing influence on nerve cells. However, even a considerable excess of external potassium ions produces only a slow membrane depolarization.

The development of excitation may differ in its properties in various parts of a single neuron. Thus action potentials recorded from different portions of a neuron may have unlike shapes and amplitudes. Elicited potentials picked up from dendrites exhibit a much slower rise and fall than their counterparts in the membrane of the cell body.

Tasaki attributes such variations in response to the distinct compositions of separate portions of the cell membrane. He also considers certain ionic diffusion processes to be involved (Adey, 1969).

Well-known and highly successful equations describing nerve conduction in terms of ionic conductances, ionic equilibrium potentials and the electrical attributes of the cell membrane were developed by Hodgkin and Huxley (1952). The observations and theoretical formulations stimulated by these equations are discussed in a review by Noble (1966).

The Refractory Period

The reversal of the membrane potential characterizes the nerve impulse. After this reversal in potential reaches its maximum at any locus, the following events occur there: First, the membrane's permeability to sodium ions falls again. Thereupon a large temporary increase in permeability to potassium ions develops in the membrane (Fig. 6-2). The resulting fast outward movement of the positively charged potassium ions once more makes the interior of the nerve fiber negative in respect to the outside and quickly restores the membrane's resting potential. Soon the ionic permeabilities of the nerve cell membrane return to the original, resting level. Another nerve impulse can then propagate over this region of the nerve fiber.

Immediately after the peak of the action potential has passed it, a point on the nerve fiber is left in a totally inexcitable state. Following this period, it is abnormally difficult to initiate a nerve impulse in the mentioned area until its resting condition is fully restored. The time of total inexcitability is known as the absolute refractory period, and the following time span of partial excitability as the relative refractory period. In the A fibers of mammals at body temperature, the absolute refractory period lasts 0.5 msec. The entire refractory period is over in a few milliseconds; in the frog it has a duration of almost 4 msec.

The refractory period, since it blocks nerve impulses during its existence, sets a limit to the rate at which a neuron may convey impulses.

Heat Production

During a nerve impulse an initial heat release is followed by a period of heat absorption and then by a final release of heat as-

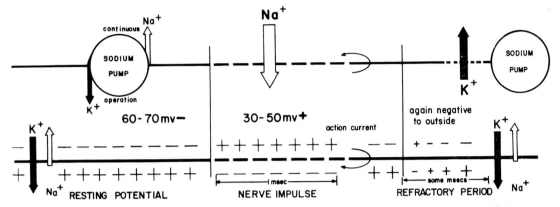

FIGURE 6-2. Diagram summarizing nerve function. The resting membrane potential is based on the outward movement of some potassium ions. A lesser amount of sodium ions also leaks into the cell, but internal concentrations of both ions are maintained by the sodium pump. The nerve impulse is marked by the inward movement of a large quantity of sodium ions. During the ensuing refractory period the permeability to sodium ions decreases again, and then a sizeable outward movement of potassium ions restores the resting condition.

sociated with the restorative processes of the refractory period.

The initial heat at 0°C has been reported to equal 9μcal/gm of nerve in the spider crab (*Maia*) and 0.8μcal/gm in the frog (Hill and Howarth, 1958). Rabbit nerve has been found to liberate an initial heat of 3μcal/gm at room temperature (Abbott, Howarth and Ritchie, 1964). The initial heat may well represent the energy which, prior to its release during the rising phase of the impulse, was stored in the capacitance of the nerve cell membrane.

The subsequent heat absorption could result from the recharging of the membrane capacitance, while the final heat release could be associated with the active transport of ions which restores the resting concentration gradients. The last phase of heat release has the greatest duration and magnitude.

Gas Exchange

The passage of an impulse causes nerve oxygen consumption and carbon dioxide release to rise to one and one-third times the normal level. Again, most of this increased gas interchange occurs at the time of the refractory period.

Maintenance of the Ionic Equilibrium

The quantity of sodium ions which enters each region of a neuron during the action potential and the amount of potassium ions which leaves it during the subsequent refractory period represent only a very minute fraction of the region's concentration of these ions. The described ion movements therefore do not noticeably change the neuron's internal ion concentrations, and even without a functioning sodium pump, the quantity of internal potassium ions suffices to permit the propagation of tens of thousands of action potentials.

The work of Chandler and Meves indicates that the membrane pores by which sodium ions enter the neuron, although they may allow some potassium ions to pass through them, are not identical with the pores by which the bulk of the potassium ions leave the neuron following the peak of the action potential. The neurotoxin produced by the puffer (*Sphaeroides maculatus*), tetrodotoxin, prevents the increase in membrane permeability to sodium ions which plays a vital role in the development of the action potential. However, tetrodotoxin does not prevent the increase in potassium ion permeability which makes the restoration of the resting potential possible.

Eyring (1967) states that in order for positive ions to traverse the lipid portion of the nerve cell membrane, they may have to jump from one nucleophyllic group to another. Such groups could be the phosphate portions of phosphatildyl substances and the anions attached to positive nitrogens. This view may be outdated by new concepts of the cell membrane.

Oscillatory Phenomena

Many investigators have electrophysiologically recorded oscillatory nerve responses.

Lickey and Strumwasser have observed unusual rhythmic responses in certain neurons of the parietovisceral ganglion of the sea hare (*Aplysia californica*). These cells, dubbed "parabolic bursters" by Strumwasser, have spontaneous cycles of discharges interrupted by hyperpolarizations. In each discharge burst the impulse rate at first rises but drops toward the end of the burst. For such a burst of firing the graph of spike intervals against time yields a parabolic shape (Adey, 1969).

The number of impulses in each burst and the rate of the bursts may vary over long time spans and also between preparations. Between 2 and 40 action potentials may develop in a burst, and the discharges may appear at a frequency of from 0.2 to 2 a minute.

The hyperpolarizations which usually intervene between bursts can reach an amplitude of 20 mV.

When tetrodotoxin is used to prevent impulses, the membrane potential of "parabolic bursters" fluctuates between −30 mV and −65 mV at the rate of the discharge-hyperpolarization cycles. Strumwasser (1968) believes that alterations between two relatively stable conditions of the membrane give rise to the discharge-hyperpolarization cycle.

The intrinsic rhythm of the "parabolic bursters" can be terminated by injecting them with chloride ions or by replacing a portion of the chloride ions in the surrounding solution with anions which cannot penetrate the cell.

The repetitive hyperpolarizations appear to result from the operation of a chloride ion-coupled sodium electrogenic pump. When excessive chloride ions, which had been injected, are expulsed into the surrounding fluid, the amplitude of the hyperpolarizations rises. That the hyperpolarizations are based on a sodium pump is shown by their effective prevention with ouabain and their absence when sodium ions are replaced with lithium ions. More sodium than chloride ions must be extruded from the neuron in order to produce hyperpolarization.

The impulse rate in the firing bursts of "parabolic bursters" follows a diurnal circadian rhythm. In most *Aplysia* the impulse frequency reaches a maximum toward sunrise at about the end of winter, while in the summer the greatest number of neurons fires at the highest rate close to noon. When 12-hour periods of light and darkness are experimentally established, the highest impulse frequency is observed in bursts which occur at about the time when the period of light begins (Adey, 1969). A diurnal rhythm is also evident in excised ganglia maintained in organ culture and appears to originate in individual neurons (Strumwasser, 1967).

The circadian rhythm of "parabolic bursters" must originate in their internal physiology, since it is not affected by impressing negative or positive potentials on the cell membrane (Strumwasser, 1965).

By treating nervous tissue with a humoral factor from the Indian scorpion, the neurons can be given a diurnal rhythm with the rate of change characteristic of the donor scorpion at the time of factor extraction (Rao and Gropalakrishnareddy, 1967).

Strumwasser (1967) discusses various aspects and models of circadian rhythms. He includes an extensive section on the circadian rhythms of the "parabolic bursters" of *Aplysia californica*.

The responses of the giant axon of the squid (*Loligo pealii*) are usually oscillatory at 20°C and lower temperatures (Sabah and Leibovic, 1969). A crustacean axon with a resistance of 700 Ωcm^2 across its membrane has been found to give responses with oscillations producing overshoots of 5 per cent. However, no oscillations were observed in similar crustacean axons having resistances approaching 2300 Ωcm^2.

Oscillatory phenomena have also been noted in other nerve tissues (see Visual System and Olfactory System, Chap. IV).

Sabah and Leibovic (1969) have mathematically analyzed the consequences of broadening the cable equation for nerve activity to include the influence of the membrane potential on ionic currents. They consider their results to suggest that, in the case of active membranes, oscillations in response may at least to some degree arise from changes in ionic conductances with membrane potential.

Coupling between neurons oscillating at different frequencies may be significant in the nervous system.

FUNDAMENTAL RELATIONS SIGNIFICANT IN NERVE PHYSIOLOGY

Threshold, Excitability and Accommodation

The minimal level of a stimulus which can produce propagated excitation in a nerve fiber is known as the threshold for a nerve impulse. This threshold level of stimulation can be seen to vary with the rate of rise of the stimulus, indicating that accommodation takes place in a nerve fiber in response to even subthreshold stimulation.

Accommodation may be defined as a reduction in sensitivity or an elevation of the threshold. If a stimulus is applied at even a quite rapid rate, the increasing subthreshold excitation it produces in a nerve region will be balanced by a progressive reduction in nerve excitability, as measured from its prestimulation level or by a rise in threshold. Whether the increasing degree of nerve excitation catches up with and reaches the threshold at any moment in time will determine if a propagated action potential is to be elicited.

A. V. Hill illustrated the above relationships in a diagram which is duplicated here (Fig. 6-3). In this diagram the line V_o—V traces the increasing excitation produced by the stimulus, while the line U_o—U represents the rise in threshold or the accommodation to this excitation. It can be seen from the two graphs on the left side of the diagram that an insufficient rate of increase in excitation, due to a too slow rise in stimulus intensity, may not result in a nerve impulse. At the right end of the diagram a fast-rising excitation, as produced by an extremely rapid condenser discharge, can be noted to reach the threshold level before much accommodation has taken place.

U_o—V_o, the gap between the original threshold (U_o) and any excitatory influences preceding stimulation (V_o), represents the reciprocal of the resting excitability of the nerve fiber. As the threshold U rises upon stimulation, the excitability of the fiber, as measured from the moment of V_o, decreases. However, U-V, the threshold at any time minus the state of excitation at this time, is normally smaller than U_o—V_o. Since U-V is the reciprocal of the excitability, the actual excitability of the nerve fiber generally increases after stimulation is initiated. Only additional excitation equivalent to U-V must be supplied at any time to reach threshold and evoke a nerve impulse.

Local Potentials and Electrotonus

A subthreshold excitation is referred to as an electrotonus or a local potential. Such local potentials are not propagated but decrement over a distance of a few millimeters at the most. In motor neurons electrotonic potentials have been calculated to effectively traverse less than 1 mm of excessively long dendrites. However, local potentials can sum to cross the threshold and give rise to an action potential.

In many neurons local potentials evoked in

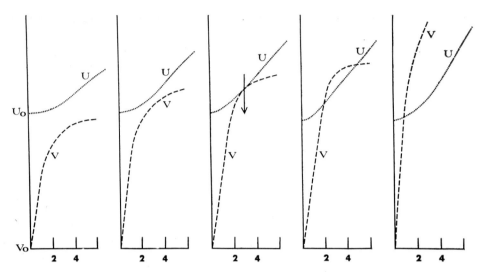

FIGURE 6-3. Relations between nerve excitation and threshold at different rates of stimulation. (V) Rise in excitation or local potential, (U) accommodation in threshold of frog nerve at 40°C, at the cathode. If V reaches or exceeds U, a nerve impulse is produced. The utilization time of the rheobase is indicated by an arrow in the middle graph. (Adapted from Mitchell, P.H.: *A Textbook of General Physiology* [Copyright 1948, McGraw-Hill Book Company, and used with their permission].)

the dendrites and on the cell soma sum to call forth an impulse at the point where the axon leaves the axon hillock. Electrotonic spread in dendrites may therefore be of the greatest importance.

Bullock (1967) differentiates between local potentials, which he considers active or associated with a change in the conductance of the cell membrane, and passive electrotonic potentials. He defines the last as alterations in membrane potential which are imposed by outside currents and which are not accompanied by changes in membrane resistance or capacity.

Dendritic Spikes

Dendritic spike propagation has been hypothesized.

According to Adey (1969), Purpura regards spike generation in mature vertebrate dendrites as an exceptional phenomenon. He states that dendritic spikes appear only when both the generation of impulses at the site of impulse origin is depressed (as by axosomatic IPSP's) and excellent axodendritic connections exist. Purpura differentiates between "partial"

spikes and spikes of full amplitude, both of which are orthodromically transmitted into the perikaryon.

It may be some time before the prevalence of dendritic spikes versus dendritic electrotonic spread can be fully ascertained, since many of the presently applicable research techniques are said to give equivocal results (Calvin, 1969).

Rheobase, Utilization Time and Chronaxie

A current which is barely able to produce enough excitation to reach the threshold and provoke an action potential, even if it is applied for infinite time, is known as the rheobase (Fig. 6-4). The intensity of such a current reflects the level of the accommodated threshold at the existing conditions and at the time when a propagated potential is initiated. The rheobase can therefore be used to roughly gauge the relative excitability of tissues.

The period over which the rheobase must be applied to evoke an action potential has been named the utilization time (Fig. 6-4).

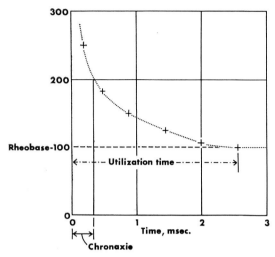

FIGURE 6-4. Strength-duration curve for the frog gastrocnemius muscle. Ordinate values, comparative current intensities necessary for response excitation, when applied for the time spans indicated on the abscissa. The rheobase (assigned a value of 100), utilization time and chronaxie are illustrated. (Adapted from Mitchell, P.H.: *A Textbook of General Physiology* [Copyright 1948, McGraw-Hill Book Company, and used with their permission].)

As can be gathered from the discussion of accommodation, impulse production with a current of greater intensity, which under standard conditions will result in a faster-rising excitation, would provide less time for an accommodative change in the threshold. Stimulation with such a stronger current will therefore supply more accurate data on the comparative excitability of tissues. Lapicque obtained more exact determinations of excitability in this way. He measured the time span required by a current having twice the intensity of the rheobase to elicit an action potential. Lapicque named this time span the chronaxie (Fig. 6-4).

The rate of increase in excitation reflects both the strength of the stimulating current and the rate of its application.

Strength-Duration Curve

The excitation produced by a stimulus is dependent both on stimulus intensity and on stimulus duration. At greater intensities less time is required to evoke a response, and vice versa. It is therefore possible to obtain a strength-duration curve for eliciting an action potential or a response from a tissue. In graphing a strength-duration curve, intensities are normally plotted along the ordinate and the required time periods along the abscissa (Fig. 6-4).

Orthodromic and Antidromic Impulses

It is possible, by stimulating axons somewhere along their course, to initiate impulse spikes which are not transmitted, as is normal, from the neuron soma toward the transmitter terminals of the axon. Instead, these action potentials, known as antidromic, travel in the opposite direction.

To differentiate spikes following the normal route from antidromic impulses, the first are referred to as orthodromic.

Studies on brain cells and spinal motor neurons indicate that in some cases antidromic impulses may enter the dendritic tree. In crustacean stretch receptors antidromic impulses have been noted to pass up the dendrites and act on the generator sites of their receptive terminals. However, in stretch receptor neurons antidromic spikes also seem to be delayed or blocked both at the junction of the axon with the cell soma and at several points in the dendrites (Edwards and Ottoson, 1958).

Antidromic impulses have been passed down the lateral olfactory tract of the mammalian olfactory system to help determine the source of its fibers. Antidromic impulses have also been stimulated in motor neurons to study their excitatory and inhibitory postsynaptic potentials (EPSP's and IPSP's). Further, dendrites have been found to propagate antidromic impulses very slowly. It has therefore been suggested that they may act as a safety device to prevent fatigue. A number of other phenomena of impulse transmission have been successfully investigated by means of antidromic spikes.

Antidromic inhibition, as occurs between motor neurons, may be produced by impulses reflexly discharged by neurons through collateral branches of their axons. Antidromic inhibition seems to represent a feedback mechanism for the control of neural activity.

SYNAPSES

Structure

Electric potentials typically must be transmitted from the end branches of the axon of one neuron to the dendrites or the body of another neuron or from a secondary receptor cell to the dendrites of a sensory neuron across a small gap. This space between adjoining cell membranes, which measures approximately 200 to 250 Å, is known in general terms as a synapse.

An interneural synapse actually consists of several parts, as determined by electron microscopy. Each terminal branch of an axon ends in a bulbous structure, the synaptic knob. The axolemma lining the synaptic knob is known as the presynaptic membrane. Beyond the presynaptic membrane lies the gap between the synapsing neurons, the synaptic cleft (200-250 Å). A substance noted in the synaptic cleft may be a mucopolysaccharide (Pappas and Purpura, 1966); it could serve to hold the membranes of the synapsing cells together while permitting diffusion. On the other side of the synaptic cleft is located a portion of the cell plasma membrane of a neuron receiving the nerve impulse, this membrane here being known as the subsynaptic (postsynaptic) membrane.

Kása (1968) reports elongated intersynaptic organelles of 70 to 150 Å diameter to pass from within the presynaptic membrane through the synaptic cleft into the postsynaptic membrane, where they give rise to a membrane thickening.

Function

General

An electric potential cannot itself jump across the synapse in the manner that an electric spark crosses the gap between two wires. This was erroneously believed some forty years ago to be the means of transmission of impulses from one neuron to another. Instead, it came to be understood that the transmission of potentials across synapses takes place by means of chemical agents. There may be many such chemical mediators.

Apparently when a nerve impulse reaches the end of an axon, it causes the axon terminals to release greatly increased quantities of a chemical mediator. The last crosses each synapse and may now initiate another impulse(s) in the adjoining dendrite(s) or cell body(ies) by interacting with sufficient receptor molecules to materially change the cell membrane's permeability.

The chemical mediator is stored in a high number of synaptic vesicles located in the axon terminals (synaptic knobs). The vesicles of different kinds of neurons are often unlike in size. The most frequently encountered synaptic vesicle ranges between 200 to 400 Å in diameter. Vesicular membranes have been found to consist of groups of globules, each containing a central osmiophilic granule (Di Carlo, 1967a).

Periodically, in the absence of a nerve impulse, a vesicle may reach the presynaptic membrane and release its contained chemical mediator into the synapse. This probably liberates thousands of mediator molecules into the synaptic cleft. Whenever such a vesicle empties at the synaptic cleft in nerve-muscle junctions, it is possible to observe a rapidly dissipating electrotonic potential in the region of the muscle cell beyond the synapse. The discharge of a single synaptic vesicle typically results in a 0.5 mV decrease within 1 msec in the resting potential of the subsynaptic muscle membrane (Katz, 1961). At nerve-muscle junctions vesicles discharge continuously at an average rate of 1/sec.

When a nerve impulse reaches the axon terminals at a nerve-muscle junction, however,

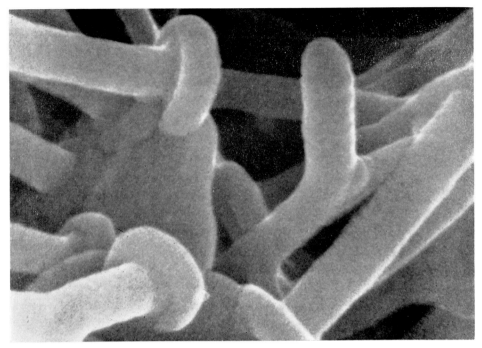

FIGURE 6-5. Fibers bearing terminal expansions converging on a laminar substrate (abdominal ganglion, *Aplysia californica*). The fibers (0.3μm to 0.5μm in diameter) may be neuronal processes and the flattened knobs (0.7um to 1.1um in diameter synaptic knobs. The laminar substrate was only 0.3μm thick. Scanning electron micrograph, ×40,000. (From Lewis, E.R., T.E. Everhart, and Y.Y. Zeevi: Studying neural organization in *Aplysia* with the scanning electron microscope. *Science, 165*:1140-1143, 1969.)

several hundred synaptic vesicles release their contents within less than a millisecond; the rate of discharge suddenly rises a millionfold. It has been calculated that the rate of vesicle discharge rises a hundredfold for every 30 mV drop in the axon terminal resting potential (Katz, 1961).

In a number of synapses currents have been observed to weaken after only approximately 1 msec; the mediator appears to no longer be sufficiently concentrated after this time. The transmitting agent acetylcholine is known to be swiftly broken down by acetylcholinesterase.

It is not yet fully understood how an action potential, upon reaching the axon terminals, causes a high number of synaptic vesicles to liberate their contents through the presynaptic membrane; nor is it known how and whether synaptic vesicles are reconstituted after opening.

Blioch *et al.* (1968) have examined parameters determining the rate of release of quanta of chemical transmitter at the presynaptic axon terminals of a frog synapse. They observed the arrival of an impulse to produce a quick rise in the frequency of vesicular discharge only if divalent cations were available whose movement through the axon membrane is enhanced by depolarization. These cations include calcium, strontium and barium. Experiments with artificial membranes indicated that internal cations may facilitate adhesion between synaptic vesicles and the terminal cell membrane.

The rate of the postsynaptic miniature end-plate potentials was also positively correlated with the axon terminal's cation concentration.

The rate of these potentials can in addition be increased by raising the osmotic pressure.

Chemical transmitters probably differ in the kinds of ionic conductances they produce in the postsynaptic membrane. Acetylcholine appears to open both sodium and potassium channels in the postsynaptic membrane of the frog (*Rana*) neuromuscular junction. Glutamate seems to be the chemical mediator released at the giant synapse of the squid (*Loligo pealii*). The function of this synapse apparently entails only a sizeable increase in postsynaptic sodium ion conductance.

An effect by glutamate on sodium channels alone should make it a more efficient transmitter than acetylcholine (Gage and Moore, 1969).

Axo-dendritic, axo-somatic, dendro-dendritic and axo-axonal synapses have all been identified. However, axo-somatic and axo-dendritic synapses are by far the most common in the central nervous system of vertebrates.

In some axo-axonal synapses there is no synaptic gap, and the general ionic environment of the postsynaptic axon appears to be affected instead (Palay, 1967). Some microneurons, the amacrine cells in the retina and certain granule cells in the olfactory bulb, form two-way synapses with adjoining neurons.

Excitatory and Inhibitory Synapses

Neurons whose axons synapse with other nerve cells may be distinguished as excitatory or as inhibitory neurons. The synaptic vesicles of these two kinds of neurons can be differentiated by diameter and shape. Presumably the kind of chemical mediator released from the synaptic knobs into the synaptic clefts determines whether a neuron tends to excite impulse formation in other neurons or whether it inhibits nerve activity. The excitation of impulses in a neuron usually requires primarily an increase in the permeability of its cell membrane to sodium ions (see Action Potentials), while synaptic inhibition instead probably normally results from a greater membrane permeability to potassium or to chloride ions.

The loss of the positively charged potassium ions from the neuron (due to a mediator from an inhibitory neuron) would make the interior (of the sensory dendrite or cell body) even more negative in respect to the exterior. Thus there would be an increase in the excess negative potential which would have to be neutralized in order to reach the threshold for the excitation of an action potential; the resting potential would be temporarily "stabilized" by the loss of potassium ions. The entrance of the negatively charged chloride ions into the cell would also temporarily increase the amplitude of the resting potential and thus make it necessary for a larger quantity of sodium ions to then enter at the neuron's synapses in order to excite a nerve impulse.

Inhibitory neurons generally call forth inhibitory potentials of less than 10 msec duration in recipient neurons.

Experimental evidence makes it appear quite possible that neuron plasma cell membranes contain larger pores for the passage of sodium ions and somewhat smaller channels for potassium and chloride ions. Chemical mediators producing excitation would combine with receptor molecules in the axolemma so as to open the sodium pores, while inhibitory chemical agents would specifically open the pores for potassium and/or chloride ions.

Typical inhibitory neurons have been shown to act by either stimulating an outflow of potassium ions or creating an inward movement of chloride ions. Which takes place may depend on the charges in the involved smaller channels of the recipient neuron. Positive charges would prevent the outward movement of potassium ions, while negative charges would inhibit the inward flow of the negatively charged chloride ions. The vagus nerve appears to inhibit the heart essentially by releasing a chemical mediator that opens negatively charged channels and permits the movement of potassium ions out of the cardiac muscle cells. On the other hand, in crustacean muscles and in snail brains an inward diffusion of chloride ions produces inhibition.

Lux and Shubert (1969) have discovered

that the equilibrium potential for inhibitory potentials can be shifted in motor neurons by the intracellular injection of any of several positively charged ions. If glycine, ammonium or hydrogen ions, and so on, are injected, a sizeable and maintained depolarizing shift in the inhibitory equilibrium potential results. None of these depolarizing shifts ever exceeds the assumed electrochemical chloride potential (60 mV). Also, injected chloride ions can still leave the cell freely. The investigators therefore attribute their observations to the specific blockage of potassium channels. Perhaps negative charges in the potassium channels are saturated.

Excitatory and Inhibitory Postsynaptic Potentials

Depolarizing potentials called forth by the transmitter substance from excitatory neurons may not reach the threshold for triggering a propagated, all-or-nothing impulse or action potential. Such potentials are known as excitatory postsynaptic potentials (EPSP's).

In many cases an EPSP of sufficient amplitude must first spread to a proximal portion of the axon, where a lower threshold permits impulse initiation.

Potentials resulting from the activities of inhibitory neurons may also range widely in amplitude and are called inhibitory postsynaptic potentials (IPSP's).

If the resting potential across a neuron cell membrane is experimentally increased, or if the internal charge is made more negative, EPSP's excited in the neuron through synapses rise more rapidly. If the resting potential is reduced, ensuing EPSP's develop abnormally slowly and reach only a lower amplitude. If the resting potential of a neuron is experimentally reversed, so that the inside of the cell is now positive to the outside, the following EPSP's are also reversed (or sodium ions flow out of the neuron). A resting potential of nearly zero millivolts marks the point at which no EPSP's are obtained, and beyond which an excess internal positive charge causes the EPSP's to be reversed.

The above results provide further evidence that the chemical mediators released by normal excitatory neurons act so as to permit ions (primarily sodium ions) at the subsynaptic membrane to follow their electrochemical gradients. This ion movement gives rise to the EPSP.

Inhibitory postsynaptic potentials (IPSP's), produced in a neuron by the chemical mediator from inhibitory neurons, also change in accordance with experimental variations of the resting potential. However, at the same maintained membrane potentials the IPSP's undergo modifications which are the converse of those shown by the EPSP's. Thus if the resting potential is reduced, the IPSP's attain a higher amplitude or reach a more negative value. On the other hand, if a greater than normal resting potential is imposed on the neuron membrane (or the interior is made more negative), the IPSP's fall to a subnormal value. IPSP's change their sign, or the direction of the ion flow producing them is reversed, when the interior of the neuron becomes more than 80 mV negative to the exterior.

Other types of postsynaptic potentials, the slow EPSP's and slow IPSP's of many seconds' duration which appear in vertebrate sympathetic ganglia, have been shown to not be accompanied by an increase in membrane conductance (Kobayashi and Libet, 1968). According to Libet and Kobayashi (1969), it is likely that an adrenergic transmitter evokes the slow IPSP and that acetylcholine elicits the slow EPSP.

Nishi and Koketsu (1967, 1968) considered the slow IPSP of sympathetic ganglia to result from the activation of an electrogenic sodium pump through the agency of a chemical transmitter. Pinsker and Kandel (1969) have discovered such a synaptic mechanism to be operative in abdominal ganglion neurons of the sea hare (*Aplysia*), where it gives rise to a lasting IPSP.

The investigations of Pinsker and Kandel (1969) revealed that an abdominal ganglion interneuron (cell L10) of *Aplysia california* can, through separate structural processes, synaptically elicit excitation, inhibition and a combination of both in different postsynaptic cells. These unlike synaptic actions seem to be called forth by the interaction of L10's chemical mediator, acetylcholine, with different receptor sites in the respective postsynaptic cells. Therefore, dissimilar ionic permeability changes are evoked in the different postsynaptic (follower) cells. In some of these cells excitation results from a rise in the conductance for sodium ions, while in others a higher chloride ion conductance is followed by inhibition. The combination of excitation and inhibition is produced in still other cells by greater transmembrane movement of both sodium and chloride ions.

Of unusual interest is the finding that L10's acetylcholine can also activate the electrogenic sodium pump of each of several follower cells. The result is the lengthening of an already 800 msec-long "early" IPSP with a "late" IPSP. The follower cell IPSP can thus be disproportionately lengthened by a series of impulses, but even a single action potential may occasionally give rise to a long-duration, "total" IPSP.

The "late" IPSP, unlike the "early" IPSP, did not invert when a hyperpolarizing current was used to increase the resting potential, even when the last was raised by over 80 mV. By demonstrating that a reduction in external potassium ions and chloride ions had no effect, Pinsker and Kandel further proved a change in conductance to have no role in "late" IPSP generation. In fact, the "late" IPSP was shown to not be accompanied by an increase in membrane conductance.

The characteristics and responses of the "late" IPSP instead indicate that it is produced by the activity of an electrogenic sodium pump. Thus the "late" IPSP falls as the temperature is lowered, and is inhibited by ouabain or the removal of external potassium ions.

The involved follower cells were also shown to have functioning electrogenic sodium pumps by the separate injection of sodium ions and potassium ions.

Acetylcholine is thought to initiate the "early" and "late" IPSP's in one cell by reacting with two types of receptor sites.

Pinsker and Kandel remark that electrogenic sodium pumps could give rise to potentials in a variety of nerve cells.

An axon may have synapses with the dendrites of a number of neurons by means of its several terminal branches; this makes possible the spread of a sensory excitation to several neurons of a higher level. Conversely, the terminals of several axons may synapse with the dendrites and body of a single neuron, producing summation. If these several axons all belong to excitatory neurons, the effects of the impulses coming down the mentioned axons add directly, and, if their combined action exceeds a threshold, an impulse is produced in the recipient neuron. If, on the other hand, both excitatory and inhibitory neurons make contact across synapses with the same recipient neuron, the result of their respectively excitatory and inhibitory actions will be the algebraic sum or net effect of the induced changes. However, there may be complex interactions, both spatial and temporal, along the nerve cell membrane.

A neuron's normal resting potential of 60 to 70 mV may be increased to 75 to 80 mV by a high number of impulses in the inhibitory neurons synapsing with it.

The nerve cells of the vertebrate central nervous system normally each receive impulses from a number, often a very high number, of other neurons, and also each synapses with numerous neurons. An impulse may be initiated in such a nerve cell through excitation by a few or only by a large number of axons. The amount of excitation required depends on the individual threshold of the neuron in question, and on the number of impulses it receives from the inhibitory neurons whose axons synapse with it.

Strychnine and tetanus toxin, if administered to the spinal cord, produce convulsions because they specifically interfere with the function of inhibitory neurons. This removes the inhibition required to counterbalance the activity of the excitatory neurons.

Amplification

Amplification seems to take place at a number of synapses, including some at electro-receptors and other receptors which develop only small generator potentials (Bennett, 1968).

Impulse Distribution in Sensory Systems

Barlow has espoused the view that as sensory nerve activity ascends sensory pathways, it becomes distributed over increasingly greater numbers of nerve fibers, so that a larger number of fibers each transmits fewer impulses (Leibovic, 1969).

Invertebrate Neurons

In many invertebrate neurons the cell plasma membrane of the perikaryon cannot easily be excited. Impulses are produced in proximal processes or in the chief axon by interaction between postsynaptic potentials and propagated action potentials which have developed in some processes. In general, arthropod neurons are characterized by more local autonomy and differentiation than the investigated vertebrate neurons. Large processes of arthropod neurons often independently give rise to action potentials.

In mollusks there are no synaptic connections on the cell bodies of ganglionic neurons. However, action potentials do pass over these somata, while in the lateral giant fibers of the crayfish an axonal action potential is accompanied by only a 5 mV fluctuation in the soma.

The neurons of invertebrate central nervous networks are large and often readily identifiable. They lend themselves to penetration with microelectrodes and to individual staining. Some invertebrate neural networks, like that of the mollusk *Aplysia*, have already yielded much information.

The properties of invertebrate neural networks are reviewed by Kennedy, Selverston and Remler (1969).

ELECTROTONIC JUNCTIONS

Basic Structure and Properties

Although the early concept that impulses can jump across the synapse like electric sparks can cross a small gap between two wires was incorrect, recent investigations have demonstrated the existence, between certain fish neurons (and other cells) of junctions which impulses traverse electrically. Such electrotonic junctions are formed by the union of the cell plasma membranes of adjacent neurons, and no synaptic cleft is present. Electrotonic junctions have a cross-membrane width of approximately 140 Å, and in many such junctions transverse, repetitive striations, found at 90 Å intervals, and a middle dense line have been seen (inset, Fig. 6-6). The striations, if they are indeed the transverse structures they appear to be, may perhaps represent water-containing pores in the fused membranes.

In the cases in which the axons of neurons have electrotonic junctions with the dendrites or bodies of other neurons, the portion of the axon adjacent to the junction contains synaptic vesicles. However, these vesicles are not as numerous as in axon terminals at synapses, nor are they as concentrated at the junction itself (Pappas and Bennett, 1966). Structures resembling desmosomes have also been noted.

Electrotonically mediated potentials have a shorter latency than is found at chemically mediated synapses in the same animal group. In the swim bladder motor neurons of the toadfish (*Opsanus*) antidromic stimulation produces electrotonically mediated potentials with a latency of 0.3 to 0.4 msec (Pappas and Bennett, 1966). The functional significance of the electrotonic junctions present in escape systems (at giant motor synapses of the crayfish, septate axons, Mauthner cells, etc.) may lie in their more rapid impulse transmission. The electrotonic junctions found in cardiac muscle may also be of importance in permitting faster transmission (Bennett, 1966).

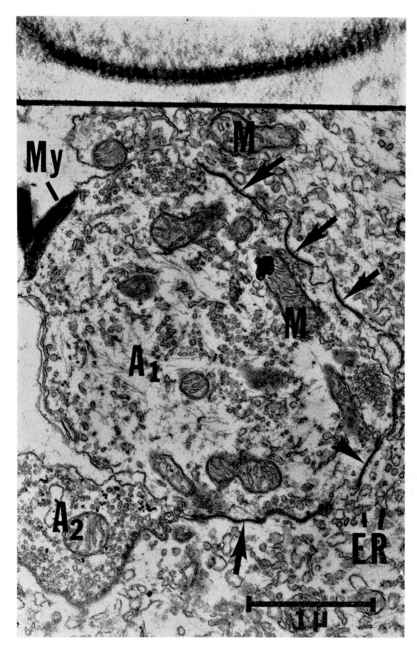

FIGURE 6-6. Electron micrograph of a surface portion of a giant neuron innervating the electric organ of the electric catfish (*Malapterurus electricus*). Two axons (A_1, A_2) adjoin this neuron. The junction with axon A_1 appears to be electrotonic, since the plasma membranes are fused at intervals (arrows). In a tangential section of such a junction (inset), repetitive striae at 90 Å intervals and an intermediate dense line can be seen. The junction with A_2 seems to be a normal axo-somatic synapse, although the synaptic cleft is poorly visible in this oblique section. In A_2 synaptic vesicles are concentrated at the presynaptic membrane. (*ER*) Endoplasmic reticulum, (*My*) myelin, (*M*) mitochondria. ×22,500, inset ×270,000. (From Pappas, G.D., and M.V.L. Bennett [presently at Albert Einstein College of Medicine]: Specialized junctions in-

volved in electrical transmission between neurons. *Ann. N.Y. Acad. Sci.,* 137:495-508, 1966 [Copyright, The New York Academy of Sciences; 1966; reprinted by permission].)

A lower electrical resistance than is found across the adjacent cell membrane has been observed at all electrotonic junctions studied in this regard. According to Asada, Pappas and Bennett (1967), in the septate axons of the crayfish (*Procambarus*) the resistance of the nonjunctional membranes exceeds 1,000 Ωcm² (it has been estimated at between 1,000-3,000 Ωcm²), whereas the resistance at the junctions lies near 1 Ωcm².

The crayfish possesses so-called septate axons, which each actually consist of a row of cells joined together endwise. There is one cell per somite, and two cells adjoin at an oblique septum in every ganglion. Over most of the septal area a dense fibrillar (collagen) layer coated by thin sheets of Schwann cell processes is interposed between the two adjacent axon segments. However, there are a number of small regions of the septum where the two axon segments come into intimate contact. These regions, each a few microns in diameter, are considered to be the actual electrotonic junctions between the axon cells (Asada, Pappas and Bennett, 1967).

The junctions between the cells of septate axons have been discovered to be quite permeable to fluorescein, a dye of large molecular size, suggesting that the low electrical resistance of electrotonic junctions is due to an unusually great membrane permeability, or to cross-junctional channels. However, fluorescein can also penetrate nonjunctional membranes.

Of outstanding significance in this regard is the work of Payton, Bennett and Pappas (1969a). They showed that the dye Procion Yellow M4RS, which cannot penetrate the normal cell plasma membranes of septate axon cells, passes through the junctions between them. This proves that there is a qualitative difference between the permeability of the junctions and that of other parts of the cell membranes.

Payton, Bennett and Pappas (1969a) also obtained evidence that extracellular Procion Yellow can move along the junctional plane between the axon cells, although it cannot pass into the cells. The fixative lanthanum hydroxide as well only penetrated in between the cells and was distributed in a seemingly hexagonal network.

Their findings lead Payton, Bennett and Pappas (1969a) to conclude that channels run from one cell cytoplasm to another, presumably at the "gap junctions" of the septum where the axons come into close contact. These scattered "gap junctions" must also be the points of electrotonic transmission. Further, they visualize the described cross-septal channels to each run through the center of a hexagonal configuration of intrajunctional channels. These hexagons would lie in the plane of the septum and at right angles to the cross-septal channels, and would be interconnected. There are no connections between the cross-septal and the intrajunctional channels.

Polar groups are considered to lie within the cross-septal channels. The last would be responsible for the low resistance of the junctional membrane by permitting the intercellular movement of potassium ions.

The intercellular resistance across the junctional membranes of the lateral giant axon of the crayfish is inversely related to temperature, and varies greatly with temperature changes. The resistance has a Q_{10} of approximately 3 between 5° and 20°C (Payton, Bennett and Pappas, 1969b).

Junctional membranes generally seem to be electrically inexcitable. Thus the electrotonic junction of the crayfish septate axon shows only a linear change in resistance with a more than 25 mV variation in potential. This linearity has so far been observed to not hold true for only one electrotonic junction, that located at the motor giant synapse of the crayfish. This junction displays great resistance at rest. However, if a 20 mV potential is imposed across it so that the protoplasm preceding the junction is positively charged to that beyond it, the junctional resistance falls considerably. Thus large rectifying capacities are demonstrated here.

Electrotonic junctions have been found in a variety of electric fish, the toadfish, the puffer, in the ciliary ganglion of the chicken, in the leech, in the lobster, and on Mauthner cells. They also exist in nonnervous tissues such as cardiac and visceral muscle and in epithelium.

Types and Their Functions

In Mormyrid fish the dendrites of the spinal electromotor neurons are electrotonically joined (Bennett, Aljure, Nakajima and Pappas, 1963), and there are also wide dendro-dendritic electrotonic junctions between the medullary relay neurons. The spinal electromotor neurons are electrotonically coupled to each other as are the medullary relay neurons (Bennett, Pappas, Aljure and Nakajima, 1967).

Three impulses are transmitted from the spinal electromotor neurons to produce an electric organ discharge. This grouping of three action potentials appears to arise from the peculiar properties of the cell membrane, since a postjunctional potential or a short direct stimulus also call forth three impulses. In an analogous manner the medullary relay neurons characteristically discharge groups of two impulses.

Both dendro-somatic and axo-somatic junctions appear to exist in the toadfish (*Opsanus*). Only junctions between axons and the cell bodies of other neurons have been observed in the electric catfish (*Malapterurus electricus*) and the electric eel (*Electrophorus*). The axo-somatic junctions of these two fish are formed between afferent fibers and the motor neurons which produce the discharge of the electric organ (Bennett, Nakajima, and Pappas, 1967a; Bennett, Giménez, Nakajima and Pappas, 1964). It has been suggested that by means of their axo-somatic junctions (Fig. 6-6) the afferent fibers act to couple the motor neurons and synchronize their activity.

Kriebel *et al.* (1969) report that axo-somatic electrotonic junctions couple oculomotor neurons in three teleost fish. The significance of this coupling may lie in the synchronization of action potentials to muscles, resulting in synchronous contractions. The involved muscles are fast effectors which play a role in retraction of the eye and possibly also in saccadic eye movements.

There are electrotonic junctions between the axons of the supramedullary neurons of the puffer (*Sphaeroides maculatus*) and of the Sargassum fish (*Histrio sp.*). These axons form compact bundles, and membrane fusions between adjacent axons are present. Furthermore, axon terminals synapse on supramedullary axons. The junctions between the axons electrotonically couple the supramedullary neurons (Bennett, Nakajima and Pappas, 1967b).

In Gymnotid fish it is possible to slow or increase the rate of discharge of the electric organ by degrees by experimentally varying respectively the degree of hyperpolarization or the degree of depolarization of one cell in the pacemaker nuclei (Bennett, Pappas, Giménez and Nakajima, 1967). This strongly suggests that the cells of the pacemaker nuclei are electrotonically coupled. The development, after an unusually brief latent period, of potentials following antidromic stimulation also indicates electrotonic coupling.

The synchronization of nerve discharges appears to be the primary function of many kinds of electrotonic junctions.

Leeches (*Hirudo medicinalis* and *Aulastoma gulo*) possess an electrotonically linked pair of giant cells in each ganglion of their ventral nerve cord. The soma cell membranes of these giant cells are inexcitable.

Tereshkov, Fomina and Gurin (1969) state that in *Aulastoma gulo* action potentials are electrotonically transmitted to a dendrite or perhaps the perikaryon of a giant cell. The duration of an action potential in *Aulastoma gulo* is 8 to 20 msec, and there is an attenuation coefficient of 5-12 for transmission of polarization between the giant cells of this species. These values are approximately twice those previously determined for *Hirudo medicinalis.* The given attenuation coefficient indicates that the electrotonic junction between the giant cells of *Aulastoma gulo* has a resistance in the range of tens of megohms. Delays of up to 15 to 20 msec occurred between synchronized spikes in the two cells.

Spatial Summation

As in the case of synapses, a number of neurons may have electrotonic junctions with the same recipient neuron. In some of these arrangements the postjunctional neuron can be excited only if two or more of the other neurons fire impulses. Such spatial summation has been studied in electric catfish (Bennett, Nakajima and Pappas, 1967a), the coupled neurons of the swim bladder nuclei of toadfish (Pappas and Bennett, 1966), Gymnotids (Bennett, Pappas, Giménez and Nakajima, 1967), the cardiac ganglia of lobsters and Mauthner cells.

Neurons of various nuclei are electrotonically joined in complex arrangements (Bennett, 1966).

Temporal Summation

Temporal summation occurs when repeated impulses from a single prejunctional cell sum to produce an impulse in a postjunctional cell. It takes place where the refractory period of the prejunctional cell, following an impulse, is sufficiently short compared to the excited subimpulse potential in the postjunctional cell. Temporal summation has been observed in the supramedullary neurons of the puffer (*Sphaeroides maculatus*) and the swim bladder motor neurons of the toadfish by Bennett (1966). In the puffer's supramedullary neurons impulse formation may be facilitated by excitation produced 150 msec previously. Lasting afterpotentials appear to be responsible for this effect.

Inhibition

Inhibitory neurons act on motor neurons in the electric catfish and the toadfish through normal synapses with synaptic clefts. Electro-tonic inhibition has only been observed in the Mauthner cells of the goldfish (Furukawa and Furshpan, 1963).

Since no propagated hyperpolarization is known, the means by which Mauthner cells may be electrotonically inhibited is interesting. Bennett (1968) indicates that the presynaptic fiber terminals end around the proximal portion of the Mauthner cell axon, the axonal region where impulses originate. A gap is assumed to exist between the presynaptic fiber terminals and the axon. When an impulse reaches the presynaptic terminals an outward current emanates from these terminals and makes the environment of the initial portion of the axon comparatively positive. Current therefore passes inward through the axon cell membrane, hyperpolarizing it. This raises the threshold of the region where the axon membrane normally has the lowest threshold and where impulses are initiated, producing impulse inhibition. It is true that there must also be a depolarizing outward flow of current through the axonal membrane, but this is assumed not to take place in the immediate zone of impulse initiation.

The described electrotonic inhibition has a lesser amplitude than certain chemically mediated inhibitions. There should be only a small conductance change in the axon, and a good part of the current flow in the fluid surrounding the axon is ineffective. However, the electrotonic inhibition does not involve a synaptic delay, and this may be significant, since the Mauthner cells evoke an escape movement of the goldfish's tail (Bennett, 1968).

Chemical Versus Electrotonic Transmission

While normal synaptic transmission is characterized by lower speed and cannot convey potentials below the threshold for an impulse, it also will not give rise to antidromic potentials; antidromic potentials probably can arise at electrotonic junctions. Amplification has not been found at electrotonic junctions and is theoretically unlikely at such junctions, although it seems to occur at some chemical synapses (see Synapse).

Electrotonic nerve junctions have so far been chiefly identified in specialized systems.

Since electrotonic junctions between neurons may show the primary characteristics of synapses, and so on, Bennett and his associates

now prefer the term *electrotonic synapses* for such junctions.

Literature

Bennett (1968) reviews the properties of chemical and electrotonic transmission across synapses. Pages 161-300 of volume 30 (1967) of the *Journal of Neurophysiology* are devoted to studies of fish electrotonic junctions performed by Bennett and his co-workers.

A PARTIAL SURVEY OF LITERATURE

Structure

The morphology of important aspects of the nervous system is described in *Nerve as a Tissue,* edited by Rodahl and Issekutz, Jr. (1966). This book consists of the proceedings of the 1964 Lankenau Hospital conference. Included are membrane structure (especially myelin and synaptic membranes), neuroglia, synapses and synaptic vesicles, and electrotonic junctions. *Neurosciences Research Symposium Summaries,* volume 1, edited by Schmitt and Melnechuk (1966), contains outstanding treatments of the structure of cell membranes. There is also a section on the synapse in which morphology is emphasized. Details of the ultrastructure of neurons, glial cells and synapses are presented in well-illustrated chapters of the book *The Neuron,* edited by Hydén (1967). One chapter, by Taxi, is restricted to the neurons, glial cells and synapses of the frog's sympathetic ganglia. In *The Neurosciences—A Study Program,* edited by Quarton, Melnechuk and Schmitt (1967), one can find a good description of various types of nerve cells and neuroglia and the structural relations of these cells in the section titled "Components of the Nervous System." Mitochondria and ribosomes are treated in "Molecular Biology," and the ultrastructure of neuronal membranes under "Molecular Biology of Brain Cells." The morphological aspects of synapses which are related to inhibition are extensively described in the book *Structure and Function of Inhibitory Neuronal Mechanisms,* edited by von Euler, Skoglund and Söderberg (1968). This work consists of

the proceedings of the fourth international meeting of neurobiologists, held at Stockholm in 1966. Membrane structure is discussed in *The Molecular Basis of Membrane Function* (1969), which provides the proceedings of the symposium held at Duke University in 1968. The editor of this volume is Tosteson.

Function

Nervous and receptor activity is based on the properties of excitable membranes. A section of *The Molecular Basis of Membrane Function* (Tosteson, 1969) is devoted to the characteristics and functions of excitable membranes, and it includes a discussion of models of such membranes by Goldman.

In *Nobel Symposium 5, Fast Reactions and Primary Processes in Chemical Kinetics,* edited by Claesson (1967), can be found a good quantitative examination of some essentials of nerve function by Eyring entitled "The Physical Chemistry Of Nerve Action." Eyring emphasizes the Hodgkin-Huxley equations for nerve conduction. Since their formulation by Hodgkin and Huxley (1952), these equations have been the basis of numerous further studies which are summarized in a review by Noble (1966). Cole (1968), in his book *Membranes, Ions and Impulses,* comprehensively deals with the processes associated with the nerve action potential. Models of nerve function and the electrical characteristics of nerve activity are covered by Deutsch (1967) in his work *Models of the Nervous System.*

The activities of nervous tissue *in vitro* (including axoplasmic flow) and the functional relationships of glial cells and neurons are included in *The Neuron,* by Hydén (1967). Neural biochemistry is emphasized in *Nerve as a Tissue,* edited by Rodahl and Issekutz, Jr. (1966). The physiology of glial cells is treated by Galambos in *Neurosciences Research Symposium Summaries,* volume 1.

The structure and function of chemical synapses and electrotonic junctions form the subject matter of *The Physiology of Synapses,* by Eccles (1964). This book provides a good background on chemical transmitters and on inhibition. More recent detail on inhibitory neuronal processes should be sought in *Structure and Function of Inhibitory Neuronal Mechanisms* (von Euler, Skoglund and Söderberg, Eds., 1968).

Physiological and Biochemical Aspects of Nervous Integration, edited by Carlson (1968), comprises the papers delivered at the 1967 Woods Hole symposium of the Society of General Physiologists. The first section of this volume is largely devoted to the physiology of synapses. Also included are a contribution by Strumwasser concerning the spontaneous activity of *Aplysia* neurons, an article by Hubel on the organization of vertebrate visual cortex cells, and several papers on the function of invertebrate nerve nets. *The Neurosciences—A Study Program* (Quarton, Melnechuk and Schmitt, Eds., 1967) contains, in the section entitled "Neuronal Physiology," material on synapses, electrotonic junctions, chemical transmitters, dendrites, postsynaptic inhibition and neural coding. Horridge (1968), in his work *Interneurons—Their Origin, Action, Specificity, Growth, and Plasticity,* deals with the properties of interneurons, inhibitory circuits, glial cells, the function of synapses and neuronal impulse patterns. Horridge's book is well worth reading, even if only for its excellent coverage of the role of interneurons in sensory systems.

REFERENCES

Abbott, B.C., J.V. Howarth, and J.M. Ritchie: The positive and negative heat production associated with the passage of a single impulse in mammalian non-myelinated nerve fibres. *J. Physiol. (London),* 175:42P, 1964.

Adey, W.R.: Slow electrical phenomena in the central nervous system (report on NRP work session, Jan. 1966). *Neurosci. Res. Progr. Bull.,* 7:75-180, 1969.

Asada, Y., G.D. Pappas, and M.V.L. Bennett: Alteration of resistance at an electrotonic junction and morphological correlates. *Fed. Proc.,* 26:330, 1967.

Baker, P.F.: Phosphorous metabolism of intact crab nerve and its relation to the active transport of ions. *J. Physiol. (London),* 180:383-423, 1965.

Baker, P.F.: The nerve axon. *Sci. Amer., 214*:74-82, 1966.

Bennett, M.V.L.: Physiology of electrotonic junctions. *Ann. N.Y. Acad. Sci., 137*:509-539, 1966.

Bennett, M.V.L.: Similarities Between Chemically and Electrically Mediated Transmission. In Carlson, F.D. (Ed.): *Physiological and Biochemical Aspects of Nervous Integration.* Englewood Cliffs, Prentice-Hall, 1968, pp. 73-128.

Bennett, M.V.L., E. Aljure, Y. Nakajima, and G.D. Pappas: Electrotonic junctions between teleost spinal neurons: electrophysiology and ultrastructure. *Science, 141*:262-264, 1963.

Bennett, M.V.L., M. Giménez, Y. Nakajima, and G.D. Pappas: Spinal and medullary nuclei controlling electric organ in the eel, *Electrophorus. Biol. Bull., 127*:362, 1964.

Bennett, M.V.L., Y. Nakajima, and G.D. Pappas: Physiology and ultrastructure of electrotonic junctions. III. Giant electromotor neurons of *Malapterurus electricus. J. Neurophysiol., 30*: 209-235, 1967a.

Bennett, M.V.L., Y. Nakajima, and G.D. Pappas: Physiology and ultrastructure of electrotonic junctions. I. Supramedullary neurons. *J. Neurophysiol., 30*:161-179, 1967b.

Bennett, M.V.L., G.D. Pappas, E. Aljure, and Y. Nakajima: Physiology and ultrastructure of electrotonic junctions. II. Spinal and medullary electromotor nuclei in Mormyrid fish. *J. Neurophysiol., 30*:180-208, 1967.

Bennett, M.V.L., G.D. Pappas, M. Giménez, and Y. Nakajima: Physiology and ultrastructure of electrotonic junctions. IV. Medullary electromotor nuclei in Gymnotid fish. *J. Neurophysiol.*, 30:236-300, 1967.

Birks, R.I., and M.W. Cohen: The action of sodium pump inhibitors on neuromuscular transmission. *Proc. Roy. Soc. [Biol.]*, 170:381-399, 1968.

Blioch, Z.L., I.M. Glagoleva, E.A. Liberman, and V.A. Nenashev: A study of the mechanism of quantal transmitter release at a chemical synapse. *J. Physiol. (London)*, 199:11-35, 1968.

Bodian, D.: Neurons, Circuits, and Neuroglia. In Quarton, G.C., T. Melnechuk, and F.O. Schmitt (Eds.): *The Neurosciences—A Study Program.* New York, Rockefeller U. Pr., 1967, pp. 6-24.

Bullock, T.H.: Signals and Neuronal Coding. In Quarton, G.C., T. Melnechuk, and F.O. Schmitt (Eds.): *The Neurosciences—A Study Program.* New York, Rockefeller U. Pr., 1967, pp. 347-352.

Calvin, W.H.: Dendritic spikes revisited. *Science*, 166:637-638, 1969.

Carlson, F.D. (Ed.): *Physiological and Biochemical Aspects of Nervous Integration.* Englewood Cliffs, Prentice-Hall, 1968.

Carpenter, D.O., and B.O. Alving: A contribution of an electrogenic Na+ pump to membrane potential in *Aplysia* neurons. *J. Gen. Physiol.*, 52:1-21, 1968.

Claesson, S. (Ed.): *Nobel Symposium 5. Fast Reactions and Primary Processes in Chemical Kinetics.* Stockholm, Almquist and Wiksell, 1967.

Cole, K.S.: *Membranes, Ions and Impulses.* Biophysics Series, Berkeley, U. of California Pr., 1968, vol. 1.

Dahlström, A.: Effect of colchicine on transport of amine storage granules in sympathetic nerves of rat. *Europ. J. Pharmacol.*, 5:111-113, 1968.

Deutsch, S.: *Models Of The Nervous System.* New York, John Wiley, 1967.

Di Carlo, V.: Ultrastructure of the membrane of synaptic vesicles. *Nature*, 213:833-835, 1967a.

Di Carlo, V.: Electron microscopical aspects of myelin ultrastructure. *Experientia*, 23:462-471, 1967b.

Eccles, J.C.: *The Physiology of Synapses.* Berlin, Springer-Verlag, 1964.

Edwards, C., and D. Ottoson: The site of impulse initiation in a nerve cell of a crustacean stretch

receptor. *J. Physiol. (London)*, 143:138-148, 1958.

Euler, C. von, S. Skoglund, and U. Söderberg (Eds.): *Structure and Function of Inhibitory Neuronal Mechanisms.* Oxford, Pergamon, 1968.

Eyring, H.: The Physical Chemistry of Nerve Action. In Claesson, S. (Ed.): *Nobel Symposium 5.* Stockholm, Almquist and Wiksell, 1967, pp. 401-412.

Furukawa, T., and E.J. Furshpan: Two inhibitory mechanisms in the Mauthner neurons of goldfish. *J. Neurophysiol.*, 26:140-176, 1963.

Gage, P.W., and J.W. Moore: Synaptic current at the squid giant synapse. *Science*, 166:510-512, 1969.

Geren, B.B.: The formation from the Schwann cell surface of myelin in the peripheral nerves of chick embryos. *Exp. Cell Res.*, 7:558-562, 1954.

Hild, W.J., and F.D. Walker: Neuroglia electrically coupled to neurons. *Science*, 165:602-603, 1969.

Hill, A.V., and J.V. Howarth: The initial heat production of stimulated nerve. *Proc. Roy Soc. [Biol.]*, 149:167-175, 1958.

Hodgkin, A.L.: *The Conduction of the Nervous Impulse.* Springfield, Charles C Thomas, 1965.

Hodgkin, A.L., and A.F. Huxley: A quantitative description of membrane current and its application to conductance and excitation in nerve. *J. Physiol. (London)*, 117:500-544, 1952.

Horridge, G.A.: *Interneurons—Their Origin, Action, Specificity, Growth, and Plasticity.* San Francisco, W. H. Freeman, 1968.

Hydén, H. (Ed.): *The Neuron.* Amsterdam, Elsevier, 1967.

Karlsson, J.O., and J. Sjöstrand: The effect of colchicine on the axonal transport of protein in the optic nerve and tract of the rabbit. *Brain Res.*, 13:617-619, 1969.

Kása, P.: Ultrastructural localization of acetylcholinesterase in the cerebellar cortex with special reference to the intersynaptic organelles. *Histochemie*, 14:161-167, 1968.

Katz, B.: How cells communicate. *Sci. Amer.*, 205:209-220, 1961.

Kennedy, D., A.I. Selverston, and M.P. Remler: Analysis of restricted neural networks. *Science*, 164:1488-1496, 1969.

Kerkut, G.A., and R.C. Thomas: An electrogenic

sodium pump in snail nerve cells. *Comp. Biochem. Physiol.*, *14*:167-183, 1965.

Kobayashi, H., and B. Libet: Generation of slow postsynaptic potentials without increases in ionic conductance. *Proc. Nat. Acad. Sci. USA*, *60*:1304-1311, 1968.

Kriebel, M.E., M.V.L. Bennett, S.G. Waxman, and G.D. Pappas: Oculomotor neurons in fish: Electrotonic coupling and multiple sites of impulse initiation. *Science, 166*:520-524, 1969.

Leibovic, K.N.: Information processing in the nervous system. *Science, 164*:457-460, 1969.

Libet, B., and H. Kobayashi: Generation of adrenergic and cholinergic potentials in sympathetic ganglion cells. *Science, 164*:1530-1532, 1969.

Lux, H.D., and P. Schubert: Postsynaptic inhibition: Intracellular effects of various ions in spinal motoneurons. *Science, 166*:625-626, 1969.

Marmor, M.F., and A.L.F. Gorman: Membrane potential as the sum of ionic and metabolic components. *Science, 167*:65-67, 1970.

Moreton, R.B.: An application of the constant-field theory to the behaviour of giant neurons of the snail, *Helix aspersa. J. Exp. Biol., 48*: 611-623, 1968.

Nakajima, S., and K. Takahashi: Post-tetanic hyperpolarization and electrogenic Na pump in stretch receptor neurone of crayfish. *J. Physiol. (London), 187*:105-127, 1966.

Nishi, S., and K. Koketsu: Origin of ganglionic inhibitory postsynaptic potential. *Life Sci., 6*: 2049-2055, 1967.

Nishi, S., and K. Koketsu: Analysis of slow inhibitory postsynaptic potential of bullfrog sympathetic ganglion. *J. Neurophysiol., 31*: 717-728, 1968.

Noble, D.: Applications of Hodgkin-Huxley equations to excitable tissues. *Physiol. Revs., 46*:1-50, 1966.

Palay, S.L.: Principles of Cellular Organization in the Nervous System. In Quarton, G.C., T. Melnechuk, and F.O. Schmitt (Eds.): *The Neurosciences—A Study Program.* New York, Rockefeller U. Pr., 1967, pp. 24-31.

Pappas, G.D., and M.V.L. Bennett: Specialized junctions involved in electrical transmission between neurons. *Ann. N.Y. Acad. Sci., 137*: 495-508, 1966.

Pappas, G.D., and D.P. Purpura: Distribution of colloidal particles in extracellular space and synaptic cleft substance of mammalian cerebral cortex. *Nature, 210*:1391-1392, 1966.

Payton, B.W., M.V.L. Bennett, and G.D. Pappas: Permeability and structure of junctional membranes at an electrotonic synapse. *Science, 166*:1641-1643, 1969a.

Payton, B.W., M.V.L. Bennett, and G.D. Pappas: Temperature-dependence of resistance at an electrotonic synapse. *Science, 165*:594-597, 1969b.

Pinsker, H., and E.R. Kandel: Synaptic activation of an electrogenic sodium pump. *Science, 163*: 931-935, 1969.

Quarton, G.C., T. Melnechuk, and F.O. Schmitt (Eds.): *The Neurosciences—A Study Program.* New York, Rockefeller U. Pr., 1967.

Rang, H.P., and J. M. Ritchie: On the electrogenic sodium pump in mammalian non-myelinated nerve fibres and its activation by various external cations. *J. Physiol. (London), 196*:183-221, 1968.

Rao, K.P., and T. Gropalakrishnareddy: Blood borne factors in circadian rhythms of activity. *Nature, 213*:1047-1048, 1967.

Rodahl, K., and B. Issekutz, Jr. (Eds.): *Nerve as a Tissue.* New York, Harper and Row, 1966.

Sabah, N.H., and K.N. Leibovic: Subthreshold oscillatory responses of the Hodgkin-Huxley cable model for the squid giant axon. *Biophys. J., 9*:1206-1222, 1969.

Schmitt, F.O., and T. Melnechuk (Eds.): *Neurosciences Research Symposium Summaries.* Cambridge, M.I.T. Pr., 1966, vol. 1.

Senft, J.P.: Effects of some inhibitors on the temperature-dependent component of resting potential in lobster axon. *J. Gen. Physiol., 50*: 1835-1847, 1967.

Strumwasser, F.: The Demonstration and Manipulation of a Circadian Rhythm in a Single Neuron. In Aschoff, J. (Ed.): *Circadian Clocks.* Amsterdam, North-Holland, 1965, pp. 442-462.

Strumwasser, F.: Neurophysiological Aspects of Rhythms. In Quarton, G.C., T. Melnechuk, and F.O. Schmitt (Eds.): *The Neurosciences—A Study Program.* New York, Rockefeller U. Pr., 1967, pp. 516-528.

Strumwasser, F.: Membrane and Intracellular Mechanisms Governing Endogenous Activity in Neurons. In Carlson, F.D. (Ed.): *Physiological and Biochemical Aspects of Nervous*

Integration. Englewood Cliffs, Prentice-Hall, 1968, pp. 329-341.

Tereshkov, O.D., M.S. Fomina, and S.S. Gurin: Electrophysiological properties of paired giant cells of the leech *Aulastoma gulo. Biofizika, 14*:86-90, 1969.

Tosteson, D.C. (Ed.): *The Molecular Basis of Membrane Function.* Englewood Cliffs, Prentice-Hall, 1969.

Walker, F.D., and W.J. Hild: Neuroglia electrically coupled to neurons. *Science, 165*:602-603, 1969.

SUGGESTED READING

Adey, W.R.: Slow electrical phenomena in the central nervous system. *Neurosci. Res. Progr. Bull., 7*:75-180, 1969.

Bennett, M.V.L.: Mechanisms of Electroreception. In Cahn, P. (Ed.): *Lateral Line Detectors.* Bloomington, Indiana U. Pr., 1967, pp. 313-393.

Bennett, M.V.L.: Similarities Between Chemically and Electrically Mediated Transmission. In Carlson, F.D. (Ed.): *Physiological and Biochemical Aspects of Nervous Integration,* Englewood Cliffs. Prentice-Hall, 1968, pp. 73-128.

Brazier, M.A.B., and V.E. Hall (Eds.): *The Interneuron.* Berkeley, U. of California Pr., 1969.

Cole, K.S.: *Membranes, Ions and Impulses.* Biophysics Series. Berkeley, U. of California Pr., 1968, vol. 1.

Eccles, J.C.: *The Physiology of Synapses.* Berlin, Springer-Verlag, 1964.

Eyring, H.: The Physical Chemistry of Nerve Action. In Claesson, S. (Ed.): *Nobel Symposium 5. Fast Reactions and Primary Processes in Chemical Kinetics.* Stockholm, Almquist and Wiksell, 1967, pp. 401-412.

Horridge, G.A.: *Interneurons—Their Origin, Action, Specificity, Growth, and Plasticity.* San Francisco, W. H. Freeman, 1968.

Noble, D.: Applications of Hodgkin-Huxley equations to excitable tissues. *Physiol. Revs., 46*: 1-50, 1966.

Quarton, G.C., T. Melnechuk, and F.O. Schmitt (Eds.): *The Neurosciences—A Study Program.* New York, Rockefeller U. Pr., 1967.

Robertson, J.D.: The Synapse: Morphological and Chemical Correlates of Function. In Schmitt, F.O., and T. Melnechuk (Eds.): *Neurosciences Research Symposium Summaries.* Cambridge, M.I.T. Pr., 1966, pp. 463-541.

Rodahl, K., and B. Issekutz, Jr. (Eds.): *Nerve as a Tissue.* New York, Harper and Row, 1966.

Schmitt, F.O., G.C. Quarton, T. Melnechuk, and G. Adelman (Eds.): *The Neurosciences— Second Study Program.* New York, Rockefeller U. Pr., 1970.

Author Index

Subject Index

Italicized numbers represent the pages of figures which appear apart from the related subject matter.

Dendrodendritic synaptic pathways, 209, 210
  efferents to olfactory bulb and, 219
  significance of, 210, 213, 215, 219
Dense bodies, taste nerve fibers, 101
Depolarization
  differing responses with degree of, 178
Depolarization, neural membrane, *see also* Action potential, neuron; Nerve impulses; Neurons
  and extracellular potassium, 328
  partial, 326
Diencephalon
  connections, olfactory, 207, 213
Direct absorption of taste substances, 197, 265
Directional sensitivity, ear
  by asymmetrical apertures, owl, 108, *109*
  by interaural distance, owl, 108
  by pinna, bats, 108
Discs, visual receptors, 245, *246*, 247, 248
  development of, 38
Dorsal tegmental nucleus
  connections, olfactory, 213
Duodenal chemoreceptors, 200
Duplexity theory of taste, 301, 302

E

Early receptor potential, *see also* Receptor potential, visual
  action spectra and pigment absorption spectrum, 244
  adaptation of, 252
  amplification of, 252, 254
  and ATP reconstitution, 249
  and ion movement, 249, 250, 252
  and pH, 247, 248
  and receptor membranes, 248, 249
  conduction of, 252
  duration of, 244
  effect of temperature, anoxia, potassium chloride, 244
  generation from dipoles, 251
  orientation of source, 251
  origin of, *241*, 244, 245, 247, 249–251, 254
  peak amplitude, 244
  phenomena similar to, 247–251
  properties of, 252
  reference for, 250
  rod eyes versus cone eyes
    cooling, effect on R2, 245
    duration of R2, 245
    ERP amplitude, 245
    excess light, effect of, 245
    threshold, 245
  saturation of, 244
  significance of, 250, 254
  similarity to various biological pigment responses, 251
  stimulus required, 244
  time of appearance, 243
  unusual origin in frog, 251, 252

Early receptor potential, R1 phase of, 243, 244
  and pH, 244
  latency, 244
  linearity with pigment excited, 244, 255
  origin of, 244, 247, 254
  temperature resistance, 244
  time of peak strength, 244
Early receptor potential, R2 phase of, 243, 244
  abolition by light, 244
  and pH, 244
  linearity with pigment excited, 244, 255
  origin of, *241*, 244, 245, 247, 254
  peak, time of, 244
  temperature resistance, 244
Early receptor potential, third phase of, 244
Early receptor potential, squid
  fast photovoltage, source of, 248, *249*
  orientation, created dipoles, 248, *249*
  transretinal voltage, cause of, 248
Early visual potential, horseshoe crab
  amplitude of, 248
  experimental changes in, 248
  latency of, 248
  other cells observed in, 248
  sources of, 248–250
    function of, 248
Eccentric cell, *Limulus,* 248
  inhibition of, 126
  self-inhibition in, 130, 131
  sensitivity of, to ethyl alcohol, 126
  structure, 124, 125
Echolocation, bat
  role of cochlear nuclei in, 168
EEG waves
  and inhibition, 187
  effect of LSD on, 220
  in olfactory bulb, 219
  locations of, 220
  source of, 219, 220
Efferent cochlear bundle, pigeon
  action of, 176
  functional difference from olivocochlear bundle, 176
  homology with olivocochlear bundle, mammal, 176
Efferent fibers, auditory, *see also* Centrifugal fibers, auditory
  to auditory hair cells
    activation
      by habituation and conditioning, 159
      by nonauditory stimuli, 159
Efferent fibers, gustatory system
  effects of, reference for, 201
  fish
    structure of, 196
  frog
    effects of, 197, 200
      parasympathetic impulses, 197–200
      stimulating lingual nerve, 199
      sympathetic impulses, 197–200

receptors for dilute electrolytes
    eliciting and inhibiting agents, 284
  salt concentration and time to peak, 284
in cat, 283, 284, 300
in dog, 283, 284
in flesh fly, 268
in frog, 283, 284
in opossum, 281, 283
in rabbit, 283
in rat, 284
species observed in, 282, 283

Water-sensitive neuron, blowfly
  effect of alcohols and amines on, 285
  responses of, qualitatively different, 115
Wavelengths, light, different
  quantum emission by, 8
  quantum, relative energy in, 8
Weber fraction, 8
  defects of, 8
    explanation for a defect, 8, 9
  vision, applicability to, 9
    basis of, 9